REVIEW AND RESOURCE MANUAL

Gerontological Nurse Practitioner

3rd Edition

Published by American Nurses Credentialing Center
Vaunette Fay, PhD, RN, FNP-BC, GNP-BC; Katherine Tardiff, MSN, GNP-BC, ACHPN;
MJ Henderson, MS, RN, GNP-BC; and Michaelene Jansen, PhD, RN, GNP-BC, NP-C

CONTINUING EDUCATION SOURCE

NURSING CERTIFICATION REVIEW MANUAL

CLINICAL PRACTICE RESOURCE

3RD EDITION

Library of Congress Cataloging-in-Publication Data

Gerontological nurse practitioner review and resource manual / by Katherine Tardiff ... [et al.]. — 3rd ed.

   p. ; cm.

  Rev. ed. of: Gerontological nurse practitioner review and resource manual / Maren S. Mayhew, Marilyn W. Edmunds. 2nd ed. c2005.

  Includes index.

  ISBN 978-1-935213-05-5

  1. Geriatric nursing—Examinations, questions, etc. 2. Nurse practitioners-- Examinations, questions, etc. 3. Nurses—Licenses--United States--Examinations— Study guides. I. Tardiff, Katherine. II. Mayhew, Maren Stewart. Gerontological nurse practitioner review and resource manual. III. American Nurses Credentialing Center.

  [DNLM: 1. Geriatric Nursing--Examination Questions. 2. Nurse Practitioners— Examination Questions. WY 18.2]

  RC954.M39 2010

  618.97'0231076--dc22

                                2010027595

The American Nurses Credentialing Center (ANCC), a subsidiary of the American Nurses Association (ANA), provides individuals and organizations throughout the nursing profession with the resources they need to achieve practice excellence. ANCC's internationally renowned credentialing programs certify nurses in specialty practice areas; recognize healthcare organizations for promoting safe, positive work environments through the Magnet Recognition Program® and the Pathway to Excellence ® Program; and accredit providers of continuing nursing education. In addition, ANCC's Institute for Credentialing Innovation provides leading-edge information and education services and products to support its core credentialing programs.

ISBN 13: 9781935213055

© 2010 American Nurses Credentialing Center.

8515 Georgia Ave., Suite 400

Silver Spring, MD 20910

Gerontological Nurse Practitioner Review and Resource Manual, 3rd Edition

AUGUST 2010

Please direct your comments and/or queries to: revmanuals@ana.org

The healthcare services delivery system is a volatile marketplace demanding superior knowledge, clinical skills, and competencies from all registered nurses. Nursing autonomy of practice and nurse career marketability and mobility in the new century hinge on affirming the profession's formative philosophy, which places a priority on a lifelong commitment to the principles of education and professional development. The knowledge base of nursing theory and practice is expanding, and while care has been taken to ensure the accuracy and timeliness of the information presented in the *Gerontological Nurse Practitioner Review and Resource Manual, 3rd Edition,* clinicians are advised to always verify the most current national guidelines and recommendations and to practice in accordance with professional standards of care used with regard to the unique circumstances that apply in each practice situation. In addition, every effort has been made in this text to ensure accuracy and, in particular, to confirm that drug selections and dosages are in accordance with current recommendations and practice, including the ongoing research, changes to government regulations, and the developments in product information provided by pharmaceutical manufacturers. However, it is the responsibility of each nurse practitioner to verify drug product information and to practice in accordance with professional standards of care. In addition, the editors wish to note that provision of information in this text does not imply an endorsement of any particular products, procedures or services.

Therefore, the authors, editors, American Nurses Association (ANA), American Nurses Association's Publishing (ANP), American Nurses Credentialing Center (ANCC), and the Institute for Credentialing Innovation cannot accept responsibility for errors or omissions, or for any consequences or liability, injury, and/or damages to persons or property from application of the information in this manual and make no warranty, express or implied, with respect to the contents of the *Gerontological Nurse Practitioner Review and Resource Manual, 3rd Edition.* Completion of this manual does not guarantee that the reader will pass the certification exam.

Published by:
American Nurses Credentialing Center
The Institute for Credentialing Innovation
8515 Georgia Avenue, Suite 400
Silver Spring, MD 20910-3402
www.nursecredentialing.org

Introduction to the Continuing Education (CE) Contact Hour Application Process for *Gerontological Nurse Practitioner Review and Resource Manual, 3rd Edition*

The Institute for Credentialing Innovation now offers the continuing education contact hours for this manual online at www.NursingWorld.org, the American Nurses Association's Web site. This process involves answering approximately 25–30 questions that test knowledge of the information contained within this manual. The continuing education contact hours can be completed at any time and a certificate can be printed from the Web site immediately upon successful completion of the test.

After studying the manual and given an online multiple-choice test, the exam candidate will be able to:

- Pass the posttest with at least 75% of the answers correct.

- Select responses to test questions based on key principles, standards of practice, and theoretical basis of nursing practice.

- Choose accepted therapeutic interventions in answering questions related to quality nursing practice.

- Utilize direct and indirect professional role responsibilities and applications regarding nursing practice in answering test questions.

Upon completion of this manual *and* the online CE test, a nurse can receive a total of 43 continuing education contact hours at a price of $86, only $2 per CE. (ANA members receive a discount on CEs.) **The entire process—online test and evaluation form—must be completed by December 31, 2012 in order to receive credit.** To begin the process, please e-mail **revmanuals@ana.org**. Your patience with this process is greatly appreciated.

Inquiries or Comments

If you have any questions about the CE contact hours, please e-mail The Institute at revmanuals@ana.org. You may also mail any comments to Editor/Project Manager at the address listed below.

Duplicate CE Certificates

Once you have successfully passed the CE test on NursingWorld, you may go back and re-print your certificate as often as you wish.

Conflicts of Interest

A conflict of interest occurs when an individual has an opportunity to affect educational content about health-care products or services of a commercial company with which she/he has a financial relationship.

The planners and presenters of this CNE activity have disclosed no relevant financial relationships with any commercial companies pertaining to this activity.

The Institute for Credentialing Innovation
American Nurses Credentialing Center
Attn: Editor/Project Manager
8515 Georgia Avenue, Suite 400
Silver Spring, MD 20910-3492
Fax: (301) 628-5342

A maximum of 43 contact hours may be earned by learners who successfully complete this continuing nursing education activity.

The American Nurses Association Center for Continuing Education and Professional Development is accredited as a provider of continuing nursing education by the American Nurses Credentialing Center's Commission on Accreditation.

ANCC Provider Number 0023

ANA is approved by the California Board of Registered Nursing, Provider Number 6178.

The ANA Center for Continuing Education and Professional Development includes ANCC's Institute for Credentialing Innovation.

Acknowledgments

The editors also gratefully acknowledge the foundational work provided by the editors of the previous edition:

Maren S. Mayhew, MSN, ANP/GNP
Suburban Hospital
Bethesda, MD

Marilyn W. Edmunds, PhD, ANP/GNP
NP Alternatives in Education, Inc.
Ellicott City, MD

Contents

REVIEW AND RESOURCE MANUAL

Gerontological Nurse Practitioner

3rd Edition

Taking the Certification Examination

When you sign up to take a national certification exam, you will be instructed to go online and review the testing and review handbook (www.nursecredentialing.org/documents/certification/application/generaltestingandreviewhandbook.aspx). Review it carefully and be sure to bookmark the site so you can refer to it frequently. It contains information on test content and sample questions. This is critical information; it will give you insight into the nature of the test. The agency will send you information about the test site; keep this in a safe place until needed.

GENERAL SUGGESTIONS FOR PREPARING FOR THE EXAM

Step One: Control Your Anxiety

Everyone experiences anxiety when faced with the certification exam.
- Remember, your program was designed to prepare you to take this exam.
- Your instructors took a similar exam, and have probably talked to students who took exams more recently, so they know how to help you prepare.
- Taking a review course or setting up your own study plan will help you feel more confident about taking the exam.

Step Two: Do Not Listen to Gossip About the Exam

A large volume of information exists about the tests based on reports from people who have taken the exams in the past. Because information from the testing facilities is limited, it is hard not to listen to this gossip.
- Remember that gossip about the exam that you hear from others is not verifiable.
- Because this gossip is based on the imperfect memory of people in a very stressful situation, it may not be very accurate.

- People tend to remember those items testing content with which they are less comfortable; for instance, those with a limited background in women's health may say that the exam was "all women's health." In fact, the exam blueprint ensures that the exam covers multiple content areas without overemphasizing any one.

Step Three: Set Reasonable Expectations for Yourself

- Do not expect to know everything.
- Do not try to know everything in great detail.
- You do not need a perfect score to pass the exam.
- The exam is designed for a beginner level—it is testing readiness for *entry-level* practice.
- Learn the general rules, not the exceptions.
- The most likely diagnoses will be on the exam, not questions on rare diseases or atypical cases.
- Think about the most likely presentation and most common therapy.

Step Four: Prepare Mentally and Physically

- While you are getting ready to take the exam, take good physical care of yourself.
- Get plenty of sleep, exercise, and eat well while preparing for the exam.
- These things are especially important while you are studying and immediately before you take the exam.

Step Five: Access Current Knowledge

General Content

You will be given a list of general topics that will be on the exam when you register to take the exam. In addition, examine the table of contents of this book and the test content outline, available at www.nursecredentialing.org/cert/TCOs.html.

- What content do you need to know?
- How well do you know these subjects?

Take a Review Course

- Taking a review course is an excellent method of assessing your knowledge of the content that will be included in the exam.
- If you plan to take a review course, take it well before the exam so you will have plenty of time to master any areas of weakness the course uncovers.
- If you are prepared for the exam, you will not hear anything new in the course. You will be familiar with everything that is taught.
- If some topics in the review course are new to you, concentrate on these in your studies.
- People have a tendency to study what they know; it is rewarding to study something and feel a mastery of it! Unfortunately, this will not help you master unfamiliar content. Be sure to use a review course to identify your areas of strength and weakness, then concentrate on the weaknesses.

Depth of Knowledge

How much do you need to know about a subject?

- You cannot know everything about a topic.
- Remember that the depth of knowledge required to pass the exam is for entry-level performance.
- Study the information sent to you from the testing agency, what you were taught in school, what is covered in this text, and the general guidelines given in this chapter.

- Look at practice tests designed for the exam. Practice tests for other exams will not be helpful.
- Consult your class notes or clinical diagnosis and management textbook for the major points about a disease. Additional reference books can be found online at www.nursecredentialing.org/cert/refs.html.
- For example, with regard to medications, know the drug categories and the major medications in each. Assume all drugs in a category are generally alike, and then focus on the differences among common drugs. Know the most important indications, contraindications, and side effects. Emphasize safety. The questions usually do not require you to know the exact dosage of a drug.

Step Six: Institute a Systematic Study Plan

Develop Your Study Plan

- Write up a formal plan of study.
  - Include topics for study, timetable, resources, and methods of study that work for you.
  - Decide whether you want to organize a study group or work alone.
  - Schedule regular times to study.
  - Avoid cramming; it is counterproductive. Try to schedule your study periods in 1-hour increments.
- Identify resources to use for studying. To prepare for the examination, on your shelf you should have:
  - A good pathophysiology text.
  - This review book.
  - A physical assessment text.
  - Your class notes.
  - Other important sources, including: information from the testing facility, a clinical diagnosis textbook, favorite journal articles, notes from a review course, and practice tests.
  - Know the important national standards of care for major illnesses.
  - Consult the bibliography on the test blueprint. When studying less familiar material, it is helpful to study using the same references that the testing center uses.
- Study the body systems from head to toe.
- The exams emphasize health promotion, assessment, differential diagnosis, and plan of care for common problems.
- You will need to know facts and be able to interpret and analyze this information utilizing critical thinking.

Personalize Your Study Plan

- How do you learn best?
  - If you learn best by listening or talking, attend a review course or discuss topics with a colleague.
- Read everything the test facility sends you as soon as you receive it and several times during your preparation period. It will give you valuable information to help guide your study.
- Have a specific place with good lighting set aside for studying. Find a place with no noise or distractions. Assemble your study materials.

Implement Your Study Plan

You must have basic content knowledge. In addition, you must be able to use this information to think critically and make decisions based on facts.

- Refer to your study plan regularly.
- Stick to your schedule.
- Take breaks when you get tired.
- If you start procrastinating, get help from a friend or reorganize your study plan.
- It is not necessary to follow your plan rigidly. Adjust as you learn where you need to spend more time.
- Memorize the basics of the content areas you will be required to know.

Focus on General Material
- Most of what you need to know is basic material that does not require constant updating.
- You do not need to worry about the latest information being published as you are studying for the exam. Remember, it can take 6 to 12 months for new information to be incorporated into test questions.

Pace Your Studying
- Stop studying for the examination when you are starting to feel overwhelmed and look at what is bothering you. Then make changes.
- Break overwhelming tasks into smaller tasks that you know you can do.
- Stop and take breaks while studying.

Work With Others
- Talk with classmates about your preparation for the exam.
- Keep in touch with classmates, and help each other stick to your study plans.
- If your classmates start having anxiety attacks, do not let their anxiety affect you. Walk away if you need to.
- Do not believe bad stories you hear about other people's experiences with previous exams.
- Remember, you know as much as anyone about what will be on the next exam!

Consider a Study Group
- Study groups can provide practice in analyzing cases, interpreting questions, and critical thinking.
    - You can discuss a topic and take turns presenting cases for the group to analyze.
    - Study groups can also provide moral support and help you keep studying.

Step Seven: Strategies Immediately Before the Exam
Final Preparation Suggestions
- Use practice exams when studying to get accustomed to the exam format and time restrictions.
    - Many books that are labeled as review books are simply a collection of examination questions.
    - If you have test anxiety, such practice tests may help alleviate the anxiety.
    - Practice tests can help you learn to judge the time you should take during an exam.
    - Practice tests are useful for gaining experience in analyzing questions.
    - Books of questions may not uncover the gaps in your knowledge that a more systematic content review text will reveal.
    - If you feel that you don't know enough about a topic, refer to a text to learn more. After you feel that you have learned the topic, practice questions are a wonderful tool to help improve your test-taking skill.

- Know your test-taking style.
  - Do you rush through the exam without reading the questions thoroughly?
  - Do you get stuck and dwell on a question for a long time?
  - You should spend about 45 to 60 seconds per question and finish with time to review the questions you were not sure about.
  - Be sure to read the question completely, including all four answer choices. Choice "a" may be good, but "d" may be best.

The Night Before the Exam
- Be prepared to get to the exam on time.
  - Know the test site location and how long it takes to get there.
  - Take a "dry run" beforehand to make sure you know how to get to the testing site, if necessary.
  - Get good night's sleep.
  - Eat sensibly.
  - Avoid alcohol the night before.
  - Assemble the required material—two forms of identification, admission card, pencil, and watch. Both IDs must match the name on the application, and at least one photo ID is preferred.
  - Know the exam room rules.
    - You will be given scratch paper, which will be collected at the end of the exam.
    - Nothing else is allowed in the exam room.
    - You will be required to put papers, backpacks, etc., in a corner of the room, or in a locker.
    - No water or food will be allowed.
    - You will be allowed to walk to a water fountain and go to the bathroom one at a time.

The Day of the Exam
- Get there early. If you are late, you may not be admitted.
- Think positively. You have studied hard and are well-prepared.
- Remember your anxiety reduction strategies.

Specific Tips for Dealing With Anxiety
Test anxiety is a specific type of anxiety. Symptoms include upset stomach, sweaty palms, tachycardia, trouble concentrating, and a feeling of dread. But there are ways to cope with test anxiety.
- There is no substitute for being well-prepared.
- Practice relaxation techniques.
- Avoid alcohol, excess coffee, caffeine, and any new medications that might sedate you, dull your senses, or make you feel agitated.
- Take a few deep breaths and concentrate on the task at hand.

Focus on Specific Test-Taking Skills
To do well on the exam, you need good test-taking skills in addition to knowledge of the content and ability to use critical thinking.

All Certification Exams Are Multiple Choice
- Multiple choice tests have specific rules for test construction.

- A multiple choice question consists of three parts: the information (or stem), the question, and the four possible answers (one correct and three distracters).
- Careful analysis of each part is necessary. Read the entire question before answering.
- Practice your test-taking skills by analyzing the practice questions in this book and on the ANCC website

Analyze the Information Given

- Do not assume you have more information than is given.
- Do not overanalyze.
- Remember, the writer of the question assumes this is all of the information needed to answer the question.
- If information is not given, it is not relevant and will not affect the answer.
- Do not make the question more complicated than it is.

What Kind of Question Is Asked?

- Are you supposed to recall a fact, apply facts to a situation, or understand and differentiate between options?
  - Read the question thinking about what the writer is asking.
  - Look for key words or phrases that lead you (see Figure 1–1). These help determine what kind of answer the question requires.

Figure 1–1. Examples of Key Words and Phrases

- avoid
- best
- except
- not

- initial
- first
- contributing to
- appropriate

- most
- significant
- likely
- of the following
- most consistent with

Read All of the Answers

- If you are absolutely certain that answer "a" is correct as you read it, mark it, but read the rest of the question so you do not trick yourself into missing a better answer.
- If you are absolutely sure answer "a" is wrong, cross it off or make a note on your scratch paper and continue reading the question.
- After reading the entire question, go back, analyze the question, and select the best answer.
- Do not jump ahead.
- If the question asks you for an assessment, the best answer will be an assessment. Do not be distracted by an intervention that sounds appropriate.
- If the question asks you for an intervention, do not answer with an assessment.
- When two answer choices sound very good, the best one is usually the least expensive, least invasive way to achieve the goal. For example, if your answer choices include a physical exam maneuver or imaging, the physical exam maneuver is probably the better choice provided it will give the information needed.
- If the answers include two options that are the opposite of each other, one of the two is probably the correct answer.
- When numeric answers cover a wide range, a number in the middle is more likely to be correct.

- Watch out for distracters that are correct but do not answer the question, combine true and false information, or contain a word or phrase that is similar to the correct answer.
- Err on the side of caution.

Only One Answer Can Be Correct
- When more than one suggested answer is correct, you must identify the one that best answers the question asked.
- If you cannot choose between two answers, you have a 50% chance of getting it right if you guess.

Avoid Changing Answers
- Change an answer only if you have a compelling reason, such as you remembered something additional, or you understand the question better after rereading it.
- People change to a wrong answer more often than to a right answer.

Time Yourself to Complete the Whole Exam
- Do not spend a large amount of time on one question.
- If you cannot answer a question quickly, mark it and continue the exam.
- If time is left at the end, return to the difficult questions.
- Make educated guesses by eliminating the obviously wrong answers and choosing a likely answer even if you are not certain.
- Trust your instinct.
- Answer every question. There is no penalty for a wrong answer.
- Occasionally a question will remind you of something that helps you with a question earlier in the test. Look back at that question to see if what you are remembering affects how you would answer that question.

ABOUT THE CERTIFICATION EXAMS
The American Nurses Credentialing Center Computerized Exam
The ANCC examination is given only as a computer exam, and each exam is different.

The order of the questions is scrambled for every test, so even if two people are taking the same exam, the questions will be in a different order. The exam consists of 175 multiple-choice questions.
- 150 of the 175 questions are part of the test and how you answer will count toward your score, 25 are included to refine questions and will not be scored. You will not know which ones count, so treat all questions the same.
- You will need to know how to use a mouse, scroll by either clicking arrows on the scroll bar or using the up and down arrow keys, and perform other basic computer tasks.
- The exam does not require computer expertise
- However, if you are not comfortable with using a computer, you should practice using a mouse and computer beforehand so you do not waste time on the mechanics of using the computer.

Know what to expect during the test.
- Each ANCC test question is independent of the other questions.
  - For each case study, there is only one question. This means that a correct answer on any question does not depend on the correct answer to any other question.
  - Each question has four possible answers. There are no questions asking for combinations of correct answers (such as "a and c") or multiple-multiples.

- You can skip a question and go back to it at the end of the exam.
- You cannot mark key words in the question or right or wrong answers. If you want to do this, use the scratch paper.
- You will get your results immediately, and a grade report will be provided upon leaving the testing site.

OTHER RESOURCES:

ANCC Web site: www.nursecredentialing.org

ANA Web site: www.nursesbooks.org. Catalog of ANA nursing scope and standards publications and other titles that may be listed on your test content outline

National Guideline Clearinghouse—www.ngc.gov

Dimensions of the NP Role

Michaelene Jansen, PhD, RN, GNP-BC, NP-C

HISTORY OF THE NP ROLE

The nurse practitioner (NP) role began in 1965 at the University of Colorado, the brainchild of Henry K. Silver, MD, of the School of Medicine, and Loretta C. Ford, PhD, of the School of Nursing. Dr. Ford, who taught within the community health program at the School of Nursing, designed the original continuing education (CE) program for experienced community health nurses. Drs. Silver and Ford published extensively about their success in having experienced registered nurses with advanced training and skills perform some of the clinical duties traditionally reserved for physicians. The Colorado program was established in the same year that the physician assistant role was being developed at Duke University. These early pediatric nurse practitioner (PNP) programs were the prototype for all NP educational programs.

Early certificate-level NP programs were typically 16 weeks in length. Many schools offered a NP certificate as part of a broader master's in nursing (MS) curriculum. However, these CE programs were open to RNs with all types of preparation, including RNs with diploma and associate's degrees who would not have been eligible for the MS programs. The first guidelines for PNP programs were published in a joint document from the American Nurses Association and the American Academy of Pediatrics in 1970. The National Board of Pediatric Nurse Practitioner Accreditation (PNP/A) established an accreditation mechanism in 1973; the ANA quickly followed with moves to accredit these CE programs. Both organizations recognized the importance of achieving some standardization and control over quality.

The first certification exams for PNPs were offered by the American Nurses Association in the fall of 1976. Later, the American Nurses Credentialing Center (www.nursecredentialing.org) was established to write exams for nurses in most areas of practice.

The NP role gained momentum as a wide variety of programs were established in the late 1970s and early 1980s fueled by the federal government's concern about the "shortage" of physicians and the realization that nurses were an underutilized resource in primary health care. This led to funding by Health Resources and Service Administration, Bureau of Health Professions— Division of Nursing for the development of the first NP programs in schools of nursing. In addition, the Robert Wood Johnson Foundation fully funded "gold star" NP programs throughout the United States in 1980 and provided additional funding for "gold star" faculty to attend these programs. Most of these early programs were joint efforts of schools of medicine and nursing.

The role of the gerontological nurse practitioner (GNP) was developed through projects that emphasized the role of the GNP in nursing homes. The Mountain States Health Corporation project received funding from the W.K. Kellogg Foundation in 1976 to build a GNP program. The purpose was to improve the quality of care to elderly clients in long-term care facilities and other community settings. The impact of GNPs from this project was studied extensively, including patient care outcomes and the career paths of the graduates. The Teaching Nursing Home Project funded by the Robert Wood Johnson Foundation emphasized improvement of care and use of GNPs in isolated healthcare institutions. As the GNP moved from the nursing home to other settings, the GNP model of practice became more varied.

NPs have worked to have the nurse practice acts revised or replaced in all 50 states in order to recognize the diagnostic and treatment functions of the role. The Advanced Practice Consensus Group developed a Consensus Model for APRN Regulation: Licensure, Accreditation, Certification, and Education in 2008. In this model, APRNs would be licensed as adult/gerontology advanced practice nurses through their state regulating bodies and also could be certified in a specialty area (APRN Joint Dialogue Group, 2008). GNPs are prepared to provide a wide variety of services in a variety of clinical settings. GNPs can now be found in many settings, including nursing homes, rehabilitation centers, primary care practices, clinics, Programs for All-Inclusive Care of the Elderly (PACE), Veteran's Administration Medical Centers, life care retirement communities, assisted living facilities, adult day care centers, homecare, and hospitals.

Nurse practitioners rely heavily on their nursing education and background, integrating new assessment skills and diagnostic and treatment knowledge to develop a totally new role. Their level of competence has brought growing acceptance of the NP role into the healthcare system. The number of certified gerontological nurse practitioners is small compared to other types of nurse practitioners, although the older population in growing. In an effort to increase the number of qualified and certified gerontological nurse practitioners, the American Nurses Credentialing Center developed alternative eligibility criteria for acute, adult, and family nurse practitioners who wish to become certified GNPs. These criteria include current licensure in the individual's state, 2000 hours of clinical practice with older adults within the last 3 years, and 75 hours of continuing education or academic credit in specified areas (see http://www. nursecredentialing.org/Documents/Certification/Application/NursingSpecialty/ GerontologicalNursePractitionerAlternativeCritiera.aspx).

CLINICAL PRACTICE OF GERONTOLOGICAL NURSE PRACTITIONERS

In 2003, the National Conference of Gerontological Nurse Practitioners (NCGNP), renamed Gerontological Advanced Practice Nurses Association (GAPNA) in 2008, developed a position paper on GNP practice. This paper (NCGNP, 2003) defines gerontological nurse practitioners (GNPs) as "advanced practice nurses with specialized education in the diagnosis, treatment and management of acute and chronic conditions often found among older adults and generally associated with aging. Many such conditions lead to functional decline requiring therapeutic interventions to restore or maintain an optimal level of function, or when appropriate, palliative care. Such chronic or debilitating conditions are often complex and can occur in younger adults. The GNP has the clinical expertise to care for such aging persons."

"Practice sites of Gerontological Nurse Practitioners include traditional ambulatory care clinics, care management companies, acute and sub-acute hospitals, private homes, and all levels of long-term care. The GNP may treat adults of any age who have acute and chronic conditions. Other GNPs work in specialty areas with expanded scopes of practice that require specialized education and close collaboration with other health care providers.

"Gerontological Nurse Practitioners have been subjected to various age related practice restrictions. Such restrictions are based upon the perception that practice scopes are defined by certification category rather than by education, ability, experience, and collaborative practice agreements. The National Council of State Boards of Nursing (1993) concluded that certification did not include a defined scope of practice. The Council stated, 'while different requirements for various areas of nursing may be acceptable for professional certification, inconsistency becomes problematic when attempts are made to apply professional certification requirements to regulatory systems'.

"NCGNP (now GAPNA) supports the position that the scope of practice of Gerontological Nurse Practitioners is concerned with the health problems of older adults that are generally associated with aging. Further, NCGNP supports the ANA (1996) position that 'the individual advanced practice registered nurse is responsible for identifying the scope of practice permitted by state and federal laws and regulations, the professional code of ethics, and professional practice standards'. Furthermore, the GNP's competence is circumscribed by his or her experience, education, knowledge, and abilities." (NCGNP, 2003)

The Gerontological Advanced Practice Nurses Association position paper includes the following positions taken:
- Gerontological nurse practitioners (GNPs) are educated through nurse practitioner programs at the master's or post-master's level to meet the medical, bio-psycho-social, and functional needs of aging persons with acute and chronic illnesses through appropriate assessment, diagnostic, and management activities.
- GNPs have received advanced nursing education and training in the health problems of adults. All GNPs have received specialized education and training in the diagnosis, treatment, and management of acute and chronic conditions commonly found among older adults and generally associated with aging. The GNP may treat adults of any age who have acute and chronic conditions. The diversity of client groups served by GNPs is reflected in their varied practice settings and individualized scopes of practice.

- GNPs are recognized as advanced practice nurses in accordance with individual state rules and regulations concerning advanced practice nursing. Generally, GNPs are required to have specialty certification through a nationally recognized credentialing center.
- The GNP scope of practice may be limited to a particular client group as delineated by the GNP's individualized scope of practice and/or collaborative practice agreements with other healthcare providers based on experience, education, knowledge, and abilities. See www.gapna.org for more information.

IMPORTANT FACTORS INFLUENCING THE NP ROLE

Legal Dimensions of the Role

I. Legal Authority for Practice

State Nurse Practice Act—Rules and Regulations

- Authority for NP practice is found in state legislative statutes and in rules and regulations. The Nurse Practice Act of every state customarily authorizes the Board of Nursing to establish statutory authority to define who may be called a nurse practitioner (title protection); what they may do (scope of practice); restrictions on their practice; the requirements an NP must meet in order to be credentialed within the state as an NP (educational, certification, etc.); and disciplinary grounds for infraction of regulations. (See http://www.ncsbn.org for a listing of state nursing board requirements.) In many states, legislative acts may specifically require that an NP develop a collaborative agreement with a physician, describe what types of drugs might be prescribed, or define some form of oversight board for NP practice.
- Statutory law is implemented in regulatory language. The rules and regulations for each state may further define scope of practice and practice requirements and/or restrictions.
- Beginning in 1999, the National Council State Boards of Nursing (NCSBN) began implementation of an interstate compact for nursing practice to reduce state-to-state discrepancies in nursing requirements to practice. The Advanced Practice Registered Nurse (APRN) Compact addresses the need to promote consistent access to high-quality advanced practice nursing care within states and across state lines. The Uniform APRN Licensure/Authority to Practice Requirements, developed by NCSBN with APRN stakeholders in 2000, establishes the foundation for this APRN Compact. Similar to the existing Nurse Licensure Compact for recognition of RN and LPN licenses, the APRN Compact offers states the mechanism for mutually recognizing APRN licenses/authority to practice. A state must either be a member of the current nurse licensure compact for RN and LPN, or choose to enter into both compacts simultaneously to be eligible for the APRN Compact. To determine which states participate, view the state compact map at www.ncsbn.org/158.htm.
- The APRN Joint Dialogue Group, consisting of an APRN Consensus Work Group and the National Council of State Boards of Nursing Advanced Practice Advisory Committee, forwarded a consensus model for APRN regulation in 2008. The model identifies APRN roles and population foci for licensure and specialty areas where the focus of practice extends beyond the population and role linked to health needs. The model identifies adult/gerontology as one population with older adults as a potential specialty. A copy of the consensus statement and regulatory model can be found at http://www.aacn.nche.edu/education/pdf/APRNReport.pdf.

II. Nurse Practitioner Professional Practice

Licensure

- The U.S. Department of Health, Education and Welfare (DHEW) in 1971 defined licensure as "a process by which an agency of state government grants permission to individuals accountable for the practice of a profession to engage in the practice of that profession and prohibits all others from legally doing so."
- The purpose is to protect the public by ensuring a minimum level of professional competence. "This regulatory method is used when regulated activities are complex, require specialized knowledge, skill and independent decision-making. The licensure process includes the predetermination of qualifications necessary to perform a legally defined scope of practice safely and an evaluation of licensure applications to determine that the qualifications are met. Licensure provides that a specified scope of practice may only be performed legally by licensed individuals. Licensure provides title protection for those roles. It also provides authority to take disciplinary action should the licensee violate provision of the law or rules in order to assure that the public health, safety and welfare will be reasonably well protected" (NCSBN, https://www.ncsbn.org/170.htm).

Certification

- "A process by which a non-governmental agency or association certifies that an individual licensed to practice as a professional has met certain predetermined standards specified by that profession for specialty practice" (DHEW, 1971).
- The purpose is to assure the public that an individual has mastery of a body of knowledge and has acquired the skills necessary to function in a particular specialty. Some certifications are required for entry into practice (e.g., required for licensure within a state, and they thus have a regulatory function); some certifications denote professional competence and recognize excellence.

Accreditation

- "The process by which a voluntary, non-governmental agency or organization appraises and grants accreditation status to institutions and/or programs or services which meet predetermined structure, process and outcome criteria" (DHEW, 1971).
- The purpose is to assure that the organization has met specific standards.

Scope of Practice

- Defines a specific legal scope determined by state statues, boards of nursing, educational preparation, and common practice within a community. For example, adult nurse practitioners are not legally authorized to care for children. The state might require a NP to have formal educational preparation in pediatrics. Broad variation exists from state to state.
- General scope of practice is specified in many published professional documents (e.g., *Nursing: Scope and Standards*, ANA, 2004; *Nursing Social Policy Statement*, ANA, 2009). In addition, many organizations have completed role-delineation studies that attempt to qualify the core behaviors that all APNs must possess, as well as the core knowledge and behaviors required of individuals in a particular specialty. For example, core knowledge for a PNP will be inherently different from that of a GNP. It is critical that these statements about specific scope and standards exist so that everyone—including nurses—will have access to materials that they can refer to when there are specific questions related to role. This is especially important when the traditional role of nurses is being changed or "advanced" at an uneven rate through changes in state law. As the nurse practitioner role has expanded into new practice settings, including hospice,

hospitals, and home care, it is important that core knowledge as well as state law protecting NPs in these practice settings expand also, providing the legal authorization and title protection necessary for these practice settings.

- Prescriptive authority is recognized as being within the scope of practice for nurse practitioners in all 50 states, though there is significant variability from state to state. This variability has created inherent difficulty in collecting data related to NP prescribing practices. A comprehensive update of legislative requirements and recent changes known as the Pearson report is published each year by the *American Journal of Nurse Practitioners* (available at www.pearsonreport.com). Data collected by Nurse Practitioner Alternatives, Inc., since 1996 have documented stability within prescribing patterns by NPs. Data from 2004 show that the majority of NPs possess their own Drug Enforcement Administration (DEA) number (72%), write between 6 and 25 prescriptions in an average clinical day (79%), recommend between 1 and 20 over-the-counter (OTC) preparations in an average clinical day (90%) and manage between 25% and 100% of their patient encounters independently (97%; www.npedu.com).

Standards of Practice

- Authoritative statements by which the quality of practice, service, or education can be judged, such as *Nursing: Scope and Standards* (ANA, 2004); *Scope and Standards of Gerontological Nursing Practice* (ANA, 2001).
- Professional standards focus on the minimum levels of acceptable performance as a way of providing consumers with a means of measuring the quality of care they receive. They may be written at the generic level to apply to all nurses (for example, standards regarding following universal precautions), as well as to define practice by each specialty.
- The presence of accepted standards of practice may be used to legally describe the standard of care that must be met by a provider. These standards may be precise protocols that must be followed, or recommendations for more general guidelines.
- Healthy People 2020 Objectives and WHO "Health for All" are, respectively, national and international policy statements that describe the objectives to be met to help all persons to obtain a level of health that will permit them to lead socially and economically productive lives. It is anticipated that over time, these objectives will form the basis for international standards of practice.

III. Client Rights

Confidentiality

- The patient and family have a right to assume that information given to the healthcare provider will not be disclosed. This practice has several dimensions:
  - Verbal information: The healthcare provider shall not discuss any information given to him or her during the healthcare encounter with anyone not directly involved in providing this care without the patient or family's permission.
  - Written information: Confidentiality of the healthcare encounter is protected under federal statute through the Health Insurance Portability and Accountability Act of 1996 (HIPAA). The Administrative Simplification provisions of HIPAA require the Department of Health and Human Services to establish national standards for electronic healthcare transactions and national identifiers for providers, health plans, and employers. It also addresses the security and privacy of health data. Information may be accessed at http://www.hhs.gov/ocr/privacy/hipaa/understanding/summary/.
  - The individual's right to privacy is respected when requesting or responding to a request for patient's medical record.

- The statute requires that the provider discuss confidentiality issues with patients (or parents in the case of a minor), establish consent, and clarify any questions about disclosure of information.
  - The provider is required to obtain a signed medical authorization and consent form to release medical records and information.
- Exceptions to guaranteed confidentiality occur when society determines that the need for information outweighs the principle of confidentiality. Examples might be when records are released to insurance companies; to attorneys involved in litigation, answering court orders, subpoenas, summonses; in meeting state requirements for mandatory reporting of diseases or conditions; in cases of suspected child abuse; or if a patient reveals an intent to harm someone.

Informed Consent
- The clinician has the duty to explain relevant information to the patient and family so that they can make an appropriate decision. This information usually includes diagnosis, nature and purpose of proposed treatment or procedure, risks and benefits, prognosis, alternative methods of treatment and their risks and benefits, and even the remote possibility of serious harm.
- It must be documented in medical records that this information has been provided.

Decisional Capacity
- The clinician must determine the client's ability to cognitively process information provided. *Decision-making capability* is the ability to cognitively process information and render a decision.
- *Competence* is a legal term referring to the determination by a court that an individual does or does not possess sufficient cognitive function to make decisions regarding health care and other legal matters. If an individual is declared not to be competent, a legal guardian is appointed and this results in limitations in the individual's exercise of basic rights.

Advance Directives
- When a patient is incapable of making decisions, a person's preferences may be expressed by way of a written living will or a health care durable power of attorney when that person is still able to make healthcare decision.
- *Living wills* are written documents prepared in advance in case of terminal illness or nonreversible loss of consciousness.
  - Their provisions go into effect when:
    - The individual lacks capacity to make healthcare decisions
    - The patient is declared terminally ill
    - No further interventions will alter the patient's course to a reasonable degree of medical certainty
- Durable power of attorney for health care
  - Individuals can identify in writing an agent to act on their behalf, should they become mentally incapacitated. The decisions of the designated agent are:
    - Binding
    - Not limited to the circumstances of terminal illness
    - Flexible enough to carry out patient's wishes throughout the course of an illness
    - Often accompanied by a durable power of attorney over financial issues, as well

Ethical Decision-Making
- Moral concepts such as advocacy, accountability, loyalty, caring, compassion, and human dignity are the foundations of ethical behavior.
- The ethical behavior of nurses has been defined for professional nursing in an American Nurses Association policy statement (ANA, 2008).
- Autonomy: Ethical behavior incorporates respect for the individual and respect for his or her right of self-determination. Thus, no decision is truly ethical if the caregiver does not involve the patient in decision-making to the full extent of the patient's capacity.
- Duty to treat patients fairly (*justice*), can be viewed as both access (those who are entitled to health care can obtain it) and allocation (how resources are distributed).
- Duty to help others (*beneficence*) and avoidance of harmful behavior (*nonmaleficence*) are also foundational components of ethical behavior.

Quality Assurance
- Quality assurance is a system to evaluate and monitor the quality of patient care and the quality of facility management.
- Formal programs provide a framework for systematic, deliberate, and continuous evaluation and monitoring of individual clinical practice. Programs promote responsibility and accountability to deliver high-quality care, assist in the evaluation and improvement of patient care, and provide for an organized means of problem solving. Thus, a good program identifies educational needs, improves the documentation of care, and overall reduces the clinician's exposure to liability.
- Programs identify components of structure, process, and outcomes of care. They also look at organization effectiveness, efficiency, and client and provider interactions.
- Programs may be implemented through audits, utilization review, peer review, outcome studies, and measurements of patient satisfaction.

IV. Nurse Practitioner Legal And Financial Issues
Liability
- Sources of legal risk
  - Patients, procedures
  - Quality of medical records
- Risk reduction or management
  - Activities or systems designed to recognize and intervene to reduce the risk of injury to patients and subsequent claims against healthcare providers
  - Malpractice insurance: does not protect a clinician from charges of practicing outside his or her legal scope of practice. It is universally recommended that all clinicians carry their own liability insurance coverage so they will have their own legal representation and attorney to advocate for them.
  - A mindset and practice that emphasizes patient safety and quality (see Agency for Health Care, Research, and Quality)
- Malpractice
  - Negligent professional acts of individuals engaged in professions requiring highly technical or professional skills
  - The plaintiff has the burden of proving four elements of malpractice
    - Duty: The clinician has the duty to exercise reasonable care when undertaking and providing treatment to the patient when a patient-clinician relationship exists.
    - Breach of duty: The clinician violates the applicable standard of care in treating the patient's condition.

- Proximate cause: There is a causal relationship between the breach in the standard of care and the patient's injuries.
- Damages: There are permanent and substantial damages to the patient as a result of the malpractice.
- National Practitioner Databank (NPDB)
  - The Health Care Quality Improvement Act of 1986 (amended in 1998) established a databank to scrutinize members of the healthcare profession and list those practitioners who have had a malpractice claim asserted against them.
  - NPDB proactive disclosure service (PDS), an online service since 2007, offers providers and agencies the opportunity to monitor practitioners.
  - Diagnosis-related problems account for almost 46% of payments for NPs. Although the number of lawsuits against NPs has risen in recent years, there is still very little history of successful litigation against NPs (www.npdb-hipdb.com/pubs/stats/2006_NPDB_annual_report.pdf).

Reimbursement

- NPs are reimbursed as primary care providers in some form for their services under Medicare, Medicaid, Federal Employee Benefit Plan, Champus, veterans and military programs, and federally funded school-based clinics.
- Private insurance plans may elect to reimburse for NP services even if not mandated to do so by state law. In some states, the insurance code may be interpreted rigidly to exclude reimbursement of NPs.
- Managed care organizations (MCOs) have frequently excluded NPs from being designated as primary care providers and allowing their own caseload. Thus, in many MCOs the only employment arrangement left open to NPs is that of being a salaried employee. As a salaried employee, the NP contributions are often not visible and may be credited to their collaborating physicians, giving them a "ghost" provider status. Without a legitimate method to document services provided and revenue generated, NP job security is often at risk. A recent focus of legislative activity by many state NP organizations has been to enact state law that allows for NPs to be impaneled as primary care providers in both health maintenance organizations (HMOs) and preferred provider organizations (PPOs). These efforts have led to opposition from state medical organizations.
- The concept of the medical home is a new model for patient care. Efforts are underway by professional nursing organizations to include nurse practitioners as primary care providers.
- There is considerable flux in state and national policy on what services and procedures NPs may bill for and whether they will be paid directly. Incorrect billing places the healthcare provider at risk for fraud and abuse charges whether they knowingly violate the law or are just ignorant of the regulations.
- NPs must be aware of specific regulations and policies for patient care services. Resources include Center for Medicare & Medicaid Services (CMS), at www.cms.hhs.gov.

Performance Assessment

- The National Practitioner Data Bank (NPDB) and Health Integrity and Protection Data Bank (HIPDB) are maintained by the U.S. Department of Health and Human Services (HHS), Health Resources and Services Administration (HRSA), Bureau of Health Professions (BHP), Division of Practitioner Data Banks (DPDB). Developed as a result of the Health Care Quality and Improvement Act of 1986 and amended in 1998, the NPDB/HIPDB is a flagging system intended to facilitate a comprehensive review of healthcare practitioners' professional credentials. The information contained in the NPDB is intended to direct inquiry into a practitioner's licensure, professional society memberships, malpractice payment history, and record of clinical privileges, with a goal of improving the quality of health care. NPs may perform a self-query by visiting the site at www.npdb-hipdb.hrsa.gov.

- Other programs monitoring and comparing health quality include the Health Plan Employer Data and Information Set (HEDIS®) developed by the National Committee on Quality Assurance (NCQA). HEDIS is a set of standardized performance measures designed to ensure that purchasers and consumers have the information they need to reliably compare the performance of managed healthcare plans (http://www.ncqa.org).

V. Current Trends

Some of the topics dominating NP discussions about their future involve:

1. Fiscal Issues

- Growing competition in the job market for NPs, as numbers of NPs have increased and NPs have begun to directly compete with physicians and physician assistants
- Reimbursement struggles with CMS, private insurance
- Increasing costs for malpractice insurance; many states have launched legislative initiatives in the area of medical tort reform in an attempt to hold down malpractice premiums
- All providers must obtain a National Provider Identifier (NPI). All healthcare providers are eligible to be assigned an NPI. Information may be obtained at http://www.cms.hhs. gov/NationalProvIdentStand/01_overview.asp
- Growing concerns over reimbursement fraud and abuse issues as well as coding issues, both in the area of overbilling and underbilling, particularly for Medicare patients

2. NP Education

- Recognition of the need to ensure the quality of NP education, faculty, and curriculum has led to efforts by the National Organization of Nurse Practitioner Faculties (NONPF) and the American Association of Colleges of Nursing (AACN) to promulgate core competency statements (2006) and specialty competencies, including those for gerontology (2002). These statements can be viewed at www.nonpf.org.
- In addition, NONPF and AACN, along with numerous NP professional organizations, NP accrediting bodies, and educational organizations, have jointly promulgated criteria for evaluation of nurse practitioner programs. In combination with accreditation standards for graduate programs and for specialty areas, the criteria provide a basis for evaluating the quality of nurse practitioner programs.

3. As an alternative to research-focused doctoral degrees, AACN in collaboration with NONPF and other nursing organizations have developed an essentials document for a Practice Doctorate in Nursing that will be the degree associated with practice-focused doctoral nursing education (available at http://www.aacn.nche.edu/DNP/pdf/Essentials. pdf). The practice doctorate will be the graduate degree for advanced nursing practice preparation by 2015.

4. Practice Environment

- Health Disparities: There is growing recognition of disparities in the health services and outcomes of different populations in the United States. The National Center on Minority Health and Health Disparities (NCMHD) at the National Institutes of Health (NIH) is a government organization with a mission to promote minority health and to lead, coordinate, support, and assess the NIH effort to reduce and ultimately eliminate health disparities (http://ncmhd.nih.gov/).
- Health Literacy: It is now recognized that one of the largest contributors to health outcomes is the ability of a patient and family to understand and act on health information. Both the Institute of Medicine (IOM) and the Agency for Health Care Research and Quality (AHRQ) have launched efforts to quantify and offer solutions to the problems that result from inadequate health literacy. The IOM report may be viewed at www.iom.edu/ CMS/3775/3827/19723.aspx; the AHRQ study can be found at http://www.ahrq.gov/news/press/pr2004/litpr.htm.
- Patient Bill of Rights: In 2004, the U.S. Senate and House of Representatives passed different versions of a Patient Bill of Rights. These bills are an attempt to ensure that patients have access to their provider of choice and have access to an independent external appeals process to address health plan grievances. The bills have not yet been approved by a joint committee or been sent to the Office of the President for signature. It is critical that NPs monitor legislation in this area to insure that the rights of nonphysician providers are protected.
- There is increasing attention being paid to preparing registered nurses to gain disaster education so they might be prepared to assume emergency roles during a time of mass casualties from either natural disasters or terrorist attacks. Because some other countries have had more experience with dealing with terrorism, the Nursing Emergency Preparedness Education Coalition (formerly the International Nursing Coalition for Mass Casualty Education) was established and headquartered at Vanderbilt School of Nursing to help U.S. nurses profit from their experience and to identify the educational competencies for registered nurses responding to mass casualty incidents. They desire to improve the ability of all nurses to respond safely and effectively to mass casualty incidents through identification of existing and emerging roles of nurses, ensuring appropriateness of education in mass casualty incidents, and helping to understand response frameworks and ensure collaborative efforts. All NPs are expected to prepare themselves to play a larger role in delivery of care during a time of disaster. Information of the objectives and work that has been done toward a uniform curriculum in this area may be obtained at www.nursing.vanderbilt.edu/incmce/.
- Direct-to-consumer advertising: Patients frequently present to the office already having formed their diagnosis and wanting specific treatments, in part because of the influence of direct-to-consumer advertising. NPs are required to become knowledgeable about the newest products on the market in order to appropriately counsel and treat patients.
- There is greater recognition of the use of complementary and alternative medicine by consumers. Research suggests that 40% to 50% of patients are currently using a form of complementary or alternative (CAM) therapy today, despite the fact that there is little research on which to base treatment regimens. NPs as providers need to learn about common CAM treatments and particularly about how some herbal products interact adversely with prescription drugs. The National Institutes of Health have established a center to begin research on these popular preparations. Until more is known, it is suggested that providers move cautiously in prescribing these preparations for their patients. See http://nccam.nih.gov/.

- Since release of the Institute of Medicine's report *To Err is Human: Building A Safer Health System* (available at www.iom.edu/Reports/1999/To-Err-is-Human-Building-A-Safer-Health-System.aspx), there has been increased attention on changes all healthcare providers should make to decrease medical errors. In response, the Joint Commission (www.jointcommission.org) has issued a list of abbreviations that should not be used in health care, and the Institute for Safe Medication Practices (ISMP) has published a list of dangerous abbreviations related to medication use that it recommends should be explicitly prohibited (available at www.ismp.org/). The list of banned abbreviations includes many symbols traditionally used on patient charts and in writing prescriptions.

VI. Professional Organizations
- Participation in professional organizations is important because nurse practitioners acting as a group can have more influence over the profession.
- State organizations: Every NP should belong to his or her state NP organization. Often these organizations are associated or affiliated with the state professional nursing organization. State organizations work diligently to monitor and affect laws and regulations affecting NP practice. In addition, these associations provide a group of peers for discussion and continuing educations.
- The American College of Nurse Practitioners (ACNP) is focused on advocacy and keeping NPs current on legislative, regulatory, and clinical practice issues that effect NPs in the rapidly changing healthcare arena. See www.acnpweb.org.
- The Gerontological Advanced Practice Nurses Association (GAPNA), formerly the National Conference of Gerontological Nurse Practitioners (NCGNP), is the professional organization that advocates for gerontological nurse practitioners who deliver health care in a variety of settings.
- The National Organization of Nurse Practitioner Faculties (NONPF) is an organization of nurse practitioner educators who are instrumental in setting standards for nurse practitioner education. NONPF has developed Core Competencies describing the domains of practice with critical behaviors that should be exhibited by all entry-level NPs.

CASE STUDIES

Case 1. Your 92-year-old female patient who lives alone at home has fallen several times in the past few months. She refuses to have physical therapy or to move to an assisted living or nursing home. Her daughter, who has not talked to her for the past 10 years, wants you to sign a document stating her mother is not competent so she can put her in a nursing home. The daughter also wants a copy of her mother's chart.

1. What are the legal issues involved?
2. Should you tell the daughter about the patient's condition or give her a copy of the chart?
3. Can you determine from the information given that the patient lacks the capacity to make healthcare decisions?

Case 2. An 82-year-old man is found to have lung cancer. This was an incidental finding on chest x-ray for admission to assisted living. He has no symptoms. He is a widower with one son.

1. What healthcare documents would you ask the patient about?
2. What healthcare decisions would you look for on his durable power of attorney?
3. How would you decide how aggressively to manage this patient?
4. The patient becomes incompetent without writing down his wishes. You need to decide whether or not to put in a feeding tube. What question do you pose to the son?

Case 3. You just graduated from your nurse practitioner program.

1. What additional qualifications do you need in order to practice?

REFERENCES

Agency for Health Care, Research and Quality. (2008). *Patient safety and quality.* Retrieved from www.ahrq.gov/qual/nurseshdbk/

American Nurses Association. (2004). *Nursing: Scope and standards.* Washington, DC: Author.

American Nurses Association. (2009). *Nursing's social policy statement: The essence of the profession.* Washington, DC: Author.

American Nurses Credentialing Center. (2009). *ANCC certification.* Silver Spring, MD: Author.

APRN Joint Dialogue Group. (2008). *Consensus model for APRN regulation: Licensure, accreditation, certification and education.* Retrieved from http://www.aacn.nche.edu/education/pdf/APRNReport.pdf

Baxter, M. L. (1999). Ethical issues. In J. T. Stone, J. F. Wyman, & S. A. Salisbury (Eds.), *Clinical gerontological nursing* (2nd ed., pp. 45–61). Philadelphia: W. B. Saunders.

Birren, J. E., & Schaie, K. W. (Eds). (2001). *Handbook of the psychology of aging* (5th ed.). San Diego: Academic Press.

Buppert, C. (2005). *The primary care providers guide to compensation and quality: How to get paid and not get sued* (2nd ed). Sudbury, MA: Jones & Bartlett.

Buppert, C. (2007). *Nurse practitioners' business practice and legal guide* (3rd ed.). Sudbury, MA: Jones & Bartlett.

Burggraf, V. (1999). Advanced practice of gerontological nursing. In J. T. Stone, J. F. Wyman, & S. A. Salisbury (Eds.), *Clinical gerontological nursing* (2nd ed., pp. 3–16). Philadelphia: W. B. Saunders.

Ebersole, P. (1985). Geriatric nurse practitioners past and present. *Geriatric Nursing, 6,* 219–222.

Edmunds, M. W., & Mayhew, M. S. (2004). *Pharmacology for primary care providers* (2nd ed.). St. Louis, MO: Mosby.

Federation of State Medical Boards of the United States. (1988). *Non-physician duties and scope of practice.* Position Statement 210.003. Dallas, TX: Author.

Ford, L. C. (1992). Advanced nursing practice: Future of the nurse practitioner. In L. H. Aiken, & C. M. Fagin (Eds.), *Charting nursing's future: Agenda for the 1990s* (pp. 287–299). Philadelphia: JB Lippincott.

Fowler, M. (2008). *ANA code of ethics for nurses.* Silver Spring, MD: American Nurses Association.

The Institute for the Future. (2000). *Health & health care 2010: The forecast, the challenge.* San Francisco: Jossey-Bass.

The Institute of Medicine. (1999). *To err is human: Building a safe healthcare system.* Retrieved from http://www.iom.edu/report.asp?id=5575

Kane, R. A., Kane, R. L., Arnold, S., Garrard, J., McDermont, S., & Keperele, L. (1988). Geriatric nurse practitioners as nursing home employees: Implementing the role. *The Gerontologist, 28*(4), 469–477.

McDougall, G. J., & Roberts, B. (1993). A gerontologic nurse practitioner in every nursing home: A necessary expenditure. *Geriatric Nursing, 14*(4), 218–220.

Mullen, F., Plitzer, R. M., Lewis, C. T., Bastacky, S., Rodak, Jr., J., & Harmon, R. G. (1992). The National Practitioner Data Bank: Report from the first year. *JAMA, 268,* 73–79.

Munden, J. (Ed.). (2001). *Nurse practitioner's legal reference.* North Wales, PA: Springhouse.

National Conference of Gerontological Nurse Practitioners. (2003). *Position statement: Clinical practice of gerontological nurse practitioners.* Retrieved from https://www.gapna.org/download/PositionStatements/ClinicalPracticeGNPs

National Council of State Boards of Nursing. (1993). *Regulation of advanced nursing practice.* National Council Position Paper. Chicago: Author.

National Organization of Nurse Practitioner Faculties. (2002). *Nurse practitioner primary care competencies in specialty areas: Adult, family, gerontological, pediatric, and women's health.* Washington, DC: Author.

National Organization of Nurse Practitioner Faculties. (2006). *Domains and core competencies.* Washington, DC: Author

Pearson, L. J. (2008). *The Pearson report.* Retrieved from http://www.pearsonreport.com

Radosevich, D. M., Kane, R. L., Garrard, J., Skay, C. L., McDermott, S., Kepferle, L., et al. (1990). Career paths of geriatric nurse practitioners employed in nursing homes. *Public Health Reports, 105*(1), 65–71.

Safreit, B. (Summer, 1992). Health care dollars and regulatory sense: The role of advanced practice nursing. *Yale Journal of Regulation, 9*(2), 417–488.

U.S. Department of Health, Education, and Welfare. (1971). *Report on licensure and related health personnel credentials.* Washington, DC: Author. (DHEW Pub No. (HSM) 72-11).

U.S. Department of Health and Human Services, Division of Nursing. (2002). *Nurse practitioner primary care competencies in specialty areas: Adult, family, gerontological, pediatric, and women's health.* Washington, DC: U.S. Department of Health and Human Services, Health Resources and Services Administration, Bureau of Health Professions.

U.S. Office of Technology Assessment. (1986). *Nurse practitioners, physician's assistants and certified nurse midwives: A policy analysis.* Washington, DC: U.S. Government Printing Office.

Walker, L., & Wetle, T. (1999). Ethical issues. In S. L. Molony, C. M. Waszynski, & C. H. Lyder (Eds.), *Gerontological nursing: An advanced practice approach* (pp. 545–557). Stamford, CT: Appleton & Lange.

Healthcare Issues

Vaunette Fay, PhD, RN, FNP-BC, GNP-BC

GERIATRICS

- Most people use the age 65 to mark the beginning of geriatrics.
- Perhaps the most important public health concern of the early 21st century is the increasing number of individuals age 65 and older; by 2020 it is estimated that 20% of the population will be over 65.
- Not only will this number double in the next 20 years, but individuals who are currently 65 years of age will, on average, live for another 20 years.
- Often geriatrics is divided into the *young old* (65–74), the *old* (75–84), the *oldest old* (85 and above), and *elite old* (over 100 years).
- Within those older than 65, the fastest growing subgroup is those over age 85.
- Variability between patients increases with age. This book presents many generalizations about older adults. Just remember that every patient is unique.
- Cultural diversity continues to be an important factor in the assessment and management of older adults.
- Older Americans are becoming increasingly more ethnically diverse.

ASSESSMENT

Nonspecific Presentation of Illness

- A crucial aspect of geriatrics is that the older adult often presents with vague complaints or deterioration of functional independence as an early, subtle sign of illness.

- This presentation generally occurs in the absence of classic (typical) symptoms and signs of disease.
- When older adults get acutely ill they most often present with the following:
  - Confusion, delirium, and mental status changes: altered attention and orientation
  - Worsening dementia or delirium superimposed on dementia
  - Increased difficulty or taking longer to perform activities of daily living
  - Incontinence
  - Falls
  - Dizziness
  - Vague, generalized, nonspecific pain
  - Decreased appetite, weight loss, failure to thrive
  - May not have high fever or increased WBC in presence of severe infection

Assessment of the Elderly

- **Functional status determines quality of life to an older adult patient.**
- Older adults define health in terms of independent function, not medical diagnosis.
- Older adults often have multiple chronic medical conditions that cannot be cured; therefore, care is focused on maintaining function while managing illness.
- An important difference from adult medicine is the need for systematic assessment of the complex and multisystem problems of the geriatric patient, encompassing both medical and social needs.
- It is advisable to use appropriate standardized assessment instruments to measure factors relevant to patients' abilities.
- Assessment tools provide standardized data for following trends and evaluating response to treatment.
- Cognitive and functional assessment is the keystone of geriatrics.
- Each GNP should have a set of assessment tools appropriate to his or her practice. Components of a complete assessment of the older adult are:
  - Physiologic: normal changes of aging, medical diagnoses
  - Cognitive (mental status): Folstein mini-mental state (MMSE), Mini-Cog, Clock Drawing Test (CDT)
  - Functional: activities of daily living (ADLs), instrumental activities of daily living (IADLs), mobility, activities, get up and go test, observe gait and balance
  - Social: relationships, support systems, elder mistreatment
  - Psychological: anxiety, hope, depression, Geriatric Depression Scale
  - Nutritional: appropriate weight and adequate intake of nutrients, nutritional assessment tool
  - Economic: ability to pay for medications and health insurance as well as basic needs of food, housing, and utilities
  - Other: alcohol abuse, physical environment, stressors, coping skills, spiritual, values, quality of life

Cognitive Function

- Essential to differentiate between normal changes of cognitive function and dementia and delirium
- Many assessment tools have been developed
- MMSE is the most famous, used as a screening test but is not highly sensitive (be aware of copyright issues and cost)

- Other good dementia screening tools are the short portable mental status questionnaire, Mini-Cog, and the CDT
- Consider culture and education when interpreting score
- Cognitive function is divided into domains:
  - Attention: maintenance of alertness over time
  - Memory: ability to collect, store, and retrieve information
  - Orientation: memory of person, place, and time
  - Language: use and understand oral and written communication
  - Visual–spatial abilities: perceive objects and spatial relationships
  - Psychomotor speed: rate of cognitive processing
  - Executive/problem solving: higher cognitive skills (judgment, insight and abstract thinking); difficult to describe or assess
  - Intelligence: global levels of general cognitive functioning
- Memory is further divided:
  - Working memory: ability to manipulate remembered items
  - Recent memory: memory of events within the last 24 hours; the first type of memory to go in dementia
  - Remote memory: memory of events that occurred in the distant past; often preserved late in dementia
  - Implicit and procedural memory: memory without awareness; memory of how to do a previously learned task such as dressing and eating

Function Assessment
- Activities of daily living are those necessary to survive in society
- They are usually divided into three categories:
  - Activities of daily living (ADL) include bathing, dressing, eating, grooming, toileting, continence of bowel and bladder, and transferring
    - Essential element of the assessment of the older adult
    - Many assessment tools available
  - Instrumental activities of daily living (IADL) include cooking, money management, use of transportation, use of telephone, and medication administration, more complex tasks than the ADL
    - Common scales used are: Lawton & Brody Instrumental Activities of Daily Living Scale, Older Americans Resource Scale for Instrumental Activities of Daily Living (OARS-IADL)
  - Mobility includes walking, gait and balance, stairs, balance and transferring; the "get up and go" test is a common assessment tool
- When using one of the functional assessment tools, judge:
  - Amount of human assistance required: independent, supervision, cueing/organization, hands-on help, dependent (total help)
  - Speed of performance
  - Degree of pain during performance; endurance
  - Quality of performance
  - Safety
- When relying on self-report, patients tend to over estimate ability while families and caregivers tend to underestimate
- Assistive devices help the patient prolong independence; these include hearing aids, glasses, respiratory equipment, and mobility aids such as canes and walkers

Demographics/Epidemiology

- Population
  - The older population is large, growing fast, and becoming more diverse
    - 13% of population is 65 or older; in 2020, 20% will be 65 or older
    - Includes 2% who are 85+; age 85+ category growing fastest
    - Still largely white; other groups growing faster
    - More women than men: 59% at 65+; 71% at 85+
    - Nursing homes: 5% reside in nursing homes; 1% of those ages 65–74; 20% of 85+
    - 33% are living alone
    - 85% of informal caregiving is done by families
    - 10% live in poverty; percentage is higher for Black and Hispanic people
- Life expectancy
  - At birth: women, 79.4 years; men, 73.6 years
  - People age 65 can expect to live an average of 18.7 more years; women age 85 can expect to live an average of 7.2 more years and men an average of 6.1 more years
  - Women live longer than men
  - Shorter life expectancy for Black and Hispanic people
- Mortality
  - Leading causes of death
    - Heart disease   35%
    - Cancer   35%
    - Stroke   10%
    - COPD   6%
    - Pneumonia/influenza 7%
    - Other: diabetes, Alzheimer's disease, nephritis, accidents, septicemia
- Morbidity
  - Chronic conditions are prolonged illnesses that are generally never cured completely
  - Chronic disease is the nation's greatest healthcare problem
  - 80% of older adults in United States have at least one chronic health condition
  - 95% of healthcare expenditures are for chronic disease
  - In noninstitutionalized persons 65 years of age and older, 79% had at least one of the seven chronic conditions common among the elderly in 2005–2006
    - Arthritis   54% of women, 43% of men
    - Hypertension   54%
    - Heart disease   26% of women, 37% of men
    - Respiratory illnesses 11%
    - Diabetes   18%
    - Stroke   9%
    - Cancer of any kind   24% of men, 19% of women
- Impairments that commonly occur in older adults
  - Visual impairment
  - Hearing impairment: 62% of people 85+ have hearing loss
  - Tooth loss: 23% of people 65–74 year of age have no natural teeth
  - Decreased functional abilities
    - 3% over age 65 and 11% over age 75 report having some difficulty with at least one ADL
    - 7% over age 65 and 22% over age 75 report needing assistance with at least IADL
    - Approximately 15% are unable to walk 1/4 mile
  - There has been a decline in disability among older people in recent years

Health Insurance

Medicare

- The federal health insurance program for people age 65 and over, disabled people, and those with end-stage renal disease
- It is run by HCFA, the Health Care Financing Administration, which can be found at http://www.hhs.gov/about/opdivs/hcfa.html
- It covers 98% of older adults
- Medicare programs
  - Part A, Hospital Insurance
    - Covers payments for inpatient hospital care, skilled nursing facility care, hospice care, home health services, and other health services and supplies
    - Eligibility is automatic once work requirements are met
    - The Hospice benefit may be selected instead of this benefit
  - Part B, Supplementary Medical Insurance
    - A voluntary plan; approximately 90% choose to enroll; monthly premium
    - Covers physician services including office visits, clinical laboratory tests, durable medical equipment, flu vaccinations, drugs that cannot be self-administered, medical supplies, diagnostic tests, ambulance services, and some therapeutic services
    - Pays the physician 80% of the allowable cost, as determined by Medicare
  - Part D, Prescription coverage
    - Part D coverage is not provided within the traditional Medicare program
    - Instead, beneficiaries must affirmatively enroll in one of many hundreds of Part D plans offered by private companies
- Standard benefit includes an initial $275 deductible; after meeting the deductible the beneficiaries pay 25% of the cost of covered Part D prescription drugs
- Medicare does not cover custodial care (assistance with ADLs and IADLs), nonskilled care in nursing homes, or assisted living facilities
- Many have a secondary insurance (medi-gap), which is designed to pay the 20% that Medicare does not pay
- About 15% of Medicare recipients are enrolled in HMOs

Medicaid is a state program for the poor
- It will fill in the gaps for certain qualifying older people
- It covers payment for medications

Long-Term Care Insurance

- Private insurance policy purchased in advance; depending on the policy, may reimburse for nursing home care, assisted living, or home health care
- Policies vary on the amount and time of reimbursement, a length of stay may be required before insurance becomes effective
- Currently covers less then 2% of all nursing home expenses and is unlikely to lead to substantial reduction in out-of-pocket expenses and decreased Medicaid use

Social Support

- Social isolation is a common problem with older people
  - Their friends and family die
  - They often live alone in their own home, unable to drive or use public transportation
  - People engage in fewer social activities as they age
  - Contact with family is the most common social activity

- Women are more socially active than men
- Disability limits social interaction
- High-quality interactions with others helps individuals maintain or regain health
- Types of supporting behaviors
  - Instrumental support gives direct assistance and service
  - Informational support uses advice, suggestions, and information in solving problems
  - Emotional support comes when love, care, empathy, and trust are provided through a relationship
  - Appraisal support uses feedback and affirmation to help a person evaluate himself or herself
- Caregivers are important to older adults
  - 35% of older adults have caregivers
  - 90% are unpaid family members; many are over 65 themselves (spouses, children, other relatives, or friends)
  - Many older adults have unmet needs because of lack of adequate help—44% of those who need help lack enough assistance

Normal Changes of Aging

- What is normal becomes less uniform as patients age
- Many physiologic functions decline with aging. Within an individual, different systems will age more rapidly than others. Mental function is often most affected.
- It is often difficult to discern what is normal aging versus what is the effect of chronic disease, medication, or disuse.
- Normal changes of aging usually mean less functional reserve: the patient or specific organ system fails when stressed. Stress may be physical (such as infection) or psychological (such as death of spouse). Specific changes in each system will be discussed in the appropriate chapter.
- Chronological age as a marker of functional capacity becomes less accurate as the patient ages. As patients age, their functional status becomes more important and can tell you more about patients than their medical diagnoses. A patient with congestive heart failure (CHF) can be functioning normally or unable to get out of bed. A 65-year-old with CHF may be less functional than a 90-year-old with CHF.
- Geriatric patients are more heterogeneous as a group than younger patients, including varying responses to the same medications for the same illness in patients of the same age and sex.

THE PRACTICE OF GERIATRICS

- Caring for older adults can be a challenging but rewarding experience.
- Older adults often have multiple comorbid conditions, complex medication regimens, and nonstandard presentation of illness.
- Not all older adults patients are medically complex, but many are.
- Assessment of older adult, especially the frail older adult, should include assessment of functional status, social support, mental health, physical health, and economic resources.
- Medications should be reviewed at first visit and at all subsequent visits.
- How to obtain a history
  - Take time to review old medical record prior to seeing patient
  - Compensate for the normal sensory changes of aging
    - Make sure patient can see and hear you—face the patient
    - Eliminate background noise

- Assure adequate lighting
- Use multiple sources of information: visual, auditory and sensory
  - Establish a respectful relationship
- Allow sufficient time with patient so encounter is not rushed
- Do not conduct the interview with a family member to the exclusion of the patient
  - Get information from patient, family, caregivers, and old records
  - Even those with cognitive impairment can provide information about symptoms
  - Observe for symptoms as you ask about them
  - Use open-ended questions to expand on current problems; geriatric patients may require more yes/no questions to get specific information.
  - Repeat questions to confirm findings and ask questions that require different answers to make sure the patient understands the question.

The Physical Examination of the Older Adult

- Taking the health history provides the clinician with opportunity to observe the older adult—it provides valuable information about functional status, cognitive status, and presence of symptoms such as pain and shortness of breath.
- Observing patients as they come into exam room gives information of gait and balance, functional status.
- Establish the baseline (asking caregiver if necessary) and look for a change from baseline.
- Observe behavior—look for changes from baseline and watch for consistency.
- Facilitate exam by organizing evaluation so the patient does not have to change position frequently.
- Focus on important, essential elements first in case the patient fatigues or become agitated.
- Modify instructions—make things as simple as possible.
- Box 3–1 provides ideas for a senior-friendly setting

Box 3–1. Guidelines for Senior-Friendly Settings

- Keep the temperature between 70° and 80° F
- Use bright lights and avoid glare by having blinds or shades on windows
- Avoid any background noise (such as radios)
- Use higher-than-standard chairs for the waiting room and office rooms
- Waiting area that will accommodate assistive devices (walkers and wheelchairs) and family members
- Have available a wide step stool with handrail for transfers to the exam table
- Have available exam tables that mechanically lift the patient from lying to sitting position
- Raise the back on the exam table and provide support for sitting
- Have weight scale with bar for stability when getting on and off
- Bathrooms that are wheelchair accessible and have raised toilet seats and grab bars
- Ease of access to facility such as wheelchair ramps, large letters on signage, automatic doors

Diagnostic Tests

- Does the proposed diagnostic test meet the "so what" test? That is, would the results change how you would treat the patient?
- Explore the risks versus benefits of the test.
- Currently there are no evidence-based protocols for determining appropriate lab studies for older adults.

- Explore with the patient his or her willingness and ability to participate in diagnostic tests.
- Ask the older adults if they would consider additional treatment based on the findings of the test.

Management

- Explore with the patient and caregiver treatment options and the impact of each.
- Focus is often on maximizing the medical management of chronic conditions.
- Will the treatment improve quality of life and decrease suffering?
- Will the treatment have an impact on outcomes? That is, increase length of life? Improve function? Decrease pain?
- Will the treatment be difficult or unpleasant to tolerate or recover from?
- What is the monetary cost of treatment or prescription? Can the patient pay for the treatment or service? Is there a source of financial assistance? Many pharmaceutical companies have programs to assist with the cost of their medications. See www.NeedyMeds. com for a listing of programs.

Pharmacology

"Start low, go slow."
- Polypharmacy is common
  - 85% of those over 65 take medications
  - With multiple drug use, the number of drug interactions increases considerably
  - Drug interactions tend to be more frequent and serious in older adults
  - The effects of alcohol use must be considered
  - Discontinue drugs as appropriate; evaluate at each visit
- Drug toxicities more common and more serious in the elderly
  - Drug dosage guidelines are usually based on studies in younger people
  - Recommended adult dosage guidelines are often too high for older patients
  - Monitor blood levels when appropriate
  - Behavioral side effects are more common in older people because the blood-brain barrier becomes less effective
  - When there is an acute change in mental status, medication should always be considered a possible cause
  - The patient presents with fewer classic symptoms
  - The adverse reaction may take longer to develop, even months
  - The reaction may be more pronounced once it occurs
- Over-the-counter (OTC) drugs can cause problems
  - Medications considered safe in the adult can cause adverse reactions in older adults
  - Patients take OTC medications in part because they think they are safe and cheap
  - Patients forget to tell the provider they are taking OTC medications
  - There has been an increase in use of herbal remedies and dietary supplements
    - They are not FDA regulated
    - Purity and quality of products may vary
    - There are few controlled studies to support safety and efficacy of supplements
- Noncompliance is very common
  - Intentional
    - Patients cannot afford the medication but do not tell you
    - Because of cost, they medicate with borrowed or old medications
    - Information about drugs from other sources such as advertisements or friends and family often confuses them

- Patients read the package insert and get scared
  - Unintentional
    - Drug regimen is overly complicated and confusing
    - Related to impaired mental status, normal age-associated forgetfulness
- Strategies to increase compliance
  - Check ability to comply
    - Patients bring all medications, including OTCs in original containers, to every visit
    - Prescribe once-a-day medications whenever possible
    - Provide readable written instructions including dose and time; use large print
    - Coordinate medication regimen with task or event such as meals
    - Medication boxes should be filled by appropriate individual or pharmacy
    - Reinforce regimens with responsible family members or caregivers

Table 3-1. Age-Related Changes That Affect Pharmacotherapy

Pharmaco-kinetics	Definition	Age Changes	Implications
Absorption	Receptor-coupled or diffusional uptake of a drug into tissue	Increased GI pH Decreased GI motility Decreased absorptive surface area Decreased splanchnic blood flow Decreased first-pass effect	Slower absorption and delayed onset Greater bioavailability of drugs with high hepatic extraction (first pass)
Distribution	Movement of the drug into the tissue or body compartment	Decreased total body fluid Increased body fat Decreased lean muscle mass Decreased albumin	Small older adults are more sensitive to usual doses Lipophilic drugs have increased half-life Hydrophilic drugs have increased peak concentrations Increased free drug Drug levels are difficult to interpret
Metabolism	Chemical change in a drug that causes it to be active or inactive	Decreased liver and kidney blood flow Decreased glomerular filtration rate Alteration in Phase I reactions and P450 system	Increased effect and toxicity of drugs metabolized by Phase I or P450 No change in drugs metabolized by conjugation
Excretion	Removal of a drug through the kidney, or via bile, feces, the saliva, or the lungs	Decreased renal blood flow and filtration rate Decreased distal renal tubular secretory function Unchanged biliary excretion	Accumulation of drug eliminated unchanged Accumulation of metabolites Increased effect and toxicity of renally eliminated drugs

Communicating With the Demented Patient

- Get his or her attention. Speak to the patient; if the patient does not respond, touch shoulder gently and position yourself so he or she can see you.
- Assess hearing. Does the patient react to what you say?
- Communicate nonverbally; smile, use friendly body language
- Keep it simple; one thought per sentence
- Repeat; in exact same words at first, then rephrase
- Give the patient time to respond; wait several seconds before asking another question
- Monitor the reaction; are they getting upset or confused?
- Continually adjust your approach
  - If the patient reacts quickly, you can speed up
  - If the patient gets upset, slow down, relax, move back a little, wait until he or she has calmed down, and then try something simpler

THEORY

Theories of Aging

- Aging is a multifactorial process. Theories of aging include biological, sociological, psychological, and medical theories. These theories can aid understanding of age-related changes and direct the care of older adults.
- Biological theories include:
  - Accumulation of oxidative damage to DNA, RNA, proteins, and lipids
  - Regulation of aging by specific genes; the regenerative ability of cells is genetically determined
- Sociological theories include:
  - Disengagement theory, which suggests that with age there is a mutually beneficial process of reciprocal withdrawal between society and older adults
  - Activity theory, which focuses on the belief that the way to age successfully is to keep active
  - Continuity theory, which posulates that the personality remains stable over time and helps direct behavior
  - Subculture theory, which suggests that older adults have their own norms, expectations, beliefs, and habits
  - Age-stratification theory, which differentiates between those who age and the impact of age on society
  - Person-environment-fit theory, which considers the relationship between personal competence and the environment
- Psychological theories include
  - Human needs theories, which focus on the relationship between motivation and need
  - Life-course and personality development theories, which identify personality types as predictive forces for successful/unsuccessful aging

Developmental Theory

- All development is patterned, orderly, and predictable, with both a purpose and a direction
- Development is continuous throughout life
- Development may occur simultaneously in several areas, such as the physical and social, but the rate of change in each area varies
- Development proceeds from the simple to the complex
- The pace of development varies among individuals

- Physical and mental stress during periods of critical developmental change, such as old age, may make a person particularly susceptible to outside stressors
- Developmental tasks are challenges that must be met and adjustments made in response to life experiences

Critical Age-Related Stresses
- Interpersonal loss, loss of social support such as loss of spouse, family, friends
- Physical disability, loss of strength
- Loss of youthful appearance and beauty
- Change in social role, such as children caring for parent
- Forced reliance on caregivers
- Change in living arrangements such as loss of house
- Confrontation with death

Stressors in Older Adults
- A common myth about older adults is that they do not tolerate change.
- However, they are faced with major life changes, especially losses—loss of spouse and friends to death, loss of home or job, decline or loss of ability to do many activities, and so on.
- These changes are a major cause of stress in older adults.
- Stress is the emotional and physical response to an increase in the environmental demands beyond the resources of an individual to cope with those demands.
- Small amounts of stress may add excitement and variety and increase the quality of life. Large amounts of stress may be overwhelming and lead to disease.
- The goal is to find the right balance of stress in life.
- Individuals often seem to have vulnerability in one system to stress (hypertension, ulcer, mental problems).
- Stress can be managed through various techniques or coping strategies:
  - Avoid unnecessary change during stressful times.
  - Manage time by keeping to predetermined goals and priorities.
  - Avoid stressful triggers when possible: people, activities, etc.
  - Create habits or routines to decrease stress.
  - Develop alternative activities or friendships that increase pleasure.
  - Exercise to help decrease stress.
  - Participate in religious, motivational, or service activities that increase self-esteem or change focus to helping others.
  - Use biofeedback, tension-relaxation exercise, yoga, or imagery to control stress reactions.

HEALTH MAINTENANCE
Models and Theories Related to Health Care
Health Belief Model
- Model to explain why healthy people do or do not take advantage of screening programs
- Involves variables such as perceptions of susceptibility and seriousness of a disease, benefits of treatment, perceived barriers to change, and expectations of efficacy

Trans-Theoretical Model of Change (Prochashka & DiClemente, 1984)
- Six predictable stages of change
  - Pre-contemplation
  - Contemplation
  - Preparation

– Action
– Maintenance
– Termination

Self-Efficacy or Social Cognitive Theory Model (Bandura, 1986, 1997)
- Self-efficacy is the perception of one's ability to perform a certain task at a certain level of accomplishment.
- Outcome expectations are the beliefs that if the behavior is performed there will be a specific outcome (e.g., If I exercise, I will get stronger).
- Behavior change and maintenance are a function of outcome expectations and efficacy expectations.
- Verbal encouragement, actually performing the activity, seeing role models perform, and physiological feedback (sensations associated with the activity such as pain or fear) all influence self-efficacy and outcome expectations.

Epidemiologic Principles

Etiology: defines the cause or the web of causation of a disease or problem
- Prevalence rates describe a group at a certain point in time and the number within a group that has a particular disease or problem. It is like a snapshot in time
- Incidence rates describe the rate of development of a disease in a group over a period of time. It describes the continuing occurrence of new cases of disease. This information is based on large-scale data collection from the Centers for Disease Control.

Natural History of Disease: the course of disease development, expression, and progression
- Several stages appear to be universally descriptive for a disease process:
  – Stage of susceptibility
  – Stage of presymptomatic disease
  – Stage of clinical disease
  – Stage of disability
- Goal is to intervene as early as possible to prevent disease or disability

Risk Factors

- Age, sex, social, cultural, familial, occupational, and lifestyle history represent potential sources of problems and diseases, and they may be difficult or impossible to alter
- Risk-reduction programs may be established to decrease the vulnerability of individuals to some problems by modifying some risks

Communicable/Infectious Diseases: patterns in which organisms attack and invade vulnerable individuals
- Intervention involves identification of causative agents
- Relies on microbiology principles in understanding life cycle of organism
- Focuses on intervention at vulnerable phases in course or disease or life cycle of organism to limit or eradicate disease

Epidemiologic Concepts

Host–Parasite Relations
- Pathogenicity
- Virulence

Reservoirs of Infection
- Cases
- Carriers

Mechanisms of Transmission of Infection
- Direct
- Indirect through vehicle, vector, or air

Concepts of Epidemic vs. Endemic Infections
- Person-to-person transmission
- Generation time: time between receipt of infection and maximal communicability of that infection
- Herd immunity: resistance of a group to invasion and spread of an infectious agent

Control Measures
- Measures directed against the reservoir: isolation, quarantine
- Measures that interrupt the transmission of organisms: water purification, pasteurization of milk, inspection procedures
- Measures that reduce host susceptibility: immunization

Factors Supporting Greater Emphasis on Health Maintenance
- Increased emphasis on disease prevention and promotion of health as infectious disease has diminished as a major cause of morbidity and mortality
- Changing demographics means that more people living longer and with less disease and dysfunction
- Emphasis on containing costs means that primary prevention is preferred over secondary and secondary prevention preferred over tertiary (see Levels of Prevention, below)
- Healthy People 2010 is the prevention agenda for the United States. The program sets national health objectives designed to identify the most significant preventable threats to health and to establish national goals to reduce the threats. The complete documents can be found at www.healthypeople.gov. New Healthy People 2020 guidelines will be released in 2010.
- Healthy People leading health indicators most relevant to geriatrics are:
  - Physical activity
  - Overweight and obesity
  - Tobacco use
  - Mental health
  - Injury and violence
  - Access to health care

Health Maintenance in Older Adults
- Goal is to preserve function and quality of life in the elderly, as well as reduction of morbidity and mortality
- Most research in this area has been done on much younger adults; most organizations that recommend preventive measures use a cutoff age of 65
- Screening is unlikely to be of benefit if the individual has less than a 10-year life expectancy.
- Prevention and screening must be individualized in the elderly, based on risk factors, potential for benefit, and on patient willingness to undergo treatment
- Emphasis should be on prevention of discomfort and maintaining quality of life
- Screening is less likely to be useful if patient:
  - Has had consistently negative screening results in the past
  - Is frail or demented
  - Has limited remaining quality and quantity of life

    – Would not be a candidate for treatment

    – Is unable or unwilling to cooperate with the intervention

Levels of Prevention

Primary Prevention

- Emphasis is on reducing incidence of disease or problems by generalized health promotion and specific disease protection
- Important examples are exercise and nutrition
- Older adults can benefit from primary prevention, which can improve quality of life even at very old ages
- Cardiovascular disease (atherosclerotic cardiovascular and cerebrovascular disease), the most common cause of death, is amenable to primary prevention

Secondary Prevention

- Emphasis is on early detection of an illness or problem while the outcome can be favorably altered
- Examples include PSA tests, breast exams, smoking cessation programs, cholesterol screening
- Must explore with older adult the pros and cons of screening and determine willingness to have further evaluation and treatment of identified disease

Tertiary Prevention

- Emphasis is on treatment and rehabilitation of the illness or problem to return the patient to the highest level of functioning and to avoid or postpone complications
- Example: post-stroke or post–myocardial infarction rehabilitation programs
- Becomes very important with older adults

Effective Health Promotion Interventions

Exercise

- Exercise can be of benefit to almost every patient; research has included people in their 90s
- The main exception is patients with an unstable cardiac condition such as angina or arrhythmia
- Caution in needed, particularly in patients with musculoskeletal disorders
- Recommendations are for 30 minutes of moderate physical activity of different types 5 to 6 days a week (150 minutes per week)
- It is not necessary to achieve this goal to receive benefit from exercise
- Older adults should be encouraged to combine both aerobic exercise and resistance training
  - Walking, swimming, water walking, biking (stationary bike, recumbent bicycle)
  - Muscle strengthening
  - Stretching, including yoga, Tai chi
  - Less strenuous activity is also beneficial, such as gardening, slow walking
- Health benefits include
  - Reduced risk of chronic disease
  - Improved bone and muscle strength
  - Decreased risk of falling
- Improved function
- Improved quality of life

- Improved bowel function
- Decreased depression
- Improved sleep
- Improved overall sense of well-being

Table 3-2. Specific Health Behaviors Amenable to Intervention

Behavior	Strength of Evidence	Benefit(s)	Age for Which Recommended	Recommendation
Exercise	Good evidence	Many, including cardiac disease, death	All ages; proven in men in their 90s	Individualize
Nutrition	Simple, focused intervention can be effective	Helps with many chronic conditions	No upper limit	Counseling about adequate diet
Calcium Supplementation	Good evidence in high risk patients	Reduces risk for osteoporosis	Postmenopausal in women	1,200–1,500 mg/day; no recommendations for men
Cholesterol Reduction	Diet not proven to be sufficient to reduce cholesterol level; normal levels proven to protect in young to middle aged men	Reduces hyperlipidemia, atherosclerotic cardiovascular disease	No support for screening and treatment over age 75	Maintain total cholesterol under 200; LDL recommendation depends on risk factors
Weight Loss	Well documented in adults up to 65	Excess weight is an independent risk factor for atherosclerotic cardiovascular disease	Not studied in older adults	Maintain ideal body weight
Smoking Cessation	Strongest recommendation, simple interventions can have 5%–10% quit rate	Cardiovascular, pulmonary, gastrointestinal diseases and malignancies	Quitting at any time improves pulmonary function and risk for MI and death	Ask about, encourage cessation at each visit
Alcohol Treatment	Cessation difficult to achieve in alcoholics; 2/3 started drinking in younger years; 1/3 are late-onset drinkers	Alcoholism puts elderly at risk for falls and confusion	No age limit to improved safety	Ask about, counsel to use in moderation

continued

Table 3–2. Specific Health Behaviors Amenable to Intervention (cont.)

Behavior	Strength of Evidence	Benefit(s)	Age for Which Recommended	Recommendation
Drug Treatment	Well documented	Polypharmacy has many risks or adverse reactions, drug interactions, a cause of death in the elderly	Never too late	Check medications at each visit, ask about OTC and herbal remedies; use only medications that are medically necessary
Safety/ Injury/Abuse Prevention	Little data on effectiveness of prevention	Falls are 6th leading cause of death	Different focus for the older adult	Home safety evaluation
Aspirin Therapy	Effectiveness proven in middle aged men; few studies in elderly	Primary and secondary prevention of cardiovascular and cerebrovascular disease	Recommended for over 40 or 50	Low-dose 81–325 mg/day for cardiovascular health
Immunizations				
Influenza	Well documented	Influenza	65+	Annually
Pneumonia	60% efficacy	*Streptococcus pneumoniae* infection	65+	Once; may repeat in 5 years
Tetanus	Well proven	Tetanus	Indicated in the elderly	Every 10 years
Herpes Zoster Vaccination		Shingles	60+	Once

Nutrition

- Supply all essential nutrients to maintain or regain health
- Maintain, gain, or lose weight if necessary, ideal body weight (IBW)—see Obesity in Endocrine Chapter 17
- Risk factors for malnutrition include: drugs, chronic disease, depression, dental problems, decreased taste and smell, poverty, physical weakness, and isolation
- Recommended calcium intake from the Institute of Medicine for 51+ years, 1,200 to 1,500 mg a day
- Adequate vitamin D intake, 800 IU a day
- Diet moderate in fat content to keep cholesterol within normal limits
- Protein should be 12% to 20% of total calories
- Adequate fluid intake 6 to 8 glasses water per day
- Adequate fiber (from grains, fruits, and vegetables); current recommendations, 14 g dietary fiber per 1,000 calories

- Avoiding excess sodium is most important in CHF, hypertension; older people are at risk for low sodium because of severe restriction of salt in their diet.
- Frail elderly at risk for malnutrition; low albumin levels

Smoking Cessation
- One of the most important preventive interventions
- Older adults can benefit from smoking cessation programs
- Usually safe to use nicotine replacement therapy or bupropion (Wellbutrin)

Safety: Injury Prevention
- Fall prevention with home safety evaluation
  - Bathrooms are the site of most falls
  - Throw rugs are dangerous
  - Sufficient lighting is needed both inside and outside the home
  - Safe and appropriate assistive devices must be made available
- Driving evaluations for safety
  - Driving essential for independence; patients reluctant to give it up
  - Driving can be impaired because of dementia, impaired vision, slowed reflexes, musculoskeletal disorders, etc.
- Seat belts
- Smoke detectors
- Safety lock on firearms

Violence and Abuse (see section in Chapter 18)
- An estimated 1.5 to 2 million older adults in the United States are abused annually
- Anticipate problems in the care of older adults and help caregivers cope with these problems (such as urinary incontinence, short-term memory changes)
- Clinicians should ask about and watch for signs of physical abuse during encounters with clients
- Patients will often admit to problems but only if they are asked
- Talk to caregivers about stress, coping, support systems, and respite care
- Know and apply state laws in determining requirements to report suspected abuse

Alcohol (see section in Chapter 18)
- Depression is highly associated with alcohol abuse
- In older adults, signs and symptoms of alcohol abuse might include falls, changes in functional status or cognition, weight loss or malnutrition, abnormal lab values, and recent losses
- Older adults may have had a prior history of drinking, or drinking may be new in older age
- Individuals may begin or resume drinking as part of grief reaction to loss or isolation/decreased social contact
- Screening should be done by assuming there is regular alcohol use and asking the older adult not whether they drink, but how much

Drugs
- See section on pharmacology in this chapter for a discussion of prescription and OTC drugs in the elderly
- Dependency is a common tendency that in its extreme form causes an individual to rely on other individuals, or activities such as eating food, drinking alcohol, having sex, gambling, or some other behavioral component to try to satisfy an emotional hunger

- Action begun voluntarily that, through repetition, becomes involuntary
- Dependency becomes an addiction when there is loss of control (compulsivity), continuation despite adverse consequences, and obsession or preoccupation with the activity

Estrogen
- For postmenopausal women to prevent osteoporosis
- See Chapter 12, Gynecologic Disorders, for discussion of risks versus benefits

Aspirin
- To prevent strokes and MI
- Most effective in high-risk patients

Immunizations
- To obtain up-to-date standards for adult immunization practices go to http://www.cdc.gov/vaccines/recs/schedules/adult-schedule.htm#chgs
- Many older adults remain without adequate immunization
- Influenza and pneumonia vaccines are underutilized
- Tetanus is a hidden risk
    - The largest age group acquiring tetanus infections is older adults
    - Men often have not had booster since they were in the military
    - Women may have never had full immunization series

To obtain Quick Reference Information for Medicare Preventive Services, go to www.cms.hhs.gov/MLNProducts/downloads/MPS_QuickReferenceChart_1.pdf

Geriatric Screening Guidelines

Table 3-3. Geriatric Screening Recommendations

Screening Procedure	Strength of Evidence	Screen for	Age for Which Recommended	Recommendations
Blood Pressure	Excellent, especially in elderly	Hypertension, isolated systolic hypertension	No age cutoff; important in the elderly	Every 1–2 years
Height and Weight	No data	Obesity	No age stated	Periodic
Clinical Breast Exam	Excellent	Breast cancer	Over age 40	Annually
Mammogram	Excellent	Breast cancer	Annually for age 50–69; continue in willing/ appropriate patients up to 80 years of age Patients with dementia up to 70 years of age	Continue every 1–3 years

continued

Table 3–3. Geriatric Screening Recommendations (cont.)

Screening Procedure	Strength of Evidence	Screen for	Age for Which Recommended	Recommendations
Papanicolau Test	Excellent in adults	Cervical cancer	Adult Not recommended in frail (significant functional impairment, life expectancy < 5 years), moderately demented patients	Can decrease to test every 2–3 years after age 65–69, if 3 consecutive negative Pap tests unless immunocompromised
Rectal Exam / PSA	Good for rectal exam; PSA now discredited	Colorectal cancer; prostate cancer	Less likely to benefit older adult	Annually
Oral Cavity Exam	Good in high risk patients	Cancer, gingivitis	No upper age limit	Annual exam and counseling
Cholesterol Level	Less certain for older adults	Cardiovascular, cerebrovascular disease	Robust 65- to 75-year-olds with additional risk factors Do not perform on patient with moderate dementia and at end of life	Every 5 years
Fecal Occult Blood	Good data	Colorectal cancer	No upper limit established	Annually
Sigmoidoscopy	Significant benefit for adults, especially with risk factors, no data spefically for older adults	Colorectal cancer	No specific recommendations over 65; into old age if healthy and willing	Every 5 years
TSH	Some data	Thyroid disorder	Older adults, especially women	Annually
Glucose	Treatment shown to reduce complications	Diabetes mellitus	Those at increased risk	If patient has symptoms or every 3 years

continued

Table 3-3. Geriatric Screening Recommendations (cont.)

Screening Procedure	Strength of Evidence	Screen for	Age for Which Recommended	Recommendations
Bone Density	Good data	Osteoporosis	Women age 65 and older with increased risk for osteoporosis, or those on FDA-approved osteoporosis drug therapy; no recommendations for men	Every 2 years
Skin Exam	No data	Skin cancer	Older adults, no upper age limit	Periodic, depends on risk
Vision	Some evidence	Vision loss, glaucoma, cataracts	Many recommend exam for patient 65 and older	Screen visual acuity of older adult with Snellen testing and refer persons at high risk for glaucoma to eye specialists
Hearing	Some evidence	Hearing loss	Over age 65	Assess hearing through physical exam and refer as needed
Urinalysis	Some evidence	Infection, cancer	Older patients and others at high risk, such as those with diabetes mellitus	Periodically
EKG	Some evidence	Heart disease	Over age 40–50	Periodically
Cognitive and Functional Assessment	Insufficient evidence	Functional status, Dementia	Some recommend screening patients over age 65 or 75	Periodic assessment
Depression	Some data	Depression	Some recommend in the older adult	Periodic assessment

Health Care and Treatment Considerations

Cultural Influences

A healthcare provider who is sensitive to issues surrounding the patient's traditions and beliefs can often provide more comprehensive health care.

- **Family:** The concept should be broadened beyond the traditional husband-wife-children pattern seen in the United States. The family initially teaches the belief patterns, religion, culture, and mores of a society.
- **Ethnicity:** The race, tribe, or nation with which a person or group identifies and which influences beliefs and behavior; the cultural background of an individual.

- **Culture:** The learned beliefs and behaviors or socially inherited characteristics that are common among all members of a group and have both practical and symbolic components.
- **Individual:** One member of a family, community, or cultural group.

Evidence-Based Medicine

- To reduce conflicting or varying recommendations for the diagnosis and treatment of common problems, the trend is to base decisions on evidence from randomized controlled research trials. Meta-analyses of these trials, together with individual trials, have gained acceptance as valid foundations on which care can be provided. Information about the status of research in these areas is growing.
- In this type of practice, outcome studies should take precedence over tradition, intuition, and individual preference in how different clinical problems are handled. NPs should have sufficient research skills to be able to critically evaluate and participate in outcome studies that will relate to their clinical practice.
- There is frequently no research that has been done on older adult patient; this severely limits evidence-based geriatric medicine. Older adults are different from younger adults and research done on younger adults must be interpreted with caution with reference to the elderly population. Age-related changes as well as more co-morbid conditions may affect treatment outcomes in the elderly.

Clinical Guidelines

- Standards of practice are derived from research by experts in the field to guide and standardize practice across the country. NPs should know how to analyze clinical guidelines to determine which are written by objective scholars and are without organizational, professional, or pharmaceutical bias. See the National Guideline Clearinghouse at www.guideline.gov.
- Factors to consider in evaluating guidelines include: the source of guideline, appropriateness of methodology used to develop guideline; use of expert opinion/clinical experience in decision-making; public policy considerations; feasibility issues; use of peer review; congruence with other practice guidelines; timeliness; and funding source.

Critical Thinking/Decision-Making

- Critical thinking involves acquisition of knowledge with an attitude of deliberate inquiry. Part of critical thinking may be innate, but most people can learn to think critically.
- Decision-making is a higher level of critical thinking. It involves making decisions based on an understanding of the different options, and the possible desirability of the outcomes of each option in the mind of the clinician and the patient.
- Pattern recognition, similarity recognition, commonsense understanding, skilled know-how, sense of importance, and deliberative rationality are all-important aspects that influence decision-making.

Communication

The written and oral transfer of information regarding the structure, process, and outcome of healthcare encounters. Healthcare providers are required to have good communication skills in interviewing and teaching patients, recording information and decisions, sharing or clarifying information with others involved in the patient's care. All communication is privileged and confidential and written documentation is subject to specific standards and audits.

- Types of special communication
  - **Triage:** The prioritization and sorting of patients according to a pre-existing standard. Used in disaster and emergency settings.
  - **Case management**
    - Case management is a system of controlled oversight and authorization of services and benefits provided to clients.
    - The case manager is an advocate in the managed care environment for both consumers and providers, where managing can also mean balancing key issues of access, cost, and outcomes.
  - **Team management**
    - Older people have many multisystem problems that require the involvement of care providers from different disciplines.
    - The different specialties must communicate with each other to provide a unified plan of care.

Interpersonal Relationships

NPs work closely with many other types of healthcare providers. The NP role boundaries are not always clear and may vary from state to state or even institution to institution. Some principles in establishing and maintaining relationships with others include:
- Flexibility
- Willingness to listen
- Respect for others views, beliefs, traditions
- Assertiveness in clarifying your own opinion, belief, traditions
- Tolerance
- Patience
- Ability to make change

CASE STUDIES

Case 1. You are asked to assess an 82-year-old man for admission to an assisted living facility.

1. What chronic conditions is he likely to have?
2. What impairments is he likely to have?
3. What kind of health insurance is he likely to have?
4. What cause is he most likely to die from?

Case 2. A 94-year-old nursing home patient with moderate dementia has had four falls in the past 2 days. She had not fallen in the past year.

1. What is this problem an example of?
2. How would you begin the evaluation of this problem?
3. What other aspects of the functional assessment would be important in this patient?

Case 3. You have a new patient in the nursing home, a 78-year-old woman with moderate dementia, impaired hearing, and impaired vision.

1. What would your initial approach be?
2. How would you alter the environment to improve communication?
3. How would you adjust your physical exam?

REFERENCES

Andersen, E., Rothenberg, B., & Zimmer, J. G. (1997). *Assessing the health status of older adults.* New York: Springer

Bandura, A. (1986). *Social foundations of thought and action.* Englewood Cliffs, NJ: Prentice-Hall.

Bandura, A. (1997). *Self-efficacy: The exercise of control.* New York: W.H. Freeman.

Becker, M. (1972). The health believe model and personal health behavior. *Health Education Monographs, 2,* 326–327.

Borson, S., Scanlan, J. M., Watanabe, J., Tu, S. P., & Lessig, M. (2006). Improving identification of cognitive impairment in primary care. *International Journal of Geriatric Psychiatry, 21*(4), 349–355.

Brownson, R. C. (1998). *Applied epidemiology: Theory to practice.* London: Oxford University Press.

Caloras, D. (1999, November). The virtues of hospice. *Patient Care for the Nurse Practitioner,* pp. 6–30.

Center for Disease Control and Prevention. (2009). *Recommended adult immunization schedule United States 2009.* Retrieved from http://www.cdc.gov/vaccines/recs/schedules/adult-schedule.htm

Draye, M. A. (2000). Health promotion, health maintenance, and disease prevention. In P. V. Meredith & N. M. Horan (Eds.), *Adult primary care.* St. Louis, MO: Harcourt Brace.

Edmunds, M. W., & Mayhew, M. S. (2004). *Pharmacology for primary care providers* (2nd ed.). St. Louis, MO: Mosby.

Emanuel, E. (2000, November). A detailed examination of advance directives. *Patient Care for the Nurse Practitioner,* pp. 31–51.

Erikson, E. (1963). *Childhood and society* (2nd ed.). New York: Norton.

Finkel, T., & Holbrook, N. J. (2000). Oxidants, oxidative stress and the biology of ageing. *Nature, 408,* 239–247.

Freedman, V. A., Martin, L. G., & Schoeni, R. F. (2002). Recent trends in disability and functioning among older adults in the United States. *JAMA, 288,* 3137–3146.

Friedman, M. (1998). *Family nursing: Research, theory and practice* (4th ed.). Stamford, CT: Appleton & Lange.

Ham, R. J., Slone, P. D., Warshaw, G. A., Bernard, M. A., & Flahety, M. (2007). *Primary care geriatrics: A case based approach* (5th ed.). Philadelphia: Mosby Elsevier.

Kane, R. A. (2001). Long term care and a good quality of life: Bringing them closer together. *Gerontologist, 41*(30), 293–304.

Kane, R. L., & Kane, R. A. (2000). *Assessing older persons.* New York: Oxford University Press.

Kerlikowske, K., Salzmann, P., Phillips, K. A., Cauley, J. A., & Cummings, S. R. (1999). Continuing screening mammography in women aged 70 to 79 years. *JAMA, 282,* 2156–2163.

Lenburg, C. B. (1995). *Promoting cultural competence in and through nursing education: A critical review and comprehensive plan for action.* Washington, DC: American Academy of Nursing.

Moon, M. (1996). What Medicare has meant to older Americans. *Health Care Financial Review, 18*(2), 49–59.

National Center for Health Statistics. (n.d.). *Aging stats 2008 report.* Retrieved from http://www.agingstats.gov/agingstatsdotnet/Main_Site/Data/Data_2008.aspx

National Institute of Health, Office of Dietary Supplements. (n.d.). *Dietary supplement facts sheet: Calcium, Vitamin D.* Retrieved from http://ods.od.nih.gov/Health_Information/Information_About_Individual_Dietary_Supplements.aspx

Pender, N. (1996). *Health promotion in nursing practice* (3rd ed.). Norwalk, CT: Appleton & Lange.

Prochaska, J. O., & DiClemente, C. C. (1984). *The trans-theoretical approach: Crossing traditional boundaries of change.* Homewood, IL: Dow-Jones-Irwin.

Resnick, B. (2007). Health maintenance, exercise and nutrition. In R. J. Ham, P. D. Sloane, G. A. Warshaw, M. A. Bernard, & M. Flahety (Eds.), *Primary care geriatirics: A case based approach* (5th ed.). Philadelphia: Mosby Elsevier.

Sadavoy, J., & Lesczc, M. (Eds.). (1987). *Treating the elderly with psychotherapy: The scope for change in later life.* Madison, CT: International Universities Press.

Selye, H. (1974). *Stress without distress.* Philadelphia: JB Lippincott.

Spalding, M. C., & Sebesta, S. C. (2008). Geriatric screening and preventive care. *American Family Physician, 78*(2), 206–215.

U.S. Census Bureau. (1999). Statistical Abstract of the United States. Retrieved from www.census.gov

United States Department of Health and Human Services. (1996). *Healthy People 2000.* Washington, DC: U.S. Public Health Service.

United States Department of Health and Human Services. (2000). *Healthy People 2010.* Washington, DC: U.S. Public Health Service.

United States Department of Health and Human Services. (n.d.) *Physical activity guidelines for Americans.* Retrieved from http://www.health.gov/paguidelines/guidelines/default.aspx

United States Preventive Services Task Force. (2002). *Guide to clinical preventive services* (3rd ed.). McLean, VA: International Medical Publishing

Vladeck, B. C. (2001) Medicare: Can its benefits be sustained as cost of coverage grows? *Geriatrics, 56*(5), 50–53.

Web Sites for Geriatrics

Administration on Aging, www.aoa.gov

AgeNet Eldercare Network, www.caregivers.com

American Association of Homes and Services for the Aging, www.aahsa.org

American Association of Retired Persons, www.aarp.org

American Geriatrics Society, www.americangeriatrics.org

American Health Care Association, www.ahca.org

American Medical Directors Association, www.amda.com

American Society of Consultant Pharmacists, www.ascp.com

CMS Medicare Learning Network, www.cms.hhs.gov,
    http://www.cms.hhs.gov/MLNProducts/downloads/MPS_QuickReferenceChart_1.pdf

Gerontological Advanced Practice Nurses Association, https://www.gapna.org/

Gerontological Society of America, www.geron.org

National Association of Area Agencies on Aging, www.n4a.org

National Council on the Aging, www.ncoa.org

National Guidelines Clearinghouse, www.guideline.gov

NCOA Benefits Checkup, www.benefitscheckup.org

Web Resources for Advance Directive

Aging With Dignity, www.agingwithdignity.org

American Academy of Family Physicians, www.familydoctor.org/handouts/003.html

Choice in Dying, www.choices.org

Healthwatch, www.healthwatch.com

Living Wills and Values History Project, www.euthanasia.cc/lwvh.html

The Medical Directive from JAMA, www.medicaldirective.org

Geriatric Multisystem Syndromes

Katherine Tardiff, MSN, GNP-BC, ACHPN

GENERAL APPROACH

Nonspecific Presentation of Illness in Older Adults

- Older adults often have multiple chronic illnesses.
- Presentation of illness often does not reflect the system causing the problem.
  - Healthcare providers must evaluate older patients using a multisystem approach
  - Comprehensive geriatric evaluation is essential to understand the patient's healthcare needs
  - Team approach is ideal

RED FLAGS

- Sudden onset of change in mental status
- Onset of acute pain

COMMON MULTISYSTEM SYNDROMES

Dementia

Description

- Disorder characterized by impairment of memory and at least one other cognitive domain, including aphasia, agnosia, apraxia, and executive function
  - Must represent a decline from previous level of functioning and interfere with daily functioning

- Major dementia syndromes include: Alzheimer's disease (AD), vascular dementia, dementia with Lewy bodies (DLB), Parkinson's disease (PD) with dementia, frontotemporal lobar degeneration (FTLD), and reversible dementias (see Table 4–1)
- Normal age-related changes in cognitive function include mild changes in memory and rate of information processing; changes are not progressive and do not affect daily function

Table 4–1. Major Dementia Syndromes

Type of Dementia	Alzheimer's Disease	Vascular Dementia	Dementia With Lewy Bodies	Frontotemporal Lobar Degeneration	Potentially Reversible Dementias
Subtypes			PD-associated dementia, DLB, progressive supranuclear palsy (PSP)	Pick disease, corticobasal degeneration, progressive aphasia, semantic dementia, FTDP-17	Metabolic dementias, normal pressure hydrocephalus (NPH)
Etiology	Findings on autopsy include extracellular buildup of amyloid-beta protein, intracellular neurofibrillary tangles, and loss of neurons	Large-artery infarctions (typically cortical or subcortical); subcortical small artery infarctions or lacunae; chronic subcortical ischemia	Cortical Lewy bodies; amyloid plaques and neurofibrillary tangles are common	Focal atrophy of temporal and frontal lobes; may be associated with abnormalities in the protein tau that is present in neurons	Medications, alcohol, metabolic disorders (e.g., thyroid, B_{12} deficiency), depression, CNS neoplasm, NPH; impaired absorption of cerebrospinal fluid
Incidence and Demographics	60%–80% of cases; estimated 5.2 million cases in U.S.; 6th leading cause of death; women > men	10%–20% of cases; more common in patients who have had a stroke	DLB: 10%–20% of cases; PD-associated dementia: 5% of cases; men > women	Rare > age 75; mean age of onset in 60's; male = female; familial occurrence in 20%–40% of cases	Uncommon; metabolic causes more common in younger adults

continued

Table 4-1. Major Dementia Syndromes (cont.)

Type of Dementia	Alzheimer's Disease	Vascular Dementia	Dementia With Lewy Bodies	Frontotemporal Lobar Degeneration	Potentially Reversible Dementias
Clinical Features	Progressive memory loss, behavior and personality changes, global cognitive dysfunction, functional impairments; prominent loss of short-term memory early in disease, functional dependency later	Depends on nature and location of ischemia; onset may be abrupt or gradual; progression may be stepwise; gait disturbance and executive dysfunction common early in disease	Progressive cognitive decline; fluctuating cognition early in disease process; recurrent visual hallucinations; features of Parkinsonism	Behavioral or personality changes with less memory loss early in disease; executive dysfunction, disinhibition, and inappropriate social behavior; language deficits; often misdiagnosed as personality or psychiatric disorder	Depends on underlying etiology
Diagnosis	Mainly clinical; no labs can confirm or refute diagnosis; MRI with hippocampal atrophy is suggestive of AD	Patients with stroke history or vascular risk factors: CT or MRI identify vascular pathology	History and physical to rule out treatable causes; MRI supports diagnosis	Mainly clinical; CT or MRI often reveals atrophy of frontal and/or temporal lobes	Medical evaluation to determine underlying cause

Risk Factors
- Age
- Family history
- Genetic factors
- Mild cognitive impairment (MCI)
- Atherosclerotic risk factors: hyperlipidemia, diabetes mellitus, hypertension
- Sedentary lifestyle
- Lower education level

Prevention and Screening
- Maintain or increase physical activity
- Encourage cognitive leisure activities and social interactions
- Educate families to be aware of early symptoms in order to facilitate early assessment and recognition

- Those over 65 should have cognitive and functional evaluation at least every 3 years
- Screen for depression in patients with dementia

Table 4-2. Stages of Alzheimer's Disease

Stage	Characteristics	Interventions
Mild dementia FAST stages 2–4	Short-term memory loss Impaired organizational, decision-making, and judgment skills Difficulty learning new skills and following directions Difficulty with driving, cooking, managing finances, and medications May get lost Decreased attention span Attempts to hide memory loss May exhibit anxiety, depression, agitation, or paranoia	Calm, structured environment with moderate stimulation in familiar surroundings Maintain a routine including meal and sleep patterns Clocks, calendars, and to-do lists Avoid distraction Simple one-step commands Repeat and rephrase Cholinesterase inhibitors Treat depression Advanced directive and long-term care planning Consider cholinesterase inhibitor
Moderate dementia FAST stages 5–6	Problems recalling major current life events Increased problems following directions Word-finding difficulty Difficulty choosing appropriate clothing Verbal or physical agitation and aggression Delusions and hallucinations Wandering and pacing Purposeless and repetitive behavior Motor apraxia	Maintain safe independent function for as long as possible Plan for and determine when patient is no longer competent to make legal, financial, and medical decisions Avoid background noise Avoid arguing Try distraction, redirection Provide reassurance Avoid new or distressing social situations Consider cholinesterase inhibitor and/or NMDA antagonist
Severe dementia FAST stage 7	Lose ability to communicate, become nonverbal Become chairbound or bedridden Totally dependent for care	Provide comfort care Consider long-term-care placement Continue to speak to, touch, and maintain eye contact with patient Consider cholinesterase inhibitor and/or NMDA antagonist

Note. FAST = Functional Assessment Staging.

Assessment

History
- Initial diagnostic approach should focus on history; validate history with family member and/or caregiver
- History of present illness, including time frame and progression, and any associated neurologic symptoms such as vision loss, aphasia, unilateral weakness
- Past medical history: hypertension, strokes, head trauma, psychiatric illness (depression, anxiety, schizophrenia)

- Medication history: including over-the-counter, supplements, and home remedies
  - Drugs that may impair cognition: analgesics, anticholinergics, psychotropics, sedative-hypnotics
- Social history: present living situation, marital status, occupation, education, alcohol, tobacco, illicit drug use
- Functional and behavioral assessments:
  - Katz Index of Independence in Activities of Daily Living, Global Deterioration Scale (GDS), and Functional Assessment Staging (FAST)
- Cognitive testing: Mini-Mental State Examination (MMSE) most commonly used
  - Tests orientation, recall, attention, calculation, language manipulation, and constructional praxis
  - Results are not diagnostic; serve as baseline for assessing trends in cognitive impairment
  - Consider impact of visual, sensory, language, and physical disabilities and education level

Physical Exam
- Thorough and complete physical exam to rule out medical illness with attention to neurological deficits
  - Consider hearing and visual impairments
- AD: typically no motor deficits or focal neurological findings
- Vascular: focal motor weakness or impaired sensation, reflex asymmetry, positive Babinski
- PD-associated dementia: cogwheel rigidity, tremors
- Normal pressure hydrocephalus (NPH): ataxia and incontinence

Diagnostic Studies
- Laboratory testing:
  - Thyroid function tests and B_{12} level recommended by the American Academy of Neurology (AAN)
  - Consider CBC, electrolytes, glucose, and renal and liver function testing if clinically indicated
  - Consider screening for neurosyphilis if high clinical suspicion
  - Urinalysis if urinary tract infection suspected
- Neuroimaging recommended by AAN in routine initial evaluation of all patients with dementia
  - Noncontrast head CT
  - MRI
- Neuropsychological testing is recommended under certain circumstances:
  - Abnormal mental status testing with normal function
  - Differentiate depression, stroke, or delirium in unusual presentations
  - Identify areas of preserved cognitive function to develop a care plan

Differential Diagnosis
- Delirium
  - Other dementias: DLB, Pick disease, etc.
- Parkinson's disease
- Depression and/or anxiety
- Hearing loss
- B_{12} and folate deficiency

- Trauma: consider subdural hematoma, history of falls may be forgotten if not witnessed
- Tumor
- Hypothyroidism
- Infectious process: chronic infection, AIDS, tertiary syphilis
- Cerebral vascular accident (CVA)
- Myocardial infarction
  - Medications: polypharmacy, interactions
- Alcohol intoxication

Management
- Rule out or treat any conditions that may contribute to cognitive impairment
- Discontinue all unnecessary medications, especially sedatives and hypnotics
- Vascular dementia: nonpharmacologic and pharmacologic reduction of stroke risks (see management of TIA and stroke)
- Surgical shunting for NPH; approximately 50% improve; improvement may be immediate or take weeks, and may be temporary

Nonpharmacologic
- Educate patient and family about the illness, treatment, community resources
- Assist with long-term planning, including financial, legal, and advance directives
- Educate about home and driving safety
- Behavior therapy identifies causes of problem behaviors and changes the environment to reduce the behavior
- Reminiscence, recreational, art, music, and pet therapy create pleasurable experiences for the patient
- Identify events or stimuli that result in agitation or aggression, anticipate unmet needs, and avoid environmental triggers to reduce agitation
- Maintain a simple daily routine for bathing, dressing, eating, toileting, and bedtime
- Remain sensitive to cultural and spiritual needs of the patient and family

Pharmacologic

MILD-TO-MODERATE COGNITIVE SYMPTOMS
- Cholinesterase inhibitors
  - Donepezil (Aricept) 5–10 mg once a day
  - Rivastigmine (Exelon) 1.5 mg–6 mg twice a day; increase gradually
  - Galantamine (Razadyne) 4–12 mg b.i.d.; increase gradually as tolerated
    » Indicated for Alzheimer's disease; may also be effective in patients with vascular dementia, DLB
    » Not disease-modifying; treats symptoms and may improve agitated behaviors, but does not prevent pathological progression of disease
    » Common adverse effects: nausea, vomiting, and diarrhea; also weight loss, insomnia, abnormal dreams, muscle cramps, bradycardia, syncope, and fatigue

MODERATE-TO-SEVERE COGNITIVE SYMPTOMS
- Donepezil may be beneficial in advanced disease
- N-methyl-D-aspartate (NMDA) antagonist
  - Memantine (Namenda) 5 mg q.d. to 10 mg p.o. b.i.d.; increase gradually as tolerated
    » Adverse reactions: dizziness, headache, constipation, hypertension, pain, GI upset, somnolence, hallucination, dyspnea

» Disease-modifying; may slow progression of disease

» May be used in combination with cholinesterase inhibitors

PSYCHOSIS AND AGITATION

- Antipsychotics
  - Atypical antipsychotics have been drugs of choice for treating psychic disturbances such as paranoia, delusions, and hallucinations
    » May increase mortality
    » Not FDA-approved for the treatment of behaviors in the person with dementia
    » Benefit may outweigh risks; use lowest effective dose and attempt to wean periodically
    » Somnolence is a concern and may limit the dose
  - Olanzapine: initially 2.5 mg daily, up to 5 mg twice daily
    » Modest effect for neuropsychiatric symptoms of AD or vascular dementia
    » Incidence of extrapyramidal symptoms is low at this dose
  - Quetiapine: initially 25 mg at bedtime, up to 75 mg twice daily
  - Risperidone: up to 1 mg daily; higher doses are associated with increased adverse effects

DEPRESSION (SEE ALSO CHAPTER 18)

- Use of a selective serotonin reuptake inhibitor (SSRI) recommended:
  - Citalopram (Celexa) 20–40 mg/day
  - Sertraline HCl (Zoloft) 25–200 mg/day
  - Escitalopram (Lexapro) 5–20 mg/day
- Tricyclic antidepressants (TCAs) may worsen confusion (anticholinergic effect); less well tolerated than SSRIs
  - Nortriptyline HCl (Pamelor) 30–50 mg/day (also may improve insomnia and neuropathic pain)
  - Mirtazapine (Remeron) 7.5–45 mg at bedtime (also may improve insomnia)
- Attempt to wean after 6–12 months; patients may become less depressed as their dementia progresses and they are less aware of their circumstances

SLEEP DISTURBANCES

- See Sleep section of this chapter
- Trazodone (Desyrel) initially 25–50 mg at bedtime; may increase by 25–50 mg/day once weekly up to 75–150 mg/day

Special Considerations

- Self-reported memory loss commonly does not correlate with development of dementia; concerns about memory loss and dementia are often addressed by a spouse or family member, not the patient
- Mild cognitive impairment (MCI): presence of memory problems and objective memory impairment with preserved functional ability in daily life; these patients appear to be at increased risk for dementia

When to Consult, Refer, Hospitalize

- Neurology: unusual presentation
- Psychiatry: unable to differentiate from depression, intractable behaviors
- Social work for long-term planning

- Hospitalize if unable to manage at home for delirium, complications of comorbid or infectious conditions, or trauma with injury (CHF, COPD exacerbations, dehydration, pneumonia, hip fracture)
- Avoid hospitalization when possible
- Demented patients are likely to become more confused and delirious and fall when hospitalized

Follow-up
Expected Course
- AD: slowly and steadily progressive downhill course leading to complications and death
- Vascular dementia: stepwise with new focal deficits and decline with each stroke; patient often declines at a faster rate as the dementia progresses
- NPH: poor outcomes if dementia is severe or precedes ataxia

Complications
- 60%–90% of patients with dementia will develop neuropsychiatric symptoms (agitation, aggression, delusions, hallucinations, wandering) as the disease progresses
- Incontinence, distressing behaviors, and inability to provide self-care often lead to institutionalization
- Depression is common, suicide is a risk when the patient is aware of the condition
- Complications related to comorbidity or complications due to immobility with severe end-stage dementia include pneumonia, decubiti, dehydration and injury due to falls, and death
- NPH: 30% complications with shunting including subdural hematomas, stroke, seizures, and shunt malfunction

Delirium
Description
- Acute disorder of cognition that is characterized by the following:
  - Change in consciousness with reduced attention
  - Disturbance in cognition not accounted for by dementia
  - Development over a short time (hours to days), fluctuating throughout the day
  - Evidence that the cause is reversible (e.g., medical condition, substance intoxication, medication side effect)
  - Other associated features may include: psychomotor behavioral disturbances (e.g., hypo- or hyperactivity, changes in sleep patterns) and emotional disturbances (e.g., fear, depression, euphoria)
- Frequently is a presenting symptom of illness in older adults
- Often occurs in the presence of an underlying dementia

Etiology
- Pathophysiology is poorly understood, with many different etiologies:
  - *Medications:* polypharmacy, opioids, sedative-hypnotics, antipsychotics, lithium, muscle relaxants, antihistamines, drugs of abuse; also withdrawal from alcohol or benzodiazepines
  - *Infections:* sepsis, urinary tract infection, pneumonia, fever
  - *Metabolic disturbances:* electrolyte imbalance (sodium, calcium, magnesium, phosphate), endocrine disturbance (thyroid, parathyroid, pancreas, pituitary, adrenal), hyper- or hypoglycemia, hypoxemia

– *Intracranial conditions:* dementia, CNS infections, head trauma, seizures
– *Systemic disease:* cardiac disease (heart failure, myocardial infarction), liver failure, pulmonary disease, renal failure

Incidence and Demographics

- Highest incidence in hospitalized older adults; approximately 30% of older adults will experience delirium during hospitalization
  - More common in older adults who are frail and those undergoing complicated surgical procedures (e.g., orthopedic or cardiac surgery)
  - Highest incidence in intensive care, emergency department, palliative care units, long-term care

Risk Factors

- See Etiology
- Underlying brain disorders: dementia, stroke, Parkinson's disease
- Infection
- Dehydration
- Malnutrition
- Immobility (restraint use)
- Bladder catheter use
- Polypharmacy
- Medications associated with increased incidence of delirium
  - Analgesics: NSAIDs, opioids (especially meperidine)
  - Antibiotics and antivirals: acyclovir, aminoglycosides, cephalosporins, fluoroquinolones, linezolid, macrolides, penicillins, rifampin, sulfonamides
  - Anticholinergics: atropine, benztropine, diphenhydramine, scopolamine
  - Anticonvulsants: carbamazepine, phenytoin, valproate
  - Antidepressants: tricyclic antidepressants (amitriptyline, doxepin, mirtazapine)
  - Cardiovascular drugs: antiarrhythmics, beta blockers, clonidine, digoxin, diuretics
  - Corticosteroids
  - Dopamine agonists: amantadine, bromocriptine, levodopa, pergolide, pramipexole, ropinirole
  - Gastrointestinal agents: antiemetics, antispasmodics, histamine-2 receptor blockers (especially cimetidine), loperamide
  - Herbal preparations: *Atropa belladonna* extract, henbane, mandrake, jimson weed, St. John's wort, valerian
  - Hypoglycemics
  - Hypnotics and sedatives: barbiturates, benzodiazepines
  - Muscle relaxants: baclofen, cyclobenzaprine
  - Other CNS-active medications: disulfiram, donepezil, interleukin-2, lithium, phenothiazines

Prevention and Screening

- Avoid factors known to cause delirium (see Etiology/Risk Factors)
- Identify and treat underlying infection or acute illness
- Eliminate unnecessary medications
- Maintain adequate hydration, nutrition, and oxygenation
- Monitor bowels, avoid constipation
- Correct visual and auditory deficits
- Continuity of care and environment

Assessment

History

- Confusion assessment method (CAM)
- Detailed history of present illness, including cognition, time frame, and progression
- Comprehensive review of systems to identify underlying etiology
- Functional history and assessment
- Validate history with family member and/or caregiver
- Mini-Mental State Examination
- Geriatric Depression Scale

Physical Exam

- Often difficult in the patient with acute delirium; may be necessary to treat agitation with an antipsychotic in order to be able to adequately examine the patient
- Complete physical exam if possible with attention to neurologic exam
  - Assess level of consciousness, attention or inattention, visual fields, cranial nerves, and motor deficits
  - Important to identify individuals with possible focal neurologic disease and rule out stroke
- Attention to hearing and visual impairments
- Possible findings include: cardiac findings (murmurs, arrhythmias, heart enlargement), pulmonary findings, evidence of infectious processes, signs of trauma, orthostatic hypotension, urinary retention, fecal impaction

Diagnostic Studies

- Depends on suspected underlying etiology
- Urinalysis if urinary tract infection is suspected
- Chest x-ray if pneumonia is suspected
- CBC, chemistry profile, thyroid function tests, B_{12} level, folate level to identify a reversible cause for cognitive impairment or etiology of delirium
- Other tests to consider:
  - Computed tomography to identify infarcts, space-occupying lesions
  - Syphilis, HIV, and drug toxicity if indicated by history
  - Arterial oxygen or pulse oximetry if hypoxemia is considered
  - EKG to identify cardiopulmonary cause
  - EEG to rule out seizure
  - Lumbar puncture for suspected encephalopathy or meningitis

Differential Diagnosis

- Dementia
- Psychiatric illness
- Depression
- Nonconvulsive status epilepticus

Management

- Identify and treat underlying cause

Nonpharmacologic

- Medication review; discontinue unnecessary medications
- Mobilize patient
- Reduce noise

- Provide orienting stimuli (windows, clocks, calendars)
- Provide eye glasses or hearing aids
- Maintain hydration, nutrition, oxygenation
- Adequate bowel and bladder regimen
- Avoid physical restraints and any unnecessary IV lines and bladder catheters

Pharmacologic
- When patient is at risk for harming themselves or others or disrupting essential therapy, treat agitation with psychotropic medications:
  - Haloperidol 0.5–1 mg PO or IM every 2–6 hours for agitation
    - Drug of choice for acute delirium
    - If patient has underlying parkinsonism, atypical antipsychotics should be used:
  - Risperidone 0.25–2.5 mg once or twice/day
  - Olanzapine 2.5–5 mg/day
  - Quetiapine (Seroquel) 25–200 mg/day in divided doses
  - Lorazepam 0.25–0.5 mg only in cases of alcohol or sedative-hypnotic withdrawal
  - Short-term use of all antipsychotics is recommended because these medications are associated with a higher risk of mortality and stroke in patients with dementia
  - Monitor for extrapyramidal symptoms, prolonged QT interval, and neuroleptic malignant syndrome
- Appropriate treatment of cause

Special Considerations
- Terms "acute confusional state," "acute brain syndrome," and "toxic or metabolic encephalopathy" are often used when describing delirium

When to Consult, Refer, Hospitalize
- Consult physician for any primary care patient with suspected delirium
- Keep patient at home if patient has adequate supervision to ensure that the condition can be adequately treated and patient can be kept safe
- Delirious patients become more confused and agitated in the hospital setting
- Hospitalize when necessary to ensure patient safety, adequate hydration, and prescribed treatment

Follow-up
Expected Outcomes
- Delirium generally resolves when etiology is adequately treated
- Depends on etiology, signs may persist for a year or longer, especially if underlying dementia is involved

Complications
- Prolonged hospitalization, functional decline, falls with injury, institutionalization
- Associated with increased morbidity and mortality
- If the delirium is not diagnosed and treated, death may result

Dizziness
Description
- Nonspecific term used to describe a multitude of symptoms with various etiologies, most commonly vertigo, nonspecific "dizziness," disequilibrium, and presyncope

Etiology
- Multifactorial etiology in older adults
- See Table 4–3
- Many medications can cause dizziness; consider polypharmacy:
  - Cardiac: antihypertensives (especially beta blockers, calcium channel blockers, ACE inhibitors), vasodilators, adrenergic blocking agents, diuretics, antiarrhythmics, nitrates, digoxin
  - Sedative hypnotics: benzodiazepines
  - Antibiotics: aminoglycosides, erythromycin, ethambutol, griseofulvin, isoniazid, nitrofurantoin, polymyxin, rifampin, streptomycin, sulfonamides, trimethoprim, vancomycin
  - Antihistamines, OTC cold preparations
  - Muscle relaxants
  - Neuroleptics: phenothiazine
  - Antidiabetics: insulin, oral hypoglycemic agents
  - Seizure medications: phenytoin (Dilantin), carbamazepine (Tegretol), gabapentin (Neurontin)
  - Antidepressants
  - Opioids
  - NSAIDs

Table 4-3. Common Causes of Dizziness

	Vertigo (see Chapter 7)	Disequilibrium	Syncope/ Presyncope	Nonspecific Dizziness
Cause	Acute asymmetry in vestibular system: benign paroxysmal positional vertigo (BPPV), acute vestibular neuronitis or labyrinthitis, Ménière disease, migraine, acoustic neuroma; rarely due to stroke, cerebral hemorrhage, multiple sclerosis	Peripheral neuropathy, musculoskeletal disorders interfering with gait, vestibular disorders, cervical spondylosis, visual impairment, med effects	Commonly caused by orthostatic hypotension, cardiac arrhythmias, atherosclerosis, cardiomyopathy, vasovagal episodes	Psychiatric disorders (major depression, generalized anxiety or panic disorder, somatization disorder, alcohol dependence, personality disorder); also hypoglycemia, head trauma or whiplash injury, medication effects

continued

Table 4-3. Common Causes of Dizziness (cont.)

	Vertigo (see Chapter 7)	Disequilibrium	Syncope/ Presyncope	Nonspecific Dizziness
History	Sensation of motion of self or environment: spinning, whirling, tilting, moving; may have nausea and vomiting	Sense of imbalance primarily with walking	"Wooziness," faint-feeling or "near-fainting"; witnesses may report pallor; usually occurs while standing or sitting upright	Difficult for patient to describe; lightheadedness; dizziness that accompanies hyperventilation, anxiety, or depression
Time Course	Intermittent, never continuous	Intermittent	Intermittent; increasing frequency often heralds a serious underlying disorder	Constant or episodic; when related to psychiatric disorders, gradually builds, waxes and wanes over approximately 20 minutes (or longer), then gradually resolves
Provoking/ Aggravating Factors	Change in head position; change in ear pressure (sneeze, cough, Valsalva)	Ambulation; visual impairment typically exacerbates the sense of imbalance	Symptoms upon standing, coughing, swallowing, urinating, defecating; warm, crowded places, prolonged orthostasis, pain, emotion, fear	Stress
Associated Signs and Symptoms	Nystagmus, postural instability, hearing loss	Often associated with Parkinson's disease	Possibly lightheadedness, diaphoresis, nausea, visual blurring, palpitations, chest pain, dyspnea	Hyperventilation, anxiety, depression

Incidence and Demographics
- One of the most common complaints in older adults
- Older adults have a higher incidence of central vestibular causes of vertigo (nearly 20% of cases), most often due to stroke

Risk Factors
- Risk of dizziness 68% in patients with five or more of the following characteristics
  - Anxiety
  - Depressive symptoms
  - Past myocardial infarction

– Use of more than 4 medications
– Impaired balance
– Postural hypotension
– Impaired hearing

Prevention and Screening

Review fall risks and prevention

- Eliminate all unnecessary medications, including OTC and herbal
- Manage medical illnesses closely
- Maintain adequate fluid intake

Assessment

- Most important to determine if acute or chronic, or if condition is unstable

History

- Description
  - Have the patient describe the feeling without using the word "dizzy"
  - Interview family member or witness
  - Was event exertional?
  - Does dizziness interfere with routine activities?
  - Aggravating/alleviating factors
  - Precipitating factors: rapid head movements, change in position
  - Associated symptoms: diaphoresis, blurred vision, nausea, hearing loss, tinnitus, associated cardiac or neurological symptoms (chest pain, palpitations, headache, diplopia, aphasia, unilateral motor weakness, paresthesia), incontinence of bladder or bowel
- Course/timing
  - Detailed history of event, frequency, when it occurs, prodromal symptoms
  - Length of loss of consciousness, seizure activity, fall hard or soft, any injuries including to tongue
  - Confusion or drowsiness after event
- Past medical history: cardiac, neurologic
- Family history: heart disease, seizures
- Medication review

Physical Exam

- Evaluate for positional changes in symptoms, orthostatic blood pressure, and pulse changes (orthostatic hypotension)
- Observe gait
- Assess for nystagmus (vertigo)
- Depending on suspected etiology, look for:
  - Cardiac abnormalities: orthostatic hypotension, arrhythmia, murmurs, cardiomegaly, bruits
  - Neurological abnormalities: focal deficits
  - Abnormal vestibular function by rotational testing
  - Otologic evaluation
  - Evaluate vision and hearing
  - Respiratory exam

Diagnostic Studies
- CBC, metabolic panel including fasting blood sugar
- Thyroid function test if hypothyroidism suspected
- If cardiac cause suspected:
  - Echocardiography to rule out valvular disease
  - Stress testing if exertional syncope to rule out ischemia
  - Holter or event monitoring to rule out arrhythmia
- If neurologic cause suspected:
  - Head CT or MRI if brain lesion suspected or focal neurologic signs
  - Tilt table to evaluate autonomic dysfunction
  - Electroencephalography if seizure history or seizures suspected
- Electronystagmography if vestibular origin is suspected
- Carotid or transcranial Doppler studies if bruits or rule out vertebrobasilar insufficiency

Differential Diagnosis
- See Table 4–3
- Need to differentiate between the types of dizziness as well as the causes of dizziness

Management
- Treat underlying cause

Nonpharmacologic
- Manage orthostatic hypotension
  - Change position slowly
  - Exercise feet before standing
  - Elastic stockings (put on before rising)
  - Elevate head of bed
- Avoid activity in hot weather
- Exercise
- Ensure adequate fluid and appropriate nutritional intake

Pharmacologic
- Discontinue unnecessary medications; use smallest doses of medications that have an effect for the patient
- Treatment depends on underlying etiology

Special Considerations
- Most causes of dizziness are benign; however, serious life-threatening conditions may present as dizziness in older adults

When to Consult, Refer, Hospitalize
- Hospitalize for unstable condition
- Refer to cardiology for suspected cardiac cause
- Refer to neurology for neurological cause, focal neurological signs
- Refer to psychiatry if symptoms interfering with function and cannot be managed with first-line medications
- Refer older adults that cannot be safely managed in their present living environment

Follow-up

Expected Course
- Depends on etiology

Complications
- Functional disability
- Falls, fractures, fear of falling
- Immobility
- Social isolation
- Long-term-care placement
- Depression
- Death

Disequilibrium

Description
- Sensation of imbalance or unsteadiness when standing or walking, "dizziness in the feet"

Etiology
- Peripheral neuropathy, a musculoskeletal disorder interfering with gait, vestibular disorder, and/or cervical spondylosis
- *Vestibular:* loss of vestibular function (see Chapter 7 under Vertigo) due to otoxic drugs, cerumen impaction, labyrinthitis, acoustic neuroma
- *Proprioceptive and somatosensory:* peripheral neuropathy secondary to alcohol, DM, renal failure
- *Motor and cerebellar lesions:* Parkinson's disease, cerebellar atrophy, tumors, infarcts, hydrocephalus
- *Normal changes of aging:* slowing of motor responses, weakness of support muscles, decreased proprioception

Incidence and Demographics
- Approximately one-third of older adults report balance symptoms

Risk Factors
- Advanced age
- Female
- Peripheral neuropathy
- Depressive symptoms

Prevention and Screening
Review fall risks and prevention
- Eliminate all unnecessary medications, including OTC and herbal
- Manage medical illnesses closely

Assessment
History
- Occurs in standing position, with movement, or turning head
- Associated symptoms may differ depending on cause of disequilibrium:

- Proprioceptive or somatosensory causes: numbness, weakness, bowel and bladder dysfunction
- Motor and cerebellar lesions: gait disturbances, ataxia
- Medication review
- Family history of dizziness or disequilibrium

Physical Exam
- Complete physical exam with emphasis on:
  - Vision assessment
  - Otologic exam
  - Cardiovascular exam including orthostatic vital signs
  - Musculoskeletal exam
  - Neurologic exam (cranial nerves, motor system, sensory testing—especially vibratory, nystagmus)
- Observe rising from chair and gait

Diagnostic Studies
- See Dizziness Diagnostic Studies

Differential Diagnosis
- See Table 4–3

Management
Nonpharmacologic
- Support with cane or walker
- Physical therapy with gait retraining, strengthening, and balance training
- Fall-prevention strategies
- Tai chi

Pharmacologic
- Depends on underlying etiology
- Manage diabetes, B_{12} and folate deficiency
- Discontinue offending medications

When to Consult, Refer, Hospitalize
- Refer to neurology if etiology in doubt, treatment not effective, patient unable to function

Follow-up
- See Dizziness Follow-Up

Syncope
Description
- Transient, sudden loss of consciousness and postural tone
- Due to impaired cerebral circulation with spontaneous recovery
- Occurs from standing position, occasionally from seated position but not lying down
- Patient is neurologically baseline upon recovery
- Near-syncope: sensation of impending faint may be caused by all of causes of dizziness, especially psychogenic etiologies and hyperventilation

Etiology
- Cause is unknown in approximately one-third of cases
- Primary bradyarrhythmias due to sinus and atrial node dysfunctions (e.g., sick sinus syndrome)
- Hypertrophic cardiomyopathy
- Aortic stenosis
- Neurocardiogenic mechanisms: vasovagal and vasodepressor episodes, urination, swallowing, cough
- Carotid hypersensitivity syndrome: an exaggerated response to carotid sinus stimulation
- Orthostatic hypotension due to dysautonomias, fluid depletion, illness, bedrest, deconditioning, medications

Incidence and Demographics
- Much more common in adults > age 70
- 30% of adults will experience at least one episode of syncope
- 3% of all emergency department visits and 1%–6% of hospitalizations

Risk Factors
- Cardiovascular disease
- History of stroke, transient ischemic attack (TIA), or hypertension
- Lower body mass index (BMI)
- Diabetes
- Increased alcohol intake
- Polypharmacy: vasodilators, diuretics, adrenergic blocking agents
- Age-related cardiovascular changes, autonomic and neuroendocrine changes
- Cardiovascular deconditioning

Prevention and Screening
- Adequate hydration
- Reduction of cardiac risk factors

Assessment
History
- Number of episodes, associated symptoms, presence of prodrome, sudden onset, position when event occurs (supine vs. erect), preceding events (e.g., coughing, urinating), duration of symptoms
- Medication history
- Depends on etiology:
  - *Neurocardiogenic (vasovagal) syncope:* precipitating events (fear, severe pain, emotional distress, or prolonged standing), occurrence of premonitory autonomic nervous system signs and symptoms preceding vasovagal episode (sweating, pallor, nausea, palpitations, shortness of breath); typically occurs while standing
  - *Orthostatic hypotension:* symptoms upon standing; may be related to start of medication or change in dosing, prolonged standing, presence of autonomic neuropathy, or Parkinson's disease
  - *Cardiac syncope:* sudden onset; presence of structural heart disease; occurs during exertion or while supine; preceded by palpitations; family history of sudden death; may report blurred vision
  - *Situational syncope:* occurs during or immediately after urination, defecation, cough, or swallowing

Physical Exam
- Orthostatic vital signs
- Focused cardiovascular exam (arrhythmia, murmur)
- Focused neurologic exam
- Stool for guaiac test (GI bleeding may be implicated)

Diagnostic Studies
- Electrocardiogram (ECG) in all patients
- Cardiac evaluation in patients with suspected or confirmed cardiac disease includes echocardiography, stress testing, prolonged ECG monitoring (Holter), and possibly electrophysiologic studies
- If cardiac evaluation is negative, test to rule out neurally mediated syncope with tilt testing and carotid massage

Differential Diagnosis
- Neurocardiogenic (vasovagal) syncope
- Orthostatic hypotension
- Pulmonary embolism
- Subarachnoid hemorrhage
- Seizure disorder
- Alcohol abuse
- Cardiovascular disease with obstruction
- Cardiac arrhythmias
- TIA
- Concussion
- Hypovolemia
- Hypoglycemia
- Anemia
- Hypoxia
- Medication toxicity
- Panic or anxiety attack

Management
- Treatment is based on the underlying etiology

Nonpharmacologic
- In cases of neurocardiogenic (vasovagal) syncope explain etiology to patient; advise to lie down when prodromal symptoms occur; compression stockings may be beneficial
- Pacemaker or implantable cardiac defibrillator may be indicated in patients with arrhythmias
- Radiofrequency ablation for supraventricular arrhythmias

Pharmacologic
- Correct metabolic disturbances
- Discontinue offending medications

Special Considerations
Workup can be expensive

When to Consult, Refer, Hospitalize
- Refer to cardiology for evaluation

- Hospitalize if hemodynamically unstable, suspected or known significant heart disease, family history of sudden death, syncope occurring during exercise, or new-onset atrial fibrillation

Follow-up
- Patient with syncope from unknown cause should be followed closely

Expected Outcomes
- Unless the cause is vasovagal, syncope is associated with decreased survival; approximately half of patients > age 85 hospitalized with syncope survive > 3 years
  - Patients with syncope from vasovagal, orthostatic, or medication have no increased risk for death or MI

Complications
Associated with high morbidity and mortality and falls

Fatigue
Description
- Fatigue is a nonspecific symptom that consists of three components:
  - Difficulty initiating activity; may be perceived as generalized weakness without evidence of objective findings
  - Difficulty maintaining activity; easily fatigued
  - Difficulty with concentration, memory, and emotional stability (mental fatigue)
- Distinguishable from somnolence, dyspnea, and muscle weakness, although these symptoms may be associated
- Three categories: recent (< 1 month), prolonged (1–6 months), chronic (> 6 months)

Etiology
Medications
- Sedative hypnotics
- Antihistamines
- Muscle relaxants
- Alcohol and drug use or withdrawal
- Antidepressants
- Beta blockers
- Opioids

Physical
- Deconditioning, sedentary lifestyle
- Sleep disorders, insomnia, sleep apnea
- GU: cancer of bladder, uterus, and prostate, renal failure
- Hematopoietic: anemia, chronic leukemias, lymphoma, multiple myeloma
- Infection: acute or chronic
- Respiratory: chronic obstructive pulmonary disease (COPD), asthma
- Cardiac disease: coronary artery disease (CAD), heart failure (HF)
- Endocrine disorders: DM, thyroid, parathyroid, and Cushing disease
- GI: pancreatic or colon cancer, chronic hepatitis, irritable bowel syndrome
- Neurological disease: neuromuscular, dementia, delirium, CVA
- Pain
- Rheumatic disease: temporal arteritis, rheumatoid arthritis, polymyalgia rheumatica
- Other malignancies

Psychological
- Depression
- Somatization disorder
- Anxiety or panic disorder

Incidence and Demographics
- Very common in older adults, common presenting symptom in primary care
- Females > males
- Psychiatric illness is present in 60%–80% of patients with chronic fatigue (major depression most common)

Risk Factors
- Chronic disease
- Psychiatric illness
- Medications, polypharmacy

Prevention and Screening
- Specific to etiology

Assessment
History
- Onset, course, duration, daily pattern, exacerbating/relieving factors
- Impact on function and ability to complete activities of daily living
- Recent weight changes
- Impact of sleep or rest on symptoms (improvement with rest points to a sleep disorder as cause)
- Medication review including prescription, over-the-counter, and alcohol/drug use
- Patient may report overall, systemic, generalized lack of energy, fatigue, nonspecific malaise; also trouble concentrating, lack of interest in activities
- Family may report weakness, decreased activity, or change in sleep patterns

Physical Exam
- General appearance: level of alertness, psychomotor agitation or retardation, grooming
- Thorough physical exam with assessment for presence of lymphadenopathy, evidence of thyroid disease, weight loss
- Cardiovascular exam: evidence of heart failure
- Pulmonary exam: evidence of chronic lung disease
- Neurologic exam: muscle bulk, tone and strength, deep tendon reflexes, sensory and cranial nerve evaluation
- Functional assessment
- Geriatric Depression Scale

Diagnostic Studies
- Laboratory studies rarely elucidate the cause of fatigue; may be reasonable to check the following:
  - CBC, ESR, chemistry panel including electrolytes, glucose, renal and liver function tests, TSH
  - CK if evidence of muscle weakness or pain
  - Consider HIV testing or PPD placement depending on patient's history
- If evidence of infection, obtain urine for urinalysis and culture and sensitivity, CXR

Differential Diagnosis
- See Etiology

Management
Treatment specific to etiology

Nonpharmacologic
- Therapeutic goal setting: accomplish activities of daily living, maintain social relationships, daily exercise routine
- Cognitive behavioral therapy
- Graded exercise therapy
- Education regarding appropriate sleep hygiene
- Referral to support groups

Pharmacologic
- Antidepressant trial in patients with depressive symptoms; discontinue if no symptomatic improvement within 6–8 weeks

When to Consult, Refer, Hospitalize
- Appropriate consultant for underlying etiology; consider referral to physical/occupational therapy, dietitian
- Hospitalize if underlying etiology or acute exacerbation of etiology cannot be managed safely on an outpatient basis

Follow-up
Expected outcomes
Full recovery is not common; depends on etiology
- Risk factors for a poor prognosis include older age and comorbid chronic medical or psychiatric illness

Complications
- Functional declines, psychiatric illness

Falls

Description
- Unintentional lowering to rest from a higher to a lower position, not due to loss of consciousness or violent impact

Etiology
- Multifactorial; often results from a threat to normal homeostatic mechanisms (e.g., infection, medication changes, environmental conditions) in combination with age-related declines in balance, ambulatory function, and changes in the cardiovascular system

Incidence and Demographics
- Incidence increases with age
  - 30%–40% of adults over age 65 living at home fall each year; increases to 50% in adults over age 80
  - 50% of older adults living in long-term care fall each year
- Equally common in men and women, though women are more likely to suffer injury
  - 5%–10% result in major injury: fractures, head trauma, major lacerations
  - Major injuries more common in long-term-care populations

- Fall-related complications are the leading cause of death from injury in older adults (5th leading cause of death)

Risk Factors
- Intrinsic risk factors:
  - Gait disorder and balance impairment
  - Peripheral neuropathy
  - Vestibular dysfunction
  - Muscle weakness
  - Vision impairment
  - Medical comorbidities
  - Advanced age
  - Impaired activities of daily living (ADL)
  - Orthostatic hypotension
  - Cognitive impairment
  - Medications: sedatives, anxiolytics (especially benzodiazepines), diuretics, laxatives, alcohol
- Extrinsic risk factors
  - Environmental hazards
  - Improper footwear
  - Restraint use

Prevention and Screening
Muscle-strengthening and balance-retraining programs (including Tai chi) shown to reduce fall risk
Multidisciplinary risk factor screening/intervention programs; variety of assessment tools, choice often depends on setting (home, nursing home, hospital)
- Vitamin D supplementation
- Avoid restraints
- Discontinue unnecessary medications

Assessment
- Fall risk assessment should be incorporated into the annual history and physical of all geriatric patients

History
- Medical and fall history, including:
  - Past medical history, medication review
  - History of previous falls
  - Risk factors for falls
  - Circumstances of the fall: time of day, events, symptoms prior to and following the fall, loss of consciousness, ability to get up under own power or required assistance, length of time on the floor
  - Perception of the cause of the fall

Physical Exam
- Neurologic exam including cognitive testing
- Musculoskeletal function:
  - "Get up and go" test: observe patient stand up from a chair, walk 10 feet, turn around, come back, and sit down; tests leg strength, balance, vestibular function, and gait

– "Functional reach" test: patient stands with fist extended alongside a wall and leans forward as far as possible; length of fist movement is measured (distance < 6 inches indicates increased fall risk)
- Cardiovascular exam including orthostatic vital signs
- Visual acuity and hearing evaluation
- Examine feet

Diagnostic Studies
- Based on history and physical exam
- Lab studies that may be indicated include: CBC to rule out anemia; electrolytes and renal function testing to rule out dehydration; and glucose rule out dehydration and autonomic neuropathy related to diabetes
- X-rays, Holter monitoring, echocardiography, and other imaging as appropriate

Differential Diagnosis
- See Etiology and Risk Factors

Management
Nonpharmacologic
- See Prevention and Screening
- Goal is to prevent falls and the complications of falls
- Personal response services to activate 911 when patient falls

Pharmacologic
- Discontinue unnecessary or offending medications
- Vitamin D intake of at least 800 IU per day (dietary or supplemental)

Special Considerations
Long periods down on floor before being found are associated with increased morbidity

When to Consult, Refer, Hospitalize
- Emergency department for serious injuries or life threatening underlying condition
- Consult with appropriate specialty (cardiology, neurology, orthopedics) if underlying condition suspected

Follow-up
Expected Outcomes
- 60% of older adults with a history of a fall in the previous year will fall again

Complications
- Fractures
- Painful soft tissue injuries
- Subdural hematoma
- Impaired mobility because of physical injury
- Fear of falling with decreased activity
- Social isolation
- Decreased independence

Fractures
Description
- A break in a bone

- Most common fractures in older adults are hip, vertebral compression, and distal radius (Colles fracture)

Etiology
- Falls
- Osteoporosis
- Tumor
- Osteomyelitis
- Osteomalacia

Incidence and Demographics
- Hip fractures are most common, estimated to account for approximately 140,000 nursing home admissions annually
- Incidence of fractures increase with age
- Fewer than 30% regain pre-fracture level of physical functioning
- White women over age 60 have a higher incidence of fracture than for men and for other races because of osteoporosis

Risk Factors
- Falls
- History of fracture
- Osteoporosis and risk factors for osteoporosis: advanced age, female, low body mass index (BMI), corticosteroid use, family history of osteoporosis, reduced lifetime exposure to estrogen
- Behavioral risk factors: low calcium intake, physical inactivity, vitamin D deficiency, smoking, excessive alcohol consumption
- Pathologic bone disorders: tumor, osteomyelitis, osteomalacia

Prevention and Screening
- Maximize bone density during adolescence/young adulthood
- Treatment of osteoporosis/osteopenia
- Weight-bearing physical activity and balance training
- Adequate dietary intake of calcium and vitamin D
- Avoidance of smoking, excessive alcohol intake
- Fall-prevention strategies

Assessment
History
- Pain is predominant symptom, often worse with movement
- May be associated with swelling, bruising, decreased range of motion, and variable degrees of deformity
- Hip fracture: may occur with a fall or occur spontaneously because of osteoporosis, hip pain
- Vertebral compression fracture: may occur with sudden move such as sneezing, coughing, lifting, or stretching
  - Most are asymptomatic, may present with acute back pain that radiates bilaterally to the abdomen
- Colles fracture of distal radius: occurs with falling on an outstretched hand (FOOSH); wrist pain

Physical Exam
- Point tenderness over bone; muscle weakness/pain with movement; deformity
- Hip fracture: leg shortened, externally rotated; severe pain with weight bearing
- Vertebra: back pain, kyphosis
- Colles' fracture of distal radius: exquisite tenderness to touch; assess neurovascular status including motor and sensory function of the ulnar, radial, and median nerves (acute median nerve compression is common); assess radial pulse and capillary refill

Diagnostic Studies
- X-ray: most cost-effective; usually adequate for showing fracture; in older adults, may take days for fracture to appear on x-ray
- Bone scan: useful for identifying occult/stress fracture
- CT: for evaluating degree of displacement, compression of fracture
- MRI: identifying lesions that may affect bone
- Laboratory studies not usually indicated

Differential Diagnosis
- Sprain
- Hematoma
- Tumor
- Torn ligament
- Tendinitis

Management
Nonpharmacologic
- Lifestyle changes to reduce risk factors for osteoporosis (quitting smoking, avoiding excessive alcohol intake, ensuring intake of calcium and vitamin D and physical exercise)
- Falls prevention program
- *Hip fracture*: surgery usually necessary
  - Intertrochanteric: pin; associated with bleeding, instability, deformity
  - Femoral neck: prosthesis; associated with avascular necrosis, infection
- *Vertebral compression fracture*: resume activity as quickly as possible to prevent further deconditioning and fractures; vertebroplasty and kyphoplasty may be considered in some patients
- *Colles fracture of distal radius*: if fracture is nondisplaced, wrist should be splinted and not casted; elevation, ice, and active range of motion of the shoulder and fingers should be performed
  - For displaced fractures, surgical intervention is often necessary

Pharmacologic
- Pain management
- Treat osteoporosis if present (see Chapter 14, Musculoskeletal Disorders)

How Long to Treat
- Primary care treatment is immobilization and referral to orthopedic surgeon

Special Considerations
- If x-ray initially negative for fracture and pain does not begin to improve after 1 to 2 weeks, re-x-ray or consider CT or bone scan to rule out occult fracture

Follow-up
Expected Course
- Fracture healing should occur in 6 to 12 weeks
- Persistent but gradual decrease in swelling and improved strength may take another 4 to 6 weeks to resolve

Complications
- Persistent deformity, arthritis, compression neuropathy, fibrous union
- Failure to heal secondary to osteoporosis
- Functional decline and loss of independence with increased health care utilization and institutionalization
- Chronic pain
- Death

Sleep Disorders
Description
- A group of syndromes characterized by disturbance in the patient's amount of sleep, quality or timing of sleep, or in behaviors or physiological conditions associated with sleep
- The American Academy of Sleep Medicine categorizes sleep disorders into eight major groups: insomnia, sleep-related breathing disorders, hypersomnias of central origin, circadian rhythm sleep disorders, parasomnias, sleep-related movement disorders, isolated symptoms and normal variants, and other sleep disorders
  - *Insomnia:* subjective problem of insufficient or nonrestorative sleep despite adequate time and opportunity to sleep that results in impaired daytime function
  - *Sleep-related breathing disorders:* abnormal respiration during sleep
    - Obstructive sleep apnea-hypopnea (OSAH): irregular respiratory patterns that disrupt sleep structure resulting in daytime symptoms (fatigue, poor concentration); snoring and restlessness during sleep is common
  - *Sleep-related movement disorders:* movements that disturb sleep
    - Restless leg syndrome (RLS): spontaneous, continuous leg movements associated with unpleasant sensations in the legs; occur at rest and relieved by movement

Etiology
- Insomnia
  - Acute insomnia:
    - Acute stress
    - Acute or chronic illness, often with pain
    - Environmental changes
    - Consumption of or withdrawal from caffeine, nicotine, alcohol
    - Medications or illicit drugs that have stimulant properties (theophylline, beta blockers, glucocorticoids, thyroxine, bronchodilators, amphetamines)
    - Withdrawal from medications with central nervous system depressant properties (benzodiazepines)
  - Long-term insomnia:
    - Inadequate sleep hygiene
    - Psychiatric disorders: depression (early morning awakening), anxiety, substance abuse, post-traumatic stress disorder

- Medical disorders: pulmonary disease, pain, heart failure are most common
- Neurological diseases: Parkinson's disease, Alzheimer's disease
- Medications: central nervous system stimulants (caffeine), respiratory stimulants (theophylline), appetite suppressants, calcium channel blockers, antidepressants, beta antagonists (propranolol, metoprolol), glucocorticoids (prednisone, cortisol)
- Sleep disorders:
    - RLS: characterized by an urge to move the legs
    - Periodic limb movement disorder (PLMD): characterized by rhythmic limb movements during sleep
    - Sleep apnea: central (failure to initiate breathing); obstructive upper-airway occlusion (usually accompanied by periods of snoring and restlessness)
    - Circadian rhythm sleep disorders
- OSAH: upper airway collapse occurs because of reduced neural output to upper airway musculature during sleep and reduced upper airway size; this results in partial or complete obstruction
- RLS: cause is unknown in most cases; may be related to underlying medical condition including iron deficiency, uremia, diabetes mellitus, rheumatic disease, and venous insufficiency

Incidence and Demographics

- Insomnia is the most common sleep disorder in older adults; up to 40% of all older adults report insomnia and approximately 20% report severe insomnia
    - More prevalent with increasing age
    - Women > men
- OSAH risk increases with age; men are more likely to be affected than women
- RLS is twice as common in women than men; risk increases with age

Risk Factors

- Insomnia: see Etiology
- OSAH: obesity, craniofacial or upper airway soft tissue abnormalities, heredity, smoking, and nasal congestion
- RLS: see Etiology

Prevention and Screening

- Public and patient education concerning the causes and risk factors associated with primary sleep disorders
- Regular bedtime routines
- Normalized daily routines and waking hours
- Physical exercise regime
- Stable interpersonal relations
- Family and social support systems

Assessment
History
- Medical, psychiatric, medication, and substance history
- Sleep history: timing (onset, duration), time it takes to fall asleep, frequency of awakenings, difficulty going back to asleep after awakening, aggravating/relieving factors

- Ask about symptoms during day/consequences of insomnia: sleepy, lethargic during day, poor performance in demanding situations, difficulty concentrating, fatigue, irritability
- Sleep diary for 1 to 2 weeks
- Obtain history from the patient's bed partner to look for snoring, apnea, jerking, restlessness

Physical Exam
- Specific to suspected etiology
- Physical exam should be tailored to the presenting symptoms, as primary insomnia is an illness of exclusion of other underlying medical conditions

Diagnostic Studies
- Depends on suspected etiology
- CBC, chemistry profile, electrolytes
- Sleep study, polysomnography if sleep apnea is suspected

Differential Diagnosis
- See Etiology

Management
- Specific to condition
- Treat short-term insomnia to avoid long-term insomnia

Nonpharmacologic
- Treat underlying cause; however, sleep disorder may not resolve with treatment of underlying disorder
- Insomnia:
  - Sleep hygiene: sleep only as much as necessary to feel rested, then get out of bed; go to bed and wake up same time every day; avoid long periods of wakefulness in bed; use bed only for sleep (and sex); avoid napping during the day; avoid caffeine after lunch and avoid alcohol near bedtime; avoid smoking near bedtime; do not go to bed hungry; regular exercise (not too close to bedtime)
  - Relaxation: progressive muscle relaxation and the relaxation response
  - Cognitive behavioral therapy
- OSAH:
  - Weight control
  - Avoidance of drugs and alcohol
  - Continuous positive airway pressure (CPAP) device
  - Oral appliances (OA)
- RLS:
  - Iron replacement therapy if serum ferritin < 45–50
  - Mental alerting activities (e.g., crossword puzzles) if symptoms occur during times of boredom
  - Avoidance of aggravating factors such as caffeine, nicotine, and alcohol

Pharmacologic
- Insomnia:
  - Benzodiazepines improve sleep onset and reduce awakenings; however, they are associated with increased risk of adverse effects and falls in older adults

– Nonbenzodiazepines: improve sleep onset, reduce awakenings, improve sleep duration and quality; side effects include headache, dizziness, and somnolence
  • Zaleplon (Sonata) 5 mg at bedtime; good for difficulty with sleep onset; for short-term use; may be habit forming
  • Zolpidem (Ambien) 5 mg at bedtime (Ambien CR 6.25 mg at bedtime); for short-term use; may be habit forming
  • Eszopiclone (Lunesta) 1 mg at bedtime; effective for both sleep-onset insomnia and sleep-maintenance insomnia; for short-term use; may be habit forming
– Antidepressants such as as trazodone, mirtazapine (Remeron), and doxepin are sedating; may be indicated if depression is associated
– Antihistamines: many over-the-counter sleep aids contain diphenhydramine, a sedating antihistamine that has a high risk for adverse effects in older adults, including sedation, decreased alertness, diminished cognitive function, delirium, dry mouth, blurred vision, urinary retention, constipation
– When using medications to treat insomnia:
  • Weigh risks and benefits of pharmacologic therapy in older adults
  • Discontinue gradually
  • Rebound insomnia may occur when medications are discontinued
  • Be aware of potential for drug tolerance, dependence, and withdrawal with benzodiazepines
  • Do not prescribe for patients with a history of substance abuse or mental illness
• RLS:
– Dopamine agonists: pramipexole (Mirapex) 0.125 mg or ropinirole (Requip) 0.25 mg one hour before the usual time of symptom onset
– If patient is unable to tolerate dopamine agonist, levodopa/carbidopa 25/100 mg before symptom onset

Special Considerations
• Habituation/tolerance is a major problem with benzodiazepines
• Older adults are very vulnerable to the effects of sedative-hypnotics, especially confusion, delirium, sleep apnea, falls with fractures

When to Consult, Refer, Hospitalize
• When symptoms continue to occur for longer than one month, refer to a sleep disorder specialist, psychiatrist, or other qualified mental health practitioner
• Refer suspected OSAH to specialist
• Consider ENT consult for upper airway evaluation

Follow-up
Expected Course
• Most patients have chronic lifelong insomnia that is best managed by nonpharmacologic treatment

Complications
• Chronic sleep disorders can lead to chronic fatigue and decreased activity
• OSAH associated with increased risk of all-cause mortality; can cause hypertension and has been associated with myocardial infarction, cerebrovascular disease, and cardiac arrhythmias

Frailty

Description

- Syndrome marked by functional decline, loss of physiologic reserve and strength, and increased risk for morbidity and mortality
- One definition describes frailty as meeting three or more of the following criteria:
  - Weight loss of ≥ 5% of body weight in last year
  - Exhaustion as defined by subjective response to questions regarding effort required for activity
  - Weakness as defined by decreased grip strength
  - Slow walking speed
  - Decreased physical activity

Etiology

- Complex and multifactorial etiology
- Endocrine function
  - Age-related decline in muscle function
  - Related to decline in sex hormone and growth hormone levels, higher cortisol levels, and low vitamin D levels
- Immune system
  - Elevated serum levels of proinflammatory biomarkers
  - Activation of innate immune system may trigger clotting cascade
- Sarcopenia
- Many disease states are implicated in the cause of frailty, including:
  - Malignancy
  - Gastrointestinal disease
  - Cardiac disease: heart failure, coronary artery disease
  - Pulmonary disease: COPD, interstitial lung disease
  - Infections: tuberculosis, aspiration pneumonia
  - Neurologic disease: dementia, stroke, Parkinson's disease
  - Endocrine disorders: diabetes, hypothyroidism
  - Renal disease
  - Psychiatric illness: depression, mania, psychosis
  - Rheumatic disease

Incidence and Demographics

- Prevalence increases with age; 3% to 7% of adults age 65–75 are frail, while up to 30% of older adults meet frailty criteria by age 90
- More common in women who are older, less educated, and current smokers or hormone therapy users
- More common in men who are single and less educated

Risk Factors

- Chronic disease (see Etiology)
- Inactivity
- Poor nutritional intake
- Stress
- Advanced age

Prevention and Screening
- Manage medical conditions that may lead to frailty
- Exercise, stretching, resistance training, and Tai chi
- Nutritional program in combination with exercise program

Assessment
History
- Functional history including fall history
- Social history
- Past medical and psychiatric history
- Medication review
- Comprehensive review of systems including factors that may contribute to frailty:
  - Vision and hearing loss
  - Musculoskeletal changes
  - Weight loss, difficulty eating, GI symptoms, dietary history

Physical Exam
- Vital signs, including orthostatic blood pressure measurements
- Comprehensive physical exam
- Functional evaluation ("get up and go" test)

Diagnostic Studies
- Depends on suspected underlying cause; rule out infection, malignancy, organ failure
- CBC with differential
- Basic metabolic panel (electrolytes, BUN, creatinine, glucose)
- Liver function tests
- Calcium and phosphate (calcium may be elevated in cancer)
- TSH
- Vitamin B_{12} and folate
- Albumin, total protein (low in protein malnutrition)
- Total cholesterol (low in malnutrition)
- Urinalysis
- Stool hemoccult
- Chest x-ray to rule out tuberculosis, malignancy, infection

Differential Diagnosis
- See Etiology

Management
Nonpharmacologic
- Interdisciplinary team management
- Exercise, resistance training, ambulation program
- Weight loss: nutritional supplementation between meals (monitor for decreased meal intake)

Pharmacologic
- Vitamin D supplementation in deficient individuals may reduce fall risk and improve balance
- Hormonal supplementation has not demonstrated benefit
- Weight loss: use of appetite stimulants (megestrol acetate, dronabinol) may be considered, though have been shown to have minimal benefit and considerable adverse effects in the frail older adult population

Special Considerations
- Although age, chronic illness, and disability are associated with frailty, frailty can exist independently of these factors

When to Consult, Refer, Hospitalize
- Speech therapist and dietitian for evaluation of unexplained weight loss or malnutrition; nutrition consult recommended for most patients
- Physical and occupational therapy for therapeutic exercise and functional mobility
- Social work for referral to community resources, patient and family support

Follow-up
Expected Course
- Depends on etiology; expected trajectory is ongoing decline
- Weight loss is a marker for a poor prognosis

Complications
- Falls
- Decreased mobility
- Worsening ADL function
- Institutionalization
- Death

Pain
Description
- Common unpleasant sensation that may or may not be associated with tissue damage
- Complex phenomenon that is both a sensory and an emotional experience
- May be acute, chronic, or acute and chronic

Etiology
- Nociceptive pain occurs in response to tissue damage or inflammation, may be somatic or visceral
  - Somatic: due to stimulation of the somatic nervous system and involves skin, soft tissue, muscle, and bone
  - Visceral: due to stimulation of the autonomic nervous system and involves the cardiac, lung, gastrointestinal, and genitourinary tracts
- Neuropathic pain results from damage to the central or peripheral nervous system
  - May be due to compression, transaction, infiltration, ischemia, metabolic injury

Risk Factors
- Multiple comorbid conditions
- Limited mobility
- Lack of exercise
- Psychiatric illness

Prevention and Screening
- Patients should be asked about pain at every visit
- For prevention, see Management

Incidence and Demographics
- 80%–85% of older adults will have a pain problem during their lifetime
- 25%–50% will experience significant pain that impairs functional status

- 45%–80% of nursing home patients will have significant pain
- 74% of older adults with metastatic disease experience pain

Assessment
- Challenging in presence of multiple sources of pain; assessment may be complicated by communication difficulties, atypical illness presentations

History
- Pain is subjective and is measured according to the patient's self-report or careful observation if the patient unable to self-report pain because of cognitive impairment
- Older adults may underreport pain for many reasons (e.g., fear of medication side effects, fear of worsening disease processes); more likely to report pain if they feel report will be taken seriously
- Thorough pain history is essential:
  - Use validated pain scales: Faces Pain Scale, Numeric Rating Scale, Verbal Descriptor Scale
  - Rate pain intensity at present, worst, and best in past 24 hours, as well as acceptable level of pain
  - Chronology and pattern of pain
  - Pain description: throbbing, shooting, stabbing, aching, sharp, dull, etc.
    - Musculoskeletal: aching
    - Visceral: cramping
    - Neuropathic: burning or tingling
  - Aggravating/relieving factors, response to previous therapies
  - Effect that pain has on mood, activity, sleep, bowels, nutrition, social interactions, self image, sexuality
  - Associated symptoms: nausea, vomiting, anorexia, anxiety, depression, fatigue, insomnia, etc.
- Past medical history
- For patients with cognitive impairment, assess pain behaviors:
  - Facial expressions: e.g., frowning, frightened face, grimacing
  - Verbalizations/vocalizations: e.g., sighing, moaning, chanting
  - Body movements: e.g., tense posture, guarding, gait/mobility changes
  - Changes in interpersonal interactions: e.g., aggressiveness, combativeness, withdrawal
  - Changes in activity patterns or routines: e.g., appetite changes, changes in sleep periods, wandering
  - Mental status changes: e.g., crying, increased confusion, irritability

Physical Exam
- Careful musculoskeletal exam
- Detailed neurologic exam
- Functional assessment

Diagnostic Studies
- Specific to suspected etiology
- X-rays, CT scan, MRI

Management
- Usually requires multidisciplinary approach; continuity of care is necessary

- Treat the underlying cause of the pain if possible; also, manage associated conditions such as muscle spasm, depression, insomnia

Nonpharmacologic

- Physical therapy for development of a safe and effective exercise program
  - Exercise increases conditioning, endurance, flexibility, blood flow, strength
  - May also provide ultrasound, massage, hot and cold packs
  - Transcutaneous electrical nerve stimulation (TENS): low-voltage electrical stimulation causes counterirritation
- Acupuncture: neurostimulatory technique that treats pain by the insertion of small, solid needles into the skin at varying depths, typically penetrating the underlying musculature
- Psychosocial interventions/coping strategies
  - Counseling, biofeedback, imagery, hypnosis, relaxation
  - Manage daily routine; allow patient as much control over routine as feasible
  - Social interactions: communicating with family and friends, avoiding isolation, maintaining outside interests
  - Treat depression: counseling and/or medications
    - Complex relationship between chronic pain and depression
    - Certain medications treat both depression and pain and can be very effective

Pharmacologic Treatment

Table 4–4. Choice of Pain Medication

	Musculoskeletal	Visceral	Neuropathic
Mild	Topical, acetaminophen, NSAIDs	Acetaminophen	Topical, acetaminophen
Moderate	NSAIDs/mild opioid	Opioid	Adjuvant
Severe	Opioid, adjuvant	Opioid	Adjuvant/opioid

- Principles of pain management
  - Expect to relieve the pain; pain can be successfully treated in older adults
  - Monitor for and treat side effects of medications that frequently limit medication usefulness
  - Administer medications around the clock with regular dosing, not on a PRN basis; give short-acting, immediate-release oral preparations as needed for breakthrough pain or pain associated with activity or procedures
  - Medications should be given by mouth if possible; if not, consider topical, transdermal, rectal, SQ, IM
  - Monitor effectiveness, individualize regimen
  - Adequate treatment of pain allows for quality of life, ability to function
  - Gradually increase dosages, increase dosing intervals, add medicines as needed to control pain
  - World Health Organization (WHO) "Pain Relief Ladder":
    - Step 1, Mild pain: nonopioid pain medications (e.g., acetaminophen, NSAIDs) +/– adjuvant
    - Step 2, Mild-moderate pain: opioid for mild to moderate pain +/– adjuvant
    - Step 3, Moderate-severe pain: opioid for moderate to severe pain +/– adjuvant

- Non-opioids:
  - Acetaminophen (Tylenol) 500 mg two tabs q4h (up to 4000 mg in 24 hours)
    - Safe in older adults with normal renal and hepatic function
  - NSAIDs
    - Ibuprofen (Motrin) 200–800 mg p.o. 2 to 4 times daily
    - Significant risk for adverse effects of GI bleed, renal failure in older adults; prolonged use not recommended
    - Cyclooxygenase-2 (COX-2) inhibitors: increased risk for cardiovascular events
  - Tramadol (Ultram)
    - Centrally acting; similar adverse effects as with opioids (dizziness, nausea, headache)
- Opioids
  - Mainstay of moderate-severe pain in older adults
  - Can be used for long periods of time without risk of organ damage
  - May be given by a variety of routes
  - Physical dependence over time will necessitate increased doses
  - No upper limits of narcotics dosing as needed to treat severe pain
    - Caution with acetaminophen/narcotic combination tablets
    - Limited by dose of acetaminophen; not to exceed 4000 mg in 24 hours
  - Give patient continuous long-acting opioid for chronic pain management
  - Provide a fast acting rescue medication for "breakthrough" pain
  - Start with low dose, progress with caution
  - Monitor for common adverse effects: constipation, sedation, respiratory depression (often multifactorial etiology), nausea, vomiting, myoclonus, pruritus
    - Treat adverse effects at first sign
    - Treat preventatively for constipation at onset of opioid therapy
    - Reduce dosage if possible
    - May require opioid rotation
  - Listed from weakest to strongest, with starting dose and comments:
    - Codeine with acetaminophen (Tylenol #3) 30–60 mg p.o. q3–4h
    - Hydrocodone 5–10 mg p.o. q3–4h
    - Oxycodone 5–10 mg p.o. q3–4h
    - Sustained release oxycodone (OxyContin) 10–20 mg p.o. q12h
    - Morphine sulfate (Roxanol, MSIR) 15–30 mg p.o. q4–6 h used as breakthrough medication
    - Sustained-release morphine (MS Contin) 15–30 mg p.o. q12h
    - Transdermal fentanyl (Duragesic) 25 mcg/hr change patch q3days
      - Never to be used in opioid-naïve patients
      - Caution in persons who are malnourished
    - Hydromorphone (Dilaudid) should not be used in older adults because of potential to cause confusion or seizures and accumulation of a toxic metabolite
- Topical
  - Rubs and liniments: use on intact skin
  - Counterirritants: camphor, capsicum, cloves, menthol, methyl salicylate, etc.
  - Antiseptics: chloroxylenol, eugenol, thymol
  - Local anesthetic: benzocaine, lidocaine
- Adjuvant analgesic drugs
  - Tricyclic antidepressants: neuropathic pain, insomnia
    - Amitriptyline (Elavil), nortriptyline (Pamelor) 10–25 mg p.o. at night

- Side effects include: anticholinergic, sedation, postural hypotension
- Anticonvulsants: neuropathic pain
  - Carbamazepine (Tegretol) 100–200 mg at night
    - Side effects include: dizziness, drowsiness, nausea, vomiting, bone marrow suppression
  - Gabapentin (Neurontin) 100 mg-1200 mg t.i.d.—excellent for pain from many causes, titrate up slowly
    - Side effects include: somnolence, dizziness, ataxia, fatigue, nystagmus, visual disturbances
- Other medications
  - Prednisone 2.5–5 mg p.o. qd for inflammation
  - Baclofen (Lioresal) 5 mg p.o. qd for muscle spasms, neuropathic pain

When to Consult, Refer, Hospitalize
- Complicated pain, pain with difficult psychosocial issues
- Team approach for pain management (palliative care team, anesthesia pain specialist)
- Hospitalize for uncontrolled pain syndromes (cancer-related, compression fracture, traumatic)
- Neurosurgeon for neuropathic pain unrelieved by management
- Palliative radiation and chemotherapy for cancer-related pain
- Hospice for pain management of terminally ill patients

Special Considerations
- Pain is a contributing factor to delirium and depression

Follow-up
- Monitor efficacy of pain regimen at regular intervals
- New pain or change in pattern: diagnostic workup, modify treatment plan
- Teach patient/family assessment tools for effective home management

Expected Course
- Most chronic pain is chronic and progressive

Complications
- Impaired function
- Depression, anxiety
- Insomnia
- Cognitive impairment, delirium
- Unacceptable quality of life and suicide risk

CARE AT THE END OF LIFE

Description
- Most older adults are more concerned about how they will die than about death itself
- There is no universally accepted definition of a "good death"
- *Palliative care:* interdisciplinary team-based care focused on the relief of suffering in an attempt to achieve the best possible quality of life for patients with serious illness and their families

- May be delivered regardless of the stage of the disease or the need for curative therapies
- Can be delivered concurrently with life-prolonging care or as the main focus of care
- *Hospice:* support and care for persons in the last phase of terminal illness so that they may live as fully and comfortably as possible
- Must have an expected prognosis of less than 6 months to live if the disease runs its natural course
- Care and comfort over aggressive medical intervention
- Multidisciplinary team including nurses, volunteers, chaplains, therapists, social workers, bereavement counselors, and clinicians
- Continues beyond death of the patient to provide bereavement support for family and friends

Etiology
- See Chapter 3 for causes of death in older adults

Incidence and Demographics
- Many patients die prolonged and painful deaths
- Many receive unwanted, painful, and invasive care that impairs the quality of life during last days with needless suffering and emotional distress
- Most deaths still occur in hospitals: 50% of Americans die in hospitals, 25% in long-term-care facilities, 20% at home or the home of a loved one, and 5% in other settings, including inpatient hospices

Core Principles of Care at the End of Life
- Communicate effectively with the patient, family, and healthcare team members
- Display sensitivity and respect for individual, cultural, and spiritual beliefs and customs
- Recognize one's own attitudes, feelings, values, and expectations about death
- Alleviate pain and symptoms and promoting comfort
- Assess, manage, and refer psychological, social, and spiritual problems
- Collaborate with the interdisciplinary team while promoting the nursing role
- Provide access to and evaluate the impact of traditional, complementary, and technological therapies that may improve the quality of the patient's life
- Provide access to palliative care and hospice services
- Respect the right of patients and families to refuse treatment
- Promote and support evidence-based clinical research in practice

Assessment
- Disease/symptom status; prognosis
- Emotional/spiritual aspects of care
- Patient/family goals/preferences
- Family support/needs
- Therapeutic options (benefits/burdens)
- Available resources

History
- Symptom and conditions near death that cause discomfort; common symptoms/conditions in older adults:
  - Pain assessment extremely important (see pain management section, this chapter)
  - GI: dry mouth, nausea, vomiting, anorexia, abdominal pain, constipation

- Respiratory: shortness of breath, cough
- Skin: pressure ulcers
- Psychosocial: delirium, anxiety, fear, family wishes, and knowledge of what is happening
- Generalized: fatigue, cachexia

Physical
- Frequent assessments necessary to ensure adequate pain and symptom control

Diagnostic Studies
- Avoid unnecessary procedures to avoid discomfort
- Weigh benefits vs. burden of diagnostic testing, consider whether abnormal results will be treated

Management
Nonpharmacologic
- Pain management (see pain management section, this chapter)
- Dyspnea:
  - Elevate head of bed
  - Provide fan or open window
- Mucosal and conjunctival care:
  - Frequent mouth care: avoid products containing alcohol, perfume, lemon, or glycerin (drying)
  - Salt-soda solution (1 teaspoon salt, 1 teaspoon baking soda, 1 quart tepid water) or artificial saliva every 30 minutes to minimize dry mouth and sensation of thirst
  - Ice chips if swallowing reflex present
  - Artificial tears or ophthalmic saline solutions to prevent drying of the eyes
- Anorexia and dehydration:
  - Educate family members: common and normal at the end of life; most experts believe it is not uncomfortable and may cause release of endorphins; also decreases risk of respiratory congestion
  - Initiation of parenteral or enteral nutrition at this time does not improve symptom control or lengthen life
- Skin care:
  - Frequent turning and positioning
  - Gentle massage over uncompromised skin
  - Incontinence care
- Delirium:
  - Identify and treat underlying cause if possible and in accordance with patient/family wishes
  - Reduce environmental stimuli, provide a safe environment, reduce anxiety
  - Discontinue nonessential medications

Pharmacologic
- Symptom management
  - Pain control: see Pain Management section of this chapter
    - Oral administration preferred (tablets or liquids); if unable to tolerate, consider:
    - Intravenous: infusion, intermittent injection, or both
    - Subcutaneous: continuous infusion, intermittent injection, or both
    - Transdermal: fentanyl patch
    - Intramuscular injections should not be used

- Constipation: identify and manage causative factors
  - Stimulants: prune juice, senna, or lactulose
  - Avoid bulking agents (psyllium) in patients with inadequate fluid intake to avoid impaction
- Nausea and vomiting: assess and treat cause if possible (e.g., constipation, CNS disease, pain)
  - Prochlorperazine (Compazine)
  - Haloperidol (Haldol)
  - Ondansetron (Zofran): good for chemotherapy- and radiation-induced nausea and vomiting
  - Metoclopramide (Reglan): not to be given if bowel obstruction is present
- Dyspnea:
  - Opioids are first-line therapy: morphine 2.5–5 mg p.o., titrate for comfort; liquid easier to swallow
  - Add anxiolytics (benzodiazepines) if anxiety component
  - Oxygen if hypoxia present
- Excessive secretions:
  - Atropine 0.4 mg SQ q 15 minutes p.r.n.
  - Scopolamine transdermal patch 1.5 mg (4-hour onset of action)
  - Hyoscyamine (Levsin) 0.125 mg liquid (p.o. or SL)
- Delirium and agitation:
  - Halperidol 1 mg p.o., IV, or SQ q 6 hours
  - Lorazepam 0.5 mg p.o., SL, or IV q 4 hours p.r.n.

Special Considerations
- Encourage communication
- Counsel family regarding bereavement
- Help family plan for death, make arrangements

When to Consult, Refer, Hospitalize
- Hospice if patient appears to be within the last 6 months of life
- Palliative care is appropriate for all patients with life-limiting condition for symptom management

Follow-up
- Be available to family and patient
- Have emergency backup plan
- Follow up with family after death

Expected Course
- A good death

Complications
- Unnecessary suffering

CASE STUDIES

Case 1: 82-year-old female comes to clinic reporting "nearly fainting" 3 times in the last month
History: States that several times in past month she has had episodes when she feels like she
is going to faint. The spell lasts maybe a few minutes, and then she slowly feels better. If she is
at home, she eats something then goes to lie down, relieving the sensation. She had a spell at
church last Sunday and her friends insisted she come to the clinic for an evaluation.
PMH: Type 2 diabetes, osteoarthritis, hypertension, hypothyroidism, rheumatic fever as a child
Medications: glipizide (Glucotrol XL) 10 mg q.d., hydrochlorothiazide 25 mg q.d., metoprolol
(Lopressor) 100 mg q.d., levothyroxine sodium (Synthroid) 125 mg q.d., naproxen (Naprosyn)
250 mg b.i.d.

1. What part of the physical exam is appropriate?
2. List the possible causes and contributing factors.
3. What diagnostic tests would you order?

Case 2. An 87-year-old man comes to your office reporting fatigue. Patient lives in an assisted
living facility, needs help with bathing and dressing, walks with difficulty with walker, and
becomes SOB walking 20 feet. He feels too tired to eat. Diagnoses include hypertension,
depression, COPD, HF, Parkinson's disease, and osteoarthritis. He is on 10 medications
including atenolol 25 mg daily for hypertension, paroxetine 40 mg daily for depression, and
oxycodone/acetaminophen (Percocet) 5/325 mg every 6 hours p.r.n. for pain related to
osteoarthritis.

1. What further history would you want to assess?
2. What diagnostic testing would you consider?
3. List your differential diagnoses.

Physical exam and diagnostic testing show patient has advanced colon cancer with metastasis to
bone. The patient declines treatment and starts preparing to die. He reports that the pain in his
low back will not let him sleep. You determine that he is competent to make his own decisions.

4. What is your initial plan?

Over the next month, the pain becomes severe and the patient becomes bedbound. Because of
the Parkinson's disease, he is having trouble handling his secretions. He is still able to take sips
of p.o. liquids.

5. What is your next plan?
6. What issues are likely to be the most important to this patient?

Case 3. A daughter brings her 80-year-old mother with moderate Alzheimer's disease for a
routine checkup. The daughter reports her mother is more easily distracted, increasingly
irritable, and less aware of her surroundings. The daughter is not sure how long this has been
going on. The patient is on multiple medications for cardiac disease and Alzheimer's disease.

1. What part of the history would be most important?
2. What would you look for on physical examination?
3. What laboratory and diagnostic tests would you consider?
4. What are your differential diagnoses?

REFERENCES

AGS Panel of Persistent Pain in Older Persons. (2002). The management of persistent pain in older persons. *Journal of the American Geriatrics Society, 50,* S205–S224.

Ahmed, N., Mandel, R., Fain, M. J. (2007). Frailty: An emerging geriatric syndrome. *American Journal of Medicine, 120*(9), 748–753.

Alzheimer's Association. (2008). *2008 Alzheimer's disease facts and figures.* Retrieved from http://www.alz.org/national/documents/report_alzfactsfigures2008.pdf

American Academy of Sleep Medicine. (2005). *International classification of sleep disorders, 2nd ed: Diagnostic and coding manual.* Westchester, IL: American Academy of Sleep Medicine.

American Association of Colleges of Nursing. (2004). *Peaceful death: Recommended competencies and curricular guidelines for end of life nursing care.* Retrieved from www.aacn.nche.edu

American Geriatrics Society, British Geriatrics Society, & American Academy of Orthopaedic Surgeons Panel of Falls Prevention. (2001). Guideline for the prevention of falls in older persons. *Journal of the American Geriatrics Society, 49,* 664–672.

American Nurses Association. (2003). *Position statement on pain management and control of distressing symptoms in dying patients.* Washington, DC: Author.

American Psychological Association. (2000). *Diagnostic and statistical manual of mental disorders* (4th ed., text rev.). Washington, DC: American Psychiatric Publishing.

Ayalon, L., Gum, A. M., Feliciano, L., & Arean, P. A. (2006). Effectiveness of nonpharmacological interventions for the management of neuropsychiatric symptoms in patients with dementia: A systematic review. *Archives of Internal Medicine, 166*(20), 2182–2188.

Berenson, S. (2006). Complementary and alternative therapies in palliative care. In F. Ferrell & N. Coyle (Eds.), *Textbook of palliative nursing* (pp. 491–509). New York: Oxford University Press.

Birath, J. B., & Martin, J. L. (2007). Common sleep problems affecting older adults. *Annals of Long Term Care, 15*(12), 20–26.

Bishop, T. F., & Morrison, S. (2007). Geriatric palliative care—part I: Pain and symptom management. *Clinical Geriatrics, 15*(1), 25–32.

Bluic, D., Nguyen, N. D., Milch, V. E., Nguyen, T. V., Eisman, J. A., & Center, J. R. (2009). Mortality risk associated with low-trauma osteoporotic fracture and subsequent fracture in men and women. *Journal of the American Medical Association, 301*(5), 513–521.

Boustani, M., Peterson, B., Hanson, L., Harris, R., Lohr, K. N., & U.S. Preventive Services Task Force. (2003). Screening for dementia in primary care: a summary of the evidence for the U. S. Preventive Services Task Force. *Annals of Internal Medicine, 138,* 927–937.

Brayne, C., Fox, C., & Boustani, M. (2008). Dementia screening in primary care. *Journal of the American Medical Association, 298*(20), 2409–2411.

Cavalieri, T. A. (2005). Pain management at the end of life. *Clinical Geriatrics, 14*(3), 44–52.

Cawthon, P. M., Marshall, L. M., Michael, Y., Dam, T. T., Ensrud, K. E., Barrett-Connor, E., et al. (2007). Frailty in older men: prevalence, progression, and relationship with mortality. *Journal of the American Geriatrics Society, 55*(8), 1216–1223.

Centers for Disease Control and Prevention. (2008). Self-reported falls and fall-related injuries among persons aged ≥ 65 years—United States, 2006. *Morbidity and Mortality Weekly Report, 57,* 225.

Chang, J. T., Morton, S. C., Rubenstein, L. Z., Mojica, W. A., Maglione, M., Suttorp, M. J., et al. (2004). Interventions for the prevention of falls in older adults: Systematic review and meta-analysis of randomized clinical trials. *British Medical Journal, 328*(7441), 680–683.

Chawla, N.,& Olshaker, J. S. (2006). Diagnosis and management of dizziness and vertigo. *Medical Clinics of North America, 90*(2), 291–304.

Cuellar, N. G., Strumpf, N. E., & Ratcliffe, S. J. (2007). Symptoms of restless legs syndrome in older adults: Outcomes on sleep quality, sleepiness, fatigue, depression, and quality of life. *Journal of the American Geriatrics Society, 55*(9), 1387–1392.

Cummings, J. L. (2004). Alzheimer's disease. *New England Journal of Medicine, 351*(1), 56–67.

Derby, S., & O'Mahony, S. (2006). Elderly patients. In B. R. Ferrell & N. Coyle (Eds.), *Textbook of palliative nursing* (pp. 635–659). New York: Oxford University Press.

Emanuel, L., Ferris, F. D., von Gunten, C. F., & Von Roenn, J. H. (2006). *The last hours of living: Practical advice for clinicians.* Retrieved from http://cme.medscape.com/viewprogram/5808

End of Life Nursing Education Consortium. (2006). *Promoting advanced practice nursing in palliative care.* Duarte, CA: City of Hope National Medical Center and Washington, D.C.: American Association of Colleges of Nursing.

Ensrud, K. E., Ewing, S. K., Taylor, B. C., Fink, H. A., Cawthon, P. M., Stone, K. L., et al. (2008). Comparison of 2 frailty indexes for prediction of falls, disability, fractures, and death in older women. *Archives of Internal Medicine, 168*(4), 382–389.

Ferrucci, L., Guralnik, J. M., Studenski, S., Fried, L. P., Cutler, Jr., G. B., Walston, J. D., et al. (2004). Designing randomized, controlled trials aimed at preventing or delaying functional decline and disability in frail, older persons: A consensus report. *Journal of the American Geriatrics Society, 52*(4), 625–634.

Field, M., & Cassel, C. (1997). *Approaching death: Improving care at the end of life.* Report of the Institute of Medicine Task Force. Washington, DC: National Academy Press.

Fink, R., & Gates, R. (2006). Pain assessment. In F. Ferrell & N. Coyle (Eds.), *Textbook of palliative nursing* (pp. 97–129). New York: Oxford University Press.

Ganz, D. A., Bao, Y., Shekelle, P. G., & Rubenstein, L. Z. (2007). Will my patient fall? *Journal of the American Medical Association, 297*(1), 77–86.

Goldstein, N. E., & Morrison, R. S. (2005). The intersection between geriatrics and palliative care: A call for a new research agenda. *Journal of the American Geriatrics Society, 53,* 1593–1598.

Hadjistavropolous, T. (Ed.). (2007). An interdisciplinary expert consensus statement on assessment of pain in older persons. *Clinical Journal of Pain, 23*(1 supp).

Hahn, J. E. (2005). Exploring alternative therapies for chronic pain. *Arthritis Practitioner, 1*(2), 15–19.

Hartford Institute for Geriatric Nursing. (2007). Pain assessment for older adults. *Try this: Best practices in nursing care to older adults.* Retrieved from www.hartfordign.org

Herr, K., Bjoro, K., & Decker, S. (2006). Tools for assessment of pain in nonverbal older adults with dementia: A state-of-the-science review. *Journal of Pain and Symptom Management, 31*(2), 170–192.

Hospice and Palliative Nurses Association. (2003). *HPNA position statement: Artificial nutrition and hydration in end of life care.* Pittsburgh: Author.

Inouye, S. K., Zhang, Y., Jones, R. N., Kiely, D. K., Yang, F., & Marcantonio, E. R. (2007). Risk factors for delirium at discharge: Development and validation of a predictive model. *Archives of Internal Medicine, 167*(13), 1406–1413.

Kapo, J., Morrison, L. J., & Liao, S. (2007). Palliative care for the older adult. *Journal of Palliative Medicine, 10*(1), 185–209.

Katsarkus, A. (2008). Dizziness in aging: the clinical experience. *Geriatrics, 63*(11), 18–20.

Kerber, K. A., & Baloh, R. W. (2006). Disequilibrium and gait disorders in older people. *Reviews in Clinical Gerontology, 16,* 243–254.

Kovar, M., Jepson, T., & Jones, S. (2006). Diagnosing and treating benign paroxysmal positional vertigo. *Journal of Gerontological Nursing, 32*(12), 22–27.

Lamarre-Cliche, M. (2007). Syncope in older adults. *Geriatrics & Aging, 10*(4), 236–240.

Last Acts. (2002). *Means to a better end: A report on dying in America.* Retrieved from http://www.rwjf.org/files/publications/other/meansbetterend.pdf

Lewis, C. R., de Vedia, A., Reuer, B., Schwan, R., & Tourin, C. (2003). Integrating complementary and alternative medicine (CAM) into standard hospice and palliative care. *American Journal of Hospice and Palliative Medicine, 20*(3), 221–228.

Lonergan, E., Britton, A. M., Luxenberg, J., & Wyller, T. (2007). Antipsychotics for delirium. *Cochrane Database Syst Rev,* CD005594.

Marcantonio, E. R., Kiely, D. K., Simon, S. E., John Orav, E., Jones, R. N., Murphy, K. M., et al. (2005). Outcomes of older people admitted to postacute facilities with delirium. *Journal of the American Geriatrics Society, 53*(6), 963–969.

Markowitz, A. J., & Rabow, M. W. (2007). Palliative management of fatigue at the close of life: "It feels like my body is just worn out." *Journal of the American Medical Association, 298,* 217.

McCurry, S. M., Logsdon, R. G., Teri, L., & Vitiello, M. V. (2007). Evidence-based psychological treatments for insomnia in older adults. *Psychology and Aging, 22*(1), 18–27.

Miller, M. O. (2008). Evaluation and management of delirium in hospitalized older patients. *American Family Physician, 78*(11), 1265.

Muangpaisan, W. (2006). Clinical differences among four common dementia syndromes. *Geriatrics and Aging, 10*(7), 425–429.

National Consensus Project for Quality Palliative Care. (2009). *Clinical practice guidelines for quality palliative care* (2nd ed.). Retrieved from http://www.nationalconsensusproject.org/guideline.pdf

Nijrolder, I., van der Windt, D., & van der Horst, H. E. (2008). Prognosis of fatigue and functioning in primary care: A 1-year follow-up study. *Annals of Family Medicine, 6*(6), 519–527.

Norman, D., & Loredo, J. S. (2008). Obstructive sleep apnea in older adults. *Clinics in Geriatric Medicine, 24*(1), 151–165.

Oliver, D., Connelly, J. B., Victor, C. R., Shaw, F. E., Whitehead, A., Genc, Y., et al. (2007). Strategies to prevent falls and fractures in hospitals and care homes and effect of cognitive impairment: Systematic review and meta-analyses. *British Medical Journal, 334*(7584), 82.

Paice, J. A., & Fine, P. G. (2006). Pain at the end of life. In B. R. Ferrell & N. Coyle (Eds.), *Textbook of palliative nursing* (pp. 131–153). New York: Oxford University Press.

Pisani, M. A., Murphy, T. E., Van Ness, P. H., Araujo, K. L., & Inouye, S. K. (2007). Characteristics associated with delirium in older patients in a medical intensive care unit. *Archives of Internal Medicine, 167*(15), 1629–1634.

Reisberg, B., Doody, R., Stoffler, A., Schmitt, F., Ferris, S., & Mobius, H. J. (2003). Memantine in moderate-to-severe Alzheimer's disease. *New England Journal of Medicine, 348,* 1333–1341.

Rochon, P. A., Normand, S. L., Gomes, T., Gill, S. S., Anderson, G. M., Melo, M., et al. (2008). Antipsychotic therapy and short-term serious events in older adults with dementia. *Archives of Internal Medicine, 168*(10), 1090–1096.

Rubenstein, L. Z., & Josephson, K. R. (2006). Falls and their prevention in elderly people: What does the evidence show? *Medical Clinics of North America, 90*(5), 807–824.

Schneider, L. S., Tariot, P. N., Dagerman, K. S., Davis, S. M., Hsiao, J. K., Ismail, M. S., et al. (2006). Effectiveness of atypical antipsychotic drugs in patients with Alzheimer's disease. *New England Journal of Medicine, 355*(15), 1525–1538.

Silber, M. (2005). Clinical practice. Chronic insomnia. *New England Journal of Medicine, 353*(8), 803–810.

Sink, K. M., Holden, K. F., & Yaffe, K. (2005). Pharmacological treatment of neuropsychiatric symptoms of dementia: a review of the evidence. *JAMA, 293*(5), 596–608.

Smith, R. C., Lyles, J. S., Gardiner, J. C., Sirbu, C., Hodges, A., Collins, C., et al. (2006). Primary care clinicians treat patients with medically unexplained symptoms: A randomized controlled trial. *Journal of General Internal Medicine, 21*(7), 671–677.

Smythe, C. A. (2008). Evaluating sleep quality in older adults: The Pittsburgh Sleep Quality Index can be used to detect sleep disturbances or deficits. *American Journal of Nursing, 108*(5), 42–50.

Strickberger, S. A., Benson, D. W., Biaggioni, I., Callans, D. J., Cohen, M. I., Ellenbogen, K. A., et al. (2006). AHA/ACCF Scientific Statement on the evaluation of syncope: from the American Heart Association Councils on Clinical Cardiology, Cardiovascular Nursing, Cardiovascular Disease in the Young, and Stroke, and the Quality of Care and Outcomes Research Interdisciplinary Working Group; and the American College of Cardiology Foundation: in collaboration with the Heart Rhythm Society: endorsed by the American Autonomic Society. *Circulation, 113,* 316–327.

Tarasiuk, A., Greenberg-Dotan, S., Simon-Tuval, T., Oksenberg, A., & Reuveni, H. (2008). The effect of obstructive sleep apnea on morbidity and health care utilization of middle-aged and older adults. *Journal of the American Geriatrics Society, 56*(2), 247–254.

Tinetti, M. E. (2003). Preventing falls in elderly persons. *New England Journal of Medicine, 348*(1), 42–49.

Tinetti, M. E., Williams, C. S., & Gill, T. M. (2000). Dizziness among older adults; a possible geriatric syndrome. *Annals of Internal Medicine, 132*(5), 337–344.

Traccis, S., Zoroddu, G. F., Zecca, M. T., Cau, T., Solinas, M. A., & Masuri, R. (2004). Evaluating patients with vertigo: Bedside examination. *Journal of the Neurological Sciences, 25*(Suppl 1), S16.

Viggo, H. N., Jorgensen, T., & Ortenblad, L. (2006). Massage and touch for dementia. *Cochrane Database Syst Rev, 4,* CD004989.

Walke, L. M., Byers, A. L., McCorkle, R., & Fried, T. R. (2006). Symptom assessment in community-dwelling older adults with advanced chronic disease. *Journal of Pain and Symptom Management, 31*(1), 31–37.

Walston, J., Hadley, E. C., Ferrucci, L., Guralnik, J. M., Newman, A. B., Studenski, S. A., et al. (2006). Research agenda for frailty in older adults: Toward a better understanding of physiology and etiology: Summary from the American Geriatrics Society/National Institute on Aging Research Conference on Frailty in Older Adults. *Journal of the American Geriatrics Society, 54*(6), 991–1001.

Wei, L. A., Fearing, M. A., Sternberg, E. J., & Inouye, S. K. (2008). The Confusion Assessment Method: A systematic review of current usage. *Journal of the American Geriatrics Society, 56*(5), 823–830.

Wijk, H., & Grimby, A. (2008). Needs of elderly patients in palliative care. *American Journal of Hospice and Palliative Care, 25*(2), 106–111.

Winblad, B., Kilander, L., Eriksson, S., Minthon, L., Batsman, S., Wetterholm, A. L., et al. (2006). Donepezil in patients with severe Alzheimer's disease: Double-blind, parallel-group, placebo-controlled study. *Lancet, 367,* 1057–1065.

Wolff, A. D., & Akesson, K. (2003). Preventing fractures in elderly people. *British Medical Journal, 327,* 89–95.

Woods, N. F., LaCroix, A. Z., Gray, S. L., Aragaki, A., Cochrane, B. B., Brunner, R. L., et al. (2005). Frailty: Emergence and consequences in women aged 65 and older in the Women's Health Initiative Observational Study. *Journal of the American Geriatrics Society, 53*(8), 1321–1330.

Infectious Disease

Michaelene Jansen, PhD, RN, GNP-BC, NP-C

GERIATRIC APPROACH

- The incidence of infectious diseases among older adults in the United States has increased during recent years. This increase is the result of complex interactions between the aging immune system, unexpected pathogens, environmental factors, comorbidities, diagnostic challenges, and rapidly changing antibiotic tolerance and resistance.
- This chapter will discuss infections in general. It will also discuss HIV exposure, HIV/AIDS, Lyme disease, West Nile disease, and severe acute respiratory syndrome (SARS). Other specific infections will be discussed in their respective chapters. For example, urinary tract infections are discussed in the Chapter 11, Renal and Urologic Disorders.

The Immune System
From the Myeloid Stem Cell

- Monocytes move into tissue and develop into macrophages, initiate immune response, and start phagocytosis.
- Granulocytes
  - Neutrophils are phagocytes active in early inflammation.
  - Eosinophils mediate allergic reactions; they also are phagocytes and defend against parasites.
  - Basophils are found in the blood and become mast cells in the tissue. Both cause inflammatory response in allergic reactions; the mast cell is the most important activator of the inflammatory response.
  - Basophils produce histamine, bradykinin, serotonin, and heparin.
  - Mast cells produce leukotrienes and prostaglandins.

From the Lymphoid Stem Cell
- These cells (lymphocytes) require an antigen to become activated.
- B cells produce immunoglobulins (antibodies) and mediate humoral immune response.
- T cells comprise cytotoxic (killer), lymphokine-producing, helper, and suppressor cells to orchestrate cell-mediated immunity.

Plasma Protein Systems
- Inactive proteins (proenzymes) that, when activated, initiate a cascade of reactions to produce potent mediators of the inflammatory response.
- Complement system
  - Consists of at least 10 proteins
  - Components participate in almost every inflammatory response
  - Activated by nonspecific particles such as:
    - Antigen-antibody complexes (immune complexes)
    - Products released from invading bacteria
- Kinin system
  - Bradykinin causes dilation of vessels, acts with prostaglandins to induce pain, increases vascular permeability
  - Important during the prolonged phase of inflammation
- Clotting system
  - Consists of intrinsic and extrinsic pathways
  - Activated by many of the substances released during inflammation

Normal Changes of Aging
- Immune system function declines with age.
- The thymus becomes extremely small (fewer T cells).
- T-cell function and specific antibody responses decrease (decreased response to infection).
- Macrophages show a decreased ability to clear antigens and attack tumor cells.
- Complement levels decrease.
- B cells produce antibodies that do not bind antigens well, causing suboptimal antibody response to vaccines and delayed hypersensitivity response (less response to a PPD test).
- The number of autoantibodies increases.

Age-related changes in other body systems: A few of the normal changes that predispose the elderly to infection. See each individual chapter for details.
- Renal
  - Impaired bladder emptying
  - Decreased ability of the kidneys to acidify urine
  - Benign prostatic hypertrophy
  - Menopause/urogenital atrophy
- Respiratory
  - Decreased cough reflex, oxygen uptake, and mucociliary function
  - Musculoskeletal stiffness leads to decreased depth of respiration
  - Kyphosis decreases movement of diaphragm
- Skin
  - Increased skin fragility, dryness, and loss of subcutaneous tissue
  - Decreased epidermal cells (50%)
- Other
  - Decreased hydrochloric acid in the stomach and small intestine

– Decreased vascular supply to extremities
– Impaired glucose metabolism

INFECTIONS

Description
- Most common infections in older adults
  – Influenza and bacterial pneumonia: fifth leading cause of death in older adults
  – Urinary tract infections: most common infection
  – Skin infections: cellulitis
  – Methicillin-resistant *Staphylococcus aureus* (MRSA)
  – Vancomycin-resistant *Enterococcus* organisms (urinary tract and skin)
  – Sepsis
- Other important infections in older adults
  – Herpes zoster
  – Infective endocarditis: increasingly seen in older adults because of degenerative valvular disorders and prosthetic valves
  – Prosthetic device infections: joints, pacemakers, vascular grafts, intraocular lens implants, etc.
  – Human immunodeficiency virus (rare, but increasing)

Etiology
- Emergence of more virulent strains (e.g., *E. coli*, influenza)
- Re-emergence of some infections (e.g., tuberculosis)
- Gram-negative bacilli more prevalent in elderly
- Vancomycin-resistant *Enterococcus* organisms (primarily urinary tract and skin)
- Methicillin-resistant *S. aureus* organisms (treated with vancomycin, but there are reports of resistance)

Incidence and Demographics
- Account for 40% of all deaths in geriatric patients
- Pneumonia/influenza is the 5th leading cause of death in older adults
- Septicemia is the 10th leading cause of death in older adults

Risk Factors
- Normal changes of aging, decreased physiologic reserves including immune system
- Decreased activity pattern, immobility
- Decreased fluid intake
- Malnourishment
- Invasive procedures
- Medications that are immunosuppressive agents, including steroids, chemotherapy
- Nursing home residence and hospital admissions can result in nosocomial infections and increased exposure to antibiotics
- Comorbid conditions that predispose the elderly to infection
  – Diabetes mellitus
  – Chronic obstructive pulmonary disease (COPD)
  – Malignancy: leukemia, multiple myeloma, or receiving chemotherapy
  – Bladder outlet obstruction
  – Condition causing decreased vascular supply to area

Prevention and Screening
- Avoid risk factors
- Three most important general measures
  - Maintain activity pattern, avoid immobility
  - Maintain adequate fluid intake; can be very difficult, but is an absolutely crucial intervention
  - Maintain nutritional intake; see section in Chapter 3
  - Hand washing

Assessment
- As functional assessment is the key to diagnosis of infection in the elderly, standardized assessment tools are useful for detecting changes from baseline and noting changes. See Chapter 3 for discussion of functional assessment of older adults.

History
- Nonspecific presentation of illness is the most common presentation of infection in older adults
  - The most frequent symptoms are delirium or decrease in activities of daily living (ADL)
  - Also sudden onset of functional decline, falls, incontinence, fatigue, or anorexia
- Symptoms generally reflect the patient's weakest system, not the system that is infected
- Usual symptoms of the particular infection may be blunted or absent

Physical Examination
- Often no temperature; look for change from baseline; temperature may be elevated and still within normal limits
- If fever is present, consider bacterial infection
- May not have leukocytosis because of decreased immune response; severe leukocytosis indicates poor prognosis
- Tachycardia, dehydration, and altered mental status seen frequently
- Absence of classic symptoms: for example, urinary tract infection (UTI) may not produce dysuria; appendicitis may not have right lower quadrant pain; stiff neck may not be seen in meningitis
- Since the three most common infections are urinary tract, respiratory, and skin, direct your search there first
- Assess for risk factors for infections of other systems and search accordingly; for example, diabetics have a specific pattern of infections (see Chapter 17, Endocrine Disorders, for details)

Diagnostic Studies
- Cultures of affected organ system before antibiotic, if possible
- WBC count and differential—leukocytosis may be blunted
- Urinalysis
- Blood cultures if patient appears septic—ill appearance, tachycardia, fever
- Increased sedimentation rate may be seen in certain infections and inflammatory diseases but also may be elevated in healthy elderly
- Low serum albumin may indicate undernutrition as a contributing factor
- More specific studies may be required to identify source of infection, such as chest x-ray, CT scans, echocardiogram

Differential Diagnosis
- Microorganisms not a pathogen in healthy adults
- Leukemia

- Multiple myeloma
- Drug reaction
- Viral or fungal infection

Management
Nonpharmacologic Treatment
- Focus on comfort care
- Frequent rest periods without prolonged immobility
- Maintain nutritional intake/supplements
- Encourage fluid intake, at least 1500 cc/day

Pharmacologic Treatment
- Review allergy history (drugs, type of reaction), recent antibiotic use
- Review other drugs patient takes to be aware of possible drug interactions
- In general use a single agent that will reach the infected area, has a narrow spectrum and low toxicity profile, and is least expensive
- Choice of drug should be based on culture or Gram stain results when available
- Severe illness may require empiric therapy; if so, consider a third-generation cephalosporin or fluoroquinolone since Gram-negative infections are common (caution with fluorquinolone if patient is on anticoagulants)
- Avoid treating with antibiotics infections that are likely to be viral
- Age, renal function, and liver function should be considered when determining dose
- Renal function monitoring and monitoring of drug levels during therapy indicated for some antibiotics, especially aminoglycosides, to prevent toxicity
- Ensure patient/family understands instruction for administration and importance of completing course of medication
- Most antibiotics should be given on an empty stomach, 1 hour before or 2 hours after a meal

How Long to Treat
- Must complete entire course of antibiotic; length of course depends on organism and severity and location of infection
- Give specific length of treatment with antibiotic; older adults usually require a longer course of antibiotic than younger adults

Special Considerations
- Chronic illnesses that reduce circulation, such as diabetes or HF, may limit delivery of the antibiotic to the infected site
- Antibiotics can be given orally and IV at home and in nursing home, depending on support systems and severity of infection
- Blunted fever and leukocytosis responses are indicators of poor prognosis
- Decreased renal function may affect elimination of drug

When to Consult, Refer, Hospitalize
- Severe infection, sepsis
- Patient not taking adequate fluids
- Not responsive to antibiotic in 3 days

Follow-up
Expected Course
- Antibiotics take at least 2 to 3 days to have an effect

- Elderly patients take longer to recover from infections than adult patients and may experience confusion, weakness

Complications
- Sepsis more likely; higher mortality in elderly
- Great risk of mortality
- Elderly more susceptible to adverse effects of antibiotics
  - Allergy
  - Drug toxicity (ototoxicity and nephrotoxicity with aminoglycosides)
  - Altered bacterial flora of the intestinal tract—*Clostridium difficile*
  - Frequent nausea, diarrhea
- Drug resistance
  - Drug resistance causes infections that are harder to treat, last longer, and require hospitalization
  - Future infections may also prove resistant to antibiotics
  - More frequent infections with a narrowing range of therapeutic options
  - Development of resistant strains of bacteria that are then spread throughout the community
- Superinfection
  - New infection during antimicrobial treatment for the primary infection
  - Caused by altered bacterial flora of intestinal, genitourinary, and upper respiratory tracts
  - More likely to occur with broad-spectrum antibiotics or when course of treatment is prolonged
  - Example seen in elderly is *C. difficile* diarrhea
- Low therapeutic response
  - No response in 3 days or deterioration in condition (dehydration, delirium) merits consultation, change in antibiotic, or hospitalization

HIV Exposure
Description
- Exposure places patient at risk for HIV infection and therefore requires consideration for postexposure prophylaxis (PEP)
- Defined as contact with blood, tissue, or other body fluids under the following circumstances: a percutaneous injury, contact of mucous membrane or nonintact skin, or contact with intact skin when the duration of contact is prolonged (several minutes or more) or involves an extensive area

Etiology
- Fluids with known risk of HIV transmission: blood, bloody fluids, semen, and vaginal fluids
- Fluids with suspected risk of HIV transmission: pleural fluid, cerebrospinal fluid, peritoneal fluid, synovial fluid, and pericardial fluid
- Materials with doubtful risk of HIV transmission: feces, vomitus, urine, saliva, sweat, tears (unless bloody)

Incidence and Demographics
- Factors that may increase risk for HIV transmission after an exposure include: a device visibly contaminated with the patient's blood, a procedure that involved a needle placed directly in a vein or artery, or a deep injury

- Risk for HIV transmission after a percutaneous exposure to HIV-infected blood is approximately 0.3%; with mucous membrane exposure it is 0.09%; with skin exposure even less

Risk Factors
- Contact with blood or other body fluids from patients with HIV

Prevention and Screening
- Universal or standard precautions
- Wear gloves when contact with blood or bodily fluids is possible
- Use "personal protective equipment" (masks, goggles, gowns) when engaging in procedures that involve blood or bodily fluids
- For prevention of needle injuries, use of puncture-proof containers, use "safety" needles, refrain from recovering needles or post-use manipulation of needles

Assessment
History
- Evaluate exposure: type of fluid, type of exposure (needle gauge, depth of needlestick, visible blood, mucous membrane) and duration of exposure
- Evaluate exposure source person: prior HIV testing results, CD4 levels, history of possible HIV exposures and risk for HIV (IV drug use, sexual contact, acute HIV syndrome)
- If source person is HIV positive, document current HIV RNA levels, CD4 levels, and current or previous antiretroviral treatment

Physical Examination
- Assess site or wound, anxiety level of patient

Diagnostic Studies
- Source person: If HIV serologic status unknown, request HIV antibody after incident, pretest counseling, and consent form
- If consent cannot be obtained, follow local and state laws
- If source person is HIV seronegative, no testing of patient is needed
- Exposed patient: HIV antibody testing offered for baseline evaluation with consent
- Maintaining confidentiality of test results and documentation is critical

Management
Nonpharmacologic Treatment:
- Immediately following exposure:
  - Skin: wash thoroughly with soap and water
  - Eyes: rinse thoroughly with sterile saline, eye irrigate, clean water flush
  - Mouth, nose: clean water rinse/flush
  - Depending on type of fluid, source risk, and type of exposure, consider and discuss risks and benefits of postexposure prophylaxis
  - Counsel exposed patient to follow measures to prevent secondary transmission, especially the first 6 to 12 weeks: sexual abstinence or use of condoms; refrain from donating blood, plasma, organs, tissue, or semen
  - Serology for HIV antibody (baseline) with consent and 2 weeks postexposure; Hepatitis B serology for immune status
  - Serological testing on "source" for hepatitis C, hepatitis B antigen, and HIV

Pharmacological Treatment
- Tetanus vaccine (if not vaccinated within the last 5 years)
- Hepatitis B vaccine (if not already vaccinated in the past)
- Hepatitis B immune globulin (if source antigen positive or high risk for hepatitis B and patient not immune)
- After evaluation/assessment of HIV infection risk, determination made regarding need for postexposure prophylaxis
- Data supports a two-drug regimen for postexposure prophylaxis (PEP). Examples: zidovudine and lamivudine, zidovudine and emtricitabine, lopinavir and ritonavir

How Long to Treat
- Postexposure prophylaxis should be administered for 4 weeks if tolerated

When to Consult, Refer, Hospitalize
- All potentially exposed patients should have a consult with infectious disease specialist, who should determine treatment

Follow-up
- Advise exposed patient to seek medical evaluation for any acute illness occurring during the follow-up period; illness characterized by fever, rash, myalgia, fatigue, malaise or lymphadenopathy may indicate acute HIV infection
- For patients exposed to HIV+ or high-risk source: HIV antibody testing at 6 weeks, 12 weeks, and 6 months

Expected Course
- Patient to finish 4-week medication regimen

Complications
- HIV seroconversion
- Side effects from antiretroviral therapy such as nausea/vomiting, nephrolithiasis, hemolytic anemia, or hyperglycemia; patient unable to finish medication

HIV and AIDS
Description
HIV
- Infection with human retrovirus, human immunodeficiency virus (HIV)
- Invades body and enters any susceptible cell (circulating CD4 lymphocytes, macrophages, and monocytes), ultimately destroying the immune system

AIDS
- HIV-positive person with opportunistic infections, *or*
- HIV-positive person with CD4 cell counts < 200/ml or a CD4 percentage < 14%

Etiology
- Viral transmission: HIV usually transmitted through sexual intercourse (homosexual/heterosexual); IV drug use; transfusions of blood or blood products; needlestick or mucous membrane exposures to person; injections with unsterilized, used needles in situations such as acupuncture, tattooing, or medical injection
- Seroconversion: takes an average of 3 weeks from transmission; using standard serologic tests > 95% of patients seroconvert within 5.8 months following HIV transmission
- Median time from infection with HIV to AIDS is 10 years

- Stages of HIV infection include: viral transmission, primary HIV infection (acute retroviral syndrome), seroconversion, asymptomatic chronic infection, symptomatic HIV infection, AIDS, advanced HIV infection

Incidence and Demographics
- Initially seen in older adults from blood transfusions for coronary artery bypass or other surgery (given 1978 to 1985)
- Being seen with increasing frequency in older adults from prior sexual activity
- Currently 20% of HIV cases are in older people, partly because people with AIDS have been living longer
- Reported in elderly women without other risk factors who are caregivers to children and grandchildren infected with AIDS, presumably transmitted through breaks in skin of hands
- 15% of new AIDS cases occur in patients over age 50

Risk Factors
- Blood transfusion outside of the United States, or in United States from 1977 to 1985
- Unprotected sex
- Exposure of person to infected blood and body fluids through breaks in skin or mucous membranes

Prevention and Screening
- HIV antibody testing of plasma, organ, and tissue donors
- HIV education programs

Clinical Categories
Category A
- Documented HIV infection and at least one of the following:
  - Asymptomatic HIV infection
  - Persistent generalized lymphadenopathy
  - Acute (primary) infection with accompanying illness or history of HIV infection

Category B
- Symptoms present
- Meets one of the following criteria: conditions attributed to HIV infection or defect in cell-mediated immunity; conditions considered to have clinical course that is complicated by HIV infection (thrush, zoster, cervical dysplasia)

Category C
- Includes clinical conditions listed in AIDS surveillance case

AIDS: CDC Definitions
- HIV+ persons with CD4 cell counts < 200mm or a CD4 percent < 14%
- With opportunistic infection such as *Pneumocystis carinii* (now *P. jiroveci*), esophageal candidiasis, cryptococcal meningitis, or tuberculosis

History
- Unprotected sex
- Illicit IV drug use

Physical Examination
- Vital signs: fever may be present

- Weight loss, lymphadenopathy, hepatosplenomegaly
- Complete physical to look for opportunistic infections
- Neurological: signs of dementia or neuropathy

Diagnostic Studies
- CBC for lymphopenia/neutropenia, thrombocytopenia, anemia
- Comprehensive metabolic panel: evaluate renal and hepatic function

Criteria for HIV Infection
- Persons with repeatedly (2 or more) reactive screening tests (ELISA) plus specific antibodies identified by a supplemental test, such as Western blot
- Other specific methods of diagnosis of HIV-1 include virus isolation, antigen detection, and detection of HIV genetic material

Differential Diagnosis
- Cancer
- Endocrine diseases
- Tuberculosis
- Dementia
- Enterocolitis

Management
- All 50 states, Washington, DC, and U.S. territories require reporting of AIDS cases to local health authorities
- Refer to specialist for evaluation and management
- Treatment is similar to that of adults
- Pharmacologic drug classes:
    - Reverse transcriptase inhibitors (RTI)
    - Nucleoside reverse transcriptase inhibitors (NRTI)
    - Nonnucleoside reverse transcriptase inhibitors (NNRTI)
    - Protease inhibitors (PI)
    - The single fusion inhibitor enfuvirtide (Fuzeon)
- Frequent interactions between HIV drugs and other drugs the patient is taking
- Adverse reactions to medications tend to occur more frequently and be more serious

Follow-up
Expected Course
- Average progression of disease without treatment is approximately 10 to 12 years from seroconversion to death in young adults
- Older adults experience a more rapid downhill course, perhaps because of impaired T-cell replacement
- Viral burden and the CD4 count is highly predictive of prognosis; time to AIDS and death decreases with a decline of CD4 cells and higher viral burden

Complications
- Many complications occur as the immune system becomes depleted, including neuropathy, chronic diarrhea, wasting syndrome, lymphoma, cancers, opportunistic infections, and dementia, ultimately leading to death

Influenza
Description
- Acute viral illness that occurs in epidemics, usually in the fall and winter

Etiology
- Caused by an orthomyxovirus that appears as antigenic types A and B
- Frequent mutations produce new strains each flu season

Incidence and Demographics
- Very common
- Frequently leads to pneumonia in older adults, contributing to the fifth leading cause of death in older adults

Risk Factors
- Residing in a nursing home
- Residing with children

Prevention and Screening
- Influenza vaccine provides immunity to 85% of those inoculated
- Protection begins about 2 weeks after vaccination and lasts a few months
- Because of influenza virus mutation the flu vaccine is reconstituted every year and people need a flu shot every year to be protected
- Those who should be vaccinated include patients over 50 and healthcare workers
- Amantadine or rimantadine can be given shortly after exposure to influenza A
- Oseltamivir and zanamivir given after exposure in influenza A or B

Assessment
History
- Acute onset
- Malaise
- Headache
- Nausea
- Muscle aches
- Nasal stuffiness

Physical
- Fever, chills
- Mild pharyngeal infection
- Conjunctival redness

Diagnostic Studies
- CBC: leukopenia is common
- Nasal or throat swab for identifying the influenza antigen

Differential Diagnosis
- Colds
- Bronchitis
- Pneumonia
- Other acute febrile illnesses

Management
Nonpharmacological Treatment
- Rest
- Encourage fluids

Pharmacological Treatment
- Analgesics
- Cough syrup
- Antivirals must be started within 2 days of onset of symptoms to be effective
- Amantadine (Symmetrel) 100 mg daily or twice daily or rimantadine (Flumadine) 100 mg p.o. b.i.d. × 7 days for influenza A
- Oseltamivir (Tamiflu) 75 mg p.o. b.i.d. or zanamivir (Relenza) 2 inhalations b.i.d. × 5 days for influenza A or B

Follow-up
Expected Course
- Usual duration is 1 to 7 days
- Often a longer and more severe course in older adults

Complications
- Pneumonia
- Death

Author's Note: At time of publication, the H1N1 (swine flu) virus was declared a Phase 6 alert by the World Health Organization. Although the original strain was not as virulent as some feared, there may be more virulent strain in the future. The reader is referred to the Center for Disease Control for the most up-to-date screening, surveillance, and management (http://www.who.int/csr/disease/swineflu/en/index.html).

Lyme Disease
Description
- Bacterial infection that often begins with a rash (erythema migrans), then headaches, arthritis; severe neurologic complications can occur in up to 20% of patients; most do not have permanent sequelae

Etiology
- Caused by the spirochete *Borrelia burgdorferi*
- Transmitted to humans by ixodid tick (deer tick); not transmitted by larger dog tick
- Size of tick is 2 to 9 mm
- Painless bite; ticks usually drop off unnoticed in 2 to 4 days; must be embedded in skin > 24 hours to transmit disease
- No person-to-person transmission
- Incubation period from bite to appearance of erythema migrans is 3 to 31 days; usually 7 to 14 days

Incidence and Demographics
- Accuracy of diagnosis remains a problem
- Probably overreported and overtreated
- Majority of cases reported in 3 distinct geographic areas: the majority of cases occur in the northeastern United States from Massachusetts to Maryland; a lower frequency is reported in the Upper Midwest (Minnesota and Wisconsin), and cases are seen less commonly on the West Coast (northern California)
- Incidence is increasing
- Occurs during tick season, spring through the first frost

Risk Factors
- Age: middle-aged gardeners, people of all ages who are outdoors
- Live in endemic region
- Exposed skin: short pants and sleeves, no use of repellents

Prevention and Screening
- Long pants, long sleeves when working outdoors; tuck shirts into pants; wear insect repellents
- Walk in middle of path, inspect skin and scalp after spending day outside
- When a patient in an endemic area presents with a flu-like illness in the summer, consider Lyme disease
- Prophylactic antibiotics are not recommended following tick bites

Table 5-1. Stages of Lyme Disease

Stage 1: Early Localized Disease	Flu-like symptoms of fever, chills, myalgia, arthralgia, headache; 50% to 90% of patients develop a distinctive rash termed erythema migrans within about 1 week of tick bite; begins as red macule or papule, expands rapidly over several days to annular, erythematous patch with central clearing, ≥ 5 cm and may be as large as 30 cm. Resolves in 3 to 4 weeks without treatment. Usually in area of tick-bite but may occur anywhere.
Stage 2: Early Disseminated Disease	Begins roughly 3 to 5 weeks after initial infection, as spirochete spreads. Wide variety of symptoms, most notably persistent fatigue. Migratory arthralgia common. Cranial nerve palsies (especially facial nerve) common. Meningitis, conjunctivitis may occur; carditis with heart block rare. Most common manifestation is multiple erythema migrans, usually smaller than initial lesion.
Stage 3: Late Disease	Months to years after initial infection, characterized by recurrent pauciarticular arthritis, usually affecting large joints (knees). Central and peripheral nervous system affected, may develop subacute encephalopathy, distal paresthesias. Memory, mood, sleep problems may be noted. Cardiac involvement.

Assessment
History
- Most unable to identify tick bite

Physical
- Without reliable history of tick bite and presence of characteristic rash, physical examination may demonstrate findings consistent with above listed symptoms but may lead to a variety of other diagnoses

Diagnostic Studies
- Antibodies to *B. burgdorferi* can be detected by ELISA several weeks after the bite; however, false-positive rate is fairly high and false negatives are also reported
- Western blot analysis is more specific after the first few weeks of the infection
- Positive ELISA and negative Western blot indicates no Lyme disease
- If joint tap done, joint fluid will have 500 to 110,000 cells/mm^3; cells are primarily neutrophils

Differential Diagnosis

Erythema migrans:
- Tinea corporis
- Erythema multiforme
- Granuloma annulare
- Nummular eczema

Early disseminated Lyme disease:
- Rheumatoid arthritis
- Septic arthritis
- Systemic lupus erythematosus
- Postinfectious arthritis
- Fibromyalgia

Management

Nonpharmacologic Treatment
- Supportive: fluids, keep skin lubricated
- Remove tick, using firm tension and fine tweezers; be sure head is completely removed; clean site

Pharmacologic Treatment
- *Early Lyme disease*
  - Doxycycline 100 mg p.o. every 12h for 10 days
  - Amoxicillin 500 mg every 8h
  - Cefuroxime 500 mg every 12h

Follow-up

Expected Course
- Erythema migrans usually resolves within several days of initiating treatment
- Treatment of erythema migrans almost always prevents progression of disease
- Most respond promptly to treatment; complete resolution of symptoms in 4 weeks
- Retesting of Lyme titer not indicated, as it will remain elevated for months to years
- Long-term outcome unclear; depends on promptness and adequacy of treatment

Complications
- Subacute encephalopathy: memory loss, mood changes, and sleep disturbances; distal sensory paresthesias, radicular pain
- Chronic arthritis or synovitis
- Myocardiopathies (rare)

West Nile Virus (WNV)

Description
- Viral infection causing febrile illness, rash, arthritis, myalgias, weakness, lymphadenopathy, and meningoencephalitis

Etiology
- Arbovirus of family *Flaviviridae* spread by mosquitoes and birds
- Humans and horses are affected by contact with either
- Infection spread through blood transfusions, organ transplantation, and intrauterine transmission

Incidence and Demographics
- Reported in Asia, Africa, Europe, and United States (first in 1999)
- In 2003, over 3,500 cases of WNV in United States with ~60% having mild disease and ~30% severe disease; 66 deaths occurred
- Incubation period 5 to 15 days
- 20% of infected people develop mild illness lasting 3 to 6 days
- 1/150 develop severe neurological disease, encephalitis more than meningitis
- Mortality 5%, with most deaths in older adults

Risk Factors
- Outdoor workers
- Blood transfusion and organ transplant recipients
- Older age

Prevention and Screening
- Avoidance of mosquito bites: wear protective clothing, use insect repellent containing DEET, drain standing water
- Control of vectors by public health measures—spraying against mosquitoes
- Use of gloves when disposing of dead birds
- Reporting dead birds to local health department
- Blood donations screened for WNV using nucleic acid-amplification test

Assessment
History
- Determine exposure to mosquitoes
- History of blood transfusion or organ transplantation

Physical
- Nondescript fever with maculopapular or morbilliform rash on neck, trunk, arms, and legs
- Arthritis, myalgias, generalized weakness, and lymphadenopathy
- Meningitis: fever, headache, and nuchal rigidity
- Encephalitis: fever, headache, and altered mental status ranging from confusion to coma with or without additional signs of brain dysfunction (paresis, flaccid paralysis, ataxia, sensory deficits, optic neuritis, seizures, and abnormal reflexes)

Diagnostic Studies
- CSF with IgM antibody for WNV is confirmative; CSF with pleocytosis (increased number of lymphocytes)
- WNV antibody in serum is presumptive of recent infection in patients with acute CNS infection; a greater than 4-fold increase in antibody titers 2 to 4 weeks apart is confirmative

Differential Diagnosis
- California encephalitis
- Eastern equine encephalitis
- Western equine encephalitis
- Powassan encephalitis
- St. Louis encephalitis
- Colorado tick fever
- Dengue fever

Management
Nonpharmacologic Treatment
- Supportive care
- Monitor for complications

Pharmacologic Treatment
- Appropriate treatment of complications

How Long to Treat
- Continue supportive care until improvement

Special Considerations
- CDC Web site for West Nile Virus: www.cdc.gov/ncidod/dvbid/westnile/background. htm.

When to Consult, Refer, Hospitalize
- West Nile Virus encephalitis cases should be reported to the local state health department
- Patients with deteriorating mental status should be referred to a physician for hospitalization

Follow-up
- Majority have very minor illness and recover without complications

Complications
- Central nervous system abnormalities
- Death

Severe Acute Respiratory Syndrome (SARS)
Description
- Severe febrile viral lower-respiratory tract illness

Etiology
- Caused by SARS-associated coronavirus (SARS-CoV)

Incidence and Demographics
- First reported in Asia in February 2003
- Spread to North America, South America, Europe
- According to CDC: 8,089 cases of SARS and 774 deaths worldwide
- In the United States, 8 people with laboratory evidence of SARS; all had traveled to SARS-affected areas
- Incubation period 2 to 10 days with median of 4 to 6 days
- Spread by close (within 3 feet) respiratory droplet transmission or fomites

Risk Factors
- Recent travel to mainland China, Hong Kong, or Taiwan
- Close contact with persons ill with SARS
- Occupations at high risk: healthcare workers, laboratory technicians
- Cluster of atypical pneumonia without other diagnosis

Prevention and Screening
- Avoid travel to high risk areas
- Isolation of persons with possible SARS infection

Assessment
History
- History of exposure to SARS patient or SARS location

Physical
- Fever > 100.4° F, headache, body aches, mild respiratory symptoms; headache and myalgia may precede fever
- 10% to 20% have diarrhea
- After 2 to 7 days, dry cough develops with dyspnea and pneumonia

Diagnostic Studies
- No specific clinical or lab test available
- Obtain CBC with differential (70% to 90% with lymphopenia), blood cultures
- Chest x-ray or chest CT scan: chest CT may show infiltrate before CXR; obtain CT if positive epidemiological link to known SARS case and negative CXR 6 days after symptoms develop; repeat CXR on day 9 of illness
- Pulse oximetry
- Sputum for Gram stain and culture
- Viral respiratory testing for Influenza A and B and respiratory syncytial virus (RSV)
  - Lab tests available through state health department: RT-PCR for SARS-CoV on blood, stool, and respiratory secretions; serology for SARS-CoV antibodies and viral culture for SARS-CoV; signed consent should be obtained; because of the possibility of false-positive results lab studies should be obtained only on patients meeting certain criteria; see CDC Web site for information, www.cdc.gov/ncidod/sars/index.htm

Differential Diagnosis
- Influenza
- RSV
- Mycoplasma
- Bacterial pneumonia
- Viral pneumonia

Management
Nonpharmacologic Treatment
- Supportive care

Pharmacologic Treatment
- No specific treatment for SARS
- Appropriate treatment for complications

Special Considerations
- Persons with possible SARS must be quarantined in the home for 10 days or until fever resolved and free from respiratory symptoms

When to Consult, Refer, Hospitalize
- Hospitalize any patients with worsening illness

- Consult with state health department or CDC for lab testing and management of possible SARS cases

Follow-up
Expected Course
- Mild cases resolve without complication

Complications
- 10% fatality rate overall with > 50% older than 60 years

ILLNESSES OF UNKNOWN ORIGIN
Infections Caused by Bioweapons
Description
- Biological agents that have the potential for use as bioweapons are characterized as Category A agents. These agents can be easily disseminated or transmitted from person to person, cause high mortality with potential for major public health impact, and require prompt action. Numerous viruses, several bacteria, and toxins may be used as weapons, but those that are known to have been weaponized, have effective dispersal methods, and be environmentally stable include anthrax, botulism, plague, smallpox, tularemia, and viral hemorrhagic fevers (Ebola, Marburg, Lassa, dengue, yellow fever and others).

Etiology
- Naturally occurring organisms that have been altered to increase lethality

Incidence and Demographics
- Smallpox is no longer is found in wild form. All other potential bioagents occur naturally. Inhalation anthrax is rare, though dermatologic infection is still found fairly often in farm workers. Large-scale outbreaks of botulism have never occurred.

Risk Factors
- Any population can be at risk, although bioweapons attacks are more likely to occur in densely populated, urban areas or at large, crowded events such as football games.

Prevention and Screening
- Primary care providers must maintain an elevated level of suspicion.
- NPs must be aware of modes of transmission, incubation periods, and communicable periods of these diseases. An excellent source of information is the CDC Emergency Preparedness and Response Web site: http://www.bt.cdc.gov/index.asp.
- Patient and contacts must be isolated rapidly.

Assessment
History
- Symptoms for most agents can initially mimic those of common viral illnesses and include fever, fatigue, malaise, muscle aches, headache, cough, vomiting, diarrhea, rashes.
- For most agents, symptoms will quickly increase in intensity and severity.
- First indication of an unannounced biologic attack will likely be an unusual increase in number of persons seeking care.

Physical
- Ill-appearing patient, often out of proportion to degree of illness prevalent in the community

Diagnostic Studies
- Blood cultures, CBC, electrolytes
- Other studies dictated by clinical picture

Differential Diagnosis
- Common wild virus agents (fifth disease, Coxsackie, varicella)
- Other potential biological agents

Management
Nonpharmacologic Treatment
- Rapidly notify public health authorities
- Psychological and mental health problems brought on by the event will require significant expertise

Pharmacologic Treatment
- See Table 5–2
- Empiric therapy may be indicated if large numbers of individuals present with a nonspecific febrile illness in a limited time frame and location under credible threat of attack. Empiric therapy is ciprofloxacin or doxycycline PO or IV at routine recommended doses.

Table 5–2. Potential Bioweapons Agents

Biological Agent	Transmission/ Incubation	Clinical Presentation	Diagnosis	Management
Anthrax (*Bacillus anthracis*): Gram-positive spore-forming aerobic rod that causes cutaneous or pulmonary infection. Cutaneous anthrax does not have BW potential.	Inhalation of aerosolized spores. Person-to-person transmission does not occur. 1 to 7 day incubation.	Biphasic, with initial prodrome of nonspecific febrile flu-like illness. May be followed by brief period of improvement, then rapid onset of high fever, severe respiratory distress. Shock, death within 24 to 36 hours.	Chest x-ray: mediastinal widening. Gram-positive bacilli on unspun peripheral blood smear.	Ciprofloxacin or doxycycline; standard contact precautions. Prophylaxis should be offered with the same agents. A vaccine is available, but supply is limited.

continued

Table 5–2. Potential Bioweapons Agents (cont.)

Biological Agent	Transmission/ Incubation	Clinical Presentation	Diagnosis	Management
Botulism: caused by neurotoxin produced by *Clostridium botulinum*, spore-forming, obligate anaerobe found in soil. Botulinum toxin is the most lethal known natural poison.	Toxin can be aerosolized; sources of entry include wounds, GI tract, respiratory. It can also be dispensed in food. There is no person-to-person transmission. 12 to 36 hour incubation.	Symmetric cranial neuropathies (drooping eyelids, weakened jaw clench, difficulty swallowing, speaking), blurred vision or diplopia, symmetric descending weakness in a proximal-to-distal pattern, respiratory dysfunction.	Routine laboratory tests usually unremarkable. Definitive diagnostic testing for botulism available only at the CDC. Diagnosis is primarily clinical.	Supportive care, including ventilator support. Passive immunization with equine antitoxin.
Plague (*Yersinia pestis*): nonmotile bacillus	*Bubonic:* transmitted by bites from infected fleas, most common type. *Pneumonic:* inhalation of respiratory droplets from a human or animal with respiratory plague; may be aerosolized. Secondary cases would occur from contact with infected individuals. A BW attack most likely to produce pneumonic plague. 2 to 4 day incubation.	*Bubonic:* Enlarged, painful, regional lymph nodes (buboes); fever, chills, and prostration. *Pneumonic:* fever, weakness, and rapidly developing pneumonia with shortness of breath, chest pain, cough, and sometimes bloody or watery sputum.	Clinical diagnosis important as treatment must be begun in ≤ 24 hours. Large numbers of patients with severe pneumonia, particularly if accompanied by hemoptysis, must trigger prompt presumptive treatment and isolation. Prophylaxis of close contacts.	Streptomycin, gentamicin, tetracycline, or chloramphenicol begun within 24 hours greatly improves prognosis. Isolation and supportive care necessary. Prophylactic therapy begun within 7 days is very effective in preventing infection. No vaccine is available.

Table 5–2. Potential Bioweapons Agents (cont.)

Biological Agent	Transmission/ Incubation	Clinical Presentation	Diagnosis	Management
Smallpox: caused by a DNA virus in the orthopoxvirus family	Person-to-person transmission; spread by inhalation of air droplets or aerosols. Smallpox virus is specific for humans; animal infection does not occur. Weaponized smallpox can be spread by aerosol or by bombs or missiles. Secondary infection would occur from direct person-to-person spread, via both droplet and infected fomites (clothing, bedding).	High fever, malaise, severe aching pains, prostration. Later, a papular rash develops over the face and spreads to the extremities, soon becomes vesicular, and later, pustular. Rash is most dense on face. 12 to 14 day incubation.	Patients are most contagious from time of onset of rash until scabs form. Initial diagnosis must occur at a military facility. After confirmation of community disease, subsequent diagnoses made on basis of clinical presentation.	No known effective antiviral agents. Treatment is supportive. All potentially infected persons should be hospitalized in their homes. In event of widespread outbreak, specific hospitals would be designated for treatment of smallpox patients. Widespread vaccination would be indicated; smallpox vaccine is effective only if administered within 4 days of exposure. Vaccine is available, though supply is government controlled.

continued

Table 5–2. Potential Bioweapons Agents (cont.)

Biological Agent	Transmission/ Incubation	Clinical Presentation	Diagnosis	Management
Tularemia (*Francisella tularensis*): Gram-negative coccobacillus. Type A most virulent and likely to be weaponized. Very small number of organisms (10 to 50) can produce disease.	Naturally occurring in temperate areas of North America, Europe and Asia. Weaponized tularemia can be delivered via aerosol, with infection occurring secondary to inhalation, skin or mucus membrane contact, or GI exposure from contaminated soil, water, food, or animals. Person-to-person transmission is not known to occur.	Presentation dependent on route of administration. Inhalation most likely. Symptoms include abrupt onset of fever with progression to pneumonia and respiratory disease, hilar lymphadenopathy, and pleuritis. Inhalation can also cause sepsis without respiratory symptoms; this syndrome has a high fatality ratio. 1 to 4 day incubation dependent on virulence of strain, site, and size of inoculum.	No means of rapid testing is widely available. Diagnosis is initially clinical. *F. tularensis* may be identified by culture done in biological safety level (BSL) 3 labs.	Streptomycin IM or gentamicin IV for infection. Ciprofloxacin or doxycycline at usual doses recommended for mass casualties or postexposure. Vaccine is not widely available and immunity is incomplete.

Table 5-2. Potential Bioweapons Agents (cont.)

Biological Agent	Transmission/ Incubation	Clinical Presentation	Diagnosis	Management
Viral Hemorrhagic Fevers (VHF): a group of illnesses caused by several distinct RNA viruses (*Arenaviridae*, *Bunyaviridae*, *Filoviridae*, *Flaviviridae*) that include Ebola hemorrhagic fever, Marburg virus, Lassa fever, hantavirus pulmonary syndrome (HPS).	Incubation dependent on virus. Humans are not the natural reservoir of these viruses and are infected when they come into contact with secretions of infected hosts. However, with some viruses, after the accidental transmission from the host, humans can transmit the virus to one another. Naturally occurring human cases occur sporadically.	Specific signs and symptoms vary by the type of VHF; initial signs and symptoms include marked fever, fatigue, dizziness, muscle aches, loss of strength, and exhaustion. Patients often show signs of bleeding under the skin, in internal organs, or from orifices like the mouth, eyes, or ears. Full-blown VHF evolves to shock and generalized bleeding from the mucous membranes.	High index of suspicion, detailed travel history important. Lab findings supportive of infection vary; typically leukopenia, thrombocytopenia occur. Testing of ommunoglobulin (Ig) M antibody by enzyme-linked immunosorbent assay (ELISA) during the acute illness. Diagnosis by viral cultivation requires 3 to 10 days and can only be done at BSL 4 labs (CDC, military facilities).	There is no cure or established drug treatment for VHFs, although ribavirin has been tried with Lassa fever. Therapy is supportive and barrier isolation techniques should be initiated. No vaccines are available.

Special Considerations
- Appropriate management of postexposure prophylaxis and its complications will be critical in containing spread of infection

Follow-up
Complications
- Dependent on agent
- Most potential agents have high lethality, 30% to 100%

CASE STUDIES

Case 1. A 96-year-old woman resides in a nursing home. She usually gets up, dresses herself, and walks to breakfast in the dining room, but today the nursing assistant reports she won't get out of bed. She is agitated, trying to hit the staff, and crying out incoherently, and she was incontinent of urine overnight.

PMH: moderate dementia, osteoporosis, type 2 DM, CHF

Medications: metformin (Glucophage) 500 mg p.o. b.i.d., furosemide (Lasix) 20 mg p.o. q.d., lisinopril (Zestril) 10 mg p.o. q.d., digoxin (Lanoxin) 0.125 mg p.o. q.o.d., alendronate (Fosamax) 70 mg p.o. every week, donepezil (Aricept) 5 mg p.o. q.d.

1. What other history or review of systems would be needed?
2. What components of the physical exam would you perform?
3. What is your differential diagnosis?
4. What diagnostic tests are needed?

Case 2. A 68-year-old woman complains of diarrhea. It is soft to liquid and profuse. No nausea or vomiting. Patient was recently in the hospital for a cholecystectomy. Patient had Foley catheter during hospital stay. Patient was started on trimethoprim-sulfamethoxazole. Culture came back with resistance to TMP-SMZ, so patient was switched to ciprofloxacin. While on Cipro, she developed a pneumonia, so the Cipro was switched to clarithromycin (Biaxin).

1. What other history or review of system would be needed?
2. What components of the physical exam would you perform?
3. What is your differential diagnosis?
4. What diagnostic tests are needed?
5. What treatment should be instituted pending diagnosis?

Case 3. A 74-year-old female, living independently, presents with many vague complaints, including fatigue, weight loss, intermittent diarrhea, painful rash on trunk, numbness and tingling of toes, white coating in mouth. Patient's social history consists of 45 years unhappy marriage to distant husband who died of mysterious illness in 2005 at age 80.

PE: weight 108, down from 126 in past year, temporal wasting
* Rash vesicles on erythematous base in dermatome pattern on right side of trunk
* Decreased reflexes to LE
* White exudate that sticks to tongue in mouth, malodorous
* Normal abdominal and rectal exam

1. What is your differential diagnosis?
2. What diagnostic tests are needed?
3. What treatment would you initiate?

REFERENCES

Bartlett, J. G. (2002). Antibiotic-associated diarrhea. *New England Journal of Medicine, 346,* 334–339.

Cassell, G. H., & Mekalanos, J. (2001). Development of antimicrobial agents in the era of new and reemerging infectious diseases and increasing antibiotic resistance. *Journal of the American Medical Association, 285,* 601–605.

Centers for Disease Control. (2007). Updated information regarding antiretroviral agents used as HIV postexposure prophylaxis for occupational HIV exposures. *MMWR, 56*(49),1291–1292. Available at http://www.cdc.gov/mmwr/preview/mmwrhtml/mm5649a4.htm.

Chong, C. P., & Street, P. R. (2008). Pneumonia in the elderly: A review of severity assessment, prognosis, mortality, prevention and treatment. *Southern Medical Journal, 101,* 1134–1140.

Gilbert, D. N., Moellering, Jr., R. C., Eliopoulos, G. M., Chambers, H. F., & Saag, M. S. (Eds.) (2009). *Sanford guide to antimicrobial therapy.* Vienna, VA: Antimicrobial Therapy, Inc.

Gradon, J. D. (2004). HIV Infection in the older population. *Clinical Geriatrics, 12*(6), 37–45.

Heymann, D. L. (2008). *Control of communicable diseases manual* (19th ed). Washington, DC: American Public Health Association.

Jaber, M. R., Olafsson, S., Fung, W. L., & Reeves, M. E. (2008). Clinical review of fulminant clostridium difficile infection. *American Journal of Gastroenterology, 103,* 195–203.

Kaplan, J. E., Masur, H., Holmes, K. K., USPHS; Infectious Disease Society of America. (2002). Guidelines for prevention opportunistic infections among HIV infected persons—2002. Recommendations of the U.S. Public Health Service and the Infectious Diseases Society of America. *MMWR Recom Rep, 51*(RR-8): 1–52.

Mandell, G. L., Bennett, J. E., & Dolin, R. (2000). *Mandell, Douglas & Bennett's principles and practices of infectious diseases.* Philadelphia: Churchill Livingstone.

Monnet, D. L., MacKenzie, F. M., Lopez-Lozano, J. M., Beyaert, A., Camacho, M., Wilson, R., et al. (2004) Antimicrobial drug use and methicillin resistant Staphylococcus aureus, Aberdeen, 1996–2000. *Emerging Infectious Diseases, 10*(8), 1432–1441.

Mouton, C. P., Pierce, B., & Espino, D. (2001). Common infections in older adults. *American Family Physician, 63,* 257–268.

Panlilo, H. L., Cardo, D. M., Groohskopf, L. A., Heinine, W., & Ross, C. S. (2005). Updated U.S. Public Health Service Guidelines for the management of occupational exposure to HIV and recommendations for postexposure prophylaxis. *MMWR, 54*(RR09).

Wormser, G. P., Ramanathan, R., Nowakowski, J., McKenna, D., Holmgren, D., Visintainer, P., et al. (2003). Duration of antibiotic therapy for early Lyme disease: A randomized, double blind, placebo controlled trial. *Annals of Internal Medicine, 138,* 697–704.

Dermatologic Disorders

Katherine Tardiff, MSN, GNP-BC, ACHPN

GENERAL APPROACH

Skin layers include:

- Epidermis (outermost, visible layer): consists of stratum corneum (protector of underlying tissues), stratum lucidum, stratum granulosum, stratum spinosum, and stratum germinativum (producer of new skin, anchors epidermis to dermis)
- Dermis: made up of connective tissue; gives skin strength and flexibility (contains blood and lymphatic vessels, sweat and sebaceous glands; composed of fibroblasts that are responsible for formation of collagen)
- Subcutaneous layer made up of adipose and connective tissue, major blood and lymphatic vessels, and nerves; dermal accessory structures include hair, nails, and glands

Table 6-1. Morphologic Definitions for Primary Skin Lesions

Term	Definition and Example	Size
Macule	Flat, nonpalpable colored spot (freckle, lentigines)	Variable
Papule	Solid or fluid-filled, elevated, circumscribed lesion (contact dermatitis)	Up to 5 mm
Nodule	Solid, elevated, circumscribed lesion (erythema nodosum)	Larger than 5 mm
Vesicle	Fluid-filled, elevated, circumscribed lesions (herpes simplex)	Up to 5 mm
Cyst	Encapsulated, fluid-filled mass (epidermoid cyst)	Variable

continued

Table 6-1. Morphologic Definitions for Primary Skin Lesions (cont.)

Term	Definition and Example	Size
Bulla	Fluid-filled, elevated, circumscribed lesion (second degree burn, severe poison ivy)	Larger than 5 mm
Pustule	Pus-filled, elevated, circumscribed lesion (acne)	Up to 5 mm
Wheal	Circumscribed, reddening with transient elevation (mosquito bite, hives, urticaria)	0.5 to 10 cm diameter
Plaques	Elevated lesion; variety of shapes; often a close grouping of multiple papules (seborrheic dermatitis, psoriasis)	Larger than 5 mm

General dermatologic signs to be assessed and documented

- **Morphology** of lesions (macule, papule, nodule, vesicle, pustule, purpura, patch, plaque, tumor, bulla, abscess, ecchymosis, wheal, cyst, comedo, telangiectasia)
- **Secondary** lesions (sequential lesions that have evolved from other skin conditions) such as scar, erosion, ulcer, fissure, scale, crust
- **Distribution** of lesions (generalized or localized, central or peripheral, symmetric or asymmetric, predilection for certain body areas such as extensor or flexor surfaces and intertriginous areas, sun-exposed or pressure areas/bony prominences)
- **Arrangement** of lesions (discrete, confluent, scattered, linear, zosteriform, polycyclic, grouped, patchy, arcuate, reticular, scarlatiniform)
- Shape or **configuration** of the primary lesion (annular, oval, nummular, iris, pedunculated, verrucous, umbilicated, gyrate, or serpiginous)
- **Color** of lesions (erythematous, violaceous, hypomelanotic, depigmented, flesh colored, hypermelanotic; uniform or variegated)
- Borders or **margins** of lesions (well-demarcated or ill-defined)
- **Palpable** qualities (soft, firm, mobile, fixed, hard, fluctuant, tender, hot/warm/cool, smooth, rough, indurated)
- **Measure** dimensions (diameter, width, length, elevation, depression)
- **Descriptive** terms (lichenified, atrophied, sclerosed, pigmented, friable, hyperkeratotic, weeping, crusted, mobile or nonmobile, hypertrophic/keloidal, excoriations)
- **Associated symptoms** involving the hair, nails, and mucous membranes; lymphadenopathy or hepatosplenomegaly; ophthalmologic and/or neurologic

Normal Changes of Aging

- Epidermis: thinner, connection to dermis less adhesive and more easily traumatized, more susceptible to blisters and skin tears, less of a barrier; keratinocytes have lower proliferation rate, which leads to slower wound healing; fewer functioning melanocytes leads to less protection from ultraviolet light; decreased # Langerhans cells means weaker immune defense
- Dermis: about 20% thinner, skin feels thin and looks transparent; reduced capillary network leads to atrophy of skin; reduced size and number of fibroblasts
- Subcutaneous layer: thinner, less protection from trauma and cold
- Hair: graying, thinning, and loss
- Nails: rate of growth slows; thin and brittle or thick and dystrophic
- Sebaceous glands: may hypertrophy, function diminishes leading to dry skin
- Wound healing: the normal changes of aging listed above all contribute to delayed healing, and weaker scars after healing; the presence of multiple medical problems add to this compromised healing process

Table 6–2. Age-Specific Dermatologic Changes

Skin Condition	Pearl	Description	Risk Factors	Treatment
Photo-aging	Many of the undesirable skin changes associated with aging are the result of sun exposure	Wrinkling, yellowing, mottled pigmentation, atrophy, easy bruising	Changes in skin as a direct result of repeated sun exposure superimposed on normal aging of the skin	Protection from further damage still needed, and both clothing and use of sunscreen SPF 15 recommended with any sun exposure
Xerosis	Almost universal	Dry, scaly, often pruritic skin Most common on legs, may be present on back and arms	Worse during winter in heated building with low humidity	Decrease use of soaps and hot water Use skin emollient regularly If inflamed or pruritic, short-term use of low dose topical steroid, e.g., 1%–2.5% hydrocortisone ointment
Pruritus	Due to decreased inflammatory response, underlying skin disease can be difficult to detect	Localized or generalized itching that may interrupt sleep and cause scratching that excoriates skin	Xerosis often primary cause Systemic diseases, e.g., renal failure, liver disease, cancer, thyrotoxicosis, and DM may cause pruritus Need to rule out drug reaction	Treat underlying cause Use topical emollients, antipruritic agents, and oral antihistamines with caution secondary to sedative effects
Skin Tags	Benign	Found especially around neck and flexural areas, pink to brown color	Frequently found in obese patients and more common in women	Removed with scissors, cryosurgery, or light electrodesiccation if irritated or cosmetically desired

continued

Table 6-2. Age-Specific Dermatologic Changes (cont.)

Skin Condition	Pearl	Description	Risk Factors	Treatment
Cherry Angiomas	Common and benign	Typically 1–4 mm dome shaped, bright red Found principally on the trunk	More numerous, larger with age	Electro- or laser coagulation if cosmetically desired
Spider Veins	Common	Dilated, star-shaped blue veins on feet and legs	Increased number in older women	Treatment with sclerotherapy by consultant if desired

Clinical Implications

Assessment

History
- Most important part of the evaluation
- Dermatologic complaints can indicate dermatological or systemic disorder
- Dermatologic disorders can have profound impact on self image; psychological assessment needs to be included

Physical
- Physical exam best performed in well-lit room with a handheld light for illumination and shadowing, Wood lamp for fluorescing certain types of lesions, a magnifying lens (5X to 10X), glass slides for diascopy and skin scrapings, KOH solution, 5% acetic acid for acetowhitening, mineral oil for suspected scabies, Giemsa or Wright stains, and a regular and dark-field microscope
- Appearance of patient and vital signs (comfortable, agitated, toxic) with referral to an ER considered for a toxic patient
- Rule out skin cancer with any suspicious lesion

Management

Nonpharmacologic Treatment
- Care of underlying age-related xerosis often important for improvement and control of many signs and symptoms
- Consider external/functional factors when looking for cause, such as incontinence, poor self care/hygiene abilities, repeated motor activities
- Know what the patient's or family's goal of care is: cure or comfort?

Pharmacologic Treatment
- Steroid medications play a big role in treatment of many skin conditions
  - Use lowest-dosage steroid possible, starting with strength below usual standard adult dosage
  - Do not use fluorinated steroids on the face as it causes thinning of the tissue

Table 6-3. Common Topical Steroids Ranked by Potency

Class	Example
Class 1 Ultra High	Betamethasone dipropionate ointment 0.05% (Diprolene) Halobetasol propionate cream, ointment 0.05% (Ultravate)
Class 2 Very High	Desoximetasone ointment 0.25% (Topicort) Fluocinonide cream, gel, 0.05% (Lidex)
Class 3 High	Betamethasone valerate ointment 0.1% (Valisone) Triamcinolone acetonide ointment, 0.1% (Aristocort, Kenalog)
Class 4 Intermediate	Hydrocortisone valerate cream, ointment 0.2% (Westcort) Triamcinolone acetonide cream 0.025% (Aristocort, Kenalog)
Class 5 Low	Desonide ointment 0.05% (Tridesilon) Fluocinolone acetonide cream 0.01% (Synalar)
Class 6 Very Low	Hydrocortisone cream 2.5% (Hytone) Methylprednisolone cream 0.25% (Medrol)

RED FLAGS

- Generalized rash with fever, blisters, mouth lesions, vesicles, pustules, scaling
- Generalized wheals and soft tissue swelling
- Generalized purpura
- Multiple skin infarcts
- Localized skin infarcts
- Facial inflammatory edema with fever
- See Table 6–4

Table 6-4. Dermatologic Emergencies

Condition	Risk Factors	History	Phsyical	Management/ Comments
Stevens-Johnson Syndrome (SJS), Toxic Epidermal Necrolysis (TEN)	Medication use, compromised immune system	Exposure to new medications; prodromal symptoms: fever, flu-like illness; skin tenderness, conjunctival burning or itching, then skin pain, burning; mouth lesions are painful	Morbiliform eruption with initial lesions (poorly defined macules with darker centers) appear on face and upper trunk initially; may spread to extremities	**Emergency referral** for treatment in intensive care; mortality ranges from 5% in SJS to 30% in TEN

continued

Table 6-4. Dermatologic Emergencies (cont.)

Condition	Risk Factors	History	Phsyical	Management/ Comments
Necrotizing Fasciitis	Trauma (insect bite, laceration, surgical incision); advanced age, renal failure, peripheral vascular disease, diabetes, compromised immune system, use of NSAIDs	Acute redness, edema, heat, pain, most often on an extremity, the perineum, or trunk; fever is prominent; severe pain disproportionate to local findings	Signs of sepsis (tachycardia, tachypnea, oliguria, mental status changes); severe skin-color changes (initially red-purple to dusky blue), swelling, bullae, cyanosis, skin pallor, muscle weakness, foul smell or exudates, crepitus	**Emergency referral** for intravenous antibiotics; may require amputation of affected extremity
Staphylococcal Toxic Shock Syndrome	Superficial skin or surgical wound infection	Recent skin infection; 2–3 day prodromal period of malaise, then fever, chills, nausea, and abdominal pain	Diffuse erythematous, nonpruritic, maculopapular or petechial rash (initially on trunk, then spreads to palms and soles); subsequent desquamation; multisystem involvement includes arrhythmia, hepatic and renal failure, disseminated intravascular coagulation and acute respiratory distress syndrome	**Emergency referral** for treatment of hypotension and multiorgan failure

COMMON DERMATOLOGIC DISORDERS
Contact Dermatitis
Description
- An acute or chronic inflammatory reaction to substances that come in contact with the skin; results from contact with an irritant (irritant contact dermatitis [ICD]) or an allergen (allergic contact dermatitis [ACD])

Etiology
- ICD due to direct contact with an irritant that has a toxic effect on the skin (e.g., detergent); damages one of the components of the water-protein-lipid matrix of the epidermal layer of the skin
- ACD results from a delayed hypersensitivity reaction to a contact allergen; cell-mediated hypersensitivity response has two phases:

– An initial exposure to the allergen sensitizes the skin and produces proliferation of T lymphocytes

– An elicitation phase, which causes the antigen-specific T lymphocytes present in the skin to combine with the allergen to produce an inflammatory response

- Most commonly recognized allergens: Rhus plants (poison ivy, sumac, and oak), nickel (jewelry), rubber chemicals, chemicals used in personal products such as cosmetics, shampoos, drugs

Incidence and Demographics
- ICD accounts for 80% of cases of contact dermatitis
- ACD is uncommon in individuals older than 70 years

Risk Factors
- ICD:
  – History of atopic dermatitis
  – White skin
  – Living in low-temperature, low-humidity climates
  – Occupational exposure to abrasives, cleaning agents, oxidizing or reducing agents, plants
- ACD:
  – Exposure to metal salts, antibiotics, dyes, plants
  – Frequent exposure to topical medications may trigger reactions in older adults

Prevention and Screening
- Avoidance of known irritants/allergens

Assessment
- Because of decreased inflammatory response of skin in older adults, dermatitis may be mild

History
- Pruritic rash common with both ICD and ACD
- Known exposure to irritant or allergen
- May include systemic symptoms of toxicity if extensive involvement

Physical Exam
- ICD: rash is limited to area of exposure, developing within a few hours of contact with the irritant; involved areas initially erythematous and may develop vesicles, erosions, or crusting
- ACD: rash initially is limited to area of exposure, but dermatitis may spread to areas that were not exposed; eruption may become generalized; papules, vesicles, erosions, and crusts may develop
- Particular irritant or allergen may be obvious by location of symptoms
- Metal allergy: most common offender is nickel in jewelry and clothing
  – Distribution: neck, wrists, waist, strap line
  – Generally mild and chronic with scaling, pigmentation changes, and pruritus
- Plant dermatitis:
  – Distribution and arrangement: often linear pattern
  – Most commonly caused by poison ivy, oak, or sumac
  – Secondary signs: weeping, scaling, edema, crusting, and excoriations

Diagnostic Studies
- Diagnosis by history and clinical exam; patch testing may be warranted for severe or recurrent episodes with unclear etiology

Differential Diagnosis
- Atopic dermatitis
- Seborrheic dermatitis
- Psoriasis
- Candida infection
- Phytophotodermatitis
- Drug eruption
- Insect bites

Management
Nonpharmacologic
- Removal of offending irritant or allergen
- Wash potentially contacted clothing
- Bathe in tepid water with gentle soap to wash allergen/irritant off skin, followed by lubrication of the skin with colloidal oatmeal suspension (Aveeno) to treat pruritus

Pharmacologic
- Application of mid- to high-potency topical steroid ointments two or three times a day; use lowest effective potency, especially for less severe lesions or lesions covering large surface area
- Systemic (oral) steroids for severe or extensive involvement
- Oral antibiotics for impetiginized lesions
- Length of treatment determined by extent of involvement and response

When to Consult, Refer, Hospitalize
- Physician consultation is recommended for oral steroid use
- Consultation/referral to allergist for unresponsive cases
- Hospitalization should be considered for toxic or unstable patients

Follow-up
Expected Outcomes
- Course is usually dictated by irritant or allergen and extent of involvement
- Metal allergies tend to be low-level and chronic with possible lichenification and hyperpigmentation

Complications
- Toxicity and impetiginization
- Oral antihistamines for treatment of pruritus may cause excessive drowsiness or confusion in older adults and should be avoided

Nummular Eczema
Description
- Chronic, pruritic, inflammatory dermatitis in coin-shaped plaques of 4 to 5 cm

Etiology
- Cause remains unknown

Incidence and Demographics
- More common in older males and in young adults
- Patients often have an atopic background

Risk Factors
- Atopic history
- Male sex
- Xerosis

Assessment
History
- Coin-shaped rash usually on anterior aspects of lower legs but may also appear on trunk, hands, and fingers
- Pruritus often intense
- More common in winter and fall months

Physical Exam
- Morphology: round or coin-shaped plaques consisting of grouped papules and vesicles on erythematous base, well-demarcated borders, often more than 4 to 5 cm in diameter
- Distribution: lower legs (older men), trunk, hands and fingers (younger females)
- Secondary signs: exudative, crusting, scales; excoriations due to scratching; lichenification
- Frequently colonized with S. *aureus*

Diagnostic Studies
- Cultures to rule out bacterial infection

Differential Diagnosis
- Contact dermatitis
- Dermatophytosis (fungal infections)
- Psoriasis

Management
Nonpharmacologic
- Emollients to moisturize involved skin

Pharmacologic
- Mid- to high-potency topical steroids in an emollient base applied twice daily until lesions have resolved
- Systemic antibiotics if S. *aureus* is present

Special Considerations
- Black skin may be more prone to postinflammatory hyperpigmentation and keloid formation

When to Consult, Refer, Hospitalize
- Physician consultation is recommended when systemic antibiotics are needed

Follow-up
Expected Outcomes
- Chronic recurrent condition

Complications
- Bacterial superinfection
- Postinflammatory hyperpigmentation

Seborrheic Dermatitis

Description
- Chronic, recurrent, and sometimes pruritic inflammatory disease of skin where sebaceous glands are most active (face, scalp, body folds)

Etiology
- Unknown with questionable role of the yeast species *Malassezia furfur*

Incidence and Demographics
- Common chronic problem; 1% to 3% of adults
- Males > females

Risk Factors
- Family history
- HIV infection
- Zinc or niacin deficiency
- Parkinson's disease

Assessment
History
- Gradual onset of greasy, scaly rash on face and scalp (often referred to as dandruff by patient)
- Possibly associated with slight pruritus

Physical Exam
- Morphology: lesions are yellowish-red, greasy, erythematous, sharply marginated, 5 to 20 mm scaling macules and papules
- Distribution: lateral sides of nose and nasolabial folds, eyebrows and glabella, and scalp; less commonly involved are the chest, upper back, and axillae
- Secondary signs: dandruff, possible inflammatory base, sticky crusting (more common on ears), fissures (more common where ear attaches to scalp)

Diagnostic Studies
- Diagnosis is usually made clinically

Differential Diagnosis
- Psoriasis
- Rosacea
- Impetigo
- Pemphigus (bullous autoimmune disease)
- Dermatophytosis (fungal infection)
- Lupus erythematosus

Management
Nonpharmacologic
- Avoiding cold creams and moisturizers
- Removal of scaling of eyelashes with baby shampoo

Pharmacologic

- Frequent shampooing with over-the-counter shampoos containing selenium sulfide (Selsun or Exsel), tar (Polytar, T-Gel, or Tegrin) or zinc (Head and Shoulders); shampoo should be left in place for a few minutes before rinsing
- 2% ketoconazole shampoo may be used initially to treat and for maintenance therapy; lather can be used on face, chest, and intertriginous areas during shower
- Low-potency topical steroid solution, lotion, or gel following medicated shampoo (ketoconazole or tar) for more severe cases
- Chronic condition requires initial therapy until symptoms resolve, followed by maintenance therapy

Special Considerations

- Topical steroids can cause atrophy and erythema, especially on the face, and may initiate or exacerbate perioral dermatitis or rosacea; topical steroid should be tapered and discontinued if this occurs
- Most severe form is generalized and develops into erythroderma

When to Consult, Refer, Hospitalize

- Consult or refer for unresponsive cases

Follow-up

Expected Outcomes

- Chronic condition requiring initial treatment phase and then maintenance therapy
- Visits every 1 to 2 months during maintenance phase to monitor disorder and for signs of skin atrophy

Complications

- Secondary *Candida* and bacterial infections
- Skin atrophy from chronic topical steroids

Psoriasis

Description

- Chronic, erythematous papules and plaques with a silver scale in characteristic distribution on knees, elbows, and scalp

Etiology

- Alteration in cell kinetics of keratinocytes with shortening of cell turnover rate resulting in increased production of epidermal cells; autoreactive immune responses result in maintenance of psoriatic lesions

Incidence and Demographics

- Affects about 1% to 2% of population; equal incidence in males and females
- Onset and persistence in latter decades not uncommon
- Rare in West Africans, Japanese, Inuits; very rare in North and South American Indians
- Family history common

Risk Factors

- Genetic predisposition
- Physical trauma

- Infections (streptococcal) can lead to guttate psoriasis
- Stress can lead to exacerbations
- Exposure to certain medications may cause flares in existing psoriasis (systemic glucocorticoids, lithium, antimalarial drugs, interferon, beta blockers)

Prevention and Screening
- Stress management

Assessment
History
- Skin lesions usually with insidious onset but may be acute
- Lesions are typically asymptomatic; pruritus may or may not be present
- May be associated with acute systemic illness with fever and malaise
- About 7% may be associated with arthralgias/arthritis, usually affecting the distal phalanges

Physical Exam
- Plaque psoriasis (psoriasis vulgaris): 90% of cases of psoriasis manifest as plaque psoriasis:
- Morphology: erythematous plaques with sharply defined margins that are raised; a thick, silvery scale is usually present, though may have been removed by recent bathing
- Lesions may range from < 1 cm to > 10 cm in diameter
- Removal of scale results in appearance of tiny blood droplets
- Distribution: symmetrical; involves scalp, extensor elbows, knees, and back; may also involve intertriginous areas (umbilicus and intergluteal cleft)
- May involve pitting of nail plates
- Köbner phenomenon: injury or irritation of normal skin induces lesions; may occur 1 to 3 weeks after injury
- Variations:
  - Guttate psoriasis: discrete, scaly plaques beginning on trunk and spreading to the extremities; lesions 3 to 10 mm in diameter; occurs after streptococcal infection
  - Pustular psoriasis: severe form with acute onset of widespread disease; more common in older patients (> 50 years); may be precipitated by infection and recent use of systemic corticosteroids
  - Psoriatic arthritis: presentation similar to inflammatory arthritis
    - Distal interphalangeal joints are a common site for arthralgia
    - Symptoms are variable and may precede the development of skin lesions

Diagnostic Studies
- Diagnosis is usually clinical; rarely, a skin biopsy is performed to rule out other conditions
- Serum antistreptolysin titer or throat culture in evaluating guttate psoriasis
- HIV screen in the case of sudden-onset psoriasis in at-risk individuals

Differential Diagnosis
- Seborrheic dermatitis
- Atopic dermatitis
- Drug eruptions
- Lichen simplex chronicus

- Fungal infections
- Candidiasis
- Rheumatoid arthritis

Management
Nonpharmacologic
- Psychosocial support
- Avoid rubbing or scratching lesions
- Topical emollients to moisturize skin and minimize itching and tenderness

Pharmacologic
- Extent of disease guides treatment decisions; mild-to-moderate disease can often be managed with topical agents; moderate-to-severe disease may require systemic therapy
- Mild-to-moderate disease:
  - Topical high- to very high-potency steroids, applied twice daily until skin has returned to normal thickness
  - Alternatives include: tar, topical retinoids (tazarotene), and calcipotriene ointment 0.005% (vitamin D analog)
  - For facial or intertriginous areas, topical tacrolimus or pimecrolimus may be used
  - Localized phototherapy (ultraviolet B [UVB]) is another option for recurrent disease
- Moderate-to-severe disease:
  - Phototherapy (UVB, narrow-band UVB, and photochemotherapy [PUVA])
  - Systemic therapies: retinoids (vitamin A derivatives), methotrexate (folic acid antagonist), cyclosporine (T-cell suppressor), or biologic immune modifying agents (e.g., alefacept, efalizumab, etenaercept, infliximab)

Special Considerations
- Treatment decisions are complex and should involve the expertise of a dermatologist
- Financial considerations may affect treatment options

When to Consult, Refer, Hospitalize
- All patients should be referred to a dermatologist for confirmation of diagnosis and assistance in developing plan of care
- Widespread pustular disease requires aggressive treatment, possibly including hospitalization

Follow-up
Expected Outcomes
- Mild-to-moderate disease: improvement with topical therapies may be seen in one week, though several weeks of treatment may be needed to demonstrate benefit
- Moderate-to-severe disease: improvement generally seen within weeks
- Frequent follow-up may be necessary to improve adherence to treatment regimen, especially adherence to topical therapies

Complications
- Bacterial infection related to scratching
- Complications secondary to treatment include but are not limited to: atrophy of skin related to corticosteroid use; skin cancer and cataract formation with phototherapy; and adverse medication effects of antimetabolites and retinoids

FUNGAL (DERMATOPHYTE) INFECTIONS

Tinea

Description

- Superficial fungal infection of nonliving, keratinized portions of skin, including stratum corneum (epidermomycosis), nails (onychomycosis), and hair (trichomycosis)
- Infections are named by the body part involved:
  - Tinea corporis: body
  - Tinea manuum: hand
  - Tinea pedis: feet
  - Tinea cruris: groin
  - Tinea capitis: scalp (Trichomycosis)
  - Tinea barbae: beard (Trichomycosis)
  - Tinea unguium: nails (Onychomycosis)
  - Tinea versicolor: named by its multicolored appearance; usually seen on torso and neck

Etiology

- Caused by several dermatophytes with regional predominance
- In the United States, three types of fungi/dermatophytes account for the majority of infections: *Microsporum*, *Trichophyton*, and *Epidermophyton*
- Can be spread by direct contact with an infected animal or human or through indirect contact with fomites such as clothing, linens, or gym mats or rarely from the soil

Incidence and Demographics

- Common in older adults, particularly on feet, nails, and groin
- Affects all ages, races, genders; Black adults are believed to have lower incidence of dermatophytosis
- More common in tropical climates, or during warmer months in temperate climates
- More common in immunocompromised patients, including when immunocompromise is secondary to prolonged use of topical steroids, with greater risk of intractable infection
- Systemic corticosteroids decrease host resistance to fungal infection
- More common when peripheral nerve disease results in reduced blood flow to periphery

Risk Factors

- Heat and humidity
- Obesity: creates body warmth and perspiration, thus providing the hot, humid conditions that can encourage fungal growth
- Exposure to fungal infections of animals and humans with whom the person has close physical contact (pets, household members, other nursing home residents)
- Exposure to fomites in hot, humid environments
- Mechanical pressure from shoes predisposes susceptible individuals to onychomycosis

Prevention and Screening

- Climate control as appropriate: air-conditioning; loose, cotton clothing
- Management of obesity
- Air drying or using electric hair dryer to completely dry intertriginous areas prior to dressing
- Completely dry shoes between wearing

- Frequently changing shoes, white cotton socks during day; wearing sandals
- Do not share combs, brushes, and hair ornaments
- Avoid occlusive ornaments: acrylic nails, synthetic jewelry, belts, shoes

Assessment

History
- Known exposure to others with tinea or high-risk population
- Mild to moderately pruritic localized "rash" or isolated lesion

Physical Exam
- Presentation differs based on location of lesion
- Scaling erythematous plaque ranging from < 1 cm up to 20 cm
- Varying shapes: round, arciform, or polycyclic
- With or without pustules/vesicles
- Usually has elevated, sharp border with central clearing; annular configuration ("ringworm")
- Color is erythematous or hyperpigmented

TINEA CRURIS ("JOCK ITCH")
- Men > women; often begins after physical activity resulting in sweating
- Begins with an erythematous patch high on the inner aspect of one or both thighs
- Spreads centrifugally with partial clearing; slightly elevated, erythematous, sharply demarcated border
- Often coexists with tinea pedis; infection transferred from feet to groin by hands
- Maceration common in intertriginous areas

TINEA PEDIS ("ATHLETE'S FOOT")
- Most common dermatophyte infection; often accompanied by tinea infection of the hands, nails, or groin
- Slowly progressive pruritic, erythematous lesions between the toes (especially the fourth digital interspace)
    - Maceration may be seen in the digital interspaces
- Diffuse desquamation with superficial white scales and possible bulla formation
- Hyperkeratosis of soles with painful fissuring/cracking along soles and lateral borders ("moccasin ringworm")
- Usually bilateral foot involvement
- Onychomycosis is often present

TINEA MANUUM
- Erythema and mild scaling of dorsal aspect of hands or chronic, scaly hyperkeratosis of palms
- May be unilateral (50%) or bilateral (50%)
- Frequently coexists with tinea pedis or tinea cruris

TINEA CAPITIS AND TINEA BARBAE (TRICHOMYCOSIS)
- Involve dermatophyte invasion of the hair follicle by *Trichophyton* dermatophytes
- Begins with an erythematous scaling patch that slowly enlarges
- In some cases, inflammation is prominent, with painful, boggy, suppurative nodules with crusting/scabs
- Alopecia

TINEA UNGUIUM (ONYCHOMYCOSIS)
- Nails become white, brown, yellow, or black
- Nails thicken and surface becomes roughened
- Nails eventually separate from the nail bed

TINEA VERSICOLOR (PITYRIASIS VERSICOLOR)
- Superficial, benign, cutaneous fungal infection caused by *Malassezia furfur* (yeast that colonizes human skin)
- Clinically significant only in some individuals
- Distribution on trunk, back, abdomen, neck, and proximal extremities
- Numerous, well-marginated, finely scaly, oval or round macules that coalesce, forming patches of altered pigmentation
- Hypo- or hyperpigmented; color varies from white to reddish-brown or fawn colored
- Usually asymptomatic but may be mildly pruritic

Diagnostic Studies
- Wood lamp
  - Tinea capitis fluoresces greenish-yellow
  - Tinea versicolor fluoresces coppery-orange
  - Tinea cruris does not fluoresce but Wood lamp exam can identify erythrasma, a bacterial infection that fluoresces coral-red
- KOH mount: skin scrapings placed on a slide in 10% to 30% KOH solution with a coverslip; can be viewed under a microscope after warming for 30 to 60 seconds; will demonstrate mycelia and hyphae
  - Tinea capitis appears as spores invading hair follicles
  - Tinea cruris appears as mycelia with septate hyphae and scattered buds
  - Tinea versicolor appears as long hyphae and few buds ("spaghetti and meatballs")
- Fungal cultures can identify a fungus but usually take weeks to grow
  - Indicated only when an infection is resistant to treatment

Differential Diagnosis: Based on location of lesions
Tinea pedis
- Impetigo
- Psoriasis
- Erythrasma
- Candidiasis
- Contact dermatitis
- Dyshidrotic eczema

Tinea manuum
- Atopic dermatitis
- Contact dermatitis
- Psoriasis
- Lichen simplex chronicus
- *In situ* squamous cell carcinoma
- Pityriasis rubra pilari

Tinea cruris
- Erythrasma
- Inverse pattern psoriasis
- Candidiasis

Tinea corporis
- Atopic dermatitis
- Contact dermatitis
- Annular erythema
- Psoriasis
- Seborrheic dermatitis
- Erythema migrans
- Pityriasis rosea

Tinea capitis
- Seborrheic dermatitis
- Psoriasis
- Atopic dermatitis
- Alopecia areata
- Lichen simplex chronicus
- Chronic SLE
- Impetigo
- Ecthyma
- Crusted scabies

Tinea barbae
- Beard folliculitis
- Acne vulgaris
- Acne rosacea
- Furunculosis

Tinea trichomycosis
- Paronychia
- Herpetic whitlow
- Eczematous dermatitis
- Allergic contact dermatitis
- Lichen planus
- Pseudomonal nail infection (black-green coloring)
- Reiter syndrome
- Traumatic injury to the nail

Management
Nonpharmacologic
- Managing and treating predisposing conditions
  - Obesity
  - Diabetes
  - Immunosuppression
- Advise patient of need to avoid tight or occlusive clothing or ornaments
- Change shoes and socks during the day or wear sandals
- Completely dry intertriginous areas after bathing

Pharmacologic
- Tinea capitis and barbae (Trichomycosis): oral griseofulvin is the drug of choice
- Tinea corporis, manuum, pedis, cruris: use topical antifungal creams or lotions
- Topical antifungal preparations: apply to affected area including a 2 cm peripheral border and rub in

- – Clotrimazole 1% cream, solution, lotion
- – Econazole 1% cream
- – Ketoconazole 2% cream, shampoo
- – Miconazole 2% cream
- – Oxiconazole 1% cream, lotion
- – Sulconazole 1% cream, solution
- – Naftifine 1% cream or gel
- – Tolnaftate 1% cream, gel, powder, topical aerosol, solution
- – Terbinafine (Lamisil) 1% cream, gel
- Onychomycosis (tinea unguium) nails:
  - – Terbinafine 250 mg daily for 12 weeks (toenails), 6 weeks (fingernails)
  - – Topical treatments are often ineffective alone, but may help to treat difficult cases when used in conjunction with systemic antifungals
    - Ciclopirox (Penlac) 8% nail lacquer
- Tinea versicolor
  - – Selenium sulfide lotion apply from neck to waist daily, leave on 10 min, daily for 2 weeks
  - – Ketoconazole shampoo for weekly maintenance
- Oral antifungal medications: synthetic antifungal agents are effective but should be reserved for severe or extensive cases: e.g., griseofulvin, ketoconazole

Special Considerations
- Side effects from systemic antifungal agents include hepatotoxicity, lowering of serum testosterone; evaluate liver function tests (LFTs) prior to starting oral agents, then every 4 to 6 weeks
- Drug–drug interactions are possible, especially with systemic antifungal medications; careful review of the patient's medications is essential

When to Consult, Refer, Hospitalize
- Consultation and/or referral appropriate for extensive involvement or unresponsive infections
- Consider hospitalization for immunosuppressed patients with extensive disease

Follow-up
Expected Outcomes
- Follow up every 4 weeks for reevaluation and LFTs
- Resolution is slow; treatment length depends on location; all take several weeks
  - – Tinea capitis and tinea barbae: 8 to 16 weeks
  - – Tinea corporis, tinea manuum, tinea cruris: 4 to 6 weeks
  - – Tinea pedis: 4 to 12 weeks
  - – Tinea versicolor: 4 to 6 weeks, with frequent relapses
- Onychomycosis: 8 to 12 months

Complications
- Tinea capitis: because of a hypersensitivity reaction to the fungus, a kerion (boggy, exudative area on scalp) may form; may lead to permanent hair loss and scarring
- Fungal infections may be complicated by bacterial superinfections

Candidiasis

Description
- Yeast-like fungus that proliferates and causes infections on moist cutaneous and mucosal sites in susceptible individuals when local immunity is disturbed

Etiology
- *Candida* species (*Candida albicans* most common) that are normal inhabitants of mucosal surfaces and intestinal tract of healthy individuals

Incidence and Demographics
- Frequently seen in older adults, especially in diabetics, and in immunocompromised individuals
- Both sexes equally and all races can be affected

Risk Factors
- Predisposing factors that alter local immunity
- Immunocompromised states, HIV
- Chronic debilitation, inability to perform personal hygiene
- Chemotherapy
- Diabetes or polyendocrinopathy
- Systemic broad-spectrum antibiotic therapy
- Moisture from repeated immersion in water or urine
- Obesity with redundant skin folds
- Occlusive clothing that traps moisture (adult diapers, incontinence pads, rubber boots)
- Hyperhidrosis (excessive sweating)
- Corticosteroid use

Prevention and Screening
- Management of underlying predisposing factors such as obesity, DM, etc.
- Avoid occlusive clothing, repetitive moisture exposure
- Frequent toileting of incontinent older adults
- Limitation of corticosteroid use

Assessment
History
- Pruritic and or burning sensation and "rash" in characteristic locations such as intertriginous areas, anogenital region and redundant skin folds (often under pendulous breasts, in the axillae, or under redundant folds of an obese abdomen)
- Painful or sensitive white "stuck on" lesions of the oral mucosa with decreased taste and odynophagia ("thrush")
- Corners of mouth thickened with slight erythema (perlèche or angular cheilitis)
- White, curd-like vaginal discharge usually associated with pruritus, external dysuria and dyspareunia (vulvovaginitis)
- Painful fissuring of foreskin in uncircumcised males with dysuria and dyspareunia (balanoposthitis)
- Painful, inflamed nail folds, discolored nails, and a creamy discharge (paronychial candidiasis)
- Painful, congested ear canal with moist exudate (otitis externa)

Physical Exam
- Bright red, smooth macules
- Maceration is typical of all intertriginous infections
- Scaling, elevated border
- "Satellite" lesions: similar macules outside main lesion
- Oral and vaginal candidiasis; white, stuck-on but removable plaques on inflamed mucosa
- Balanoposthitis: flattened pustules, edema, erosions, fissuring on erythematous surface
- Candida otitis externa: edematous ear canal with macerated appearance and moist, white, scaly exudate

Diagnostic Studies
- Diagnosis is based on clinical appearance
- 5% KOH preparation under microscope demonstrates buds and pseudohyphae in clusters
- Fungal culture may be done; C. *albicans* will grow on fungal media within 48 to 72 hours

Differential Diagnosis
Oral candidiasis
- Hairy leukoplakia
- Pernicious anemia
- Geographic tongue
- Apthous ulcers
- Bite irritation

Genital candidiasis
- Bacterial vaginosis
- Lichen planus
- Scabies
- Condyloma acuminatum
- Erythrasma
- Inverse-pattern psoriasis

Intertriginous areas
- Eczema
- Atopic dermatitis
- Contact dermatitis
- Dermatophytosis

Paronychial candidiasis
- Herpetic whitlow
- S. *aureus* paronychia

Management
Nonpharmacologic
- Management of underlying predisposing factors such as obesity, DM, etc.
- Air exposure to affected areas in older adults who are incontinent
- Careful drying of intertriginous areas and redundant skin folds
- Wearing cotton undergarments and avoiding tight, synthetic clothing
- If incontinent, change incontinence briefs frequently

Pharmacologic

- Oral candidiasis: nystatin oral suspension 200,000 to 400,000 units, swish in mouth and swallow 5x/day, Clotrimazole 10 mg troches 5x/day, systemic fluconazole 200 mg once then 100 mg daily
- Cutaneous candidiasis: Topical antifungals:
  - Imidazoles: clotrimazole 1% cream twice daily, miconazole 2% cream twice daily, ketoconazole 2% cream once daily, econazole (Spectazole) 1% cream twice daily
  - Ciclopirox (Loprox) twice daily
  - Nystatin (Mycostatin) twice daily
- Vulvovaginal candidiasis: topical antifungals or oral fluconazole (Diflucan 150 mg) given once
- Oral antifungal treatment may be necessary in extensive or recurrent infections or when host immunity is suppressed
- Length of treatment:
  - Oral candidiasis: 10 to 14 days
  - Cutaneous candidiasis: 1 to several weeks depending on extent of the infection and the immune status of the host
  - Paronychial candidiasis: 2 to 4 weeks

Special Considerations

- Immunosuppressed patients are subject to extensive and recurrent infections and may require a daily maintenance dose to limit recurrences

When to Refer, Consult, Hospitalize

- Candidiasis may lead to fungal septicemia requiring hospitalization
- Immunosuppressed patients with extensive or severe candidiasis, particularly oral/esophageal candidiasis, may require hospitalization or home IV infusion therapy of amphotericin B and nutrition supplementation

Follow-up

Expected Outcomes

- Resolution can be expected in patients without immunosuppression; however, other predisposing factors such as obesity and poorly controlled diabetes mellitus may make recurrences common
- Patients should be seen in follow-up in 2 to 4 weeks and p.r.n. to evaluate progress

Complications

- Bacterial superinfection of excoriated lesions
- Weight loss secondary to odynophagia with esophagitis

BACTERIAL INFECTIONS OF SKIN

Cellulitis

Description

- Acute infection of the dermis and subcutaneous tissues

Etiology

- *Staphylococcus aureus* and Group A β-hemolytic streptococci most common causative agents
- *Streptococcus agalactiae* (Group B)

- Gram-negative bacilli, anaerobes such as:
  - *Escherichia coli*
  - *Pseudomonas aeruginosa*
  - *Clostridium spp.*

Incidence and Demographics
- Common in older adults, particularly those with comorbid diseases such as diabetes or those with immunodeficiency

Risk Factors
- Older adults with chronic diseases and age-related factors that delay wound healing
- Breaks in skin from trauma (lacerations, abrasions, excoriation, pressure ulcers, skin tears)
- Underlying dermatosis, stasis ulcers with dermatitis
- Diabetes mellitus
- Hematologic malignancies
- Chronic lymphedema (following mastectomy or coronary artery grafting)
- Immunocompromise
- Previous episodes of cellulitis

Prevention and Screening
- Avoid scratching; maintain short, clean nails
- Educate diabetic patient to examine feet daily for any breaks in skin, lubricate to prevent cracking of skin

Assessment
History
- May be unaware of original break in skin
- Possible history of fungal infection or dermatitis of the affected area
- Possible fever, malaise, anorexia, pain that is increased with weight bearing or dependency

Physical Exam
- Erythema, induration, and pain are the classic signs, often accompanied by systemic symptoms such as malaise, fever, chills
- Decreased age-related immune response may lessen clinical signs of infection
- Puncture wound, fissure, pressure ulcer, skin tear, or laceration may be visible
- Erythematous plaque that is edematous, hot and tender with sharply defined, irregular border
- Vesicles, bullae, abscesses may be seen within the plaque
- Lymphangitis–surrounding erythematous streaking
- Regional lymphadenopathy
- Systemic toxic signs may be present especially if involved area large, patient immunocompromised
- Necrotizing fasciitis, deep infection of subcutaneous tissue appears as a large erythematous plaque with a central area of necrosis; ß-hemolytic streptococci usually invading organism; staph may or may not be involved

Diagnostic Studies
- Cultures are usually not warranted and result in false negatives in about 75% of cases
- WBCs and sedimentation rate are indicated if the patient appears toxic

Differential Diagnosis
- Deep vein thrombosis or thrombophlebitis
- Early contact dermatitis
- Giant urticaria
- Fixed drug eruption
- Erythema migrans
- Early herpes zoster
- Necrotizing fasciitis
- Gas gangrene

Management
Nonpharmacologic
- Manage underlying conditions such as tinea pedis, lymphedema, venous insufficiency
- Rest, elevate involved extremity (bed rest if leg is involved)
- Application of moist heat (closely monitored secondary to increased risk of burn)

Pharmacologic
- Treatment decisions are based on extent of infection; patients may require IV therapy for more severe symptoms
- Antibiotics with activity against β-hemolytic streptococci and S. *aureus*
  - Dicloxacillin 250 to 500 mg 4 times daily for 7 to 10 days
  - Cephalexin 250 to 500 mg 4 times daily for 7 to 10 days
  - Erythromycin 250 to 500 mg 4 times daily for patients with penicillin allergy
- MRSA (community-acquired)
  - Clindamycin 300 to 400 mg oral every 6 to 8 hours
- Trimethoprim-sulfamethoxazole 2 double-strength tabs oral every 12 hours
- Doxycycline or minocycline 100 mg oral twice daily
  - NSAIDs p.r.n. analgesia, fever, decreased inflammation (risk of gastritis, UGI bleed)
- Treat for 7 to 10 days depending on the extent of involvement

Special Considerations
- Immunocompromised patients and patients with synthetic heart valves: greater risk of toxicity, may warrant hospitalization
- Medical management of predisposing conditions such as diabetes, IV drug use, malignancies or chronic lymphedema will augment treatment
- Immunocompromised patients as well as patients on dialysis may be more prone to develop infections from drug-resistant bacteria

When to Consult, Refer, Hospitalize
- Consult with infectious disease specialist if the patient is not responding
- A toxic patient may require transfer to a hospital
- Hospitalization and surgery may be necessary to debride the necrotic tissue and prevent further tissue damage

- Facial cellulitis (erysipelas) may require hospitalization to prevent spread of infection to brain and to monitor for and manage obstructive symptoms if they occur
- Orbital cellulitis (exopthalmos, orbital pain, restricted eye movement, visual disturbances) is an emergency and should be treated with emergency evaluation

Follow-up
Expected Outcomes
- Clinical response to treatment may be difficult to assess if initial site also has age-related changes
- Erythematous plaque should be outlined with an indelible pen on initial assessment; patient should return daily for monitoring of progression or regression of the involved area
- Incremental improvement should be noted and documented and resolution expected in 5 to 10 days depending on the initial level of involvement, and patient's compliance with therapeutic regimen of elevation, antibiotics, and moist heat compresses

Complications
- Toxicity or septicemia
- Meningitis or respiratory distress secondary to occlusion from head and neck cellulitis
- Diabetic patients may potentially require amputation because of severe cellulitis

Abscess, Furuncle, and Carbuncle
Description
- Abscess: a circumscribed collection of purulent exudate associated with tissue destruction and inflammation that may arise from any organ or structure
- Furuncle ("boil"): an infection of a hair follicle that extends through the dermis into the subcutaneous tissue where a small abscess forms; usually caused by S. *aureus*
  - Furunculosis refers to several discrete furuncles
- Carbuncle: deeper infection, arising in several contiguous inflamed follicles that are interconnected by sinus tracts; involves subcutaneous tissue; may have several pustular openings onto skin; may be associated with systemic symptoms of fever and malaise

Etiology
- Usually S. *aureus*, rarely other bacteria

Incidence and Demographics
- Often seen in older adults with chronic illness, such as DM, obesity
- Sex: male > female

Risk Factors
- Chronic staph carrier state (nares, axillae, anogenital, intestine)
- Close contact with individuals with active infection with skin abscesses, furuncles, and carbuncles
- Diabetes
- Immunodeficiency
- Poor hygiene, inability to perform hygiene
- Metabolic abnormalities (chronic granulomatosis, high serum IgE)

Prevention and Screening
- Education about good hygiene, improving the status of underlying predisposing factors such as diabetes

Assessment
History
- Painful, hot lesion developing over days
- Sometimes accompanied by systemic symptoms of fever and malaise
- Predisposing factors or history of prior abscesses, furuncles, or carbuncles

Physical Exam
- Abscess: initially tender, fluctuant, erythematous nodule that frequently is surrounded by erythematous swelling
  - Central fluctuance found in a fully developed or "ripe" abscess
- Furuncle: firm, tender nodule with a central necrotic plug, fluctuant below plug, usually with a pustule over the plug
- Carbuncle: several adjacent, coalescing furuncles with multiple, loculated abscesses, draining pustules and necrotic plugs
  - Distribution commonly on back of the neck, face, axillae, and buttocks

Diagnostic Studies
- Laboratory studies usually not indicated
- Gram staining usually demonstrates Gram-positive cocci with multiple polymorpho-nuclear neutrophils (PMNs)
- Culture and sensitivity may be done to confirm *S. aureus* or identify methicillin-resistant *S. aureus* or other bacteria that may be resistant to treatment
- Blood cultures are indicated if the patient remains febrile or appears toxic

Differential Diagnosis
- Ruptured epidermal or pilar cyst
- Folliculitis
- Hydradenitis suppurativa
- Necrotizing HSV

Management
Nonpharmacologic
- Warm moist compresses or sitz baths × 10 minutes every 2 to 3 hours for small furuncles
- Surgical treatment
  - Larger furuncles, all carbuncles and all abscesses require incision and drainage with material sent for culture and sensitivity testing
  - Sterile packing is often necessary to allow the incision to continue to drain

Pharmacologic
- Topical antibiotics are usually not effective in treating acute abscess, furuncle, or carbuncle
- Mupirocin ointment (Bactroban) 3 times daily to nares is helpful in eliminating chronic *S. aureus* carrier state
- Systemic antibiotic therapy should cover *S. aureus*:
  - Cephalexin (Keflex) 250 to 500 mg 4 times daily
  - Dicloxacillin 250 to 500 mg 4 times daily
- Empiric antibiotic therapy for abscesses, furuncles, and carbuncles should include activity against MRSA in areas of high MRSA prevalence:
  - Trimethoprim-sulfamethoxazole DS twice daily
  - Doxycycline or minocycline 100 mg twice daily
  - Clindamycin 300 to 450 mg every 6 to 8 hours

    – Vancomycin IV for severe infections

    – Treat for 7 to 10 days

Special Considerations
- Diabetic patients may have delayed wound healing
- Individuals at risk for endocarditis should receive antibiotic prophylaxis prior to incision and drainage (vancomycin 1 gm IV 1 hour before the procedure)

When to Consult, Refer, Hospitalize
- Referral to general surgery is indicated for extensive abscess involvement

Follow-up
Expected Outcomes
- Follow up daily initially to monitor response to therapy and to remove packing from surgical site

Complications
- Rarely endocarditis from manipulation of abscess
- Rare cavernous sinus thrombosis from manipulation of abscess near nasolabial folds

VIRAL SKIN INFECTIONS

Herpes Zoster
Description
- "Shingles"; acute, painful, unilateral, cutaneous infection in dermatomal distribution

Etiology
- Varicella zoster virus (VZV) usually contracted in childhood as chickenpox
- Lies dormant in a nerve ganglion until reactivation of virus causes eruption along course of the nerve
- Reactivation related to age-related declines in immune function and immunodeficiency

Incidence and Demographics
- Occurs most often in persons over 50; less than 10% of cases occur under age 20
- In those over 75 years, more than 10 cases per 1000

Risk Factors
- Found in patients without immunosuppression, but severity of disease is increased if immunocompromised, such as with decreased immunity of the aged
- Advanced age
- Stress

Prevention and Screening
- Most (90%) of adult population in the United States today is positive for anti-VZV antibodies
- Varicella vaccine now included in routine childhood immunization schedule may prevent development of herpes zoster in later life
- Varicella vaccine later in life when anti-VZV antibodies are declining may be effective in preventing development of herpes zoster

Assessment
History
- Frequently pain (piercing, stabbing, boring), paresthesias (tingling, burning, itching), and allodynia (heightened sensitivity to mild stimuli) preceding eruption by 3 to 5 days along neuronal pathway
- Generalized malaise, fever, and headache in about 5%

Physical
- Initially grouped vesicles along a unilateral dermatomal pathway followed by bullae within 2 days (more than one contiguous dermatome may be involved but noncontiguous dermatome involvement is rare)
- By day 4, bullae become pustules, followed by crusting in 7 to 10 days
- Lesions occur on erythematous, edematous cutaneous base

Diagnostic Studies
- Tzanck test, serum VZV antibodies, viral culture
- EKG to rule out cardiac etiology, x-ray to rule out pleural or abdominal etiology, ultrasound to rule out cholelithiasis/nephrolithiasis

Differential Diagnosis
Prodromal stage
- Migraine
- Cardiac or pleuritic pain
- Acute abdomen
- Disc disease

Vesicular-crusting stage
- Herpes simplex
- Contact dermatitis
- Erysipelas
- Bullous impetigo
- Necrotizing fasciitis

Management
Nonpharmacologic
- Moist dressings (water, normal saline, or Burow solution) or colloidal oatmeal suspension (Aveeno) may decrease pain

Pharmacologic
- Treatment with antivirals should begin within 72 hours of onset of symptoms; if started early, treatment can shorten the course of HZ and reduce post-herpetic neuralgia
  - Acyclovir (Zovirax) 800 mg 5 times daily
  - Valacyclovir (Valtrex) 1000 mg 3 times daily
  - Famciclovir (Famvir) 500 mg evert 8 hours
  - Antiviral therapy should continue for 7 to 10 days
- Pain management with non-narcotic and narcotic pain medications
- Gabapentin (start at 100 mg q.d.) or nortriptyline (start at 10 mg QHS) may be used to manage chronic pain of post-herpetic neuralgia
- Capsaicin ointment (0.025%–0.075%) t.i.d.-q.i.d. may be tried for postherpetic neuralgia (not to be applied to open lesions; burning sensation may be intolerable)

Special Considerations
- May become disseminated in immunocompromised patients; if so, requires hospitalization or in-home IV therapy
- Monitor hydration and renal function of frail older adults on antiviral medication

When to Consult, Refer, Hospitalize
- Disseminated disease should be evaluated for malignancy, immunodeficiency, or AIDS
- Ophthalmology consult if cranial nerve V affected

Follow-up
Expected Outcomes
- Initial course generally resolved in 2 to 3 weeks, although postherpetic neuralgia may persist for months or years

Complications
- Postherpetic neuralgia: may be long-term, need chronic pain management; older adults at greater risk, with 20% to 50% affected; severity of acute phase does not predict the risk or severity of postinfection neuralgia
- Local hemorrhage, gangrene, or superinfection
- Systemic meningoencephalitis, cerebral vascular syndrome, cranial nerve syndromes (ophthalmic, trigeminal, facial, and auditory), peripheral motor weakness

PARASITIC INFESTATIONS
Scabies
Description
- Infestation by mite, spread by direct contact leading to generalized pruritus, which is a hypersensitivity reaction to the scabies

Etiology
- *Sarcoptes scabiei* that thrive and multiply only on human skin; spread by human-to-human contact; mites may live up to 2 days on clothing and bed linens
- Sensitization to S. *scabiei* must occur prior to developing generalized pruritus associated with infestation
- In initial infestation, sensitization takes about 10 days; subsequent infestations advance to pruritic stage much more quickly

Incidence and Demographics
- Common in older adults and those living in residential facilities
- Epidemics occur in cycles

Risk Factors
- Exposure to others with scabies
- Institutional living particularly in those with neurologic disorders and dementia
- Crusted scabies
- Immunocompromised status

Prevention and Screening
- Education about the mode of transmission

Assessment

History

- Often history of family members or close contacts with similar symptoms
- Severe generalized pruritus, sparing head and neck
- Pruritus and scratching often interfere with sleep

Physical Exam

- Scattered vesicles, burrows, or nodules with excoriations
- Common distribution: axillae, anogenital region, flexures of the wrists and arms, interdigital spaces of the hands, waist, buttocks
- May develop generalized erythroderma
- May also develop lichen simplex chronicus from chronic scratching
- In atopic individuals, an eczematous dermatitis is common
- Postinflammatory hyperpigmentation may occur
- Secondary infections to denuded sites are common
- Crusted vesicles or burrows result after infestation of several months
- Classic burrow (straight or S-shaped ridge) is present < 20% of the time

Diagnostic Studies

- Serum eosinophilia
- "Scabies prep": drop of mineral oil placed over a burrow and burrow scraped with a blade; mites and their eggs or fecal droppings can be collected and placed on a slide with mineral oil and a coverslip to be examined under the microscope

Differential Diagnosis

- Drug-eruption dermatitis
- Atopic or contact dermatitis
- Pityriasis rosea
- Herpetiform dermatitis
- Pediculosis dermatitis
- Insect bites
- Delusions of parasitosis
- Metabolic pruritus

Management

Nonpharmacologic

- Not effective alone
- Wash bedding and clothing after application of medication

Pharmacologic

- Management of pruritus relies on pharmacologic eradication of mites and their eggs and pharmacologic treatment of pruritus
- Permethrin 5% cream applied from neck down and left on overnight (8 to 14 hours) once, then washed off; treatment should be repeated in 1 week
  - One-time treatment with permethrin may be effective but a repeat treatment in 1 week is often necessary to eliminate infestation
- A tapered course of systemic steroids starting at 70 to 80 mg daily and tapering by 5 mg daily is often necessary to treat widespread pruritus
  - Systemic steroids are generally tapered over 10 to 14 days
- Topical steroids may be applied twice daily to severely pruritic areas

Special Considerations
- Lesions may appear as excoriations on the back of older adults
- All household contacts and facility residents and staff should be identified and treated and all clothing and bedding must be washed in hot water and dried on the hot cycle of the dryer.

When to Consult, Refer, Hospitalize
- When resolution is not achieved with above regimen

Follow-up
Expected Outcomes
- Mites may be eradicated with one or possibly two treatments with the above medications, but the generalized pruritus may persists for several weeks since it is a hypersensitivity reaction to the mite
- Patients should be brought back for follow-up in 1 to 2 weeks and then at weekly intervals if there is extensive dermatitis

Complications
- Secondary bacterial infection, abscesses, and cellulitis are possible complications as a result of the associated scratching

MISCELLANEOUS

Rosacea
Description
- Persistent erythema of central area of face lasting at least 3 months
- Characterized by 4 subtypes: erythematotelangiectatic rosacea (ETR), papulopustular rosacea (PPR), phymatous rosacea, and ocular rosacea

Etiology
- Etiology is unknown; however, several factors likely play a role in development, including vasculature, climatic exposures, matrix degeneration, chemicals and ingested agents, pilosebaceous unit abnormalities, and microbial organisms

Incidence and Demographics
- Frequently seen in older adults
- Commonly found in fair-skinned, middle-aged to older adults
- Severe form with rhinophyma is seen almost exclusively in men over 40

Risk Factors
- Found more commonly in individuals with fair skin (skin phototypes I, II, and III; see Table 6–5) due to increased sensitivity to sun exposure
- Positive family history of rosacea is a risk factor
- Excessive ETOH consumption is associated with flares

Prevention and Screening
- Identify triggers and provide education about avoiding trigger factors such as hot or cold temperatures, wind, hot beverages, caffeine, spicy food, alcohol
- Use of sunscreen that protects against ultraviolet A and B

Assessment

History

- History of abnormal flushing of the central portion of the face after drinking hot beverages or eating spicy foods or with heat, emotion, and other causes of rapid body temperature changes
- Symptoms usually intermittent
- May report "gritty" sensation in the eyes

Table 6-5. Skin Phototype Based on Sun Sensitivity

Skin Type	Sunburn and Tanning History
I	Always burns easily; rarely tans
II	Always burns easily; tans minimally
III	Burns moderately; tans gradually and uniformly to a light brown color
IV	Burns minimally, always tans well to moderate brown color
V	Rarely burns; tans profusely to dark brown color
VI	Rarely burns; deeply pigmented black color

Physical Exam

- Variable erythema and telangectasias across cheeks and forehead
- Inflammatory 2 to 3 mm papular and pustular discrete and clustered lesions on the central portion of the face on any erythematous base
- Ocular symptoms may be associated and include blepharitis, conjunctivitis
- Chronic symptoms can lead to periorbital lymphedema causing cellulitis
- Irreversible hypertrophy of the nose, rhinophyma, is a result of chronic inflammation and is seen almost exclusively in men over 40

Diagnostic Studies

- Based on clinical presentation; culture or biopsy is not necessary

Differential Diagnosis

- Acne vulgaris
- Butterfly rash of SLE
- Folliculitis
- Pustular tinea

Management

Nonpharmacologic

- Avoid triggers that cause facial flushing such as hot beverages, alcohol, highly spicy foods, exposure to sun and wind, emotional stress, certain medications such as niacin
- Apply sunscreen that protects against ultraviolet A and B light
- Use mild cleansers

Pharmacologic

- Topical metronidazole 0.75%, erythromycin 2%, or clindamycin 1% topical gel b.i.d.
- Tetracycline 250 to 500 mg twice daily, doxycycline 50 to 100 mg once or twice daily; after 4 weeks of control, gradually attempt taper over the next 4 weeks; long-term therapy may be necessary
- Erythromycin 250 mg twice to 4 times daily is an alternative

- Treat initially for 4 to 6 weeks, but will likely require ongoing, long-term maintenance therapy

Special Considerations
- ASA may be given to lessen the flushing associated with niacin cholesterol therapy

When to Consult, Refer, Hospitalize
- If suboptimal response with above regimen, refer to dermatology
- Referral for surgical intervention if patient has rhinophyma unresponsive to topical or oral therapy

Follow-up
Expected Outcomes
- Response usually seen in 3 weeks; maximum response from one regimen usually seen by 9 weeks

Complications
- Rhinophyma as described above

Burns
Description
- Damage to the epidermis, dermis, or subcutaneous tissue caused by electrical, thermal, or chemical agents

Etiology
- Exposure to intense heat of fire or steam (thermal), chemicals, or electricity

Incidence and Demographics
- Approximately 2 million burn injuries annually in the United States; 80% are minor
- Flame and scald injuries most common in older adults
- Scald burns more common in patients with early dementia

Risk Factors
- Unsupervised older adults with dementia or progressive debilitating diseases
- Exposure to scalding liquids (steam), chemicals, or electricity at home or nursing facility

Prevention and Screening
- Fire safety and safe handling of hot liquids, chemicals, and electricity education in the community; caretakers to review home for risk factors
- Lower thermostat of water heater
- Ensure functional smoke detectors
- Educate patients and families regarding safe use of heating pads
- Practice evacuation drills in community settings, homes, and nursing facilities

Assessment
History
- Exposure to fire, chemicals, scalding liquids or electricity
- Intense pain and site of exposure (third-degree burns are usually painless)

Physical Exam
- Burns classified by extent and depth of tissue involvement, patient age, and associated illness or injury
- Extent of involvement can be measured by using the "rule of nines" (see Table 6–6)

Table 6–6. Rule of Nines

Body Part Affected	Percentage
Anterior head and neck	4.5%
Posterior head and neck	4.5%
Torso and abdomen	18%
Back	18%
Anterior arms	4.5% each
Posterior arms	4.5% each
Genitalia	1%
Anterior legs	9% each
Posterior legs	9% each

- Another estimate of extent of involvement is to equate the patient's palm size as 1% of total body surface area (TBSA)
- Depth of injury described as superficial, partial-thickness, or full-thickness burn injury
  - Superficial burns: involve the epidermis only; redness and blanching erythema (demonstrating capillary refill) of affected area with no initial blistering
  - Partial-thickness burns: involve entire epidermis and variable portions of the dermis; red, moist and edematous skin with small or large bullae
  - Full-thickness burns: involve entire dermis and subcutaneous tissue; pale, white, tan, or charred wound that may appear dry and depressed below surrounding skin; skin may feel tight and leathery
- American Burn Association Burn Injury Severity Grading System
  - Patients over 50 years of age considered "high risk"
  - Patients with underlying illnesses such as cardiac disease, respiratory disease, and diabetes are considered "low risk"
  - Minor:
    - Superficial or partial-thickness burn of < 5% TBSA in adults > age 50
    - Full-thickness burn of < 2% TBSA in all age groups
  - Moderate:
    - Superficial or partial-thickness burn of 5%–10% TBSA in adults > age 50
    - Full-thickness burn of 2%–5% TBSA in all age groups
    - High-voltage injury, suspected inhalation injury, or circumferential burn
    - Medical problem predisposing to infection (e.g., diabetes mellitus)
  - Major:
    - Superficial or partial-thickness burn of > 10 percent TBSA in adults > age 50
    - Full-thickness burn of > 5% in all age groups
    - High-voltage burn, known inhalation injury
    - Any significant burn to face, eyes, ears, genitalia, or joints
    - Significant associated injuries (fracture or other major trauma)

Diagnostic Studies
- Immediate clinical triage is essential to allow patients to be treated in most appropriate setting
- CBC, electrolytes, BUN, creatinine, glucose, urinalysis, and tissue culture may be necessary in more serious injury
- CXR indicated if suspected inhalation injury

Differential Diagnosis
- Chemical burn
- Electrical burn
- Thermal burn
- Ritter disease
- Scalded skin syndrome

Management
- Only minor burns with no associated injuries should be managed in the outpatient setting
- Emergency stabilization of patients with moderate or major burns

Nonpharmacologic
- If burn is chemical, remove offending agent and irrigate skin
- Burns involving eye should be irrigated with water, saline, or lactated Ringer solution
- Wound should be cleaned and debrided using plain soap and water or saline solution; any dead skin should be removed
- Elevate involved extremities

Pharmacologic
- Topical silver sulfadiazine (Silvadene) in a ½-inch layer over entire surface, covered with nonabsorbent gauze (Kerlix or Telfa) and wrapped in at least a three-inch-thick nonadhesive wrap
- Analgesia with narcotics
- Tetanus prophylaxis
- Antibiotic coverage for superinfection
- Dressing changes twice daily until resolution, with frequent reevaluation

Special Considerations
- Patient's age and health status is critical; even a minor burn in an older adult patient can be fatal
- Older adults or debilitated patients are at higher risk for hemodynamic compromise

When To Consult, Refer, and Hospitalize
- Emergency referral for moderate or major burns
- Emergency referral for burns that can result in functional or cosmetic impairment, have an associated injury, or affect a high-risk patient
- Emergency referral for suspected toxic epidermal necrolysis syndrome
- Consultation with a wound specialist for wounds that do not show signs of improvement with treatment
- Consultation with a psychiatrist as needed

Follow-up

Expected Outcomes
- Depends on the extent and location of the burn

Complications
- Local infection and inflammation
- Hemodynamic compromise
- Multiorgan failure
- Sepsis
- Scarring
- Posttraumatic stress disorder
- Increased photosensitivity of healed skin

TUMORS

Seborrheic Keratosis

Description
- Common benign tumors that appear in later adulthood, developing from proliferation of epidermal cells
- Normal changes with age

Etiology
- Etiology is unknown, though epidermal growth factors or their receptors have been implicated in the development of seborrheic keratoses
- Probable autosomal dominant inheritance
- Results from proliferation of keratinocytes, melanocytes, and plugged follicles

Incidence and Demographics
- Most common benign tumor in older adults
- Often seen in older adults secondary to photoaging; reticulated type may develop from solar lentigines
- Less common in populations with dark skin compared to those with white skin

Risk Factors
- Family history
- Excessive sun exposure

Prevention and Screening
- Use of sunscreen and protective clothing when in the sun
- Complete skin exam annually

Assessment
History
- Gradual onset of one or more skin lesions that appear sharply defined, brown, and flat
- "Stuck on" appearance
- Typically asymptomatic, but may be mildly pruritic or inflamed; painful if secondarily infected
- Family history may be present

Physical Exam

- Initially < 1 cm scattered and discrete, lightly tan-colored round or oval macules arising on normal skin that appear on the face, trunk, and upper extremities
- Lesions slowly develop into a slightly raised papule or plaque that has usually darkened in color to brown, gray, or black
- "Stuck on" appearance with a warty surface and multiple plugged follicles or "horny cysts"

Diagnostic Studies

- Usually not indicated
- Biopsy should be done if diagnosis is unclear; rule out carcinoma or melanoma

Differential Diagnosis

- Solar lentigo
- Actinic keratosis
- Basal cell carcinoma
- Squamous cell carcinoma
- Malignant melanoma
- Verruca vulgaris

Management

- No treatment is indicated unless lesion is symptomatic or causes cosmetic problems

Nonpharmacologic

- Electrocautery, cryosurgery, and curettage

Special Considerations

- Patients with a history of actinic keratosis or skin cancer should have lesions biopsied by an experienced clinician; special attention should be paid to excising with a margin around the borders to rule out malignant lesions

When to Consult, Refer, Hospitalize

- Dermatology consult for excision and biopsy if primary care clinician is not experienced with excision procedures or if sudden appearance of multiple pruritic seborrheic keratoses (Leser-Trélat sign)
- Oncology consult for malignant lesions

Follow-up

Expected Outcomes

- Lesions are considered benign and may continue to develop throughout a lifetime
- Lesions may recur after removal or destruction with cryosurgery
- Follow-up for patients with multiple lesions is important because malignant tumors may develop elsewhere on the body

Complications

- Inflammation
- Secondary infection

Actinic/Solar Keratosis

Description
- Discrete, dry, scaly lesions occurring on prolonged or recurrently sun-exposed skin of susceptible adults
- Often precursor to squamous cell carcinoma (SCC)

Etiology
- Recurrent or prolonged sun exposure

Incidence and Demographics:
- Common in older adults secondary to photoaging of skin
- Males more commonly than females
- Appears in middle adulthood, earlier in Australia and the southwestern United States

Risk Factors
- Fair skin
- Prolonged or recurrent unprotected sun exposure
- Outdoors work or frequent outdoor sports

Prevention and Screening
- Education about the risks of unprotected sun exposure
- Use of sunblock and protective clothing during periods of exposure

Assessment
History
- Gradual onset of light tan, brown, or red dry, roughened lesions on sun-exposed skin
- Minimal sensation but may be mildly tender
- May bleed if irritated

Physical Exam
- Single or multiple discrete adherent, hyperkeratotic, scaly papules or plaques on sun-exposed skin
- Base of lesion often erythematous
- Approximately 1 cm in size and round or oval
- Color ranges from light tan to brown with or without reddish tinge

Diagnostic Studies
- Biopsy demonstrates atypical keratinocytes

Differential Diagnosis
- Discoid lupus erythematosus
- Seborrheic keratosis
- Basal cell carcinoma
- Squamous cell carcinoma

Management
Nonpharmacologic
- Cryotherapy
- Curettage
- Photodynamic therapy

Pharmacologic
- Topical 5% 5-fluorouracil cream applied twice daily for 2 to 4 weeks
- Topical imiquimod 5% cream applied once daily, 2 to 3 days a week for 16 weeks
- Topical diclofenac 3% in hyaluronan 2.5% gel applied twice daily for 90 days

How Long to Treat
- Weeks

Special Considerations
- Identifying at-risk patients is essential

When to Consult, Refer, Hospitalize
- Dermatology for excision of large or extensive lesions or for management if primary care clinician is unfamiliar with excision and management protocols

Follow-up
Expected Outcomes
- Treatment is effective in eradicating lesions but vigilant follow-up is warranted to monitor for new lesions

Complications
- Squamous cell carcinoma in untreated lesions

Basal Cell Carcinoma (BCC)
Description
- Most commonly seen skin cancer
- Typically appears on sun-exposed skin
- Slow growing, rarely metastasizes
- Can become invasive and lead to local destruction or disfigurement if neglected

Etiology
- Excess sun exposure, particularly in fair-skinned individuals
- Tumors usually arise from basal cells in the epidermis or the outer root sheath of a hair follicle

Incidence and Demographics
- Accounts for 75% of 1 million cases of skin cancer diagnosed annually in the United States
- Basal cell carcinoma is the most common cancer in the United States today
- Age: 95% between 40 and 79 years
- Male > female
- Fair skin > dark skin (dark skin rarely affected)

Risk Factors
- Excess sun exposure (recreational or occupational)
- Fair skin with poor tanning ability
- Prior treatment with x-ray for facial acne, commonly used before 1950

Prevention and Screening
- Primary prevention involves avoiding sun exposure and using sun protection
- Secondary prevention involves screening for skin lesions with premalignant or malignant characteristics during routine health exams, referral for lesions of concern

- Tertiary prevention involves removal of precancerous lesions such as suspicious moles and actinic keratoses, usually done by dermatologist or surgeon

Assessment
History
- Slowly enlarging lesion, often on the face, that does not heal and may bleed with trauma
- Chronic sun exposure, either recreational (sunbathing, outdoor sports) or occupational (farming, construction)

Physical Exam
- 80% occur on head and neck, and 25% of lesions occur on the nose
- Firm, round, "pearly"-appearing papule with telangectasias on sun-exposed skin
- With enlargement, a central ulceration with a raised, rolled border may form ("rodent bite ulcer")
- Crusting may be present
- Pigmented lesions may be brown, blue, or black and are difficult to differentiate from melanoma
- Central umbilication possible

Diagnostic Studies
- Clinical diagnosis of suspicious lesions on sun-exposed skin
- Biopsy demonstrating atypical basal cells

Differential Diagnosis
- Molluscum contagiosum
- Solar lentigo
- Actinic keratosis
- Squamous cell carcinoma
- Malignant melanoma
- Verruca vulgaris

Management
Nonpharmacologic
- Excision, cryosurgery, or electrosurgery
- Mohs surgery: microscopically controlled surgery for lesions in the danger zones of nasolabial folds, around eyes, in ear canal, and in posterior auricular sulcus
- Radiation therapy is alternative in areas of possible cosmetic disfigurement

Pharmacologic
- Some topical treatments exist for some forms of BCC, though generally with lower cure rates than with surgery
- 5% 5-fluorouracil (superficial BCC), imiquimod cream (superficial BCC, indicated only when surgical methods are inappropriate)

Special Considerations
- Tumors on the nose or T-zone of the face have higher rates of recurrence

When to Consult, Refer, Hospitalize
- Refer to dermatologist for biopsy and excision of lesions or lesions with cosmetic disfigurement

Follow-up
Expected Outcomes
- Resolution with above therapies is the norm but at-risk patients should be monitored for new lesions
- Patients diagnosed with BCC have a 35% chance of developing another tumor within 3 years and a 50% chance of developing another BCC within 5 years

Complications
- Cosmetic disfigurement

Squamous Cell Carcinoma (SCC)

Description
- Second most common type of cutaneous carcinoma
- Capable of locally infiltrative growth, spread to regional lymph nodes, and distant metastasis

Etiology
- Malignant tumor of epithelial keratinocytes; develops on skin and mucous membranes
- Results from skin exposure to sunlight, arsenic ingestion, tobacco, ionizing radiation, HPV
- Bowen disease is a form of SCC arising de novo on any area of skin

Incidence and Demographics
- Incidence varies by location and skin color
- Estimates of annual incidence in the United States approximately 107 cases per 100,000 people
- Higher incidence in locations closer to the equator
- Age > 55
- Male > female
- More common than basal cell carcinoma in black individuals, occurring at sites of scars or chronic inflammation rather than sun-exposed areas

Risk Factors
- Fair skin with poor tanning ability
- Sun exposure, recreational or occupational
- Exposure to chemical carcinogens (e.g., arsenic, tar in tobacco)
- Exposure to ionizing radiation
- Chronic immunosuppression
- HPV infection

Prevention and Screening
- Education about the risks of unprotected sun exposure, tobacco use, arsenic ingestion, and radiation exposure
- Use of sunblock and protective clothing

Assessment
History
- Presence of one or more risk factors for SCC
- Suspicious new or enlarging skin lesion
- May be asymptomatic or have associated bleeding, weeping, pain, or tenderness

- Most often on sun-exposed skin (face, lips, hands, neck, and forearms)

Physical Exam
- Raised, firm skin-colored to erythematous papule, nodule, or plaque arising on sun-exposed skin
- Thick, adherent, keratotic scale or a cutaneous horn may be present
- Honey-colored exudate extruded from periphery
- May be eroded, crusted, ulcerated, hard, erythematous
- Isolated or multiple lesions

Diagnostic Studies
- Biopsy demonstrating atypical squamous cells
- Radiologic imaging in select patients

Differential Diagnosis
- Nummular eczema
- Psoriasis
- Paget disease
- Pyoderma gangrenosum
- Basal cell carcinoma
- Actinic keratosis

Management
Nonpharmacologic
- Surgery or radiation depending on the size, shape, and location of the tumor
- Surgical excision via cryotherapy, electrodessication and curettage, excision, or Mohs micrographic surgery

Pharmacologic
- Topical chemotherapy (5-fluorouracil), topical immune response modifiers (imiquimod), photodynamic therapy (PDT)
- Systemic chemotherapy reserved for metastatic disease

Special Considerations
- Patients who develop one SCC have a 40% risk of developing additional SCC within the next 2 years

When to Consult, Refer, Hospitalize
- Refer to dermatology for microscopically controlled surgery
- Refer to head and neck surgeons for cases involving metastases
- Adjuvant or palliative radiotherapy by a radiation oncologist may be necessary

Follow-up
Expected Outcomes
- Remission achieved in 90% of cases, though recurrence is common
- Patients with a history of SCC should be evaluated with a complete skin examination every 6 to 12 months

Complications
- Recurrence or metastasis

Malignant Melanoma (MM)

Description
- Least common but most lethal of all cutaneous carcinomas
- Malignancy of pigment-producing cells (melanocytes) located predominantly in the skin; also found in the eyes, ears, GI tract, leptomeninges, and oral and genital mucous membranes

Etiology
- Proliferation of malignant melanocytes that results from a process of progressive genetic mutations

Incidence and Demographics
- 4% of all cutaneous carcinomas in the United States
- Incidence rates rising dramatically over past 2 decades with estimated lifetime risk for developing invasive melanoma of 1 in 60 Americans
- There is greater incidence and risk for death among older adults
- Primarily a malignancy of White individuals, though mortality rates are higher in Blacks and Hispanics

Risk Factors
- Family history
- Excessive sun exposure
- Severe sunburn, particularly at an early age
- Outdoor occupations
- Fair skin

Prevention and Screening
- Education about the risks of unprotected sun exposure and genetic predisposition
- Patient information regarding the ABCDE criteria:
  - Asymmetry
  - Border irregularity
  - Color variegation
  - Diameter (> 6 mm or enlarging)
  - Evolving

Assessment
History
- New or changing mole or skin lesion
- Changes or variation in color, diameter, height, or irregular borders of skin lesion
- Bleeding, itching, ulceration, or pain are less common but may be present

Physical
- Can occur on any skin or mucosal surface
- Occurs most commonly on the trunk in White males and on the back and lower legs of White females
- Plantar surface of the foot is the most common site in Black, Hispanic, and Asian persons
- Characteristics vary by type:
  - Superficial spreading melanoma (SSM)
    - Commonly in individuals aged 30 to 50 years

- Found on the trunk in men and women and on the legs in women
- Flat or slightly elevated brown lesion with variegate pigmentation (black, blue, pink, white)
- > 6 mm in diameter, irregular borders
- Nodular melanoma (NM)
  - 15% to 30% of patients with melanoma have this subtype
  - Occurs in 5th or 6th decade, grows rapidly over weeks to months
  - Commonly found on the legs and trunk
  - Dark brown, red, or black papule or nodule with variety of shapes; frequent crusting and bleeding
- Lentigo maligna melanoma (LMM)
  - 6th or 7th decade, found on the head, neck, and arms of fair-skinned individuals
  - Starts as nonmelanoma with slow progression; better prognosis
  - Precursor lesion is brown/black color; may stay flat, often with irregular borders
  - Hypopigmented (white) areas are common within the lesion
- Acral-lentiginous melanoma (ALM)
  - Least common subtype, but most common melanoma in dark-skinned individuals
  - Seen on palms, soles, terminal phalanges (beneath nail plate), mucous membranes
  - Brown/black, usually flat; elevated lesions very aggressive

Diagnostic Studies
- Biopsy including margins and depth of invasion assessment
- Lymph node biopsy is also indicated in most cases
- If primary tumor > 1 mm in depth, chest x-ray may be indicated for staging purposes

Differential Diagnosis
- Benign nevi
- Pigmented basal cell carcinoma
- Vitiligo
- Lentigo
- Seborrheic keratosis
- Squamous cell carcinoma

Management
Nonpharmacologic
- Surgery is the main mode of therapy for localized melanoma
- Aggressive surgical management by excision with margins intact
- Lymph node dissection may be indicated

Pharmacologic
- Adjuvant interferon alpha-2b is the only adjuvant therapy currently approved by the U.S. Food and Drug Administration for high-risk melanoma

Special Considerations
- Advanced age may limit treatment options because of comorbid conditions, decreased ability to tolerate adverse medication effects or toxicity, increased risk for drug interactions

When to Consult, Refer, Hospitalize
- If a lesion is suspicious for MM, referral to a trained physician, dermatologist, or surgeon is indicated
- For confirmed MM, referral to multiple specialties may be indicated, depending on the case, including surgical, radiation and/or medical oncology, nuclear medicine, pathology, or neurosurgery

Follow-up
Expected Outcomes
- Most metastases occur within 1 to 3 years of treatment of the primary tumor; 5% of patients develop new primary melanoma
- Annual skin exams by an experienced physician or dermatologist are recommended for life
- Prognosis depends on tumor thickness, presence of histologic ulceration, and lymph node involvement (most important)

Complications
- Metastases within or around the primary site, in regional lymph nodes, or distally (remote skin or lymph nodes, viscera, skeletal, or CNS sites)

PRESSURE ULCERS

Description
- Areas of local tissue trauma caused by unrelieved pressure or pressure in combination with shear or friction of tissues that are compressed between a bony prominence and external surface
- A sign of local tissue necrosis and death

Etiology
- Mechanical injury to skin, underlying tissues; primarily caused by pressure and shear
- Increased pressure gradient over bony prominences where there is less available compressible tissue leads to more pressure ulcers at these points
- Unrelieved pressure over time occludes blood and lymphatic circulation, causing tissues to be deprived of oxygen, nutrients, and waste removal, leading to tissue breakdown and eventual tissue death

Incidence and Demographics
- Highest incidence noted in both acute-care and long-term-care facilities and private homes where a person's mobility and capability to perform self-care has been altered
- Orthopedic surgery and spinal cord injury patients have higher risk than other institutionalized patients
- Terminally ill older adults at high risk

Risk Factors
- Use validated risk assessment tool such as Braden Scale or Norton Scale
- Risk factors include:
  - Decreased mobility, activity, sensory perception/alertness, pain
  - Extrinsic factors of increased moisture (incontinence/perspiration/leakage), friction, shear
  - Intrinsic factors of increased age, poor nutrition (involuntary weight loss), and arteriolar pressure

Prevention and Screening
- Any patient at risk should have thorough skin inspection regularly
- Start program of care, which would address risk factors identified
- Diligent skin cleansing of waste, regular moisturizing, and skin barrier ointments for incontinence/leakage, etc.
- Nutritional guidance and support
- If immobility present, patient needs proper pressure-relief devices for bed and chair and proper and frequent repositioning of patient
- Provide adequate pain management to facilitate ease of movement and change of position
- Provide/arrange for education for caregivers and patient

Assessment
History
- Recent or gradual change in health, mobility, continence, self-care abilities; injury, trauma, surgery
  - Postoperative state, especially following orthopedic surgery
  - Recent or worsening of paralyzing or spastic neurological illness, such as CVA, spinal cord injury, Parkinson's disease
  - Injury or illness causing pain and secondary immobility or restlessness
  - Cognitive impairment
  - Poor nutritional or hydration status

Physical Exam
- Pressure ulcers and surrounding tissues should be examined, measured and staged regularly. Acute and long-term healthcare facilities mandated to perform assessments weekly
- Ulcer bed should be described in terms of types of tissue present, e.g., granulation, necrotic, epithelial
- Photograph if possible to assist in monitoring the healing process
- Evidence of wound infection to be monitored
- National Pressure Ulcer Advisory Panel updated the pressure ulcer staging system in 2007:
  - Suspected deep tissue injury: purple or maroon localized area of discolored intact skin or blood-filled blister; tissue may be painful, firm, mushy, boggy, warmer or cooler as compared to adjacent tissue preceding development of visible skin changes; may be difficult to detect in dark-skinned individuals
  - Stage I: nonblanchable erythema of intact skin; in individuals with darker skin, discoloration of the skin, warmth, edema, induration, or hardness may also be indicators
  - Stage II: partial thickness skin loss involving the dermis; ulcer is superficial and has a red or pink wound bed without slough or bruising; may also present as a intact or open serum-filled blister
  - Stage III: full thickness skin loss involving damage to subcutaneous tissue that may extend down to, but not through, underlying fascia (bone, muscle or tendon are not exposed); presents as a deep crater with or without undermining or tunneling; slough may be present; depth depends on anatomical location
  - Stage IV: full thickness skin loss with exposed muscle, bone, or supporting structures; slough or eschar may be seen and undermining or tunneling are often present; depth depends on anatomical location

– Unstageable: full thickness tissue loss in which the base of the ulcer is covered by slough and/or eschar, preventing appropriate staging; slough and eschar must be removed to expose the base of the wound and determine depth (and stage); stable eschar on the heels should not be removed
- Sequential monitoring of ulcer should be documented on a flow record
- Staging should never be used to describe healing (reverse staging)
- The Pressure Ulcer Scale for Healing (PUSH) tool was developed to monitor change in pressure ulcer status over time

Diagnostic Studies
- Clinical diagnosis based on precipitating factors
- Bone scans or MRI are helpful in diagnosing osteomyelitis
- Serum albumin or prealbumin levels may be useful in diagnosing undernutrition

Differential Diagnosis
- Arterial/diabetic ulcer
- Venous ulcer
- Malignancy
- Rheumatoid disease
- Pyoderma gangrenosum

Management
Nonpharmacologic
- Basics: nutritional assessment and support, management of tissue loads, ulcer care
- Nutrition: as compatible with patient's wishes, supplement diet as needed to provide at least RDA of vitamins and minerals, and a minimum of 30 to 35 calories/kg/day and 1.25 to 1.5 gms of protein/kg/day
- Tissue load management: proper positioning, frequent repositioning, adequate pressure relief devices in chair and bed to facilitate healing and comfort
- Ulcer care
  – Cleansing: adequate, nontraumatic with noncytotoxic cleanser at safe irrigation pressure (4 to 15 psi)
  – Debridement: remove devitalized tissue when appropriate, choosing method of debridement based on condition and goals (sharp, mechanical, enzymatic, autolytic)
  – Dressings: moist wound healing shown to be most physiologically ideal; e.g., hydrocolloid, hydrogel dressings; protect periulcer area from maceration with skin barrier; control excess exudate from ulcer without drying out ulcer bed

Pharmacological
- For wound infection or surrounding cellulitis, or evidence of early osteomyelitis, use antibiotic appropriate for treatment of probable *S. aureus*, Gram-negative rods (swab cultures not used to diagnose infection as pressure ulcers are usually colonized)
- Use analgesics to control pain around the clock or p.r.n. before care
- Treat until ulcer healed or if terminally ill, until death, evaluating treatment plan about every 2 weeks for progress (if healing is goal) and adjust plan as needed

Special Considerations
- Approach to care and goal of treatment must be based on wishes for cure or for comfort

When to Consult, Refer, Hospitalize
- Physical therapy for adjunctive treatments such as electrotherapy, electrical stimulation

- Nutritionist for evaluation of nutritional intake
- Plastic surgeon if surgical repair may be appropriate
- Wound care center if treatment plan is failing
- In advancing cellulitis or osteomyelitis not appropriate for outpatient treatment, consider hospitalization

Follow-up
Expected Course
- If the older patient can maintain adequate nutrition, cooperate with care, and avoid serious concurrent illnesses, healing is expected
- Slow or poor healing may be secondary to chronic physical and cognitive illnesses

Complications
- Wound infection/cellulitis
- Osteomyelitis
- Loss of extremity
- Necrotizing fasciitis
- Septicemia, death

Venous Stasis Dermatitis and Ulcers
Description
- Common inflammatory skin disease of the lower extremities resulting from chronic venous insufficiency
- Chronic venous stasis dermatitis may lead to ulcerations of the distal lower extremity

Etiology
- Sustained venous hypertension of lower extremities resulting from age-related valvular incompetence in venous system or injury from deep vein thrombosis, surgery, or trauma
- Leakage of fibrinogen from vascular system into dermis leads to decrease in oxygen and nutrients
- Trapping of WBC in microcirculation secondary to altered inflammatory mechanisms

Incidence and Demographics
- 3.5% of patients > 65 years of age
- About 70% have recurrence of ulcers
- Women slightly > men

Risk Factors
- Obesity
- Lower-extremity edema
- History of thrombophlebitis
- Multiple pregnancies
- Positive family history
- Trauma
- Advancing age
- Previous venous ulcer

Prevention and Screening
- Control of edema with elevation and compression
- Avoidance of trauma to lower extremities

- Monitor for skin color and consistency changes in gaiter area of leg (area around and proximal to ankle)
- Good moisturizing of lower legs

Assessment
History
- Insidious onset of unilateral or bilateral lower-extremity pruritus
- Reddish-brown skin discoloration, most often in the area of the medial ankle (gaiter area)
- May present with a history of lower-extremity edema, phlebitis, injury, surgery, or ulceration
- Family history

Physical
- Location: distal lower extremity, usually proximal to medial or lateral malleolus
- Skin: hyperpigmented, erythematous, eczematous, scaling patches; skin may be weeping; lichenification may occur because of chronic scratching
- Associated findings: lipodermatosclerosis, edema, palpable pulses, varicose veins
- Ulcer bed: shallow, irregular shape; beefy red and/or fibrinous necrosis; often moderate to heavy exudate
- Pain: usually mild, relieved with elevation

Diagnostic Studies
- Often diagnosis of clinical determination
- Rule out arterial insufficiency with ankle-brachial index (ABI) test; ABI test not appropriate in diabetic patients, although toe pressure studies may be helpful
- Rule out deep vein thrombosis (DVT) with ultrasound in acute, new-onset cases

Differential Diagnosis
- Arterial ulcer
- Diabetic ulcer
- Pressure ulcer
- Vasculitis
- Pyoderma gangrenosum
- Malignancy
- Osteomyelitis

Management
Nonpharmacologic
- Dermatitis: emollients, compression and elevation for edema
- Ulcers
  - Irrigate or use mild whirlpool with noncytotoxic agent at safe irrigation pressure of 4 to 15 psi
  - Select appropriate dressing that fits wound(s) and provides basis for moist wound healing; e.g., hydrocolloid or foam dressing if drainage minimal, alginate if excess drainage, hydrogel if wound dry
  - Compression is cornerstone to success: use medium-to-high (if ABI ≥ 0.8) compression if tolerated, such as with special order knee-high stockings, Unna's or Duke boot, multilayered compression wrap, pneumatic compression device

Pharmacologic
- Use topical mild steroids for acute dermatitis and antifungals for infection as needed
- Oral pentoxifylline (Trental) improves rates of complete or partial wound healing, especially in combination with compression, though gastrointestinal side effects are common
- Aspirin may accelerate healing and reduce ulcer size
- Systemic antibiotics if surrounding cellulitis; use of topical antibiotics should be avoided (excess use can lead to secondary reactive dermatitis)

How Long to Treat
- Continue until healed, altering approach as ulcer and surrounding skin changes
- If not improving in 6 to 12 weeks, consider biopsy

When to Consult, Refer, Hospitalize
- To vascular surgeon if considering evaluation of superficial venous system for possible corrective surgery
- To physical therapy if increased joint mobility and increased ambulation is needed
- To hospital for extensive cellulitis at level beyond appropriate for outpatient treatment
- To wound care center for treatment failure > 3 months if skin biopsy negative, or if considering advanced treatment such as skin substitutes, growth factors

Special Considerations
- Concurrent arterial disease makes treatment more complex and can affect healing

Follow-up
Expected Course
- Prolonged healing time of ulcers and recurrences are common
- Compression therapy needed continuously even if skin healed
- Progression of venous disease and secondary skin changes expected with age

Complications
- Cellulitis
- Woody fibrosis and nonpitting edema with secondary ankle restriction
- Lifestyle change with negative aspects of prolonged treatment, change in mobility, change in body image, and powerlessness over healing

Arterial Ulcers
Description
- Ulceration of the lower extremities resulting from peripheral arterial disease
- Occurs when arterial blood flow is insufficient to meet the metabolic demands of tissue

Etiology
- Insufficient blood supply can be caused by atherosclerosis, resulting in chronic progressive arterial ischemia, or by an embolic event, resulting in acute arterial ischemia
- Occlusion can occur in a single lower-extremity artery or in more than one vessel along the arterial tree
- Ulceration often begins with minor trauma that fails to heal because the blood supply is insufficient to meet the increased demands of the healing tissue

Incidence and Demographics
- More common in older adults; as many as 20% of Americans over age 65 are affected by peripheral arterial disease
- Arterial ulcers account for approximately 20% of all leg ulcers

Risk Factors
- Advanced age
- Diabetes
- Hyperlipidemia
- Hypertension
- Cigarette smoking

Prevention and Screening
- Control diabetes, hypertension, and hyperlipidemia
- Counsel patient to quit smoking
- Monitor for vascular changes on routine physical exams

Assessment
History
- Painful ulcers of the lower extremities
- Often associated with other manifestations of peripheral arterial disease, including rest pain, pallor, hair loss, and nail hypertrophy

Physical
- Location: sites of increased focal pressure such as the lateral malleolus, tips of toes, metatarsal heads, and bunion area
- Skin: appears shiny or taut, pale or cyanotic; can have dependent rubor
- Associated findings: foot is cool and dry, pulses are absent, capillary refill time longer than 3 seconds
- Ulcer: pale, dry base with surrounding shiny skin; "punched out" appearance with borders that have a clear demarcation from the adjacent tissue
- Pain: present, may be severe; can be absent if the patient has associated peripheral neuropathy caused by diabetes

Diagnostic Studies
- Noninvasive vascular testing:
  - Ankle-brachial index (ABI)
  - Doppler ultrasound
  - Segmental limb pressures and segmental volume plethysmography
  - Duplex ultrasound
  - Transcutaneous oxygen pressure
- Invasive arteriogram testing

Differential Diagnosis
- Venous ulcer
- Diabetic ulcer
- Pressure ulcer
- Vasculitis
- Pyoderma gangrenosum

- Malignancy
- Osteomyelitis

Management
Nonpharmacologic
- Surgical revascularization with bypass graft
- Debridement of nonviable tissue after revascularization; arterial ulcers and any dry eschar or gangrenous tissue should be kept dry until revascularization is performed to prevent development of bacterial infection

Pharmacologic
- Control hypertension, diabetes, and hyperlipidemia
- Platelet inhibitors can improve healing

When to Consult, Refer, Hospitalize
- Refer to vascular surgeon for potential revascularization procedures

Special Considerations
- Concurrent venous disease or diabetes makes treatment more complex and can affect healing
- Consider the patient's prognosis, functional ability, life expectancy, risk of the proposed treatments, arterial outflow, and lesion morphology when recommending treatment options

Follow-up
Expected Course
- Unless underlying cause is identified and treated, ischemia is expected to progress with ongoing nonhealing ulcer formation and possible limb loss
- Patient must be educated regarding proper footwear and should be taught to cleanse the feet well, dry between the toes, and inspect the feet carefully on a daily basis

Complications
- Infection and osteomyelitis
- Amputation

CASE STUDIES

Case 1. An 86-year-old female resident of long-term-care facility for 2 years secondary to advanced dementia has fallen and suffered a right hip fracture. She was sent to the hospital for open reduction–internal fixation and returned to the facility 2 days post-op. Upon readmission, she is noted to have a 3 × 3 cm bulla on her posterior right heel. Prior to the fall, she was underweight, needed assistance to ambulate, and had poor short-term memory and poor safety insight. Meds include multivitamin with minerals, docusate (Colace), and enoxaparin (Lovenox) injections.

1. What is the probable cause of the right heel bulla?
2. What were her risk factors for pressure ulcers pre- and post-op?
3. How could this heel ulcer have been prevented?
4. What are basics for treatment?
5. What are possible complications of this pressure ulcer?

Case 2. A 75-year-old blond White male, former construction worker, complains of raised lump on the back of his neck that is irritated by his shirt collar. His wife has noticed that the lesion seems to be getting larger and darker in color over the past few months. He has no other significant medical history. Medications: safety coated aspirin (Ecotrin), atorvastatin (Lipitor), lisinopril.

1. How common are skin cancers?
2. How does this patient follow the demographics and risk factors for skin cancer?
3. Does location of lesion help in assessment?
4. What diagnostic test is necessary?
5. What is the appropriate treatment for such lesions, and what is the expected outcome?

Case 3. A 95-year-old nursing home patient has advanced dementia and is no longer ambulatory. She must be fed and is incontinent of urine. Chronic conditions include: obesity, diabetes mellitus, polymyalgia rheumatica, and gastroesophageal reflux. Medications: rosiglitazone (Avandia), prednisone, omeprazole (Prilosec), and acetaminophen (Tylenol) p.r.n. The nursing assistant involved with her care noticed red, inflamed skin on her abdomen and perineal area when cleaning her today. Upon exam, you find bright red, smooth macules with maceration and satellite lesions under her breasts and in the skin folds on her abdomen and perineal area.

1. What is your most likely diagnosis?
2. What risk factors does she have?
3. What nonpharmacologic treatment would you order?
4. What pharmacologic treatment would you order?
5. How long would you expect to treat this condition?

REFERENCES

Balin, A. K. (2006). *Seborrheic keratosis*. Retrieved from http://emedicine.medscape.com/article/1059477-overview

Berger, T. G. (2005). Skin, hair and nails. In L. M. Tierney, M. A. Papadakis, & S. J. McPhee (Eds.), *Current Medical Diagnosis and Treatment* (44th ed.). New York: Lange Medical Books/McGraw Hill.

Black, J., Baharestani, M., Cuddigan, J., Dorner, B., Edsberg, L., Langemo, D., et al. (2007). National Pressure Ulcer Advisory Panel's updated pressure ulcer staging system. *Dermatology Nursing, 19*(4), 343–349.

Blount, B. W. (2002). Rosacea: A common, yet commonly overlooked, condition. *American Family Physician, 66*(3), 435–440.

Buttaro, T. M., Trybulski, J., Bailey, P. P., & Sandberg-Cook, J. (2008). *Primary care: A collaborative practice* (3rd ed.). St. Louis, MO: Mosby.

Davidge, K., & Fish, J. (2008). Older adults and burns. *Geriatrics and Aging, 11*(5), 270–275.

Davidovici, B. B., & Wolf, R. (2007). Emergencies in dermatology: Diagnosis, classification, and therapy. *Expert Review of Dermatology, 2*(5), 549–562.

Edmunds, M. W., & Mayhew, M. S. (2004). *Pharmacology for the primary care provider* (2nd ed.). St. Louis, MO: Mosby.

Goroll, A. H., & Mulley, A. G. (2005). *Primary care medicine* (5th ed.). Philadelphia: Lippincott, Williams & Wilkins.

Habif, T. P. (2003). *Clinical dermatology: A color guide to diagnosis and therapy* (4th ed.). St Louis, MO: Mosby.

Hall, J. C. (2006). *Sauer's manual of skin diseases* (9th ed.). Philadelphia: Lippincott, Williams & Wilkins.

Helfrich, Y. R., Sachs, D. L., & Voorhees, J. J. (2008). Overview of skin aging and photoaging. *Dermatology Nursing, 20*(3), 177–184.

Hirsch, A. T., Haskal, Z. J., Hertzer, N. R., Bakal, C. W., Creager, M. A., Halperin, J. L., et al. (2006). ACC/AHA 2005 Practice Guidelines for the management of patients with peripheral arterial disease (lower extremity, renal, mesenteric, and abdominal aortic): A collaborative report from the American Association for Vascular Surgery/Society for Vascular Surgery, Society for Cardiovascular Angiography and Interventions, Society for Vascular Medicine and Biology, Society of Interventional Radiology, and the ACC/AHA Task Force on Practice Guidelines (Writing Committee to Develop Guidelines for the Management of Patients With Peripheral Arterial Disease): Endorsed by the American Association of Cardiovascular and Pulmonary Rehabilitation; National Heart, Lung, and Blood Institute; Society for Vascular Nursing; TransAtlantic Inter-Society Consensus; and Vascular Disease Foundation. *Circulation, 113*, e463–e654.

Lee, M., & Kalb, R. E. (2008). Systemic therapy for psoriasis. *Dermatology Nursing, 20*(2), 105–111.

McIntyre, W. J., Down, M. R., & Bedwell, S. A. (2007). Treatment options for actinic keratoses. *American Family Physician, 76*(5), 667–671.

Norman, R. A. (2008). Common skin conditions in geriatric dermatology, *Annals of Long Term Care, 16*(6), 40–45.

Sarabi, K., & Khachemoune, A. (2007). Tinea capitis: A review. *Dermatology Nursing, 19*(6), 525–529.

Schmader, K. E., Harpaz, R., & Oxman, M. N. (2007). Current treatment and future strategies for herpes zoster and postherpetic neuralgia. Supplement to *Annals of Long-Term Care: Clinical Care and Aging and Clinical Geriatrics, 15*. Available at http://www.clinicalgeriatrics.com/article/5150

Sieggreen, M. Y., & Kline, R. A. (2004). Arterial insufficiency and ulceration: Diagnosis and treatment options. *Advances in Skin & Wound Care, 17,* 242–251.

Stulberg, D. L., Crandell, B., & Fawcett, R. S. (2004). Diagnosis and treatment of basal cell and squamous cell carcinomas. *American Family Physician, 70*(8), 1481–1488.

Swetter, S. M. (2008). *Malignant melanoma.* Retrieved from http://emedicine.medscape.com/article/1100753-overview

Tabloski, P. A. (2006). *Gerontological nursing.* Upper Saddle River, NJ: Pearson Education.

Wilson, D. (2007). Herpes zoster: Prevention, diagnosis, and treatment. *Nurse Practitioner, 32*(9), 19–24.

Wolff, K., Johnson, R. A., & Suurmond, D. (2005). *Fitzpatrick's color atlas and synopsis of clinical dermatology* (5th ed.). New York: McGraw-Hill.

Eye, Ear, Nose, and Throat Disorders

Katherine Tardiff, MSN, GNP-BC, ACHPN

GENERAL APPROACH—EYES

- Number of people with low vision or blindness is expected to nearly double by 2020
- Prevalence of low vision and blindness increases with age
- Four main causes of visual impairment and blindness in the older adult: cataracts, age-related macular degeneration (AMD), glaucoma, and diabetic retinopathy
- May lead to loss of independence, depression, decreased quality of life, and increased risk for falls
- Patients with central or severe peripheral vision loss will not be able to drive

Normal Changes of Aging

- Tear production diminishes because of atrophy of lacrimal glands, predisposing to dry eyes
- Arcus senilis, age-related gray-white ring around limbus caused by calcium deposits, no clinical significance
- Lens denser, less elastic, decreased accommodation results in presbyopia (farsightedness); dull lens may lead to glare
- Corneal sensitivity to touch decreases with age, may lead to corneal damage
- Pupil size diminishes; pupils react more slowly to light, dilate more slowly in the dark
- Liquefaction of vitreous humor leads to "floaters"
- Retina may become duller
- Retinal cell loss affects color discrimination
- Loss of neurons in the visual pathways beyond the retina

Clinical Essentials

History

- Evaluate for any visual changes since last visit, including difficulty driving (night- or daytime) or changes in reading habits
- Date of last complete ophthalmologist exam
- Glasses or contact lenses, previous ocular injury or surgery
- Medications (ocular, systemic, over-the-counter, herbal); consider ocular effects of systemic medicines such as steroids, anticholinergics, antiarrhythmics; also may identify conditions associated with ocular diseases such as diabetes, hypertension, hyperthyroidism, or vascular disorders
- Family history of glaucoma, cataracts, macular degeneration

Physical

- Test of visual acuity is keystone of exam; assess vision using the Snellen chart (placed 20 feet from the patient) or other standardized measurement of visual acuity
- Pupil should be evaluated for dilation and constriction, equality, size, and shape
- Other exam components include external examination and tests of extraocular muscle function and visual fields
- Funduscopic exam should be attempted; if lens opacities prevent visualization, the patient should be evaluated for possible cataracts

Assessment

- Many eye disorders present in a similar fashion
- Determine effects of low vision on patient and family members
- The eyes offer a unique opportunity to visualize arteries directly; arteriosclerosis visible in the retinal blood vessels mirrors arteriosclerosis elsewhere in the body; changes in arteriole wall lead to loss of transparency (see Chapter 9, Cardiovascular Disorders for details)

Treatment

- Refer immediately any sudden painless loss of vision; most eye problems require ophthalmology referral
- Monitor for effects of topical treatments on eye
  - Local: irritation, inflammation, hypersensitivity
  - Systemic effects of drug are the same as if given PO
- Because of potential for severe damage if given in the setting of undiagnosed herpes infections, steroid preparations should only be prescribed by a physician
- Contact lenses may be damaged by ophthalmologic preparations: instruct patient not to administer eye drops when wearing contacts
- Have patient demonstrate the proper administration of eye drops

RED FLAGS—THE ACUTE EYE

Table 7-1. Indicators of Vision-Threatening Disorders

Symptoms	Signs
• Blurred vision that does *not* clear with blinking • Sudden loss or decreased vision • Halos around sources of light • Flashing lights • Sudden floating spots or sensation of "cobwebs" across field of vision • Photophobia • Periocular headache • Ocular pain	• Ciliary flush • Corneal damage (opacities, trauma) • Abnormal pupils • Increased intraocular pressure • Appearance of RBC or WBC in anterior chamber • Proptosis (forward displacement of the eye globe within the orbit of the eye) • Severe green-yellow d/c, erythema, chemosis, and lid edema • Acute-onset limited ocular movement • Facial cellulitis

Table 7-2. Conditions of the Eye Requiring Emergency/Urgent Referral

Disease	Etiology	Risk Factors	History	Physical	Management/ Comments
Keratitis	Inflammation of cornea	Irritation or infection, dry eye	Acute pain, visual loss, photophobia, foreign body sensation	Red eye, ciliary flush	Refer immediately to ophthalmologist
Uveitis	Inflammation of the uveal tract: iris, ciliary body, and choroids	Caused by immune system, infection, or systemic disease	With or without pain, blurred vision, photophobia	May be inflamed, injected, small pupils, cloudy cornea	Refer immediately to ophthalmologist
Corneal Abrasion	Superficial injury of the corneal epithelium	Often due to dry eye, trauma	Pain, photophobia, foreign body sensation	Generalized redness	Refer to ophthalmology, urgency depends on severity
Angle-Closure Glaucoma	Anterior chamber drainage is blocked	Anatomically narrow anterior chamber	Sudden severe pain in or around eye, photophobia, nausea	Acute, red, hard, tender eye; IOP 40–80 mm Hg, fixed, mid-dilated pupil	**Emergency** bed rest until ophthalmologic consult, may lead to blindness

continued

Table 7-2. Conditions of the Eye Requiring Emergency/Urgent Referral (cont.)

Disease	Etiology	Risk Factors	History	Physical	Management/ Comments
Retinal Tear/ Detachment	Separation of the sensory retina from the pigment epithelium	Age, diabetes, myopia (near-sightedness), cataract surgery, ocular injury	*Tear:* new-onset light flashes, new floaters, shadows *Detachment:* "curtain coming down over my eye"	*Tear:* crescent-shaped, red or orange in color *Detachment:* gray, cloud-like, hanging in vitreous	Emergency position so gravity aids in repositioning of retina during transport
Retinal Artery Occlusion	Blockage of the arterial supply to the retina	Carotid artery atherosclerosis, diseased cardiac valves	Sudden onset of painless loss of vision in one eye	Pale swollen retina, "cherry red" spot at fovea	Emergency treatment to prevent blindness
Retinal Venous Occlusion	Obstruction of central retinal vein or its branches	Hypertension, diabetes, glaucoma	Sudden painless decrease in vision, complete or partial	Swollen disk, tortuous veins, retinal hemorrhage	Immediate referral, results in visual loss

COMMON EYE DISORDERS

- **Dry eyes:** generalized redness, dry cornea due to decreased tear production, inadequate blink, poor lid closure, medications, and environmental factors. Develops slowly. Sensation of dry, burning, foreign body. Use artificial tears.
- **Subconjunctival hemorrhage:** bright red area because of blood beneath the conjunctiva, asymptomatic, sudden onset. No precipitating event usually identified. May be associated with trauma, cough, Valsalva maneuver, hypertension, anticoagulant. Rule out hyphema. Completely benign, reassure patient. Resolves spontaneously over 2 to 3 weeks.
- **Foreign body (FB):** dust, dirt lying on the epithelium of the cornea. Sudden sharp pain, photophobia, urge to rub eyes. Complete exam, refer to ophthalmology unless superficial and resolves within 24 hours. Irrigate eye with normal saline. *Do not patch.* Recheck in 24 hours.
- **Ectropion:** eyelid turns out away from the eyeball, because of decreased tone in orbicular oculi muscles that close the eyelid and cause dry eye. Treat with artificial tears, surgery.
- **Entropion:** eyelid turns in toward eyeball, because of muscle spasm of the orbicular oculi, and causes chronic irritation from rubbing the eyeball with each blink. Artificial tears and surgical treatment.
- **Xanthelasma:** asymptomatic, benign growths, slightly raised, well-circumscribed yellowish plaques along the nasal aspect of the eyelids; occur in diabetics and those with hypercholesterolemia. These can be surgically removed for cosmetic reasons.
- **Blepharitis:** obstruction and inflammation of the sebum and sweat glands on the lid margins. Symptoms are burning and itching of eyes. Treat with warm compresses, scrub lids with baby

shampoo and water 1:1 with cotton-tipped swab and administer ophthalmic antibiotics as needed.

- **Pingueculae:** yellowed areas of thickened conjunctiva near the corneal limbus in the eyelid fissure, may be due to sunlight exposure. Bilateral, more nasally than temporally, present in a majority of older adults.
- **Chalazion:** obstructed and inflamed meibomian gland on inner aspect of eyelid, caused by infection or debris. Localized, firm nodule on inner aspect of eyelid, subacute onset, pain and tenderness. Treat with warm compresses and ophthalmic antibiotic as needed.
- **Hordeolum** (also called stye): infection of the glands that lubricate lashes and outer eyelid, similar to chalazion, except on outer aspect of eyelid. Treat as chalazion, may need systemic antibiotics.
- **Pterygium:** a triangular growth of conjunctival tissue growing from inner canthus toward pupil that vascularizes and invades cornea; may be due to sunlight exposure and genetic factors. May obstruct vision as reaches center of cornea. Refer for surgery, may recur.
- **Conjunctivitis:** commonly called "pinkeye," is dilation of the blood vessels of bulbar and palpebral layers of conjunctiva. Vision may be slightly blurry but clears with blink. May be viral or bacterial. See Table 7–3.

Table 7-3. Conjunctivitis

Condition	History	Physical	Nonpharmacologic Treatment	Pharmacologic Treatment
Allergic	Intermittent with seasons; feels itchy, gritty; associated with other allergic signs and symptoms	Generalized redness, cobblestone edema of palpebral conjunctiva; discharge thin, watery, stringy	Cool compress useful in decreasing itching	Topical vasoconstrictors or antihistamines; add local NSAID and mast cell stabilizer if needed
Viral	May have upper-respiratory infection; may begin unilaterally, spread to other eye; feels gritty	Generalized redness; if herpetic, may see cold sores; discharge is watery, mucoid	Compresses for comfort	Self-limiting; antibiotics, steroids, and vasoconstrictors should not be used
Bacterial	Acute onset; may begin unilaterally, spreads to other eye; feels gritty, burning; eye "stuck shut" upon awakening	If severe, may have palpable periauricular nodes; generalized redness; discharge mucopurulent, crusting on lids/lashes	Cool compresses for comfort, warm compresses to remove crusts; hand washing, contact precautions	Topical antibiotic with coverage for *S. pneumoniae*, *H. influenzae* or *S. aureus*; Gram-negative coverage may be needed; only ophthalmologist should prescribe steroids

Glaucoma

Description
- A heterogeneous group of eye disorders marked by damage to the optic nerve
- Irreversible damage to the optic nerve can occur if intraocular pressure (IOP) is not lowered
- There are three types of glaucoma
  - Angle-closure glaucoma (ACG), also called narrow-angle glaucoma or acute angle-closure glaucoma
  - Open-angle glaucoma (OAG), also called chronic glaucoma
  - Secondary glaucoma (SG)

Etiology
- ACG: anatomically narrow anterior chamber is suddenly blocked, resulting in an abrupt increase in IOP
- OAG: less dramatic increase in IOP related to resistance to outflow of aqueous humor
- SG obstruction of outflow tracts caused by complications of other diseases (such as diabetes and hypertension)

Incidence and Demographics
- Affects 2.2 millions Americans, with 80,000 diagnosed as legally blind
- Leading cause of irreversible blindness in the world; about 10% of all cases of blindness in the United States are related to glaucoma
- OAG is most common, comprising about 90% of cases; OAG occurs about six times more often among Blacks, in whom it is the leading cause of blindness
- ACG accounts for less than 10% of glaucoma cases; it is more common among Asian-Americans and Inuits

Risk Factors
ACG
- Family history of angle-closure glaucoma
- Age > 40–50 years
- Female
- Hyperopia (farsightedness) because of shape of eyeball, with narrowed angle
- Use of anticholinergic (atropine-like) drugs
- Anatomic small eye with shallow anterior chamber
- Pathology of the eye: cysts of the iris or ciliary bodies, cataracts, intraocular tumor

OAG
- Elevated IOP
- Advanced age
- More common in Blacks
- Family history of glaucoma
- Use of topical, oral, or inhaled corticosteroids
- Other possible risk factors include: systemic hypertension, diabetes, and cardiovascular disease

Prevention and Screening
- Ophthalmology screening every 1 to 2 years including visual acuity, visual fields, slit lamp inspection, dilated exam, and IOP measurement

Assessment

History and Physical Exam

Table 7-4. Comparison of ACG and OAG Physical Exam

ACG	OAG
Acute onset	Insidious onset
Severe pain, headache, nausea	No early symptoms, painless
Profound visual loss, halos around lights	Progressive loss of peripheral vision
Hard, red eye, ciliary flush, steamy cornea, mid-dilated pupil that reacts poorly to light	Evidence of optic nerve damage, optic nerve head pale, with increased cup-to-disc ratio

Diagnostic Studies

ACG
- Gonioscopy is gold standard

OAG
- IOP measurement
- Peripheral visual field testing
- Fundus examination

Differential Diagnosis
- See Table 7–2

Management

Nonpharmacologic

ACG
- Bed rest pending surgery
- Laser peripheral iridotomy

OAG
- Laser therapy (trabeculoplasty)
- Surgery; may involve shunt placement in advanced disease

Pharmacologic

ACG
- If more than 1 hour before patient can be evaluated by ophthalmology and suspicion of ACG is high, consider administration of pressure-lowering drops and systemic medications to control IOP

OAG
- Medical management in OAG aimed at decreasing aqueous production and increasing aqueous outflow
- Prostaglandin analogs and ß-adrenergic antagonists are the most frequently used eye drops

Special Considerations
- Patients generally do not report symptoms of glaucoma until advanced stages of the disease

- Eye drop caps are color-coded to help patients distinguish different classes of medications

When to Consult, Refer, Hospitalize
- ACG immediate referral to an ophthalmologist
- OAG less urgent referral to ophthalmologist
- Secondary glaucoma refer to ophthalmologist

Table 7–5. Pharmacologic Management of OAG

Medication Class	Examples	Mechanism of Action	Local Effects	Systemic Effects
Beta blocker (blue or yellow cap)	Timolol	Suppress aqueous production	Transient discomfort, tearing, blurred vision	Side effects of beta blockers: CHF, asthma, bradycardia, etc.
Miotic/ cholinesterase Inhibitors (green cap)	Pilocarpine	Increase aqueous outflow	Constricted pupil	Diarrhea, sweating, bronchospasm,
Adrenergic (purple cap)	Epinephrine	Decreases inflow and increases outflow	Allergic lid reaction and eye irritation	increased heart rate, palpitations, hypertension
Prostaglandin agonist	Latanoprost (Xalatan)	Increases outflow	Eye pigment change, local irritation	Rare
Carbonic anhydrase inhibitors (orange cap)	Trusopt, dorzolamide	Suppresses aqueous production	Conjunctivitis	Side effects of sulfonamides

Follow-up
Expected Outcomes
- Damage caused by uncontrolled glaucoma is permanent
- ACG surgery curative, stops vision loss
- OAG not cured, controlled by life-long administration of medications

Complications
- Loss of visual fields and visual acuity
- Damage to optic nerve, leading to blindness if left untreated
- Corneal damage: chronic edema, fibrosis, vascularization, or cataracts
- Atrophy of iris, multiple synechiae (iris adhesions to cornea)
- Malignant glaucoma, central retinal vein occlusion

Diabetic Retinopathy (DR)
Description
- Microvascular disease of the eyes related to prolonged high blood glucose in diabetes, resulting in retinal changes; frequently leads to blindness

Etiology

- Chronic hyperglycemia leads to progressive damage to blood vessels supplying the retinal tissue
- Nonproliferative DR: dilated vessels steal circulation from retinal surface; aneurysms form, leak, and bleed, resulting in macular edema and vision loss
- Proliferative DR: marked by the formation of fragile new blood vessels and the consequences of this neovascularization, including preretinal and vitreous hemorrhage, fibrosis, and retinal detachment

Incidence and Demographics

- Leading cause of impaired vision and new-onset blindness in persons aged 25 to 74 years
- Prevalence increases with duration of diabetes
- Up to 45% of adults with diabetes have some form of DR

Risk Factors

- Poor glucose control
- Proteinuria
- Hyperlipidemia
- Hypertension

Prevention and Screening

- Good control of blood sugars (A1C ≤ 7%) may delay onset and minimize severity
- Control of hypertension (< 130/80 mmHg) slows the rate of progression and decreases the risk for vitreous hemorrhage
- Regular ophthalmology exam for diabetics shortly after diagnosis and at least yearly thereafter

Assessment

History

- Most patients are asymptomatic until the very late stages
- Symptoms depend on the clinical problem: "curtain over the eye" with vitreous bleed, "floaters," spots, cloudy vision during resolution of vitreous bleeds

Physical Exam

- In nonproliferative DR, small red spots with sharp edges around the optic nerve and macula; retinal ("dot" and "blot") hemorrhages, hard (intraretinal) and soft exudates ("cotton wool spots"), and areas of dilated capillaries are later seen; macular edema indicates need for prompt action to preserve vision
- In proliferative DR, neovascularization may be seen or visualization may be obscured because of vitreous hemorrhage

Diagnostic Studies

- Glucose, hemoglobin A1C

Differential Diagnosis

- Hypertensive retinopathy
- Retinal detachment
- Glaucoma
- Macular degeneration

Management
- Treatment options are limited once sight is threatened by DR

Nonpharmacologic
- Laser photocoagulation (not curative)
- Vitrectomy for vitreous hemorrhage and tractional retinal detachment

Pharmacologic
- Optimal blood sugar and blood pressure control

Special Considerations
- Patients with macular edema, severe nonproliferative DR, or proliferative DR should be followed closely by an ophthalmologist experienced in the management of diabetic retinopathy

When to Consult, Refer, Hospitalize
- All patients with a diabetes diagnosis should be referred to ophthalmology for evaluation and monitoring of disease
- Sudden loss of vision or evidence of macular edema warrants emergent evaluation with ophthalmology

Follow-up
Expected Outcomes
- No curative therapy exists for DR; disease is progressive

Complications
- Progressive visual loss leading to blindness

Macular Degeneration
Description
- Age-related macular degeneration (AMD): a progressive degeneration of the central portion of the retina (macula) that results in loss of central vision; may be classified as dry (atrophic) or wet (exudative)

Etiology
- Disturbance of retinal pigment epithelium, which supports and nourishes the sensory retina; cause unknown
- Wet AMD: Neovascularization with hemorrhage or exudation of fluid between retinal pigment epithelium and sensory retina, death of photoreceptor cells, with a loss of central vision
- Dry AMD: Atrophy of retinal pigment epithelium and photoreceptor cells; associated with presence of drusen, but exact relationship is unclear

Incidence and Demographics
- Leading cause of blindness in older adults
- Wet AMD comprises 10% to 15% of cases, but accounts for more than 80% of cases with severe visual loss or blindness

Risk Factors
- Advanced age
- Smoking

- Cardiovascular disease
- Family history

Prevention and Screening
- Amsler grid used to screen at annual vision examination may be useful in detecting subtle visual changes
- Smoking cessation
- Control of cardiovascular risk factors

Assessment
History
- Often asymptomatic early in disease process
- Loss of central vision (may be gradual or sudden) in one or both eyes
- Difficulty driving or reading; may need bright lights or magnifying glass for tasks that require fine visual acuity
- Alteration of vision with straight lines appearing blurry, wavy, or with missing segments (e.g., grid lines, power or telephone wires), patchy or blurry vision, distorted central visual field

Physical Exam
- Decreased visual acuity and visual fields, central vision loss
- Amsler grid is seen with wavy or broken lines or open areas
- Wet AMD: neovascularization, retinal pigment change, exudation of fluid, and hemorrhage
- Dry AMD: drusen and macular pigmentary changes

Diagnostic Studies
- Dilated eye examination using a slit lamp instrument (biomicroscopy)
- Fluorescein angiography
- Optical coherence tomography

Differential Diagnoses
- Diabetic retinopathy
- Hypertensive retinopathy

Management
- Dry AMD: No proven effective treatment
- Wet AMD:
  - Vascular endothelial growth factor (VEGF)
  - Thermal laser photocoagulation

Special Considerations
- AMD may affect quality of life by affecting basic daily tasks such as reading, driving, and facial recognition
- One-third of patients with AMD have depression
- Dry AMD may progress to wet AMD

When to Consult, Refer, Hospitalize
- Acute vision loss (period of days or weeks) requires urgent evaluation by ophthalmology

Follow-up
Expected Outcomes
- Dry AMD: progressive and usually bilateral, with preservation of peripheral fields
- Wet AMD: further visual loss may be prevented in about half of those treated; however, only one-fifth retain the benefit at 5 years post-treatment
- Once advanced AMD develops in one eye, greater than 40% risk of development in the other eye within 5 years

Complications
- Blindness
- Increased risk for falls and need for placement in long-term care

Cataracts
Description
- Opacities of the lens, reducing visual acuity

Etiology
- Protein changes in the lens, causing opacity and scattering of light

Incidence and Demographics
- Increasing with aging, female > male
- Cataract surgery is the most frequently performed surgical procedure in those > 65
- > 50% of older adults have cataracts

Risk Factors
- Aging
- Smoking
- Alcohol consumption
- Low education
- Poor nutrition
- Corticosteroid use
- Atopic dermatitis
- Exposure to UV light (sunny climates)
- Trauma
- Diabetes

Prevention and Screening
- Use sunglasses with UV protection
- Smoking cessation

Assessment
History
- Progressive decrease visual acuity, without pain; loss may be complete, central, or peripheral
- "Second sight": temporary improvement in presbyopia as development of central lens opacities alters refractive power of lens and induces myopia
- Glare from bright lights, related to scattering of light by opacified lens
- Difficulty with night driving and reading signs and fine print

Physical Exam
- Opacity is a black silhouette against the red reflex, irregular, gray/brown, looks like a rock
  - More complete cataracts can be seen progressively as whitish-blue clouding through the pupil

Diagnostic Studies
- None

Differential Diagnosis
- Corneal scar
- Macular degeneration
- Retinal tear

Management
Nonpharmacologic
- Referral for surgical correction is made when vision loss is severe enough to affect function and when surgeon feels that vision can be sufficiently corrected

Pharmacologic
- None

Special Considerations
- A routine battery of tests is not indicated prior to cataract surgery; testing (e.g., EKG, blood tests) is necessary only if indicated by history and physical exam

When to Consult, Refer, Hospitalize
- In the absence of other visual symptoms, patients should be referred on a nonurgent basis to ophthalmology

Follow-up
Expected Course
- 85% to 95% of patients have excellent post-op vision; patients may resume normal activity such as reading, walking, eating, and watching television the evening of surgery
- The eye is examined by ophthalmology on the first postoperative day, then after one week, and one month; corticosteroid drops are often needed during this time

Complications
- Incomplete correction with residual decrease in visual acuity
- Disintegration of cataract material
- Retinal detachment, glaucoma, hemorrhage, infection post-op
- Blindness

GENERAL APPROACH—EARS
Normal Changes of Aging
- Presbycusis is the hearing loss of old age, caused by a combination of the normal changes of aging
- Vestibular function is also affected by the changes of aging

External Ear
- Number and activity of cerumen and apocrine glands decrease, leading to increased dryness of cerumen; men have more hair in the canal resulting in decreased movement of cerumen
- The walls of canal thin and becomes drier, possibly resulting in pruritus
- The tympanic membrane (TM) becomes thicker and wider, which may impede sound wave transmission
- Blockage of transmission through ear canal causes conductive hearing loss

Middle Ear
- The joints of ossicular chain are affected with calcification and other degenerative changes; however, studies have not demonstrated that these changes cause any related decrease in hearing

Inner Ear
- Degeneration of organ of Corti and basal end of cochlea destroys sensory cells results in sensory presbycusis, with loss of ability to hear high-frequency tones
- Decreased sensory neurons with a functional organ of Corti is associated with loss of speech discrimination: one can hear but cannot understand speech; this is the picture of neural presbycusis
- Degenerative changes in CNS may also contribute to presbycusis
- Debris collecting in ampullae of semicircular canal moves with head motion, causing neural stimulation and episodes of intense vertigo, the sensation of spinning; this can be either the feeling that patient is spinning in place, or that things are spinning around patient

Clinical Implications
History
- Obtain confirming information regarding extent of problem
- Assess for depression caused by social isolation of deafness

Physical
- External ear should be examined for any skin lesions
- Painful gouty tophi, lesions exuding chalky monosodium urate deposits, may be seen on the pinna, as well as nodules of rheumatoid arthritis

Assessment
- Ear pain (otalgia) should be carefully evaluated and etiology sought; pain may be referred from temporomandibular joint pain related to poorly fitting dentures or bruxism (teeth grinding)
- Tumors of the head and neck may also caused referred ear pain

Treatment
- A perforated eardrum is a contraindication to any use of otic drops
- Provide clearly written instructions for any medication administration; have patient demonstrate the correct use of drops
- When drops are used, the affected ear should be kept facing up (head tilted or patient lying down) for 2 minutes after instilling the medication, or a cotton plug should be inserted

- Ophthalmic drops are sometimes used in the ear; however, otic drops are never used in the eye

COMMON EAR DISORDERS

Hearing Loss

Description
- Diminished hearing, due to either mechanical obstruction of sound transmission, neurological impairment, or both
- Presbycusis is a high-frequency hearing loss and is considered a nonpathologic normal function of aging
- There are three types of hearing loss—conductive, sensorineural, and mixed
- Conductive hearing loss involves any cause that prevents external sound from accessing the inner ear
- Sensorineural involves the inner ear, the cochlea, or the auditory nerve and is further divided into:
  - Sensory degeneration of the organ of Corti
  - Neural degeneration of the higher auditory pathways

Etiology
- Conductive hearing loss involves outer- or middle-ear abnormalities that interfere with the conduction of sound waves. It is caused by a physical obstruction of the normal conduction of sound as in occlusion of external canal by wax, infection, or foreign object; perforated TM; bony growth or tumor interfering with ossicles in middle ear.
- Sensorineural hearing loss involves the inner ear. This is the usual cause of presbycusis. It is loss of transmission of sound for processing because of damage of inner ear (cochlear apparatus) and of cranial nerve VIII. Causes include:
  - Exposure to loud noises
  - Ototoxic medications
    - Antibiotics: streptomycin, gentamycin, vancomycin, aminoglycosides
    - Diuretics: ethacrynic acid and furosemide
    - Miscellaneous: salicylates, cisplatin (and other antineoplastic agents)
  - Cranial nerve VIII dysfunction
  - Neurologic disorder such as MS, syphilis, Ménière's disease

Incidence and Demographics
- Third most common major chronic disability in those older than 65 years
- 50% to 100% of those in nursing homes have significant loss of hearing
- 30% of adults age 65 to 74 and 47% of adults age 75 or older have a hearing loss
- Men more than women
- Older adults of lower economic status have poorer hearing than those of higher economic status

Risk Factors
- Family and occupational history, chronic otitis media, physical trauma
  - Worsened by other disease states: diabetes mellitus, chronic lung disease, hypothyroidism, hypertension, cerebrovascular disorders, alcohol abuse
- Contributory cardiovascular disorder such as stroke or vasculitis

Prevention and Screening

- Routine screening after age 65 (U.S. Preventive Services Task Force); specific time frame not mentioned but at least an annual exam seems prudent
- Avoidance of flying or diving (changes in barometric pressure) when ill with upper respiratory infection
- There is no specific prevention for the age-related changes leading to presbycusis

Assessment

History

- Onset and progression of hearing loss
- History of trauma (including noise) or previous ear surgery
- Hear better in certain settings (for example, hear well in quiet exam room but hear poorly on a busy street or in a room with television on)
- Family or social contacts report problems with hearing or apparent disorientation
- Associated tinnitus, disequilibrium, or vertigo

Physical

- Examination of the ear
  - Treat any conditions of the ear canal before testing hearing
  - Pneumoscopy to evaluate mobility of the tympanic membrane
- Whispered voice test for hearing impairment is a good screening device
  - Stand at arm's length behind a seated patient, whisper a combination of numbers and letters, ask patient to repeat; test each ear while covering the other
- Tuning fork assessments (Weber and Rinne tests)

Table 7–6. Characteristics of Types of Hearing Loss

Type of Loss	History	Pattern of Loss	Exam
Conductive	Unilateral loss of low tones; can produce 60–70 dB deficit; may experience tinnitus; gradual or acute decrease in hearing dependent on etiology	Good understanding (discrimination) of speech, loss of volume (can understand when volume is loud enough)	AC < BC; Weber lateralizes to affected ear May visualize cerumen or foreign body in ear canal; may see fluid level behind TM; TM may be stiff to insufflation, retracted, or bulging
Sensori-Neural	Slow onset, generally bilateral; loss of high frequency and pitch; may experience tinnitus or vertigo	Loss of both tone and discrimination; can hear but cannot understand; volume is sufficient but consonant sounds are lost; increased discrimination loss may indicate a central processing problem Sudden loss: look for acoustic neuroma	No abnormalities seen; AC ↓ BC; Weber lateralizes to better ear

continued

Table 7-6. Characteristics of Types of Hearing Loss (cont.)

Type of Loss	History	Pattern of Loss	Exam
Mixed	Bilateral sensorineural, with unilateral conductive component; may have tinnitus or vertigo; may have slow onset with acute loss	Loss for both volume and discrimination	Weber & Rinne nonconclusive; physical findings otherwise as under conductive

Note. AC= air conduction, BC= bone conduction

Diagnostic Studies
- Studies ordered by ENT/audiology for new-onset hearing loss

Differential Diagnoses
- See Etiology

Management
Nonpharmacologic Treatment
- Patient and family education:
  - Many patients will benefit from hearing aids, including those with sensorineural hearing loss
  - Hearing loss does not indicate cognitive losses
  - For many, hearing loss is permanent and must be accommodated
  - Patient may still experience difficulty hearing in certain situations such as those with increased background noise, areas with poor acoustics, or poor visualization of speaker
  - Communication strategies to improve patient's comprehension of spoken language (speech reading):
    - Face patient when speaking
    - Speak clearly and distinctly
    - Speak slightly louder without shouting
    - Lessen background noise

Pharmacologic Treatment
- Only about 5% of hearing loss (conductive) can be treated medically
- Discontinue ototoxic drugs if possible; if not, modify dosing schedule in attempt to decrease ototoxicity. Patients with decreased renal function are more at risk

Special Considerations
- Resource for patient with hearing loss and families: www.hearingexchange.com
- Information on hearing aids:
  - Healthy Hearing: www.healthyhearing.com
  - Hearing Aid Help: www.hearingaidhelp.com
- Consider the patient's personal and cultural attitudes towards hearing loss; these will determine the successful use of hearing aids, more than fit of the hearing aid or improvement of hearing
- For most, hearing loss is a way of life; hearing aids may greatly improve quality of life, but presbycusis and many sensorineural losses cannot be reversed

When to Consult, Refer, Hospitalize
- All patients with newly diagnosed or acute-onset hearing loss should be referred to ENT
- Refer to an audiologist when hearing loss becomes a problem to the patient
- Refer patient as needed for aural rehabilitation such as training in speech reading
- Refer to auditory assistive devices such as amplified doorbells and telephones; low-frequency ringers; and telecommunications devices for the deaf (TDD), which display a message on LED display or printer
- Refer to social services as needed

Follow-up
Expected Outcomes
- Presbycusis and sensorineural loss is irreversible in most cases; however, progression may be slowed or halted

Complications
- Decreased function, depression, and social isolation

Cerumen Impaction
Description
- Obstruction of ear canal by hardened wax

Etiology
- Cerumen is naturally occurring lubricant of ear canal that acts to protect the canal from water damage, infection, and trauma
- With aging, glands of the skin in the ear canal that produce cerumen atrophy, resulting in cerumen that is dry and hard and accumulates, obstructing the canal

Incidence and Demographics
- More common in older adults and those with cognitive impairment
- 20% to 60% of adults older than 65 years
- Most common cause of correctable hearing loss in older adults

Risk Factors
- Age
- Improper cleaning methods
- Hearing aids

Prevention and Screening
- Instruct patients in appropriate cleaning techniques (see Management)
- Assess on annual exam and with any new decreased hearing

Assessment
- Assess TM patency to determine treatment
- If TM is not visible, look for pain and risk factors for damaged TM

History
- Recent onset of pain, fullness, itching, tinnitus, pressure, hearing loss
- May present with acute onset pain if cotton swab broke off and became lodged in canal, resulting in swelling and pressure on sensitive canal or TM
- Significant pain indicates possible damage to TM
- History of perforation of TM
- Often bilateral

Physical Exam
- Otoscopy shows TM partially or completely obscured by dark brown cerumen in canal
- Scratch marks along canal may be present if patient has used cotton swab to clean or to remove obstruction on their own

Diagnostic Studies
- None indicated

Differential Diagnosis
- Foreign body in canal
- Tumor
- Otitis externa

Management
- Asymptomatic cerumen accumulation should not be removed
- Indications for removal: symptomatic impaction; cerumen obstructs visualization of ear canal or TM
- Presence of perforated TM is contraindication to ear drops or irrigation

Nonpharmacologic
- Ceruminolytics if no history of infections, perforations, or otologic surgery; avoid if status of TM is unknown
  - Soften ear wax with one to two drops of mineral oil daily for 5 days
  - Other OTC preparations of hydrogen peroxide and liquid docusate sodium may be used to soften wax
- If ceruminolytics are unsuccessful, then irrigate ear with solution of hydrogen peroxide and warm water
  - Avoid excess pressure, aim toward anterior wall of canal
  - Direct otoscopy following procedure to determine success
- Patient education
  - Attempts to "clean" ear canal and remove wax using cotton swab, washcloth, bobby pin, or other item may force wax medially and cause impaction or perforation of TM
  - Cleaning of ear with alcohol and water can exacerbate ear canal problems

Pharmacologic Treatment
- If no contraindications exist, ear drops containing neomycin/polymyxin B/ hydrocortisone (such as Cortisporin otic gtts), 1 to 2 drops q.i.d. for several days may be used after irrigation if ear canal is abraded

Special Considerations
- Cerumen can interfere with hearing aid function and patients with hearing aids should be regularly evaluated for cerumen impaction
- Ear candling has not been shown to be an effective method of cerumen removal and has the potential for serious injury; patients should avoid the use of ear candles for wax removal

When to Consult, Refer, Hospitalize
- Referral to otolaryngology if affected ear is only ear with intact hearing; if there is suspected perforation of the TM; or if coexisting problems of ear are present, such as severe infection, unexplained hearing loss, or hearing loss that did not clear with treatment of the impaction

Follow-up

- Patients with hearing aids should have their ears monitored for buildup of wax and have their ears and hearing aids cleaned regularly

Expected Outcomes

- Acute problem is generally resolved by irrigation
- Prophylactic mineral oil may ↓ recurrence

Complications

- Perforation of TM, infection, trauma to ear canal with bleeding
- Severe pain, fever and chills, mastoid tenderness, cellulitis, malaise, facial nerve palsy may indicate necrotizing malignant otitis externa and should be considered an emergency and urgently referred

Tinnitus

Description

- Perception of external or internal sounds in the absence of an external source; may be continuous or intermittent
- Symptom, not a disease, and reflects an underlying pathology; often associated with sensorineural hearing loss
- Two types of tinnitus:
  - Subjective tinnitus is only heard by the patient
  - Objective tinnitus is heard by others as well

Etiology

Subjective: majority have sensorineural tinnitus due to hearing loss at the cochlea or cochlear nerve level

- Cerumen obstruction
- Hearing loss
- Perforation of TM
- Serious otitis media
- Ménière's disease
- Otosclerosis
- Depression
- Caffeine
- Alcohol
- Medications: ASA, NSAIDs, antineoplastic drugs, aminoglycosides, tricyclic antidepressants, loop diuretics, oral contraceptives
- Meningitis
- Acoustic neuroma, may be unilateral

Objective: relatively rare, vascular or muscular etiology

- Vascular disorders (pulsatile quality, may be subjective) may be unilateral, resulting from:
  - Arteriovenous malformation
  - Aneurysm
  - Carotid occlusive disease
- Muscular disorders
  - Amyotrophic lateral sclerosis: deterioration of neuromuscular control over the muscles in the ear results in a repetitive flutter or myoclonus of either the stapedius or tensor tympani muscles

– Palatal myoclonus, a muscular-induced clicking tinnitus caused by a brainstem lesion due to stroke, trauma, encephalitis, multiple sclerosis (MS), or degenerative disease

Incidence and Demographics
- Incidence increases with age: 25% of older adults have tinnitus; severe in 1 of 6 and disabling in 1 of 30
- More prevalent among women than men

Risk Factors
- See Etiology

Prevention and Screening
- Avoidance of toxic medications
- Protection from noise exposure

Assessment
History
- Onset, intensity, pattern (episodic or constant, pulsatile or nonpulsatile, rhythmicity, pitch, quality)
  - May be described as high-pitched, low-pitched, clicking, buzzing, hissing, roaring
- Exacerbating and relieving factors—Is it worse in quiet room, unnoticed in noisy one?
- Effect on function—Does it interfere with concentration or sleep?
- Progression of symptoms
- History of previous ear disease, noise exposure, hearing status, head injury
- History of anemia, thyroid disorders, diabetes, cardiovascular disorder, trauma, neurologic disorder
- Medication review

Physical Exam
- Assess for hearing loss and, if present, pattern and changes and association with tinnitus
- Assess for cerumen obstructing canal, and fluid or mass behind the TM
- Focused head, neck, and CV evaluation (usually no abnormalities are found)
  - Assess for bruits over precordium, neck, and temporal bone
- Neurological exam for any focal abnormalities; cranial nerve testing and cerebellar functioning are key

Diagnostic Studies
- Pulsatile tinnitus: may require contrast CT scanning, contrast MR scanning, or angiography
- Auditory cause: audiometric testing
- Lab studies to rule out etiology as indicated

Differential Diagnosis
- See Etiology

Management
- For many patients, tinnitus is a chronic condition; goal of care should be reducing symptom burden

Nonpharmacologic
- Hearing aids may help resolve tinnitus by increasing normal sounds
  - Audiologist will determine sound frequency of tinnitus and evaluate patient for effectiveness of hearing aids or masking devices in relief of patient symptoms
- Cochlear implants may be used for patients with severe hearing loss who do not benefit from hearing aids
- A white noise generator at bedside may enable patient to sleep
- Tinnitus feedback retraining, biofeedback, and cognitive behavioral therapy have been useful in some cases

Pharmacologic
- Stop ototoxic medications
- There is no clear pharmacologic treatment for tinnitus
- Oral antidepressants have been most successful in relieving symptoms
- *Ginkgo biloba* has also been used; may not be more effective than placebo

Special Considerations
- 80% of patients with tinnitus have associated depression
- Referral to the American Tinnitus Association may provide support and education

When to Consult, Refer, Hospitalize
- Unilateral or pulsatile tinnitus should be promptly referred to rule out vascular or tumor cause
- New-onset tinnitus should be referred for evaluation if it is not promptly resolved by medication adjustment (such as addressing ASA excess) or clearing of cerumen impaction

Follow-up
Expected Outcomes
- Approximately 75% of patients with tinnitus can be helped with nonpharmacologic measures
- Tinnitus due to bilateral sensorineural hearing loss may worsen over time
- Tinnitus due to aminoglycosides and antineoplastic agents may be partially reversible; tinnitus due to ASA and loop diuretics is reversible when drug is stopped

Complications
- In severe cases, functional disruption with inability to carry out activities of daily living due to interrupted concentration and impaired sleep
- Vascular disaster (stroke) if atherosclerotic or aneurysmal etiology is not identified
- Progressive acoustic neuroma, causing deafness, disequilibrium, visual loss, chronic headache

Vertigo
(Also see Dizziness, Chapter 4)

Description
- Sensation of movement (frequently rotary) by either environment around patient or of patient within environment; may present as an exaggerated sense of motion in reaction to normal bodily movement, such as "rolling" unsteady sensation in response to walking
- Vertigo is the distinctive symptom of vestibular disease; it is not a diagnosis

- Distinguish from other forms of dizziness; see Chapter 4, Geriatric Multisystem Syndromes
- Two types: peripheral and central

Etiology
- Peripheral: arising from the ear, changes in the vestibular or labyrinthine system (80% of cases); benign paroxysmal positional vertigo, vestibular neuritis, and Ménière's disease are the most common
- Benign paroxysmal positional vertigo (BPPV): believed to be caused by free-floating calcium debris in the semicircular canals; as patient reclines or changes position, debris settles and signals are sent to brainstem, stimulating sensation of vertigo and nausea
- Vestibular neuritis (labyrinthitis): infection of inner ear, most likely viral, often following an upper respiratory infection; affects the vestibular portion of cranial nerve VIII
- Ménière's disease: peripheral vestibular disorder resulting from excess endolymphatic pressure; tears in membrane separating endolymph and perilymph allow mixing and distention, causing vertigo
- Central: CNS disturbance
  - Brainstem vascular disease: vertebrobasilar insufficiency TIA; may be caused by hypertension, atherosclerosis, embolic events
  - Multiple sclerosis (MS): 20% patients with MS have vertigo; demyelinization of nerve cells
  - Acoustic neuroma: slow-growing tumor arising from audiovestibular nerve; compresses cranial nerve VIII with resultant hearing loss and tinnitus; vertigo is a late symptom

Incidence and Demographics
- BPPV most common in those over 60
- Labyrinthitis: affects any age, usually after upper-respiratory infection
- Ménière's occurs between ages 40 and70

Risk Factors
- Age
- Upper-respiratory infection

Assessment
History
- All vertigo is made worse by head movements
- Peripheral vertigo generally has sudden onset and is fatigable, with hearing loss, nausea, and vomiting
- Central vertigo generally has gradual onset and is progressive, becomes disabling, not fatigable; exception is TIAs
- Spinning sensation is not required, may also experience sense of tilting or swaying
- Postural instability more common in central vertigo
- In older adults, vertigo may have a combination of etiologies; obtain clearest history possible, with detailed description; be careful not to lead patient by using words like "vertigo" or "dizziness"

Physical Exam
- Complete neurological exam with attention to cranial nerves
- Nystagmus is indicative of vertigo, but may be central or peripheral

- Otologic and bedside hearing exams
- Assess gait and balance
  - Romberg test: patient stands with feet together and eyes open, then closed; inability to maintain balance is failed test
- Dix-Hallpike maneuver: seat the patient with the head turned to one side, then place the patient supine rapidly, so that the head hangs over the edge of the bed; the patient is kept in this position until 30 seconds have passed if no nystagmus occurs; the patient is then returned to upright, observed for another 30 seconds for nystagmus, and the maneuver is repeated with the head turned to the other side; reproduction of symptoms and nystagmus are positive for positional vertigo

Table 7-7. Peripheral Vertigo

Disorder	History	Physical	Nonpharmacologic Treatment	Pharmacologic Treatment	Refer
Benign Paroxysmal Positional Vertigo	Severe vertigo seconds after changing head position; lasts seconds to minutes	Controlled head movements recreate symptoms; + nystagmus	Semont & Epley maneuvers; habituating exercises; vestibular rehab; self-limiting	Short course of vestibular suppressant (e.g., Meclizine 6.25–25 mg every 4–6 hrs p.r.n.)	If associated with auditory findings
Ménière's Disease	Sudden episodes vertigo, associated with tinnitus and diminished hearing lasting minutes to hours; asymptomatic between episodes	May be non-specific; + nystagmus during acute episode; may be progressive	Limit salt, caffeine, alcohol intake; rest & volume repletion if necessary; hearing aids, vestibular rehab; surgical intervention if episodes are incapacitating	Vestibular suppressants and antiemetics acutely; diuretic: HCTZ 12.5–25 mg q.d. or Triamterene 50 mg q.d. (monitor electrolytes)	To ENT for unilateral hearing loss evaluation
Vestibular Neuritis	Disabling vertigo with nausea, vomiting, gait impairment; may experience hearing loss; lasts hours to days	Symptoms: URI, sensorineural hearing loss, nystagmus first 24–48 hrs	Vestibular rehab; usually resolves in several days; Support symptomatically	Corticosteroids acutely (e.g., prednisone taper); antihistamines, antiemetics, anticholinergics in first 24–48 hrs	If any suspicion of hearing loss

Diagnostic Studies
- MRI or MRA if central lesion suspected
- Audiogram to evaluate sustained hearing loss
- Depending suspected etiology: CBC, chemistry panel, lipids, thyroid function studies, or ESR
- Unilateral hearing loss requires evaluation to rule out acoustic neuroma

Differential Diagnosis
- Otitis media
- Otitis externa
- Other causes of dizziness (see Chapter 4)
- Cerebellar disease
- Cerumen impaction

Management
Nonpharmacologic
- Rest in quiet, darkened room
- Safety precautions: change positions slowly; cane or walker during episodes
- Bland diet with small portions, fluids if nausea and vomiting present
- See Table 7–7 for specifics

Pharmacologic
- See Table 7–7
- Antihistamines can cause drowsiness, confusion, and anticholinergic symptoms of dry mouth, constipation, and urinary retention, and/or precipitate acute narrow-angle glaucoma
- Stop drugs when symptoms resolved, do not use prophylactically or as maintenance

Special Considerations
- Referral for vestibular rehab can be arranged through most physiotherapy departments or dizziness clinics
- Education about fall prevention is extremely important for older adults with vertigo; physical therapy may be beneficial

When to Consult, Refer, Hospitalize
- Hospitalize for dehydration and inability to take oral rehydration, secondary to severe nausea and vomiting
- Neurology referral if there are focal neurological deficits, severe headaches, transient neurological events, seizures, or other suggestions of central nervous system problem
- ENT for any patient with vertigo and unilateral auditory symptoms to rule out acoustic neuroma
- Urgent MRI or CT in acute sustained vertigo to rule out a vascular event in the cerebellum or brainstem in patients who are older, have vascular risk factors, and have headache

Follow-up
Expected Outcomes
- Peripheral generally lasts several days to weeks; may recur

Complications
- Hearing loss
- Falls with injury and possible long-term care placement
- Dehydration with associated nausea and vomiting

GENERAL APPROACH—NOSE

Normal Changes of Aging

- Nose becomes longer and narrower, with a sagging tip, because of influence of gravity and changes in support structures
- Cartilage of nose softens and thins and skin becomes more loose
- Nasal dryness is caused by decreased mucus production due to atrophy of mucus producing cells; mucus membrane thins and there is less submucosal tissue
- Thinned blood vessel walls leads to increased risk of epistaxis
- Changes in vasomotor secretory fibers may result in rhinorrhea when patient is exposed to some foods or cold air
- Olfaction, the sense of smell, comprises 85% of "taste"; neural degeneration causes a decrease in smell and fine taste, which may result in lack of interest in eating and poor nutrition
  - Smoking and exposure to environmental pollutants may also decrease sense of smell

Clinical Implications

History
- Acute onset of anosmia (loss of sense of smell) suggests tumor and requires investigation
- Ask about self-treatment of nasal symptoms and use of other medications that may cause dryness or rhinorrhea

Physical
- Pale, dry mucosa

Assessment

- Rhinitis, sinusitis, epistaxis, allergies, and nasal fractures are as common an occurrence in older adults as in younger adults

Management

- The anticholinergic effects of some antihistamines can cause syncope, vertigo, excessive sedation, hypotension, incoordination, constipation, and urinary retention in the patient with BPH, as well as thickening secretions and making airway clearing more difficult
- Sympathomimetics such as decongestants stimulate the cardiovascular system and can cause tachycardia, hypertension, confusion, agitation, and urinary retention
- Septal hematomas should be promptly evaluated by ENT and treated to prevent necrosis
- Nasal saline is safe and often provides comfort for rhinitis

COMMON NOSE DISORDERS

Rhinitis

Description
- An inflammation of the mucous membranes of the nose, usually accompanied by increased production of clear secretions (rhinorrhea); produces tissue inflammation of the nasal mucosa

- Defined by the presence of one or more of the following symptoms: sneezing, rhinorrhea, nasal congestion, nasal itching

Etiology
- Allergic rhinitis is an IgE-mediated hypersensitivity reaction; may be seasonal or perennial
  - Seasonal is related to inhaled seasonal pollen allergens (from trees, grasses, other sources)
  - Perennial is caused by always available allergens such as dust mites, pets dander, cockroaches, molds, and indoor pollutants
- Nonallergic rhinitis characterized by the chronic presence of one or more of the following: nasal congestion, rhinorrhea, and postnasal drainage with the absence of itching; common triggers include:
  - Tobacco smoke, diesel and car exhaust, temperature changes, fragrances, cleaning products, newsprint, and alcoholic beverages
  - Infectious rhinitis is most commonly caused by viral infections such as rhinovirus, as well as coronavirus, influenza, parainfluenza, and adenoviruses
  - Vasomotor rhinitis: etiologies are not well understood; thought to be an exaggerated autonomic response that results in vascular dilatation of the nasal submucosal vessels; influencing or triggering factors include temperature or humidity change, odors, selected drugs, emotional response, and body positions such as lying down
  - Drug-induced rhinitis: overuse of nasal decongestants (such as oxymetazoline [Afrin]) with rebound vasodilatation of the mucous membranes and nasal congestion after continuous use
  - Gustatory rhinitis: vagally mediated nasal vasodilation in response to eating spicy foods
  - Nonallergic rhinitis with eosinophilia syndrome (NARES): abnormal prostaglandin metabolism with the presence of eosinophils
  - Other types of nonallergic rhinitis include: occupational rhinitis and hormonal rhinitis
- Atrophic rhinitis: uncommon, sometimes seen after nasal surgery; more common in older adults; characterized by loss of cilia and abnormal patency of nasal passage, with formation of thick, dry, odorous crusts

Incidence and Demographics
- Allergic rhinitis: affects 10% to 30% of adults; more likely in individuals with eczema or asthma
- NARES: 20% of rhinitis diagnoses
- Mixed rhinitis: combination of allergic and nonallergic rhinitis is most common; 45% of individuals

Risk Factors
- Allergic rhinitis:
  - Family or personal history of atopy (asthma, eczema)
  - Male > female
- Nonallergic rhinitis:
  - Exposure to irritants (e.g., smog, exhaust fumes, tobacco smoke) or occupational exposure to fumes
  - Prolonged use of decongestant nasal drops or sprays

– Female > male

Prevention and Screening

- Frequent hand washing to reduce risk of infection; avoid close contact, particularly with older adults with cognitive impairment who are unable to cover their mouth and nose when sneezing or coughing
- Avoidance of known allergens and use of environmental control measures indoors such as frequent vacuuming with particulate filters, using air cleaners (HEPA filters), using mattress and pillow encasements, removing carpeting, using air conditioner, maintaining indoor humidity at least 50%, mopping tile, dusting furniture

Assessment

History and Physical Exam (see Table 7–8)

Diagnostic Studies

- Allergic rhinitis: clinical diagnosis in most cases
  - If symptoms are poorly controlled or cause is not identified, skin testing may indicate relevant IgE antibodies
- Nonallergic rhinitis: clinical diagnosis of exclusion

Table 7–8. Differentiating Rhinitis Presentations: History & Physical Exam

	Allergic Rhinitis	Viral Rhinitis (Cold)	Vasomotor Rhinitis	Atrophic Rhinitis
Onset	Any age	Anytime	Adulthood	Geriatric
Common primary symptoms	Nasal congestion, sneezing, itchy nose, clear drainage	Congestion, obstruction, nasal crusting, cloudy white to yellow drainage	Abrupt-onset congestion and pronounced watery postnasal drip, sneezing	Nasal congestion, thick postnasal drip, repeated clearing of throat, bad smell in nose
Associated symptoms	Cough, sore throat, itching and puffy eyes	Cough, sore throat, malaise, headache, fever > 100°	Watery eyes	None
Physical exam findings	Nasal mucosa pale, boggy, violaceous Enlarged turbinates, Clear watery d/c	Edema and hyperemia of mucous membranes Throat erythema Postnasal drainage Cervical lymph nodes tender, enlarged	Turbinates pale and edematous No other findings	Nasal mucosa dry, non-edematous; airway patent; no other findings
Diagnostic studies (if indicated): Hansel or Wright nasal smears	Positive for eosinophils	Positive for neutrophils Consider CBC, throat culture if suspect strep, advanced infection, or complications	Normal smears	Not indicated

Differential Diagnosis
- See Etiology

Management
Nonpharmacologic
- Identification and avoidance of triggers
- General measures: hydration, humidification, intranasal irrigations with saline solutions or OTC saline sprays
- Nonallergic rhinitis: inferior turbinectomy may be considered in patients with severe congestion that is refractory to adequate trials of medical management

Pharmacologic
- Allergic rhinitis:
  – An intranasal glucocorticoid (INGC), administered regularly or p.r.n., is first line
  – Add oral or topical second-generation antihistamines if symptoms not controlled with INGC
    • Oral: loratadine (Claritin), cetirizine (Zyrtec); topical: azelastine (Astelin)
  – Allergen injection immunotherapy if moderate-to-severe symptoms uncontrolled with the above
- Nonallergic rhinitis:
  – Combined therapy with INGC and topical antihistamine (azelastine)
    • Many formulations of INGC: fluticasone propionate (Flonase), triamcinolone acetonide (Nasacort)
      – Aqueous preparations may be more comfortable, cause less irritation; nasal inhalants may dry mucous membranes and cause irritation and bleeding
      – Azelastine HCL 0.1% (Astelin)
  – Ipratropium bromide nasal spray if prominent rhinorrhea or for patients with gustatory rhinitis
  – If nasal congestion refractory to INGC or azelastine, add OTC oral decongestants cautiously
    • Generally avoided in this age group because of high risk for adverse effects
    • In healthy older adults, give pseudoephedrine (Sudafed) 15–30 mg every 6 hours
- Specific recommendations:
  – Viral rhinitis: acetaminophen or NSAIDs for pain or fever, decongestants
    • Avoid antihistamines as they may over-dry and reduce ability to clear secretions
  – Atrophic rhinitis: guaifenesin to liquefy mucus, or intranasal saline solution spray

Special Considerations
- Monitor closely for adverse effects from medications and drug interactions with antihypertensives, antidepressants, other cardiac drugs
- Use OTC decongestants with caution in patients with diabetes, HTN, or glaucoma
- Patient education: do not combine these medication with herbal treatments as some contain the same ingredients (e.g., ephedra) that can cause side effects or overdosage if used concomitantly

When to Consult, Refer, Hospitalize
- Referral to an allergist to consider allergen immunotherapy for allergic rhinitis that is not easily managed by medications or avoidance of known allergens
- Referral to ENT for those with symptoms unmanageable with above described treatments, if complications, or if nasal polyps or other growths are seen or suspected

Follow-up
Expected Outcomes
- Viral rhinitis usually resolves within 7 to 10 days
- Allergic, vasomotor, and atrophic rhinitis are ongoing problems that are managed symptomatically and not cured

Complications
- Worsening of related pulmonary conditions such as COPD, asthma
- Development and spread of bacterial infection: acute sinusitis, bronchitis, pneumonia

Rhinosinusitis
Description
- Inflammation of the nasal cavity and maxillary, frontal, ethmoid, or sphenoid sinuses due to infection (viral, bacterial, or fungal) or allergic reaction; risk for sinusitis increased by sinus structure in some patients
- Categorized as acute, subacute, chronic, or recurrent
  - Acute: lasting < 4 weeks
  - Subacute: lasting 4–12 weeks
  - Chronic: lasting > 12 weeks; may result in irreversible damage to mucosa
  - Recurrent: ≥ 4 episodes of acute rhinosinusitis/year with resolution of symptoms between episodes

Etiology
- Three major common factors:
  - Drainage of the sinus is blocked
  - Mucus secretions accumulate, providing media for pathogenic organisms
  - Change in quality of sinus secretions
- Majority of cases are caused by viral infection (rhinovirus, coronavirus, adenovirus)
  - Acute bacterial infection occurs in only 0.5% to 2% of acute episodes
  - Most common bacterial pathogens in acute sinusitis: *Streptococcus pneumoniae*, *Haemophilus influenza*, *S. aureus*, *Enterobacteriaceae*, and *Moraxella catarrhalis*
  - Other infectious causes like fungal (*Aspergillus*) infection, especially in the immunocompromised
- Allergic rhinitis may predispose the individual

Incidence and Demographics
- 30 million cases of sinusitis diagnosed in United States each year
- Common among older adults because of dry nasal passages and airflow changes associated with aging

Risk Factors
- Advanced age
- Immunocompromise
- Asthma, allergies, upper-respiratory infections
- Nasal polyps or other obstruction
- Other risk factors: dental infections, changes in atmospheric pressure, cigarette smoking, air pollutants

Prevention and Screening
- Appropriate treatment of allergies and infections
- Correction of mechanical obstruction such as polyps, septal deviation
- Avoidance of adverse environmental factors such as known allergens, cigarette smoke, and other polluting agents

Assessment
- Differentiating between viral and bacterial rhinosinusitis is primarily clinical
  - Viral: Partial or complete resolution of symptoms within 7 to 10 days following the onset of an upper-respiratory infection
  - Bacterial: symptoms lasting ≥ 7 days with any one of the following:
    - Purulent nasal discharge
    - Maxillary tooth or facial pain, especially unilateral
    - Unilateral maxillary sinus tenderness
    - Worsening symptoms after initial improvement

History
- Acute and chronic rhinosinusitis typically present with a history of precipitants such as allergic or nonallergic rhinitis, or an upper-respiratory infection that has persisted beyond 5 to 7 days
- Classic presenting symptoms include: nasal congestion, yellow/green rhinorrhea, postnasal drainage, facial or dental pain or pressure, headache, altered sense of smell, cough that is worse at night, sinus pressure when bending over
- Other associated symptoms of fever, malaise, fatigue, sore throat, halitosis, nausea, and increased snoring may be present
- Complaints of orbital pain or vision disturbances are indicators of a more serious problem

Physical Exam
- Complete HEENT and pulmonary exam:
  - Face/sinuses: tenderness overlying the involved sinuses
  - Ears: middle ear abnormalities and eustachian tube dysfunction
  - Nose: erythema of the mucosa and purulent drainage
  - Mouth: purulent postnasal drainage on posterior pharyngeal area
  - Chest: potential for wheezing, congestion associated with asthma or URI

Diagnostic Studies
- CT scans are used to confirm the diagnosis and identify obstruction and need for surgical intervention in recurrent sinusitis; cost of CT is similar to that of standard sinus films
- MRI is most useful for assessing the presence of fungal sinusitis and tumors and for differentiating between inflammatory disease and malignant tumors
- Recurrent or chronic sinusitis may warrant bacterial culture

Differential Diagnosis
- URI
- Allergic rhinitis
- Nasal polyps
- Nasal septum deviation
- Nasopharyngeal tumor

Management
Nonpharmacologic
- Supportive care for all patients with symptoms for < 10 days unless patient experiences clinical worsening after initial improvement, patient has severe symptoms and a worsening clinical course, or patient is immunocompromised
- Watchful waiting has been recommended for patients presenting with > 10 days of symptoms with mild pain and temperature < 101° F (mild acute bacterial rhinosinusitis)
  - Close observation for 7 days after diagnosis; if no improvement, antibiotics should be initiated
  - Factors such as age, comorbid medical conditions, and overall health should be considered when choosing this option
- Comfort measures to decrease inflammation and promote drainage include: adequate rest and hydration, analgesics (NSAIDs and acetaminophen), warm facial packs, steamy showers, saline nasal sprays and irrigation, sleeping with the head of bed elevated, increased humidity in home

Pharmacologic
- Antibiotics used for 10 to 14 days
  - Amoxicillin 500 mg t.i.d. should be used first line; trimethoprim/sulfamethoxazole DS b.i.d.; first-generation macrolide (erythromycin) for patients with penicillin allergy
  - Failure to respond to first-line antibiotics within 7 days or worsening clinical status warrants switching to a new antibiotic such as amoxicillin/clavulanic acid or a fluoroquinolone
- Corticosteroids
  - Intranasal glucocorticoids for those with chronic rhinosinusitis (cornerstone of maintenance therapy), underlying rhinitis, or associated bronchial hyper-responsiveness
  - Oral corticosteroids, short-term, for those with significant anatomic obstruction, invasive nasal polyposis, or who have demonstrated marked mucosal edema radiographically
- Decongestants topically to help with drainage of sinuses

Special Considerations
- Patients with underlying allergic rhinitis with sneezing and rhinorrhea may benefit from daily use of a second-generation antihistamine

When to Consult, Refer, Hospitalize
- Serious complications requiring urgent referral and treatment
  - External facial swelling
  - Erythema
  - Cellulitis over an involved sinus
  - Vision changes (diplopia, difficulty moving eyes [extraocular muscles]; proptosis [forward displacement of eye])
  - Any abnormal neurologic signs
- Refer to ENT or allergist for treatment failure, chronic or complicated sinusitis management

Follow-up
Expected Outcomes
- Acute rhinosinusitis: improvement of symptoms within 72 hours and resolution of sinusitis within 10 days
- Chronic rhinosinusitis: cannot be cured in most cases; goal of care is reduction of symptom burden

Complications
- Asthma, bronchitis, bronchiectasis, or pneumonia
- Facial or orbital cellulitis
- Ophthalmoplegia and visual loss
- Osteomyelitis of facial bones
- Meningitis
- Subdural empyema
- Intracranial complications

Epistaxis
Description
- Hemorrhage from the nostrils, nasopharynx, or nasal cavity
- A symptom of an underlying problem or disease, not a disease of its own

Etiology
- Localized irritation secondary to rhinitis of all types, sinusitis
- Excessive drying of the membranes by low humidity or nasal oxygen
- Trauma such as nose picking, forceful blowing of nose, or nasal fracture may precipitate bleed
- Tumor
- Arteriovenous malformation (AVM)
- Hypertension a rare cause (bleed may be worsened by but not caused by HTN)
- Use of NSAIDs or aspirin (even cardioprotective baby aspirin)
- Coagulation disorders or use of medications such as warfarin

Incidence and Demographics
- Common among older adults
- Male = female
- Increased incidence in dry winter months
- Anterior bleeds most common

Risk Factors
- Age-related mucosal and vessel wall changes
- Use of anticoagulant medications
- Family history of blood dyscrasias
- Vascular disease

Prevention and Screening
- Adequate moisturizing of the mucous membranes: humidifier, saline nasal spray
- Keep nails short and away from the nose
- Apply petroleum jelly (Vaseline) or K-Y jelly to nares routinely for lubrication
- Humidify oxygen

Assessment
History
- Patients may present with actively bleeding nose, or may consult for episodes that were resolved with self-care
- Determine
  - Bleeding unilateral (which nostril) or bilateral
  - Precipitating events
  - Past history of epistaxis
  - Associated symptoms: URI, nausea and vomiting (swallowed blood), other signs/symptoms of systemic bleeding (coffee-ground emesis, hemoptysis, melena)

Table 7–9. Characteristics of Nasal Bleeding Sites

	Anterior Epistaxis	Posterior Epistaxis
Presentation	Typically unilateral, one nostril	Unilateral or bilateral
Timing	Lasts between a few to 30 min, in isolation or recurrently	Intermittent
Source of bleed	90% are venous from Kiesselbach plexus	Typically arterial from posterior nasopharynx
Miscellaneous Facts	Usually less severe, easier to treat Direct pressure frequently stops bleeding	May have nausea or coffee-ground emesis Frequently requires nasal packing More common in older adults

Physical Exam
- Inspect for site of bleed: note localized or diffuse mucosal irritation, bleeding from one or two nostrils, duration of bleeding (see Table 7–9)
- Adequate exam requires the use of a nasal speculum

Diagnostic Studies
- Only recurrent or severe cases warrant extensive evaluation
- If significant blood loss is suspected, obtain a hemoglobin and hematocrit
- If bleeding disorders are suspected, then obtain a CBC, PT, and PTT

Differential Diagnosis
- See Etiology

Management
Nonpharmacologic
- For simple nosebleed
  - Application of direct pinching pressure just below the bridge of the nose for 10 to 15 minutes will stop the bleeding
  - Keep the patient in an upright position and leaning forward, to drain blood into bowl and discourage swallowing
  - Apply ice packs over the bridge of the nose
  - See Prevention

Pharmacologic
- For anterior hemostasis, vasoconstrictors: oxymetazoline (Afrin) 0.05% with topical anesthetic agents (tetracaine and lidocaine)

- Silver nitrate stick cautery is very painful; give local anesthetic first
- If packing is necessary, coat nasal tampon with antibiotic ointment (bacitracin) to facilitate placement
- Correct any coagulopathies, iatrogenic or otherwise, so clot can form
- Acute treatment with antihypertensives if associated with an acute HTN crisis

Special Considerations
- Treatment is episodic for the actual bleeding incident
- Ongoing monitoring and treatment indicated for the associated underlying disorders
- Retained anterior gauze packing is a frequent foreign body in older adults; monitor carefully

When to Consult, Refer, Hospitalize
- Immediate referral to an ER or ENT for severe bleeding or bleeding unresponsive to first-line treatment
- Recurrent epistaxis is cause for referral to a specialist
- Patient requiring posterior packing may be admitted to hospital for respiratory monitoring

Follow-up
Expected Course
- Excellent prognosis for isolated, idiopathic epistaxis
- In other cases, variable outcome depending on underlying cause

Complications
- Sinusitis
- Nasal obstruction
- Abscess from excessive trauma during packing of nose
- Septal perforation from cauterization therapy
- Vasovagal episode during packing
- Anemia from blood loss during recurrent or severe epistaxis

GENERAL APPROACH—MOUTH
Normal Changes of Aging
- Some atrophy of oral epithelial tissue, but it remains functional and intact, with a slight decrease in salivary production
- Periodontal changes: increase in dental plaque and gingival recession and bleeding
- In larynx, muscle atrophy, decreased vibratory mass, decreased support by fibrous tissue, and squamous metaplasia are seen
- Bowing of the vocal cords (due to decreased elasticity and decreased muscle mass) combine with decreased pulmonary volume and expiratory effort to produce a high, quivery voice

Clinical Implications
History
- Problems eating, food taste
- Lumps or sores in the mouth or on the lips
- Frequency of dentist visits, wearing dentures or partials, fit
- Tobacco, alcohol use
- Medications

Physical
- Note fit of dentures
- Have patient remove dentures or partials, and using a flashlight and tongue depressor, examine thoroughly all surfaces
- Lesions in back and underside of tongue are easily missed; look carefully
- Palpate for any masses
- If any plaques are noted, see if they are fixed or if they can be scraped off
- Note the tongue; large lesions and those persisting more than 2 weeks should be referred for biopsy
- Assess for gingivitis (inflammation of gums); may lead to periodontal disease and loss of teeth

Assessment

- Decreased salivary function and decreased taste combine to put the patient at risk for decreased oral intake; carefully assess patient's nutritional status and hydration status
- Patients with a history of heavy tobacco and alcohol use are at higher risk for malignant oral lesions and should be carefully evaluated for any ulcer that is atypical in appearance or does not heal in 2 weeks

Management

- Good nutritional support and hydration are key to resolution and prevention of oral lesions; poor dentition may have led to poor nutrition, and should be referred for dental correction
- Patients should be encouraged in good dental hygiene: brushing with soft brush including gum surfaces, flossing, and use of a fluoride dentifrice or rinse
- Patient should see dentist every 6 months to 1 year

COMMON MOUTH DISORDERS

- **Oral cancer:** ulcers that do not completely heal within 2 to 3 weeks of diagnosis or treatment, or that present with no clear etiology should be referred to ENT for evaluation
  - Most common site of malignancies of the head and neck is the oral cavity
  - Extrinsic risk factors include tobacco and alcohol use
  - Oral cancer should always be included in the differential diagnosis.
- **Aphthous ulcers** (canker sores): common, benign, and generally resolve spontaneously
- **Denture sores:** appear where dentures rub the gum
  - Ill fitting dentures are common due to weight loss
  - Infected denture sores that do not heal by taking dentures out of the mouth overnight should be treated by dentist
- **Angular cheilitis:** leukoplakic fissures formed in the redundant skin of the lip commissures, usually resolves with treatment with mild topical steroid
- **Gingivitis:** the inflammation of gums with swelling, receding, easily bleeding gums, and cold sensitivity
- **Periodontal disease** is inflammation and destruction of supportive structure of tooth, causing loosening then loss of teeth
  - More common and extensive among those who have not had recent dental care, especially underserved populations such as Blacks, Hispanics, and refugees
  - Those with gingival hyperplasia are more prone to this disorder
    - Gingival hyperplasia may be seen as a side effect of some medications, including calcium channel blockers, phenytoin, and cyclosporine
  - Gingivitis and periodontitis should be managed by a dentist and oral surgeon

- **Xerostomia:** sensation of dry mouth related to decreased saliva production due to
  - Sjögren syndrome (autoimmune exocrinopathy)
  - Dehydration
  - Other oral conditions such as: infection, salivary gland obstruction (sialolith, a stone), trauma and neoplasms that may result in decreased salivary output
  - Stress (sympathetic nervous system effect)
  - Mouth breathing (nasal obstruction)
  - Medications such as: anticholinergics, antidepressants, antihistaminics, anxiolytics, diuretics, antidepressants, and antiparkinsonian agents
  - Management
    - Modify medication regimen: substitute medications that are less anticholinergic, decrease dosages, or split dosages throughout the day
    - Stimulate salivation with sugarless mints and gums
    - Moisturizing gels and rinses, artificial saliva
    - Institute good oral hygiene
    - Lubricants can be used to prevent painful lip cracking
    - Pilocarpine 5 mg t.i.d. and at night may be tried
    - Oncologic treatment: radiation therapy and cytotoxic chemotherapy
- **Decreased taste:** alteration in perceptions of flavor of food or drink due to
  - Xerostomia
  - Anticholinergic medications
  - Medical illnesses such as: chronic renal failure, diabetes mellitus
  - Places patient at risk for anorexia, malnutrition, and dehydration

Oral Candidiasis

Description
  - Local overgrowth of normally occurring *Candida* flora on mucous membranes of the mouth and esophagus
  - Oral candidiasis can manifest in several ways, including
    - Pseudomembranous candidiasis (thrush): leukoplakic plaques easily removed with an erythematous base beneath
    - Papillary hyperplasia: confluent leukoplakic plaques that cannot be removed
    - Atrophic candidiasis (denture stomatitis): smooth, diffuse erythematous mucosal lesions, often found beneath dentures

Etiology
  - Majority is caused by the fungus *Candida albicans*, which is an organism common to the oropharyngeal cavity, gastrointestinal tract, and vagina of humans
  - Opportunistic infection may occur in the following instances: disruption of normal flora, a breach of the mucocutaneous barrier, or an immunocompromised host

Incidence and Demographics
  - 60% of healthy adults carry *Candida* species as part of their normal oral flora
  - Atrophic candidiasis is most common form in older adults

Risk Factors
  - Diabetes, resulting in high blood and salivary glucose levels
  - Medications such as: antibiotics, corticosteroids, antineoplastics, and other immunosuppressants
  - Immunosuppression

Prevention and Screening
- Oral evaluation during routine physical exam and dental visits every 6 months
- Good oral hygiene
- Rinse mouth following use of inhaled corticosteroids

Assessment
History
- Many patients are asymptomatic
- Others may describe: cottony feeling in the mouth, loss of taste, or occasional pain with eating and swallowing
- Patients with dentures often have pain when wearing their dentures

Physical Exam
- Pseudomembranous candidiasis: white plaques on the buccal mucosa, palate, tongue, oropharynx, or under dentures; scraping of plaque may result in bleeding of the underlying tissue
- Atrophic candidiasis: erythema without plaques found under dentures

Diagnostic Studies
- Gram stain or KOH prep of tongue scrapings; budding yeasts with or without pseudohyphae are seen
- Testing for HIV may be appropriate depending on the patient's risk factors

Differential Diagnosis
- Oral hairy leukoplakia
- Burn
- Bacterial gingivitis
- Periodontitis
- Oral cancer

Management
Nonpharmacologic
- Rinse following use of inhaled glucocorticoids
- Good oral hygiene

Pharmacologic
- Treat underlying cause
- Treat for 7 to 14 days following resolution of symptoms
- Topical agents (successful therapy depends on contact time of at least 2 minutes with the oral mucosa):
    - Nystatin swish and swallow: 200,000 to 400,000 units 5 times daily
    - Clotrimazole troches: one 10-mg troche dissolved slowly 5 times daily
- If unsuccessful, oral antifungals may be used:
    - Fluconzaole 200 mg p.o. once, then 100 mg p.o. daily

Special Considerations
- Immunosuppressed patients with thrush often have concurrent *Candida esophagitis*
- *Candida* species also cause angular cheilitis or perleche, a painful fissuring at the corners of the mouth

When to Consult, Refer, Hospitalize
- Oral lesions that do not completely heal within 2 to 3 weeks of diagnosis or treatment or that present with no clear etiology should be referred to ENT for evaluation
- Hospitalization should be considered for patients presenting with symptoms of systemic infection or who are severely immunocompromised

Follow-up
Expected Outcomes
- Recurrence is common if underlying risk factors are still present (ongoing steroid use, chemotherapy)

Complications
- Systemic infection
- Bacterial superinfection of oral lesions

CASE STUDIES

Case 1. An 83-year-old female nursing home patient is observed to have crusting on both eyelashes in the mornings.

HPI: Patient diagnosed with Alzheimer's disease is a resident in a long-term-care (LTC) facility. You are told that there have been several cases of conjunctivitis in the facility in the past week. Patient is nonverbal, but has been observed rubbing her eyes in the past few days.

PMH: Resident in LTC for several years. Her personal care is provided by nurse aides. In general good health otherwise. Under treatment for seborrheic dermatitis. No food or drug allergies.

Medication: Hydrocortisone 1% cream sparingly to affected facial area daily; multivitamin daily.

1. Which are the most likely differential diagnoses for the presenting problem?
2. Review the risk factors for the possible diagnoses.
3. What further history would you obtain?
4. What key findings would you look for in the physical exam?

Exam: Eyelids are found to be inflamed, with broken and misdirected lashes. Scaling of lids noted. Conjunctiva is mildly injected. Golden crusting is noted along lid edges; drainage is reported to be worse in the morning, staying clear through the day.

5. What treatment plan would you develop, based on these findings?
6. What follow-up would you recommend?
7. Under what circumstances would you make a referral?

Case 2. An 82-year-old man comes to clinic accompanied by his wife. He has not been back for his routine visits for 8 months. He has no complaints, says no to every question you ask. Wife states he is driving her nuts; she thinks he is getting senile or going crazy because he has lost interest in socializing and has stopped watching TV. Chart shows patient was a construction worker. He smoked and drank heavily for many years before quitting about 15 years ago. His medical diagnoses are hypertension, osteoarthritis, and COPD; medications are atenolol (Tenormin) 50 mg p.o. q.d., enalapril (Vasotec) 5 mg p.o. q.d. theophylline sustained release (Theo-Dur) 100 mg p.o. b.i.d., and aspirin as needed for arthritis pain.

1. What part of this history suggests hearing loss?
2. What risk factors for hearing loss does he have?

Exam: Shows that the patient can hear sound but cannot understand many of the words.

3. What kind of hearing loss does this suggest?
4. Would a referral for a hearing aid be appropriate for this kind of hearing loss?

Case 3. A 65-year-old female patient presents with complaint of "a cold." States symptoms have been present for 6 days and include a "runny nose, cough, and just feel miserable." Has gotten worse in past 2 days. Gives history of "Allergies to pollen." No regular medications; has been taking ibuprofen and pseudoephedrine to control symptoms.

Exam: Patient appears mildly ill but not in distress; temp 100.2° F oral; pulse 100, respiration 20, mouth breathing, but no acute respiratory distress. Ears: canals clear, TMs bilaterally dull and retracted, nasal mucosa swollen, red, with green discharge. Palpable enlarged lymph nodes tender to palpation. Chest is clear, heart normal.

1. What further history would you like?
2. What else is included in your physical exam?
3. What is your diagnosis?
4. What would you do for the patient on this visit?

REFERENCES

Ahmad, N., & Seidman, M. (2004). Tinnitus in the older adult: Epidemiology, pathophysiology and treatment options. *Drugs and Aging, 21*(5), 297–305.

American Academy of Ophthalmology. (2005a). *Primary angle closure, preferred practice pattern.* San Francisco: American Academy of Ophthalmology.

American Academy of Ophthalmology. (2005b). *Primary open-angle glaucoma, preferred practice pattern.* San Francisco: American Academy of Ophthalmology.

Bhattacharyya, N., Baugh, R. F., Orvidas, L., Barrs, D., Bronston, L. J., Cass, S., et al. (2008). Clinical practice guideline: Benign paroxysmal positional vertigo. *Otolaryngology–Head and Neck Surgery, 139*(5S4), S47–S81.

Bourla, D. H., & Young, T. A. (2006). Age-related macular degeneration: A practical approach to a challenging disease. *Journal of the American Geriatrics Society, 54*(7), 1130–1135.

Buttaro, T. M., Trybulski, J., Bailey, P. P., & Sandberg-Cook, J. (2008). *Primary care: A collaborative practice* (3rd ed.). St. Louis, MO: Mosby.

Chibber, R., Chibber, S., & Kohner, E. M. (2008). 21st century treatment of diabetic retinopathy. *Expert Review of Endocrinology and Metabolism, 2*(5), 623–631.

Kucik, C. J., & Clenney, T. (2005). Management of epistaxis. *American Family Physician, 71*(2), 305–311.

Labuguen, R. H. (2006). Initial evaluation of vertigo. *American Family Physician, 73*(2), 244–251.

Little, D. (2005). Allergies in the aging. *Geriatrics and Aging, 8*(5), 52–53.

National Eye Institute, National Institutes of Health. (2006). *National Eye Health Education Program (NEHEP): Five-year agenda.* Retrieved from http://www.nei.nih.gov/nehep/docs/nehep_5_year_agenda_2006.pdf

Pokhrel, P. K., & Loftus, S. A. (2007). Ocular emergencies. *American Family Physician, 76*(6), 829–836.

Ramakrishnan, V. R., Meyers, A. D., & Woodall, B. S. (2008). *Nonallergic rhinitis.* Retrieved from http://emedicine.medscape.com/article/874171-overview

Regan, E. N. (2008). Diagnosing rhinitis: Viral and allergic characteristics. *Nurse Practitioner, 33*(9), 20–26.

Roland, P. S., Smith, T. L., Schwartz, S. R., Rosenfeld, R. M., Ballachanda, B., Earll, J. M., et al. (2008). Clinical practice guideline: Cerumen impaction. *Otolaryngology–Head & Neck Surgery, 139*(3S2), S1–S21

Rosenfeld, R. M., Andes, D., Bhattacharyya, N., Cheung, D., Eisenberg, S., Ganiats, T. G., et al. (2007). Clinical practice guideline: Adult sinusitis. *Otolaryngology–Head & Neck Surgery, 137*(3S), S1–S31.

Shay, K. (2006). Oral infections in the elderly part II: Fungal and viral infections: Systemic impact of oral bacterial infections. *Clinical Geriatrics, 14*(7), 37–45.

Silverman, S. J. (2007). Mucosal lesions in older adults. *Journal of the American Dental Association, 138*(S), 41–46.

Tabloski, P. A. (2006). *Gerontological nursing.* Upper Saddle River, NJ: Pearson Education, Inc.

Respiratory Disorders

Michaelene Jansen, PhD, RN, GNP-BC, NP-C

GERIATRIC APPROACH

Normal Changes of Aging

Capacity

- Total lung capacity (TLC; volume of gas in the lungs after a maximal inspiration) remains unchanged
  - Decreased elastic recoil makes it easier to expand the lungs
  - Chest wall is stiffer with aging, limiting the amount the lungs can expand (a normal musculoskeletal change of aging)
- Residual volume (RV; volume of air remaining in the respiratory system when subjects have expired as much air as possible) increases with aging
  - Vital capacity (VC) is the difference between the total lung capacity (TLC) and the residual volume (RV); this is the air that is being moved in and out of the lungs
  - Since the RV increases while the TLC stays the same, the VC (amount of air being moved in and out) decreases
- Functional residual capacity (FRC; the lung volume at the end of normal quiet respiration) increases slightly with age

Flow Rate

- Peak expiratory flow (PEF) rate decreases
  - The initial PEF rate (maximal flow) decreases slightly; correlates with forced expired volume in first second (FEV_1). The rate is determined by recoil of lung and chest wall and the speed with which the respiratory muscles generate positive pleural pressure

- The initial maximal flow decreases slightly
- FEV_1 decreases at the rate of about 30 ml per year
- The FEV_{25-75} decreases significantly (see below)
  - Major reductions in maximal expiratory flow occur at lower lung volumes
  - The maximal flow throughout the remainder of the VC after FEV_1 is determined by the intrinsic properties of the lung: elastic recoil pressure, the cross-sectional area of the airways, and airway compliance
  - Much of the decrease is caused by lung elastic recoil with aging
- Healthy Black older adults have a 10% decrease in FEV_1
- Respiratory drive is reduced because of hypoxia, elevated pCO_2 levels, and resistance changes
- Increased airway reactivity

Table 8-1. Definitions of Pulmonary Function Tests

Test	Definition
Spirometry	
FVC	Forced vital capacity—volume of gas that can be forcefully expelled from the lungs after maximal inspiration
FEV_1	Forced expiratory volume in 1 second—volume of gas expelled in the first second of the FVC
FEF_{25-75}	Forced expiratory flow from 25% to 75% of the FVC—maximal midexpiratory airflow rate
PEFR	Peak expiratory flow rate—maximal airflow rate achieved in the FVC maneuver
MVV	Maximum voluntary ventilation—the maximum volume of gas that can be breathed in 1 minute (measured in 15 seconds and multiplied by 4)
Lung volumes	
TLC	Total lung capacity—volume of gas in the lungs after a maximal inspiration
RV	Residual volume—volume of gas remaining in the lungs after maximal expiration
ERV	Expiratory reserve volume—volume of gas representing the difference between functional residual capacity and residual volume
FRC	Functional residual capacity—volume of gas into the lungs at the end of a normal tidal expiration
SVC	Slowed vital capacity—volume of gas that can be slowly exhaled after maximal inspiration

Clinical Implications

History

- Frequent nonspecific presentation of respiratory problems as confusion, decreased activities of daily living (ADL), and falls
- Obtain complete smoking history of patient and spouse
- Is cough productive or nonproductive? Note color, amount, consistency of sputum
- Exercise tolerance/activity level, how far can the patient can walk, or climb stairs before getting short of breath

Physical
- Older adult patients may have difficulty following instructions when asked to take a deep breath; subtle findings may be missed
- If patient is unable to sit up, roll patient onto side, auscultate the higher side; then roll patient onto opposite side and auscultate other side
- Respiratory and cardiac problems closely related, evaluate both systems
- Spirometry for lung status in acute illness
- Chest x-ray is frequently necessary for accurate diagnosis
- Pulse oximetry for resting and exercise oxygenation

Assessment
- Older adult patients tend to present with confusion when their pO_2 is decreased for any reason
- Majority of respiratory infections are viral, but risk for secondary bacterial infection is great
- Exacerbations in chronic obstructive pulmonary disease (COPD) symptoms are usually due to infection
- Older adults often have low baseline peak flow rates; however, monitoring may useful

Treatment
- Respiratory medications have increased adverse reactions in older adults
- Dizziness causes falls
- Older patients may not tolerate oral decongestants because of tachycardia or agitation and nervousness
- When using metered dose inhalers (MDI) instruct in proper use, use spacer, and have them give return demonstration; many older adults have difficulty manipulating inhalers
- Use nebulizers instead of inhalers for bronchodilators; steroids may be more effective
- Patients should stay well hydrated, but watch for fluid overload
- Influenza vaccination annually
- Pneumovax vaccination > 65 or otherwise indicated; one-time revaccination if older adult vaccinated 5 or more years previously and was < 65 years old at time of primary vaccination

ASTHMA

Description
Complex disorder characterized by variable and recurring symptoms, airflow obstruction, and underlying inflammation

Etiology
- Caused by allergic and nonallergic triggers
  - Allergic triggers: seasonal or environmental allergens—pollens, feathers, pet dander, dust mite and cockroach excrement, molds, food additives, preservatives such as sulfites
  - Nonallergic triggers: smoke, fumes, dyes, air pollutants
- Respiratory/cardiac diseases or infections such as chronic heart failure, bronchitis, and viral respiratory infection
- Drug induced—acetysalicylic acid (ASA), NSAIDs, topical and systemic beta-blockers

Incidence and Demographics
- Prevalence is similar to that for adults
- Usually develops in younger people, but onset in the older adult is not unusual
- Deaths three times greater among Blacks and Hispanics than among Whites

Risk Factors
- Family history asthma or allergies
- Nasal polyps
- Eczema/atopic dermatitis
- Untreated/asymptomatic gastroesophageal reflux disease (GERD)

Prevention and Screening
- Use of air filters and air conditioners
- Treat upper-respiratory infections when present
- Control GERD

Assessment
History
- Classic symptoms—episodic acute onset of wheezing (absent in severe exacerbations), chest tightness, dyspnea, chronic dry or nonproductive cough; symptoms worse at night, with exercise, and with exposure to cold temperatures and the patient's triggers
- Confusion, slight shortness of breath, decreased exercise tolerance
- Severity of symptoms (see Table 8–2)
- Asthma Therapy Assessment Questionnaire (ATAQ), Asthma Control Questionnaire (ACQ), Asthma Control Test (ACT)
- Frequency of episodes, previous treatment
- Smoking history

Physical
- General: diaphoresis, use of accessory muscles to breathe, tachycardia, tachypnea
- Lungs: decreased breath sounds, wheezing, prolonged expiration, hyperresonance
- Look for signs of chronic heart failure or dehydration
- If allergic may see nasal discharge, sinus tenderness, mucosal edema and erythema, postnasal drainage
- Severe exacerbation: cyanosis, barely audible to absent breath sounds, pulsus paradoxus (> 20 mm Hg fall in blood pressure during inspiration)

Diagnostic Studies
- Routine monitoring of pulmonary function is essential with peak flow meter (home use)
  - Peak flow meter measures peak expiratory flow (PEF)
  - Used for monitoring lung status, not to confirm diagnosis
  - Values vary with height, age, gender; with the very old patients are greatly decreased
  - Values less than 200L/min may indicate severe airflow obstruction
  - 80% to 100% of patient's "personal best"—good control, maintain treatment
  - 50% to 80%—acute exacerbation, adjust treatment
  - < 50%—severe asthma exacerbation, emergency treatment
- Pulmonary function tests (PFT)/spirometry—reveal obstructive dysfunction
  - See Table 8–1, Definitions of Pulmonary Function Tests
  - Used to diagnose obstructive and restrictive airway disease
  - Airflow obstruction indicated by reduced FEV_1/FVC ratio (< 70%)

Table 8-2. Classification and Treatment of Asthma

Step	Symptoms	Night-time Symptoms	Lung Function	Treatment
Step 6 Severe Persistent	Symptoms throughout day, most days SABA (short-acting beta$_2$-agonist) several times a day Limited activity	Most nights	FEV$_1$ < 60% predicted FEV$_1$/FVC reduced > 5%	High-dose inhaled corticosteroid (ICS) + long-acting beta$_2$ agonist (LABA) and oral corticosteroid *and* Consider omalizumab for patients who have allergies
Step 5 Severe Persistent	Symptoms throughout day, most days SABA several times a day Limited activity	Most nights	FEV$_1$ < 60% predicted FEV$_1$/FVC reduced > 5%	High-dose ICS + LABA *and* Consider omalizumab for patients who have allergies
Step 4 Severe Persistent	Symptoms throughout day, most days SABA several times a day Limited activity	Most nights	FEV$_1$ < 60% predicted FEV$_1$/FVC reduced > 5%	Medium-dose ICS + LABA Alternative: Medium-dose ICS + leukotriene receptor antagonist (LTRA), theophylline, or zileuton
Step 3 Moderate Persistent	Daily symptoms Daily use of inhaled SABA Some limitation in activity	> 1 time a week	FEV$_1$ > 60% to < 80% predicted FEV$_1$/FVC reduced 5%	Low-dose ICS +LABA *or* Medium-dose ICS Alternative: Low-dose ICS + LTRA, theophylline or zileuton
Step 2 Mild Persistent	Symptoms > 2 times a week but not daily Minor limitation in activity	3 to 4 times a month	FEV$_1$ > 80% predicted FEV$_1$/FVC normal	Low-dose ICS Alternatives: Cromolyn, LTRA, nedocromil, or theophylline
Step 1 Intermittent	Symptoms < 2 times/week No activity limitation	< 2 times a month	Normal FEV$_1$ between exacerbations FEV$_1$ > 80% predicted FEV$_1$/FVC normal	SABA as needed

*The presence of one of the features of severity is sufficient to place a patient in that category. An individual should be assigned to the most severe grade in which any feature occurs. The characteristics noted in the figure are general and may average because asthma is highly variable. Normal FEV$_1$/FVC for 60- to 70-year-olds is 70%.

Note. From Expert Panel Report 3: *Guidelines for the diagnosis and management of asthma.* 2007, by the National Asthma Education and Prevention Program, Washington, DC: U.S. Department of Health and Human Services.

– Partial reversibility: improvement in FVC or FEV_1 of at least 15% or improvement in FEF of at least 25% after bronchodilator treatment differentiates asthma from COPD
- Arterial blood gases (ABG): normal to mild hypoxia and respiratory alkalosis less likely because of higher pCO_2 level
- Complete blood count (CBC): slight increase of white blood cells during acute attack
- Chest x-ray: hyperinflation in uncomplicated episodes
- Sputum exam: if patient is allergic, mucus casts, eosinophils, and elongated rhomboid crystals are visible

Differential Diagnosis
- Chronic obstructive pulmonary disease (COPD)
- Chronic heart failure (CHF)
- Pulmonary embolism
- Bronchogenic carcinoma
- Foreign body aspiration
- Acute infections—bronchitis/pneumonia, tuberculosis, mycoplasma
- Vocal cord dysfunction/upper airway obstruction
- GERD
- Anxiety

Management
- National Heart, Lung, and Blood Institute of the National Institutes of Health revised general guidelines for the treatment of asthma in adults in 2007 (see Table 8–2)

Nonpharmacologic Treatment
- Identify and avoid factors that trigger asthma
- Avoid cigarette smoke
- Promote adequate hydration to provide adequate bronchial toilet
- Adjunctive treatment of asthma (such as yoga) has shown improvement in mechanical aspects of breathing as well as reduction in stress

Pharmacologic Treatment
- Management of acute exacerbations

  SEVERE EXACERBATION (PEF < 40% OF PREDICTED OR PERSONAL BEST)
  - Partial relief of short-acting $beta_2$ agonist
  - Send to Emergency department, possible hospitalization
  - Oral steroids
  - Adjunctive therapies

  MODERATE EXACERBATION (PEF 40% TO 60% OF PREDICTED OR PERSONAL BEST)
  - Frequent use of short-acting beta-2 agonists (inhaled, nebulized)
  - Course of oral corticosteroids may be needed
  - Office visit

  MILD EXACERBATION (PEF ≥ 70% OF PREDICTED OR PERSONAL BEST)
  - Care at home
  - Beta agonist 2 to 4 puffs every 3 to 4 hours
  - Possible short course oral corticosteroids

Quick-relief medications
- Short-acting beta agonist (SABA): onset of action 1 to 10 minutes
  - Relax the smooth muscle of the airway

- May be less effective in older asthmatics with COPD
- Albuterol (Proventil, Ventolin): 90 mcg/inhalations, 1 to 2 inhalations/nebulized 0.083% solution every 4 to 6 hours p.r.n.
- Levalbuterol (Xopenex), single-isomer albuterol: 0.63 mg via nebulizer t.i.d.
- Metaproterenol (Alupent): 0.65 mg/inhalations, 2 inhalations/nebulized 0.4% solution every 4 to 6 hours p.r.n.
- Anticholinergics: onset of action 15 minutes
  - Inhibits vagal reflex with resulting bronchial smooth muscle relaxation
  - Good choice for older asthmatics with COPD, because of activity on larger airways
  - Ipratropium bromide (Atrovent): 18 mcg/puff, 2 puffs or nebulized 0.02% solution four times daily
- Systemic corticosteroids: onset of action 12 to 36 hours
  - Need to carefully monitor use especially regarding coexisting diabetes, risk for steroid-induced hyperglycemia, greater risk for steroid-related psychosis in older adults, risk for increased osteoporosis
  - Prednisone (Liquid Pred, Deltasone): 5 to 60 mg/day in divided doses b.i.d., t.i.d., or q.i.d.; typical course ≤ 10 days
  - Prednisolone (Delta-Cortef, Prelone): 5 to 60 mg/day in divided doses

Long-Term Management
- Stepwise approach
  - Gain control quickly
  - Gradual stepwise reduction in treatment if possible
  - If control not maintained, stepwise increase in medication
- Inhaled corticosteroids (ICS): onset of action 2 to 3 days
  - Good choice for avoiding systemic corticosteroid use; large dosing range with reduced systemic effect
  - Consider calcium and vitamin D for older adults with risk factors for osteoporosis
  - Beclomethasone dipropionate (Beclovent, Vanceril, Vancenase): 42 mcg/puff, 2 puffs or 84 mcg/puff 1 to 2 puffs b.i.d. to q.i.d. not to exceed 840 mcg daily
  - Fluticasone (Flovent): 44 mcg/spray, 110 mcg/spray, 220 mcg/spray, 2 to 4 puffs b.i.d. to q.i.d., should not exceed 660 mcg daily
  - Triamcinolone acetate (Azmacort): 100 mcg/puff, 2 puffs t.i.d. to q.i.d.
- Long-acting beta$_2$ agonists (LABA)
  - Salmeterol (Serevent): aerosol 25 mcg/spray, 2 puffs every 12 hours
  - Formoterol (Foradil) 12 mcg dry powder via inhaler every12 hours
  - Caution: not for treatment of acute attacks; use with caution in patients with cardiovascular disease
  - Well-tolerated in the older adult, generally
  - Combined inhaled corticosteroids and long-acting beta$_2$ agonists
    - Fluticasone/salmeterol (Advair): diskus 100/50, 250/50, 500/50, 1 inhalation twice daily; HFA MDI 115/21, 230/21, 2 inhalations twice daily
    - Budesonide/formoterol (Symbicort): 80/4.5, 160/4.5, 2 inhalations twice daily
- Methylxanthines
  - Theophylline (Theo-Dur, Slo-bid): individualize dose—16mg/kg/24 hours or 400 mg/24 hours, whichever is less in divided doses at 6- to 8-hour intervals
  - Dose to therapeutic range of 10 to 20; most older adults have fewer side effects on lower end of range; dose must be individualized
  - Adverse reactions: arrhythmias, nausea, restlessness
  - Watch for drug interactions with other commonly used medications, such as digoxin, warfarin (Coumadin), macrolides, quinolones, beta blockers, and corticosteroids

- – Theophylline products are not interchangeable; absorption varies by brand
- – If other medications are not effective, theophylline should be used with caution in older adults because of the potential for adverse reactions and drug interactions; recommended dose < 400 mg/day
- Mast cell stabilizers
  - – Cromolyn sodium (Intal): inhalation 20 mg; 2 sprays 800 mcg/spray q.i.d.
- Leukotriene-receptor antagonists (LTRA)
  - – Zafirlukast (Accolade): 10 mg b.i.d.
  - – Zileuton (Zyflo): 600 mg q.i.d.
  - – Montelukast (Singulair): 10 mg daily
- Recombinant DNA-derived humanized IgG monoclonal antibody
  - – Inhibits binding of IgE to the high-affinity IgE receptor on surface of mast cells and basophils
  - – Omalizumab (Xolair): 150 to 375 mg subcutaneous every 2 to 4 weeks

How Long to Treat
- Dependent on the severity of the attacks.
- Goal of treatment is to gain control of asthma as quickly as possible and decrease treatment gradually to the least amount of medication needed to maintain control

When to Consult, Refer, Hospitalize
- Severe asthma exacerbation or severe persistent asthma, requiring Step 4, 5, 6 care
- Patient not meeting goals of treatment after 3 to 6 months of therapy
- Other conditions complicating asthma (infections, GERD, COPD)
- Additional diagnostic testing is indicated
- Continuous use of oral corticosteroid therapy or high-dose inhaled corticosteroids

Follow-up
Expected Course
- Patients should monitor peak flow rates regularly
- For acute exacerbations, follow up in 24 hours then in 3 to 5 days; follow-up weekly until symptoms are controlled and peak flow is consistently 80% of predicted, and then monthly
- Once stabilized follow up every 2 to 3 months
- Monitor theophylline levels 2 weeks after initiation of therapy, then every 4 months
- Use of quick-relief medications more than 2 times a week in intermittent asthma (daily, or increasing use in persistent asthma) may indicate the need to initiate (increase) long-term therapy

Complications
- Exhaustion, dehydration, cor pulmonale, airway infection, tussive syncope
- Change in mental status, frequent falls, and exacerbation of other existing illnesses
- Pneumothorax, hypercapnia, hypoxic respiratory failure, and death

CHRONIC OBSTRUCTIVE PULMONARY DISEASE (COPD)

Description
- Limitation of expiratory airflow caused by destruction of airway tissue caused by emphysema, chronic bronchitis, or chronic asthma
- The obstruction is progressive and unresponsive to bronchodilators

- Emphysema: dyspnea from abnormal remodeling of air spaces within the terminal bronchioles
- Bronchitis: produces a productive cough most days of the month for at least 3 months over a 2-year period
- Asthma produces permanent remodeling of the basement membrane resulting from chronic inflammation
- Most patients have characteristics of both emphysema and chronic bronchitis

Etiology
- Smoking 80%

Incidence and Demographics
- Seventh-ranking chronic condition
- Fourth leading cause of death in America (2007)
- Mortality rates continue to increase
- Affects patients older than age 50

Key Indicators
- Dyspnea—progressive increase with exercise
- Chronic cough
- Chronic sputum
- History of risk factors

Risk Factors
- Smoking
- Secondhand smoke
- Occupations involving high concentrations of dust and fumes are also at high risk—coal miners, metal molders, grain handlers, farmers, situations involving asbestos exposure
- Air pollution
- Allergies
- Genetic predisposition
- Male gender

Prevention and Screening
- Smoking cessation
- Reduction in secondhand smoke exposure
- Treatment and control of upper-respiratory illnesses and allergies

Assessment
History
- Presenting symptoms usually dyspnea with cough
- Duration and characteristics of cough
- Smoking history of patient and family members
- Exercise/activity tolerance, dyspnea on exertion or at rest
- Work history: disability
- Chills/fever, weight gain/loss, edema, fatigue, angina
- Sleep habits: number of pillows used
- Respiratory illness history: asthma, bronchitis, sinusitis, allergies
- Other existing illnesses: cardiovascular diseases

Physical
- General: weight loss, tachycardia, tachypnea
- Respiratory: pursed-lip breathing, use of accessory respiratory muscles with breathing, increased AP diameter of chest, decreased breath sounds with prolonged expiratory phase, poor diaphragm mobility

Diagnostic Studies
- Chest radiographs: in emphysema, hyperinflation, subpleural blebs, parenchymal bullae, flattened diaphragm; in chronic bronchitis ("dirty lungs"), nonspecific peribronchial and perivascular markings at bases
- Pulmonary function tests (PFT): typically airflow obstruction of 70% or more diffusion capacity; determine air trapping and hypercapnia
- ECG: may show sinus tachycardia; abnormalities typical of cor pulmonale in advanced disease with pulmonary hypertension; supraventricular arrhythmia; ventricular irritability; right ventricular hypertrophy
- Arterial blood gases (ABG): should be done for baseline; hypoxemia in advanced chronic bronchitis; compensated respiratory acidosis with chronic respiratory failure in chronic bronchitis

Differential Diagnosis
- Obliterative bronchiolitis
- Bronchiectasis
- Interstitial fibrosis
- Diffuse panbronchiolitis
- Tuberculosis
- Chronic heart failure
- Cardiomyopathy

Management
- See Table 8–3
- Refer to Global Initiative for Chronic Obstructive Lung Disease (GOLD) guidelines

Nonpharmacologic Treatment
- Smoking cessation
- Encourage well-balanced diet to maintain ideal body weight
- Monitored exercise program
- Avoid exposure to colds and influenza
- Avoid respiratory irritants—secondhand smoke, dust, and other air pollutants
- Increase fluids and humidification
- Breathing exercises, effective cough techniques
- Avoid outdoor activities when air pollutant concentrations are high

Pharmacologic Treatment
- Based on severity and etiology of COPD

  ANTICHOLINERGICS
  - Side effects mild: dry mouth, cough, nervousness, dizziness, GI upset

  SHORT-ACTING
  - Ipratropium bromide (Atrovent): 0.65 mg/inhalation; 2 inhalations every 6 hours; maximum 12 inhalations or 500 mcg via nebulizer every 6 to 8 hours
  - Oxitropium: 100 mcg (MDI); 1.5 mcg/mL via nebulizer

Table 8-3. Step Therapy for COPD

Stage	Function	Therapy
1 Mild	FEV_1/FVC $FEV_1 \geq 80\%$ predicted	Selective beta$_2$ agonist inhaler p.r.n. Annual influenza vaccination
2 Moderate	$FEV_1/FVC < 0.70$ $50\% \leq FEV_1 < 80\%$ predicted	Selective beta$_2$ agonist p.r.n. or on regular basis One or more long-acting bronchodilators on a regular basis Pulmonary rehabilitation (when needed) Annual influenza vaccination
3 Severe	$FEV_1/FVC < 0.70$ $30\% \leq FEV_1 < 50\%$	Selective beta$_2$ agonist p.r.n. or on regular basis One or more long-acting bronchodilators on a regular basis Add inhaled corticosteroid if repeated exacerbations Pulmonary rehabilitation (when needed) Annual influenza vaccination
4 Very severe	$FEV_1/FVC < 0.70$ $FEV_1 < 30\%$ predicted value or FEV_1 $< 50\%$ predicted plus chronic respiratory failure	Selective beta$_2$ agonist p.r.n. or on regular basis One or more long-acting bronchodilators on a regular basis Add inhaled corticosteroid if repeated exacerbations Add long-term oxygen use if chronic respiratory failure Consider surgical treatments (lung volume reduction, transplant) Annual influenza vaccination

Adapted from "Global strategy for the diagnosis, management and prevention of chronic obstructive pulmonary disease," by the American Thoracic Society, 2007, *American Journal of Respiratory Critical Care Medicine, 176,* 532–555.

LONG-ACTING
- Tiotropium (Spiriva) 18 mcg one cap via inhaler daily

BRONCHODILATORS—BETA$_2$ AGONIST
- Side effects: hypertension, nasal congestion, headache, dizziness

Short-acting
- Albuterol (Proventil, Ventolin): 90 mcg/inhalation, 2 inhalations every 4 to 6 hours *or* nebulizer 0.083% 2.5 mg 3 to 4 times a day
- Side effects: tremor, nervousness, headache, dizziness, hypokalemia, insomnia, tachycardia

Long-acting
- Formoterol (Foradil) 12 mcg dry powder via inhaler b.i.d.
- Salmeterol (Serevent Diskus or MDI) 50 mcg dry powder via inhaler b.i.d.

Combination short-acting beta$_2$-agonist plus anticholinergic
- Fenoterol/ipatropium 200/80 mcg (MDI), 1.25/0.5 mcg/mL via nebulizer
- Salbutamol/ipatropium 75/15 mcg (MDI), 0.75/4.5 mcg/mL via nebulizer

Methylxanthines
- Theophylline SR (Theo-24, Uniphyl): individualize dose; 16mg/kg/24 hr or 400 mg/24 hr, whichever is less, in divided doses 1 to 2 times a day

- Aminophylline: 200 to 600 mg daily (limit to 400 mg in older adults)
- Side effects: GI upset, headache, CNS stimulation, arrhythmias, seizures
- Theophylline has a narrow therapeutic window; close monitoring with serum levels necessary

  CORTICOSTEROIDS: INHALED
  - Beclomethasone dipropionate (Beclovent, Vanceril, Vancenase): 42 mcg/puff, 2 puffs or 84 mcg/puff, 1 to 2 puffs 3 to 4 times a day, 0.2 to 0.4 mcg/mL via nebulizer
  - Budesonide: 100, 200, 400 mcg dry powder inhaler (DPI), 0.20, 0.25, 0.5 mcg/mL via nebulizer
  - Triamcinolone (Azmacort): 100 mcg/puff, 2 to 4 puffs b.i.d. to q.i.d.
  - Fluticasone (Flovent): 50 to 500 mcg (MDI and DPI)

  COMBINATION LONG-ACTING BETA$_2$-AGONIST PLUS GLUCOCORTICOSTEROID
  - Fortometerol/budesonide (Symbicort): 4.5/160, 9/320 (DPI)
  - Salmeterol/fluticasone (Advair): 50/100, 50/250, 50/500 (DPI), 25/50, 25/125, 25/250 (MDI)

  ORAL GLUCOCORTICOSTEROIDS
  - Oral most effective for acute exacerbations
  - Approximately 10% of stable COPD patients respond to oral steroids
  - Prednisone (Liquid Pred, Deltasone): 1 mg, 2.5 mg, 5 mg, 10 mg, 20 mg, 50 mg tabs or 5 mg/5 mL oral solution, 5 to 60 mg/day in divided doses b.i.d., t.i.d., or q.i.d.
  - Methylprednisolone: 4, 8, 16 mg

  OXYGEN
  - The only drug documented to alter the natural history of COPD
  - Medicare coverage for patients with resting hypoxemia:
    - PaO$_2$ less than or equal to 55 while awake
    - During sleep (nocturnal O$_2$ only): PaO$_2$ less than or equal to 55 *or* decrease in PaO$_2$ more than 10, *or* more an 5 decrease with associated with symptoms of hypoxemia
    - During exercise (use during exercise only): PaO$_2$ less than or equal to 55 *and* evidence that O$_2$ improves the hypoxemia.
  - 1 to 3L/min via nasal cannula 15 hours/day

How Long to Treat
- Chronic condition requiring ongoing therapeutic treatments and monitoring

Special Considerations
- Acute exacerbation of COPD: characterized by an increase in baseline symptoms; increased dyspnea, cough, increased sputum production
- Bacterial infection usual underlying cause—responds well to broad-spectrum antibiotics (see pharmacologic treatment for community-acquired pneumonia [CAP]); increase of maintenance MDI; treat based on severity of symptoms
- Other possible comorbidities should be investigated—chronic heart failure, pulmonary embolus, TB, pneumothorax

When to Consult, Refer, Hospitalize
- Signs and symptoms of respiratory failure
- Severe exacerbations

- Symptoms of cor pulmonale
- Progression of disease
- Poor response to therapy

Follow-up

Expected Course
- Exacerbation should resolve within 7 to 10 days; if it persists, obtain CBC, chest x-ray, pulmonary function tests
- Degree of pulmonary dysfunction at initial visit is most important predictor of survival
- Poor prognosis especially for severe disease and emphysematous form—median survival approximately 4 years

Complications
- Acute exacerbation of COPD, pneumonia, pulmonary thromboembolism, spontaneous pneumothorax, acute bronchitis, pulmonary hypertension, cor pulmonale, chronic respiratory failure, left ventricular heart failure, death

COMMUNITY-ACQUIRED PNEUMONIA

Description
- An acute pulmonary infection with that begins outside the hospital and is associated symptoms of infection, parenchymal infiltrate on chest radiograph, and bronchial breath sounds or rales on auscultation
- Community-acquired pneumonia (CAP) may also begin within 48 hours of hospital admission in a patient who has resided < 14 days in a long-term care facility before symptom onset

Etiology
- Bacterial more common than viral
- Approximately 85% of CAP cases are caused by typical pathogens, such as S. pneumoniae, H. influenzae, or M. catarrhalis, and approximately 15% are due to the nonzoonotic atypical pathogens, such as Legionella species, Mycoplasma species, or C. pneumoniae
- Viral: influenza, adenovirus, parainfluenza, respiratory syncytial virus

Incidence and Demographics
- Common; 2 to 3 million cases/year
- Sixth leading cause of death

Risk Factors
- 65 years of age or older
- Nursing home residents
- Alcoholism
- Altered mental status—decreased gag and cough reflex
- Smoking
- Sedating drugs
- Influenza
- Poor dental hygiene
- Neurological deficits, aspiration secondary to conditions such as stroke, Parkinson's disease
- Feeding tubes

Prevention and Screening
- Influenza vaccine
- Polyvalent pneumococcal vaccine
- Good nutritional screening

Assessment
- Assess preexisting conditions that influence ability to care for patient at home
  - Hemodynamic instability
  - Acute hypoxemia
  - Chronic oxygen dependency
  - Ability to take oral medication
- Assess severity
  - Characteristics that confer increased risk include advanced age, alcoholism, comorbid diseases, altered mental status, respiratory rate of 30 or more, hypotension, and elevated BUN or sodium
  - Use Pneumonia Patient Outcomes Research Team (PORT) score
- Assess overall health and suitability for home care
  - Frail physical condition
  - Social or psychiatric problems compromising home care
  - Unstable living situation

History
- Confusion or nonspecific presentation of illness may be the only symptoms
- Classic presentation: fever, chills, sweats, rigors *and*
- Cough (productive or nonproductive), dyspnea
- Fatigue, myalgias, chest discomfort, headache, failure to thrive
- Anorexia, abdominal pain may or may not be present or may be intermittent

Physical
- Patient may only appear mildly ill, have mental confusion
- Hypothermia, fever, or normal temperature
- Tachypnea over 30, very reliable indicator of pneumonia in the older adult; tachycardia
- Abnormal breath sounds and rales present; "A to E" changes on auscultation
- Percussion dullness if effusion present

Diagnostic Studies
- Chest x-ray
- CBC
- BUN, glucose, electrolytes, liver function
- Gram stain and culture of sputum
- TB testing if atypical or at high risk

Differential Diagnosis
- Upper-respiratory tract infections
- Reactive airway disease
- Chronic heart failure
- Bronchiolitis
- Malignancy
- Myocardial infarction
- TB
- Pulmonary embolism

- Pulmonary vasculitis
- Atelectasis

Management
- Patient must be hospitalized if unable to take adequate PO fluids

Nonpharmacologic Treatment
- Rest
- Increase fluids
- Humidification
- Smoking cessation

Pharmacologic Treatment
- Treat Gram stain results if available
- Treat culture results when available
- In normal hosts do not need to cover *S. aureus, Klebsiella species*, or *P. aeruginosa*
- Most antibiotics (doxycycline, respiratory quinolones, beta lactams) are effective against community-acquired aspiration pneumonias (oral anerobes; clindamycin or moxifloxacin preferable for aerobic lung abscesses
- Coverage should include typical (*S. pneumoniae, H. influenzae, M. catarrhalis*) and atypical (*Legionella* and *Mycoplasma* species, *C. pneumoniae*) pathogens
- Avoid empiric macrolide monotherapy because approximately 25% of *S. pneumoniae* strains are naturally resistant to all macrolides
- Most highly penicillin-resistant *S. pneumoniae* infections (minimum inhibitory concentration [MIC] > 2 mcg/mL) may also be treated with beta-lactams; Alternatively, doxycycline or respiratory quinolones may be used; vancomycin is rarely, if ever, needed (Cunha, 2007)
- Monotherapy coverage of both typical and atypical pathogens in CAP is preferred over double-drug therapy

Table 8–4. Initial Empiric Therapy of Community-Acquired Pneumonia

Patient Variable Outpatient	Treatment Options
Previously healthy No risk factors No recent antibiotic therapy	Macrolide (erythromycin, azithromycin, clarithromycin) *or* doxycycline
Recent antibiotic therapy (within 3 months) Comorbidities: COPD, diabetes, renal, failure, CHF, malignancy, immunosuppression	Respiratory fluoroquinolone (moxifloxacin, levofloxacin [750 mg], or gemifloxacin) *or* Macrolide (azithromycin or clarithromycin) *plus* Beta-lactam
In regions with high rate of infection (> 25%) with macrolide-resistant *S. pneumoniae*, without morbidities	Respiratory fluoroquinolone (moxifloxacin, levofloxacin [750 mg], or gemifloxacin) *or* Macrolide (azithromycin or clarithromycin) *plus* beta-lactam

Adapted from "Infectious Diseases Society of America/American Thoracic Society Consensus Guidelines on the management of community acquired pneumonia in adults," by L. A. Mandell, R. G. Wunderink, A. Anzueto, J. G. Bartlett, G. D. Campbell, N. C. Dear, et al., 2007, *Clinical Infectious Diseases, 44*(S2), pp. 27–72.

ANTIMICROBIALS
- Macrolides
  - Erythromycin 250 to 1000 mg every 6 hours
  - Clarithromycin (Biaxin) 500 p.o. every 12 hours for 14 days
  - Azithromycin (Zithromax) 500 mg p.o. × 1 day, then 250 mg p.o. daily × 4 days
- Doxycycline: 100 mg p.o. every 12 hours
- Fluoroquinolones
  - Levofloxacin (Levaquin) 500 mg p.o. daily
  - Ciprofloxacin (Cipro) 500 mg p.o. daily
  - Gatifloxacin (Tequin) 400 mg p.o. daily
  - Moxifloxacin (Avelox) 400 mg daily
  - Gemifloxacin not yet available
- Beta-lactams
  - Cefpodoxime (Vantin) 200 mg every 12 hours
  - Cefprozil (Cefzil) 500 mg every12 hours
  - Cefuroxime (Ceftin) 250–500 every12 hours

ANTITUSSIVES
- Generally, cough should not be suppressed and antitussives should not be used
- However, in patients with severe chest discomfort and persistent cough, may consider use of non-narcotic or low-dose narcotic antitussive for night use only

How Long to Treat
- Treat bacterial infections until patient is afebrile or asymptomatic for 72 hours
- Treat for 7 to 14 days
- Most patients admitted to the hospital for CAP are treated with intravenous medications for 2 days and then complete a 12-day oral course of therapy for a total of 14 days of combined intravenous and oral therapy.

When to Consult, Refer, Hospitalize
- Refer moderate to severe pneumonias to physician
- Hospitalize patients with comorbid conditions, altered mental status, tachycardia, tachypnea, systolic blood pressure < 90 mm Hg, temperature elevated or subnormal, and institutionally acquired pneumonia

Follow-up
- After discharge should be followed weekly until clear chest x-ray and asymptomatic

Expected Course
- Dependent upon pathogen, patient response, complications

Complications
- Heart failure, renal failure, pulmonary embolism, bacteremia, acute myocardial infection, death

PRIMARY LUNG MALIGNANCIES

Description
- Bronchogenic carcinomas include two classes
  - Non-small-cell carcinoma (NSCLC): which includes squamous cell carcinoma, adenocarcinoma, and large cell carcinoma
  - Small-cell carcinoma (SCLC): also known as oat-cell carcinoma

Etiology
- Cigarette smoking
- Secondhand smoke
- Ionizing radiation (radon gas, therapeutic radiation)
- Asbestos exposure (most common occupational cause), synergistic action with smoking
- Heavy metals (nickel, chromium), industrial carcinogens

Incidence and Demographics
- Lung cancer is the leading cause of cancer death for both men and women
- Smoking causes 85% to 90% of lung cancer
- Lung cancer constitutes 25% of cancer-related deaths in women a higher percentage than for breast cancer; lung cancer accounts for 32% of cancer deaths in men
- Most cases present between ages 50 and 70
- Non-small-cell carcinomas comprise 80% of lung cancers; small-cell carcinomas comprise 20%
- High mortality and low 5-year survival rates are due to inability to diagnose at early stage

Risk Factors
- See Etiology

Prevention and Screening
- *Do not smoke*
- Annual chest x-rays and cytology as preventive screening have not had significant impact on survival
- Low-dose helical computed tomography (LDCT) is being evaluated for screening current of former heavy smokers

Assessment
History
- Initial symptoms: cough associated with smoking that persists for more than 1 month after cessation of smoking, change in characteristics of cough
- Later symptoms: chest pain, often made worse by deep breathing; hoarseness; weight loss and loss of appetite; dyspnea; fever without a known reason; recurring infections such as bronchitis, pneumonia; new onset of wheezing
- Symptoms of metastasis: bone pain; weakness or numbness of the arms or legs; dizziness; jaundice; skin tumors; lymphadenopathy, obstruction of trachea and esophagus
- Hemoptysis most frequently associated with lung cancer but can be from other causes, ranging from minor erosions to severe necrosis of mucosa due to inflammation, pulmonary infarct, or gastrointestinal bleeding; other noncancer causes include TB, coagulopathies, infection, and pulmonary edema; investigation as outlined below would be similar

Physical
- Findings vary on exam; may have none to fairly benign findings
- General: weight loss, hoarse voice
- Lung dyspnea, hemoptysis, wheezing, stridor, decreased breath sounds with effusion
- Pneumonia

Diagnostic Studies
- Chest radiographs: most important initial diagnostic test in predicting whether or not a bronchogenic carcinoma is potential cause of chronic cough
- Histologic confirmation is essential; cytology via bronchoscopy

Differential Diagnosis
- Asthma
- HF
- Tuberculosis
- COPD
- Pulmonary embolism

Management
Nonpharmacologic Treatment
- Surgical resection
- Radiation therapy
- Palliative therapy includes general care of the patient with particular attention to pain control, maintenance of adequate nutrition, and psychological support; consider hospice referral

Pharmacologic Treatment
- Multiple anticancer chemotherapeutic agents are used to treat lung cancer
- For more complete listing of specific agents, refer to American Cancer Society, www.cancer.org

How Long to Treat
- Duration of treatment depends on type and stage of cancer

When to Consult, Refer, Hospitalize
- Any patient with suspected lung malignancy should be referred to a pulmonologist and oncologist for evaluation and treatment
- Hospitalization for frank hemoptysis

Follow-up
Expected Course
- Overall 5-year survival rate is 10% to 15%
- 5-year survival rate after curative resection of squamous cell carcinoma is 35% to 40%
- 25% for adenocarcinoma and large cell carcinoma
- Patients with small-cell carcinoma rarely survive for 5 years after diagnosis

Complications
- Superior vena cava syndrome, phrenic nerve palsy, recurrent laryngeal nerve palsy, death
- Weight loss is a significant adverse indicator of prognosis; associated nausea, vomiting, and anorexia can increase this problem

TUBERCULOSIS

Description
- Chronic infectious acid-fast bacillus disease, most frequently of the lungs
- In 15% of cases, the bacilli cause disease in other regions, such as the skin, kidneys, bones, and reproductive and urinary systems

- Requires immediate respiratory isolation and reporting to a public health agency
- See Table 8–5

Table 8–5. Classification of Tuberculosis

Classification	Status	PPD
0	No TB exposure—not infected	Negative
1	TB exposure—no evidence of infection	Negative
2	TB infection—no disease	Positive
3	TB clinically active	Positive
4	TB not clinically active	Positive
5	TB suspected	Pending result

Adapted from "Diagnostic standards and classification of tuberculosis," by the American Thoracic Society, 1990, *American Review Respiratory Disease, 142,* pp. 725–735.

Etiology
- Inhalation of aerosolized droplets containing *Mycobacterium tuberculosis* causes infection
- The bacteria is ingested by macrophages and will either die or grow, depending on the effectiveness of the immune system of the patient
- If the immune system is effective, the bacteria will be walled-off in a granuloma
- The bacteria remains dormant in the granuloma until the patient's immune system weakens
- Weakening can arise from factors such as old age, chronic disease, steroids
- Most tuberculosis in older patients is from reactivation of dormant bacteria or nursing home exposure

Incidence and Demographics
- Causes more deaths worldwide than any other infectious disease
- Approximately 15 million people in the United States are infected with M. *tuberculosis*
- Persons 65 or older have the highest incidence of TB
- 75% of active TB is in the lungs of older adults
- TB of the spine is most common form of extrapulmonary TB in older adults
- In the United States, racial and ethnic minorities are disproportionately affected by TB

Risk Factors
- Diabetes mellitus
- HIV infection
- Malignancy
- Chronic renal failure
- Poor nutrition
- Immunosuppressive drugs
- Close contacts of people with newly diagnosed infectious TB
- People with positive TB skin tests
- Abnormal chest x-rays compatible with inactive TB

Prevention and Screening
- Identifying and treating infected individuals early
- Isoniazid (also called INH) prevents the disease in most people in close contact with infected people or who are infected but who do not have active TB

- Preventive therapy indicated for patients in the following groups with positive tuberculin skin test results
  - Close contacts of newly diagnosed patients with infectious TB
  - Converters: people whose skin test results have recently converted from negative to positive
  - Patients with pre-existing medical conditions such as HIV infection, diabetes mellitus, end-stage renal disease, chronic malabsorption syndromes, and hematologic malignancies
  - Patients on corticosteroid therapy, immunosuppressive therapy
  - Patients with x-ray changes without previous adequate therapy

Assessment

History
- Older adults with TB infection may have no symptoms
- Older adults with TB disease may have any, all, or none of the following symptoms: chronic productive cough, fatigue/malaise, weight loss, anorexia, fever, hemoptysis, night sweats, pleuritic chest pain, changes in functional capacity

Physical
- Chronically ill appearance, weight loss
- Chest exam: normal or reveals apical rales, increased tactile fremitus on palpation; percussion dull

Diagnostic Studies
- Tuberculin skin tests: Mantoux (PPD) test: standard test, establishes exposure to TB; 0.1 mL given intradermally on volar surface of forearm; reaction read in 48 to 72 hours (see Table 8–6, PPD Interpretation) Refer to CDC for interpretation of skin tests results for immunocompromised persons and factors causing false-negative TB skin tests (http://www.cdc.gov/mmwr/preview/mmwrhtml/rr5412a1.htm); see Table 8–6.
- Older adults require "boosting" for accurate results; the PPD should be done twice, with second test applied within 2 weeks of the first
- Chest x-ray: high incidence of atypical chest x-ray presentation in middle, lower lobes and pleura; primary TB frequently middle and lower lobes as well as hilar and mediastinal lymph nodes
- Sputum smear: suggestive of, does not confirm, diagnosis of TB
- Sputum cultures: definitive diagnosis of TB
- CBC with differential and platelets
- Bronchoscopy with bronchial washings and biopsy

Differential Diagnosis
- COPD
- Pneumonia
- Carcinoma
- Pleurisy
- Histoplasmosis
- Silicosis

Management
- Follow national treatment guidelines, protocols, and latest findings from CDC

Nonpharmacologic Treatment
- Isolation for new cases of confirmed tuberculosis

Table 8-6. PPD Interpretation

Reaction Size	Patient Characteristics
≥ 5 mm	HIV infection, or persons at risk for HIV infection
	X-rays suggestive of previous healed TB infection
	Close contacts of people with active TB
≥ 10 mm	Immigrants from Asia, Africa, Latin America
	Residents of long-term-care facilities—nursing homes, correctional institutes, or mental institutions
	Medically underserved and low-income populations
	Recent converters
	People with pre-existing medical conditions: ≥ 10% below ideal body weight, diabetes mellitus, gastrectomy, jejunoileal bypass, silicosis, chronic renal failure, immunosuppressive therapy, cancer
≥ 15 mm	All persons

Adapted from "Diagnostic standards and classification of tuberculosis," by the American Thoracic Society, 1990, *American Review Respiratory Disease, 142,* pp. 725–735.

Pharmacologic Treatment
- First-line drugs: isoniazid (INH), rifampin, rifapentin, pyrazinamide, ethambutol
- Second-line drugs: cycloserine, ethionamide, fluoroquinolones (levofloxacin, gatifloxacin, moxifloxacin are not FDA indicated for treatment of TB), p-aminosalicylic acid, streptomycin, amikacin/kanamycin, capneomycin
- Initial phase of treatment requires 3 to 4 drugs for 8 weeks, then 2-drug regimen for 18 weeks
- Most geriatric cases are reactivation of disease, thus less likely to have multiple drug resistance
- Treatment changes often with changing patterns of resistance

Treatment of Exposure to TB
- Patient who are infected with M. *tuberculosis* have tuberculosis, even if they do not have symptoms
- Recent converters should receive chemoprophylaxis
- INH prophylaxis 300 mg/day for 6 to 12 months is recommended
- This will reduce the incidence of reactivated tuberculosis
- The major risk with INH treatment is liver toxicity

How Long to Treat Person Exposed to TB
- Duration of treatment depends on medications used
- Generally, patients are treated for 6 to 12 months

When to Consult, Refer, Hospitalize
- All suspected or confirmed cases of tuberculosis should be reported to the local and state health departments
- Refer all patients to specialist for treatment
- Hospitalize patients if they are incapable of self-care, or if patient is likely to expose new susceptible individuals

Follow-up
Expected Course
- 90% cure rate with proper treatment; relapse rate less than 5% with current treatments

- Sputum culture at diagnosis and after initial phase of treatment
- Monitor liver function tests because of high risk of liver toxicity; at baseline and monthly while on medication
- Hepatic toxicity high with INH in geriatric patients

Complications
- Treatment failure most often due to noncompliance
- The death rate for untreated TB patients is between 40% and 60%
- Most deaths result from overlooked disease

PULMONARY EMBOLISM (PE)

Description
- An obstruction of a pulmonary artery caused by a blood clot (or fat, air, bone) that has traveled to the area through the circulatory system

Etiology
- Deep venous thrombosis (DVT) causes 90%; blood clot initially develops in deep venous circulation; the vessels at highest risk are the popliteal and iliofemoral
- Other sites of origin of blood clot: right atrium (due to atrial fibrillation); right ventricle; renal, pelvic, hepatic, subclavian, and jugular veins
- Sources of fat emboli: hip fractures and repairs, long bone fractures, pelvic fractures

Incidence and Demographics
- Primary cause of death in 100,000 people annually
- Contributing cause of death in additional 100,000 annually; many found only on autopsy
- Misdiagnosis in about 30% of cases, commonly in older adults because of high incidence of pulmonary and cardiovascular conditions

Risk Factors
- Venous stasis
- Estrogen use
- Immobility
- Surgery
- Injury to vessel wall
- Femoral vein catheters
- Altered clotting states

Prevention and Screening
- Prophylactic anticoagulation
- Mobility
- Anti-embolism devices: TED hose, alternating compression hose and mattresses
- If history of multiple venous clots, vena cava filter

Assessment
History
- Most common complaints: shortness of breath, chest pain with possible pleuritic component, anxiety, leg pain or swelling, hemoptysis, and syncope
- Can also see a variety of symptoms such as confusion, fever, wheezing, congestion, changes in mentation, unexplained palpitations, transient shortness of breath

Physical
- Classic presentation of dyspnea, chest pain, and hemoptysis
- Most PE will present with DVT, although symptoms may be subtle: calf tenderness, edema, increased leg temperature
- Other common findings: arrhythmias, tachycardia, chronic heart failure, pleural friction rub, fever, and cyanosis

Diagnostic Studies
- D-dimer test; if positive, CT angiography (see below)
- EKG: may show signs of right side heart failure if significant PE exists
- Arterial blood gases will show signs of hypoxia, possible lower CO_2 levels,
- Lung scan: diagnostic, noninvasive testing; will show degree of probability of embolus based on amount of perfusion defect
- Pulmonary angiography: most diagnostic, gold standard test; will show constant intraluminal filling defect and sharp cutting off of flow; low incidence of false-negative results; invasive test with use of contrast material, therefore higher risk for complications
- Venous duplex or Doppler studies: most common and quickest way to diagnosis DVT; noninvasive; may be used to monitor calf embolus if there is suspected risk of popliteal or femoral vein involvement; *not* used to diagnosis PE

Differential Diagnosis
- COPD
- Right-sided heart failure
- Heart failure
- Pulmonary hypertension
- Rib fractures
- Pneumothorax
- CAD
- Cardiac arrhythmias
- Heart valve disease

Management
Nonpharmacologic Treatment
- Education in regard to outpatient anticoagulation: foods and medications to avoid, bleeding risks, monitoring of therapeutic levels; see Chapter 9, Cardiovascular Disorders
- Exercise, antiembolism stockings if DVT involved

Pharmacologic Treatment
- Streptokinase: inpatient
- Heparin: inpatient
- Warfarin (Coumadin)
  - Generally started in hospital and continued in outpatient setting
  - Requires 3 to 5 days to achieve therapeutic range
  - Monitored by prothrombin time (PT) and international normalizing rate (INR)
  - Goal of therapy is usually an INR of 2 to 3

How Long to Treat
- Length of time varies, generally minimum of 3 to 6 months after the event

Special Considerations
- Risk for falls in older adults that may result in serious bleeding when patient is on anticoagulation therapy
- Warfarin and heparin have many drug interactions
- Coexisting diseases also affect action of heparin and warfarin

When to Consult, Refer, and Hospitalize
- Refer to physician for hospitalization for initial treatment
- Recurrence or extension of embolus with therapy
- Inability to control clotting times
- Pulmonary consult with any pulmonary embolus event with at least one outpatient follow-up
- Reaction to anticoagulant

Follow-up
- Initially should be seen within 10 days of discharge
- INR should be monitored weekly until stable within therapeutic range
- Re-evaluation of DVT with Doppler studies should be considered based on extent and location
- Length of therapy depends on severity of disease, risk of recurrence, and prior history
- Multiple events should prompt consideration of placement of filter in vena cava

Complications
- Acute respiratory failure
- Death

CASE STUDIES

Case 1. A 70-year-old male comes to clinic with productive cough, shortness of breath. Denies fever, upper-respiratory symptoms. Patient is a retired construction worker with history of asthma.

HPI: Medications include asthma medications: albuterol p.r.n., salmeterol (Serevent) 2 puffs b.i.d., triamcinolone (Azmacort) 2 puffs b.i.d., and loratadine (Claritin) p.r.n. allergies.

1. What additional history would you like?

Physical Exam: Vital signs stable. No acute respiratory distress, lungs without wheezes or rales (crackles), breath sounds are decreased bilaterally with prolonged expiration. Heart rate regular. Peak flow rate 300; his baseline is 350.

2. What is your assessment?
3. What do you think is happening?
4. What is your initial plan?

Case 2. A 75-year-old female with complaints of productive cough, fever, chills, chest discomfort, and chest congestion; fatigue and headache for 3 days.

PMH: Bronchitis. Medications: Robitussin DM and Tylenol extra strength for headache. Allergic to penicillin.

1. What additional history would you ask?

Exam: Patient appears ill; temp 100.8° F, tachypnea with exertion, skin warm to touch; ENT exam normal; chest splinting with fremitus and rales (crackles) in right lower lobe.

2. What diagnostic tests will you order?
3. What are the most likely diagnoses?
4. Based on your current impression, what treatment will you order?

Case 3. A 67-year-old male complains of shortness of breath, both at rest and on exertion. Unable to perform normal activities without becoming "winded." Notes occasional cough.

PMH: Hypertension. Former smoker, 1½ packs per day for 40 years. Medications: OTC cough medicine, enalapril (Vasotec) 5 mg daily for hypertension.

1. What additional history would you ask?

Exam: Vital signs BP 152/90; no tachypnea; ENT, normal findings; chest, increased AP diameter, hyper-resonance on percussion, decreased expansion on respiration, no abnormal breath sounds; extremities, no edema, no nail clubbing.

2. What diagnostic tests would you order?
3. What is your differential diagnosis?
4. What would you do for this patient on this visit?

REFERENCES

American College of Chest Physicians Consensus Statement. (1998). Managing cough as a defense mechanism and as a symptom. *Chest, 114*(2; suppl 2).

American Thoracic Society. (1990). Diagnostic standards and classification of tuberculosis. *American Review Respiratory Disease, 142, 725–735.*

American Thoracic Society. (2007). Global strategy for the diagnosis, management and prevention of patients with chronic obstructive pulmonary disease. GOLD executive summary. *American Journal Respiratory Critical Care Medicine, 176, 532–555.*

Bach, P. B., Brown, C., Gelfand, S. E., McCrory, D. C., American College of Physicians, American Society of Internal Medicine, & American College of Chest Physicians. (2001). Management of acute exacerbations of chronic obstructive pulmonary disease: A summary and appraisal of published evidence. *Annals of Internal Medicine, 134, 600–620.*

Bach, P. B., Niewoehner, D. E., Black, W. C., American College of Chest Physicians. (2003). Screening for lung cancer: The guidelines. *Chest, 123*(1 Suppl), 83S–88S.

Barnes, P. J. (2000). Chronic obstructive pulmonary disease. *New England Journal of Medicine, 343,* 269–280.

Bilello, K. S., Murin, S., & Matthay, R. A. (2002). Epidemiology, etiology, and prevention of lung cancer. *Clinical Chest Medicine, 23, 1–25.*

Busse, P. J., & Kilaru, K. (2009). Complexities of diagnosis and treatment of allergic respiratory disease in the elderly. *Drugs & Aging, 26, 1–22.*

Busse, W. W., & Lemanske, R. F., Jr. (2001). Asthma. *New England Journal of Medicine, 344,* 350–362.

Busse, W. W., & Lemanske, R. F., Jr. (2007). Expert Panel 3 Report: Moving forward to improved asthma care. *Journal of Allergy and Clinical Immunology, 120*(5), 1012–1014.

Center for Disease Control. (2003). American Thoracic Society, Center for Disease Control, Infectious Diseases Society of America statement: Treatment of tuberculosis. *MMWR, 52, 1–82.*

Cunha, B. A. (2007). *Pneumonia, community acquired.* Retrieved from http://emedicine.medscape. com/article/234240

Gilbert, D. (2008). *Sanford guide to antimicrobial therapy.* Hyde Park, VT: Antimicrobial Therapy, Inc.

Mandell, L. A., Wunderink, R. G., Anzueto, A., Bartlett, J. G., Campbell, G. D., Dear, N. C., et al. (2007). Infectious Diseases Society of America/American Thoracic Society Consensus Guidelines on the management of community acquired pneumonia in adults. *Clinical Infectious Diseases, 44*(S2), 27–72.

National Asthma Education and Prevention Program. (2007). Expert Panel Report 3: *Guidelines for the diagnosis and management of asthma.* NIH Publication No. 08-4051. Washington, DC: U.S. Department of Health and Human Services. Available at http://www.nhlbi.nih.gov/guidelines/ asthma/index.htm

National Cancer Institute. (2008). *Lung cancer screening.* Retrieved from http://www.cancer.gov/ cancertopics/pdq/screening/lung/HealthProfessional/

National Institute of Allergy and Infectious Disease. (March 2004). *Tuberculosis fact sheet.* Retrieved from http://www.niaid.nih.gov/factsheets/tb.htm

Small, P. M., & Fujiwara, P. I. (2001). Management of tuberculosis in the United States. *New England Journal of Medicine, 345, 189–200.*

Wenzel, S. E., Barnes, P. J., Bleecker, E. R., Bousquet, J., Busse, W., Dahlen, S. E., et al. (2009). A randomized, double-blind, placebo-controlled study of TNF-alpha blockade in severe persistent asthma. *American Journal of Respiratory and Critical Care Medicine, 179*(7), 549–558.

Cardiovascular Disorders

Michaelene Jansen, PhD, RN, GNP-BC, NP-C

GERIATRIC APPROACH
Normal Changes of Aging
- Normal changes of aging of the cardiovascular system are difficult to separate from changes related to atherosclerosis and lifestyle

Vascular structure
- The large, elastic arteries increase in wall thickness, become dilated, decrease in elastin, and increase in collagen, causing the arteries to be more stiff, less elastic
- The average systolic BP increases slightly, probably because of decreased elasticity; diastolic BP is low, stops rising around midlife, then decreases slightly

Cardiovascular function at rest
- Heart rate decreases slightly, as does the respiratory variation in heart rate
- Right side of the heart takes longer to fill: preload (amount of blood going into the heart)
  - Time between aortic valve closure and mitral valve opening becomes prolonged
  - Peak rate at which the LV fills with blood in early diastole is decreased
  - Reduced filling rate may be due to decreased speed of contraction of heart muscle
- Afterload (the force against which the ventricle must contract to eject blood)
  - Stroke volume determined by level of myocardial contractility, vascular afterload, compliance of the arteries
  - Age-related arterial stiffness increases afterload resistance against which heart works to push out the blood
  - Cardiac pump and myocardial contractile function is decreased, causing a decreased ability to compensate for increased afterload

- In conclusion, overall resting cardiac output not affected as the heart adapts to decreased elasticity of the arteries

Cardiovascular response to stress
- Slower response to change in position
- There is an age-related decrease in cardiac output during exercise; this is because the heart does not increase its rate as much as when younger because of the slowed cardiac refilling in the diastolic interval
- The stroke volume does not decline with age
- Beta-adrenergic stimulation—myocardial and vascular responses to beta-adrenergic stimulation decline with age

Clinical Implications

History
- Remember nonspecific presentation of illness in the older adult; many cardiovascular conditions present with vague symptoms in the older adult

Physical
- Supine and standing blood pressure to detect postural hypotension
- "White coat hypertension": excessive variability in BP in presence of person taking BP; if suspected obtain series of readings taken outside of office setting

Assessment
- Incidence of coronary atherosclerosis increases with age, but disease is not a universal aspect of aging
- Problems related to myocardial infarction are one of the four leading causes of malpractice lawsuits; to reduce legal liability related to a patient with chest pain, the clinician must accurately answer two questions: (1) Does the patient have a significant problem? (2) Can the patient go home today?

Treatment
Clinical practice should adhere to national guidelines such as the proceedings of JNC VII, *Report of the Joint National Committee on the Prevention, Detection, Evaluation, and Treatment of High Blood Pressure* (May 2003) and the *Third Report of the National Cholesterol Education Program Expert Panel on Detection, Evaluation, and Treatment of High Blood Cholesterol in Adults*—Adult Treatment Panel III (2001). In July 2004 NCEP published an update to ATP III—*Implications of Recent Clinical Trials for the National Cholesterol Education Program Adult Treatment Panel III Guidelines*. The ATP III update has been endorsed by the National Heart, Lung, and Blood Institute, the American Heart Association, and the American College of Cardiology. Based on a review of five clinical trials of cholesterol-lowering statin treatments that were conducted since the release of ATP III, the update offers options for more intensive cholesterol-lowering treatment for people at high risk and moderately high risk for a heart attack. JNC VIII and the ATP IV publication is anticipated in 2010. A guideline for cardiovascular risk reduction in adults is also has an anticipated publication date in 2010.
- Many cardiovascular problems respond well to nonpharmacologic measures. Educate patient to modify lifestyle risk factors. Elderly people respond well to modifications such as decreased salt intake and weight loss.
- Medications: "start low, go slow"; older adults often start at half the usual adult dose
- Medication compliance is a major problem with chronic cardiac disorders; consider dosing regimens, cost, and side effects to improve outcome

- There are many classes of cardiovascular drugs and many drugs in each class; be knowledgeable about two or three drugs from each class and prescribe these drugs Pharmacologic intervention is lifelong.

CORONARY ARTERY DISEASE (CAD)

Description
- Also called ischemic heart disease
- CAD resulting from atherosclerotic lesions may reduce blood flow to an artery, thus decreasing myocardial oxygen and possibly progressing to the subsequent chest discomfort associated with angina
  - Classic presentation: substernal pressure or heaviness associated with exertion or anxiety, resolving with rest
  - Atypical symptoms, silent ischemia are more common in older adults
  - Angina is a clinical manifestation of myocardial ischemia and CAD
- Types of angina include
  - Stable: pain duration less than 15 minutes, with no change in frequency, severity, duration of anginal episodes during the preceding 6 weeks
  - Unstable: recent change in characteristic angina symptoms
  - Variant or Prinzmetal angina: transient ST-segment elevation, at rest, with angina symptoms related to coronary spasm usually involving right coronary artery

Etiology
Atherosclerosis
- Plaque forms on the intima lining of artery; composed of lipoproteins, cellular components, and extracellular matrix molecules and causes this inner lining of the blood vessels to thicken and the blood vessel to lose elasticity
- First appears as a fatty streak for about 30 years
- Foam cells form and plaque begins to form
- These cells develop into multilayered plaque with fibrous cap
- As early as the fourth decade, the plaque becomes unstable: the foam cells necrose and rupture underneath the fibrous cap
- The fibrous cap tears and bleeds to produce a thrombus, which completely or partially occludes the blood vessel and causes decreased blood flow and ischemia or necrosis

Incidence and Demographics
- Leading cause of death and disability in the United States
- Male/female ratio before age 40 is 8:1; after age 70 is 1:1
- Male peak age 50 to 60; female peak age 60 to 70

Risk Factors
- A complex multifactorial disease with interrelated risk factors
  - Age: male gender until menopause
  - Family history of atherosclerosis (especially under age 50)
  - Elevated low density lipoprotein (LDL) cholesterol
  - Low high density lipoprotein (HDL) cholesterol
  - Diabetes mellitus, insulin resistance
  - Metabolic syndrome
  - Hypertension

– Elevated blood homocysteine levels
– Markers of inflammation such as C-reactive protein
– Cigarette smoking
– Sedentary lifestyle
– Diet high in saturated fat and cholesterol
– Obesity
– Cocaine use, especially with alcohol use

Prevention and Screening

- Smoking cessation, avoidance of secondary smoke
- LDL-C < 100 mg/dL
- BP < 130/80
- Heart-healthy diet with < 7% saturated fats
- Aerobic activity 30 to 60 minutes for a minimum of 5 days/week
- BMI 18.5 to 24.9
- Treatment of comorbid conditions—hypertension, diabetes, hyperlipidemia
- Aspirin 75 to 162 mg daily
- Elevated plasma homocysteine levels can be treated with folic acid 1 mg/day (with B_6 and B_{12}) but it is unclear whether this is effective in reducing the risk of CAD
- ACE inhibitors/angiotensin-receptor blocker (ARB) if ejection fraction < 40%
- Beta blockers if history of MI, acute coronary syndrome, or left ventricular dysfunction
- Annual influenza vaccination

Assessment

History

- Classic presentation of substernal pressure or heaviness associated with exertion or anxiety and relieved with rest
- Dyspnea most common symptom; chest pain is next most common symptoms in patients > 85
- Often asymptomatic
- Substernal pain with radiation to multiple locations: left arm, shoulder, forearm and hand, jaw, neck
- Other common symptoms: delirium, syncope, falls, weakness, nausea, anxiety
- Precipitated by exercise, stress, cold temperature, heavy meal, smoking
- Duration 15 to 20 minutes
- Discomfort relieved by rest or nitroglycerin
- Multiple subjective descriptions: tightness, squeezing, burning, pressure, heaviness
- A change in the patient's typical pattern is indicative of unstable angina

Physical

- Vital signs: elevation in BP, pulse, and respirations
- Holosystolic murmur; mitral valve prolapse may be present
- Transient S3 or S4
- Comorbid conditions: diabetes mellitus, hypertension, aortic stenosis, peripheral vascular disease

Diagnostic Studies

- Resting ECG between episodes will be normal in more than 50% of patients
- ECG at the time of the pain should show change

- Evidence of CVD is left ventricular hypertrophy or ST-T wave changes consistent with ischemia and evidence of previous Q-wave MI
- ECG unreliable in patients with bundle branch block, Wolff-Parkinson-White syndrome
- Chest x-ray to rule out heart failure
- Refer to cardiologist for relevant tests when indicated
  - Exercise stress test: ST segment depression
  - Exercise thallium imaging: hypoperfusion found in areas with diminished uptake
  - Echocardiogram to evaluate left ventricular function
- CT not recommended

Differential Diagnosis
Cardiac
- Pericarditis
- Aortic dissection
- MI
- Heart failure

Gastrointestinal
- GERD
- Cholecystitis
- Esophageal spasm
- Peptic ulcer

Respiratory
- Costochondral pain
- Pneumothorax
- Pneumonia
- Asthma
- Pulmonary emboli

Musculoskeletal
- Chest wall syndrome
- Shoulder arthropathy

Psychological
- Anxiety
- Panic disorders
- Depression

Management
Nonpharmacologic Treatment
- Addressing modifiable risk factors: weight loss, smoking cessation, increased aerobic activity, adoption of low saturated fat and sodium diet
- Careful exercise program based on stress test results
- Coronary stent placement
- Coronary artery bypass grafting (CABG)
- Percutaneous transluminal coronary angioplasty (PTCA)

Pharmacologic Treatment
- Acute: nitroglycerin sublingual tablets or buccal spray 0.3 to 0.6 once; if unrelieved after 5 minutes, call 911/emergency department

Treatment of Stable Angina

- Optimal management of comorbid conditions: hyperlipidemia, diabetes, CHF, hypertension, arrhythmias
- New American Heart Association guidelines (2007) suggest treatment in patients with symptomatic chronic stable angina to prevent MI or death and to reduce symptoms:
  - Aspirin 75 to 162 mg/day
  - Beta-blockers in patients with previous MI
  - Low-density lipoprotein (LDL) cholesterol-lowering therapy with a statin
  - Angiotensin-converting enzyme (ACE) inhibitor if ejection fraction < 40%
- Agents that should be used in patients with symptomatic chronic stable angina to reduce symptoms only are sublingual nitroglycerin or nitroglycerin spray for immediate relief of angina
- Calcium antagonists (long-acting) or long-acting nitrates when beta-blockers are clearly contraindicated
- Calcium antagonists (long-acting) or long-acting nitrates combined with beta-blockers when beta-blockers alone are unsuccessful

Drug Specifics

- Nitrates (long acting) used to promote coronary vasodilation
  - Patient education regarding storage and use of nitroglycerin so it will remain effective; when and how to take it; when to go for medical help
  - Monitor for hypotension
  - Drug tolerance develops rapidly, so patient should have a planned drug-free interval of 10 to 14 hours on a scheduled basis
  - Isosorbide dinitrate 5 to 40 mg t.i.d.
  - Isosorbide mononitrate 10 to 40 mg p.o. b.i.d. or sustained release 60 to 120 mg q.d.
  - Nitro-Dur skin patch 0.2 to 0.8 mg/hr, on for 12 hours, off for 12 hours
- Aspirin 75 to 162 mg q.d.
- Hyperlipidemic medication: lower LDL to 100 or lower; see section on hyperlipidemia
- Beta blockers: decrease heart rate, contractility, and oxygen requirements
  - Monitor bradycardia, fatigue, depression, CHF, asthma
  - Metoprolol (Lopressor) 25 to 200 mg b.i.d.; atenolol (Tenormin) 25 to 200 mg q.d.
- Calcium-channel blockers: coronary vasodilation with reduction of myocardial oxygen
  - Best drug for vasospasm
  - Monitor headache, pedal edema, constipation
  - Avoid verapamil and diltiazem in patients with arrhythmias
  - Coronary spasm: nifedipine XL (Procardia) 30 to120 mg q.d.; verapamil (Calan) 120 to 320 mg q.d.; diltiazem (Cardizem) 120 to 480 mg q.d.
  - Avoid short-acting calcium-channel blockers

When to Consult, Refer, Hospitalize

- Dial 911 for unstable angina
- Refer to physician any new diagnosis of CAD, continued symptoms, and failure of medical therapy/coronary artery bypass grafting

Follow-up

- Individualize follow-up dependent on symptoms and cardiac status (such as CAD, left ventricular function, comorbid conditions)
- See patient a minimum of every 3 months

Expected Course

- Prognosis depends of the number of vessels diseased, the severity of obstruction, degree of left ventricular function, presence of complex arrhythmias
- Course unpredictable, with sudden death occurring in half of cases
- Aggressive treatment of hyperlipidemia has been shown to decrease the incidence of further ischemic events

Complications

- MI, CHF, cardiac arrest, death

ACUTE CORONARY SYNDROMES

Non–ST-Elevation Myocardial Infarction (NSTEMI)/ Unstable Angina (UA)
ST-Elevation MI (STEMI)

Description

- Acute coronary syndrome (ACS) is an umbrella term used to cover any group of clinical symptoms associated with acute myocardial ischemia; ACS covers the spectrum of conditions ranging from unstable angina (UA) to non-Q-wave and Q-wave MI
- Myocardial muscle oxygen demand is severely compromised by thrombus formation; this leads to subsequent reduction in coronary blood flow if there is a total coronary occlusion (Q-wave transmural infarction) or non-occlusion (non-Q-wave nontransmural infarction, a patent but highly narrowed artery)
- Older adults (> 75 years) make up one-third of the population diagnosed with UA/ NSTEMI

Etiology

- CAD: coronary thrombosis secondary to ruptured atherosclerotic plaque
- Coronary spasm

Incidence and Demographics

- Global incidence with mortality 30% to 40%
- Male preponderance fourth through sixth decade, equal by age 70

Risk Factors

- See CAD risk factors

Prevention and Screening

- Enteric coated aspirin 75 to 162 mg/day

Assessment

History

- Often presents as nonspecific presentation of illness in older adults
- The older patient may have no symptoms or may present with confusion or dyspnea
- Shortness of breath, heart failure
- Pain radiates at rest or with minimal activity
- Classic: oppressive retrosternal chest pain, not relieved by nitroglycerin; nausea or vomiting; accompanied by diaphoresis

Physical
- High incidence of mortality within first hour following cardiac event
- May have obvious pain, but usually reduced sensitivity to pain in older adults—"silent MI"
- Nonspecific presentation, confusion, weakness
- Vital signs: hypotension, tachycardia, dyspnea
- General appearance: apprehensive, appears ill, ashen color
- Respiratory: shortness of breath, rales
- Heart: S3, S4, new mitral regurgitation murmur, arrhythmia
- Older adults have altered cardiovascular physiology including hypertension, hypotension, cardiac hypertrophy, heart failure, and left ventricular dysfunction

Diagnostic Studies
- ECG diagnostic in 85% of cases with ST-segment elevation, Q waves, inverted T waves
  - Subendocardial infarction: note ST-segment depression (may be the only finding)
- Cardiac enzymes
  - Creatine kinase (CK): CK-MB enzymes are released during myocardial injury. Isoforms rarely used
  - Troponin T (cTnT) or troponin I (cTnI) are not found in muscle or blood of healthy person and are more specific than CK-MB; become positive 4 to 12 hours after onset of MI; these studies confer greater sensitivity; serial changes useful
  - Myoglobin: not specific to cardiac muscle; presents 1 to 4 hours after infarct

Table 9-1. Cardiac Enzymes in the Diagnosis of MI

Lab	Onset	Comment
CK MB	3 to 4 hours; peak 24 hours	Sensitive, not specific
Troponin I and troponin T	3 to 4 hours; peak cTnI is 24 hours; cTnT is 12 hours to 2 days	Highly specific
Myoglobin	1 to 4 hours	Sensitive, not specific, used infrequently

Differential Diagnosis
- Unstable angina
- Aortic dissection
- Pericarditis
- Pulmonary embolism
- Esophageal spasm
- Biliary tract disease
- Gastroesophageal reflux disease
- Pancreatitis
- Chest wall muscle spasm

Management
Nonpharmacologic Treatment
- Acute: immediate emergency room care for evaluation and stabilization
- After infarction: diet low in saturated fat and sodium; caloric restriction if appropriate, BMI < 24; exercise 30 minutes 5 to 7 days a week

- After infarction: treat the underlying risk factors of hypertension, hyperlipidemia, smoking cessation, diabetes (A1C < 7)

Pharmacologic Treatment

ACUTE
- Nitroglycerin sublingual 0.3 to 0.6 mg, once
- Stop COX-2 inhibitors and NSAIDs
- If chest pain unrelieved, transport to nearest emergency room or chest pain center
- Aspirin 161 to 325 mg, preferably chewable (day 1)
- O_2 via nasal cannula at 2 liters per minute if available
- Percutaneous coronary intervention/fibrinolytics within 90 minutes if not contraindicated

AFTER INFARCTION
- Treatment of hyperlipidemia
- Smoking cessation
- Yearly influenza vaccination; pneumovax if not given previously
- Antiplatelet agent
- Aspirin 75 mg to 325 mg q.d. for 3 to 6 months, then 75 mg to 162 mg/day
- Clopidogrel (Plavix) 75 mg po q.d. (with ASA); reasonable up to 1 year; if drug-eluting stent placed, may need indefinitely
- Beta blockers improve survival rates
- Continue after infarction
  - Monitor bradycardia, fatigue, depression
- Metoprolol (Lopressor) 25 to 200 mg b.i.d.
- Atenolol (Tenormin) 25 to 200 mg q.d.
- Calcium-channel blockers are not effective and are indicated for secondary prevention
- ACE inhibitors should be considered for all patients
  - Decrease morbidity in patients with left ventricular dysfunction
- Heart Outcomes Prevention Evaluation (HOPE) study showed reduction of mortality in patients at low risk for heart failure
- Lisinopril 2.5 mg to 10 mg q.d.; start with small dose, titrate up
- Many other ACE inhibitors available, effective; HOPE study used ramipril
- ARB if unable to tolerate ACE inhibitors
- ARB/ACE inhibitor in systolic heart failure is reasonable
- Nitrates
  - Effective for residual ischemia and coronary atherosclerosis
  - Monitor hypotension
- Coumadin
  - Indicated for atrial fibrillation

When to Consult, Refer, Hospitalize
- Acute: immediate referral to emergency department
- Initial post-MI care and evaluation by cardiologist

Follow-up
- For long-term management, see patient at least every 3 months

Expected Course
- Two variables dictate course: status of vessel disease and ventricular damage
  - Left main CAD: 20% mortality first year; single-vessel damage has 2% mortality; double-vessel damage has 3% to 4% mortality; triple-vessel damage has 5% to 8% mortality
  - Left ventricular dysfunction: ejection fraction < 40% doubles annual mortality rate
- Overall mortality rate 10% in hospital phase, 10% mortality during first year
- 60% of deaths occur in first hour

Complications
- Death
- Chronic heart failure
- Ventricular tachycardia or ventricular fibrillation first 24 hours
- Atrial fibrillation and flutter, bradycardia, heart block
- Deep vein thrombosis, pulmonary embolism, mitral regurgitation, cardiogenic shock

MURMURS

Description
- Abnormal sounds made by turbulent blood flow due to partial obstruction (stenosis) or faulty valve closure (regurgitation, also called insufficiency) that are distinguishable from normal heart sounds

Etiology
- Atherosclerosis
- High-output state from another medical condition, such as anemia, thyrotoxicosis, fever, hypertension
- Innocent murmurs: no evidence of cardiac pathology
- Rheumatic fever is a potential contributor to all murmurs
- Infective endocarditis: regurgitation murmurs
- Other contributing factors include:
  - Aortic stenosis: differentiate between common benign lesion and one with significant obstruction associated with diabetes, hyperlipidemia, CAD
  - Aortic regurgitation: high blood pressure, aortic dissection, collagen vascular disease
  - Mitral regurgitation: left ventricular hypertrophy, CAD with ischemia
  - Mitral stenosis: rheumatic fever

Incidence and Demographics
- Murmurs are extremely common
- Aortic stenosis murmur present in more than 50% of patients older than the age of 75, usually benign

Risk Factors
- Age

Prevention and Screening
- Periodic routine cardiac examination

Assessment

History

- Low output due to valvular disease may cause delirium, fatigue, CHF, weight loss, debility

Physical

- Objective terms: guide to identifying murmurs
- Assessment of murmurs
  - Grading of intensity: see Table 9–2
  - Location: area with greatest intensity
  - Radiation: heard in direction of blood flow
  - Pitch: high, medium, low
  - Quality: soft, harsh, rumbling

Table 9-2. Grading of Murmurs

Grade	Characteristics
I/VI	Very faint, and may not be heard in all positions
II/VI	Quiet but heard immediately upon placing the stethoscope on the chest
III/VI	Moderately loud
IV/VI	Loud accompanied by palpable thrill
V/VI	Very loud, heard with a stethoscope partly off the chest, accompanied by palpable thrill
VI/VI	Heard with the stethoscope entirely off the chest, accompanied by palpable thrill

- Timing: within the cardiac cycle (systolic between S_1/S; diastolic between S_2/S_1)
  - Once auscultated, a murmur must be identified as systolic or diastolic
  - S_1 is mitral and tricuspid valve closure
  - S_2 is aortic and pulmonic valve closure
  - The period between S_1 and S_2 is systole
  - The period between S_2 and S_1 is diastole

Diastole	Systole	Diastole	Systole
S_2	S_1	S_2	S_1
A/P close	M/T close	A/P close	M/T close
M/T open	A/P close	M/T open	A/P close

- Murmurs that occur after S_1 and before S_2 are systolic murmurs
  - Mitral and tricuspid regurgitation (backflow through an incompetent valve)
  - Aortic and pulmonic stenosis (turbulent flow through a tight opening)
- Murmurs that occur after S_2 and before S_1 are diastolic murmurs
  - Aortic and pulmonic regurgitation (backflow through an incompetent valve)
  - Mitral and tricuspid stenosis (turbulent flow through a tight opening)
- Placement of murmurs
  - Once murmurs are identified as systolic or diastolic the likely valve of origin must be identified by location
  - Murmurs loudest at the second intercostal space, right sternal border, are likely aortic murmurs
  - Murmurs loudest at the second intercostal space, left sternal border, are likely pulmonic murmurs
  - Murmurs loudest at the fourth intercostal space, left sternal border, are likely tricuspid murmurs

– Murmurs loudest at the fifth intercostal space, midclavicular line, are likely mitral murmurs

Figure 9-1. Standard Chest Auscultatory Points

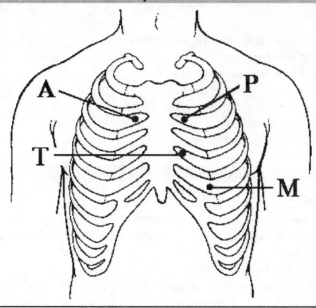

- Systolic regurgitant murmur: murmur begins with S_1 and usually lasts throughout systole (pansystolic or holosystolic); caused by blood flow from a chamber that is at a higher pressure throughout systole than the receiving chamber (associated *only* with ventricular septal defect [VSD], mitral regurgitation [MR], tricuspid regurgitation [TR])
- Diastolic: early diastolic (caused by the incompetence of the aortic or pulmonary valve—aortic regurgitation [AR], pulmonic regurgitation [PR]); mid-diastolic (caused by turbulence of the tricuspid or mitral valve); or presystolic (caused by flow through the atrioventricular valves during ventricular diastole—tricuspid stenosis [TS], mitral stenosis [MS])
- Continuous murmur: S_1 through S_2; conditions such as patent ductus arteriosus (PDA)
- Innocent heart murmurs (functional, physiologic, benign)
- Left sternal border (LSB), 2nd through 4th left interspaces and apex
  - Grade I-II/VI: low pitch; soft, short, nonradiating, midsystolic
  - Variable loudness: heard best in supine position and diminishes with upright position
- Interpretation of murmurs
  - Once timing and placement are identified, the valvular disorder is evident
  - A systolic murmur at the second intercostal space, right sternal border, is an aortic murmur occurring when the aortic valve is open: aortic stenosis
  - A diastolic murmur at the second intercostal space, right sternal border, is an aortic murmur occurring when the aortic valve is closed: aortic regurgitation
  - A systolic murmur at the fifth intercostal space, midclavicular line, is a mitral murmur occurring when the mitral valve is closed: mitral regurgitation
  - A diastolic murmur occurring at the fifth intercostal space, midclavicular line, is a mitral murmur occurring when the mitral valve is open: mitral stenosis

Table 9-3. Types of Murmurs

Systolic murmur	Occurs between S_1 and S_2 Systolic ejection murmur: interval between S_1 and the onset of the murmur (also called crescendo-decrescendo); caused by blood flow through stenotic or deformed semilunar valves or by increased blood flow through normal semilunar valves Systolic regurgitant murmur: murmur begins with S_1 and usually lasts throughout systole (pansystolic or holosystolic); caused by blood flow from a chamber that is at a higher pressure throughout systole than the receiving chamber (associated *only* with VSD, MR, and TR)
Diastolic murmur	Occurs between S_2 and S_1 Classified as: early diastolic and caused by the incompetence of the aortic or pulmonary valve, AR, PR; mid-diastolic caused by turbulence of the tricuspid or mitral valve; or presystolic, caused by flow through the atrioventricular valves during ventricular diastole (TS, MS)
Continuous murmur	Occurs with S_1 and continue through the S_2 into diastole Seen with conditions such as PDA, pulmonary artery (PA) stenosis, Blalock-Taussig shunt
Innocent heart murmur (functional murmur)	Murmurs that arise from cardiovascular structures in the absence of anatomic abnormalities (80% of children have innocent murmurs sometime throughout childhood, usually beginning at age 3 years old); also called functional, benign, or physiological murmurs

Systolic Murmurs

Aortic Stenosis

- Second intercostal space (IC) right of sternum, with patient sitting and leaning forward
- Valve is open when stenotic murmur occurs and is caused by forward flow through stenotic valve
- Begins after S_1 and is a crescendo-decrescendo or diamond-shaped ejection murmur
- Radiation into neck from aortic area
- Medium pitch with intensity variable
- Harsh; loudest at base, musical at apex
- Midsystolic
- Systolic thrill may be present
- Seen frequent in the elderly and associated with a diminished S_2

Tricuspid Regurgitation

- Lower LSB
- Begins with S_1; high-pitched, smooth, blowing quality
- Pansystolic regurgitant murmur; increases in intensity with inspiration
- Right ventricular lift
- Always associated with pathology; usually diseased right ventricle from rheumatic heart disease

Ventricular Septal Defect
- LSB (3rd to 5th ICS)
- Radiation wide over precordium but not into axilla
- Loud (particularly base), harsh, pansystolic, regurgitant murmur with thrill

Hypertrophic Obstructive Cardiomyopathy
- LSB
- No radiation
- Murmur increases with Valsalva maneuver, decreases with patient squatting
- Midsystolic

Pulmonic Stenosis
- LSB 2nd or 3rd ICS, pulmonary area
- Generally no radiation unless loud, and then toward left neck
- Variable intensity, medium pitch
- Midsystolic: begins after S_1 with crescendo-decrescendo contour
- Associated with thrill if significant pathology; usually congenital cause

Mitral Regurgitation
- Location: apex; frequently radiates to wide area of chest and to left axilla
- Intensity variable, often loud; does not increase with inspiration
- Pitch is high with a blowing quality
- S_3 usually also heard
- Pansystolic regurgitant murmur frequently accompanied by thrill
- Begins with S_1 (which may be decreased)
- Valve is closed when the murmur occurs; noise caused from backflow through incompetent valve
- Always pathologic

Diastolic Murmurs
- Always indicative of heart disease
- Often heard best with bell of the stethoscope

Mitral Stenosis
- Listen with patient in left lateral decubitus position; also with exercise
- Diastolic rumbling murmur that begins after a short period of silence after S_2
- Low in pitch; heard best with bell of stethoscope in light skin contact
- No radiation
- Loudest at apex; best heard after mild exercise

Aortic Regurgitation
- Heard at LSB with patient leaning forward and listening with *diaphragm* pressed firmly on the chest
- Early diastolic murmur that begins immediately after S_2 and diminishes in intensity
- Blowing, high-pitched, decrescendo
- Heard with rheumatic heart disease or syphilis

Pulmonary Valve Insufficiency
- LSB 2nd ICS
- Radiates mid-right sternal border

- High-pitched, loudest base, decrescendo murmur

Continuous murmurs (quality often varies when patient changes position)
- Patent ductus arteriosus
- Coarctation of the aorta
- Peripheral pulmonary stenosis

Diagnostic Studies
- Electrocardiogram to detect underlying heart disease
- CBC to look for signs of infection, anemia
- Chest x-ray to evaluate heart failure, size of heart
- Echocardiography to evaluate valve pathology and systolic/diastolic function
- Angiography for more thorough evaluation
- Fluoroscopy to demonstrate calcified aortic valve

Differential Diagnosis
- See descriptions of systolic and diastolic murmurs

Management
Nonpharmacologic Treatment
- Patient education on disease entity and lifestyle modifications for underlying disorder
- Valvular surgical repair

Pharmacologic Treatment
- Stabilize hemodynamic deficiencies
- Antibiotics for endocarditis prophylaxis as indicated

How Long to Treat
- Often a chronic condition

Special Considerations
- Aortic stenosis common in older adults

When to Consult, Refer, Hospitalize
- Consult or refer if symptomatic (signs of heart failure, syncope, cyanosis); diastolic murmur; systolic murmur that is loud (grade III/IV or with a thrill), long in duration, and transmits well to other parts of the body; abnormally strong or weak pulses; abnormal cardiac size or silhouette or pulmonary vasculature on chest x-ray
- If abnormal ECG and symptomatic, hospitalization may be necessary

Follow-up
- Asymptomatic patients should be assessed at least annually and at every visit
- No follow-up necessary for innocent murmurs

Complications
- Chronic heart failure
- Poor activity tolerance
- Progression of mitral stenosis has potential for thrombus formation and hypoxia
- Progression of mitral regurgitation is associated with dyspnea and orthopnea
- Atrial fibrillation with mitral stenosis and mitral regurgitation
- Stroke and/or TIA
- Bacterial endocarditis

Table 9-4. Characteristics of Common Murmurs

Murmur	Grade	Location	Radiation	Pitch	Quality	Timing	Significance
Systolic							
Innocent	I to III, variable	2nd to 4th ICS LSB	None	Medium	Soft	Short early to midsystolic	None
Stenosis							
Aortic	Variable	Aortic	Neck, LSB	Medium	Harsh	Crescendo decrescendo, midsystolic	Common, cause CHF, angina and syncope
Pulmonic	Variable	Pulmonic area and 3rd ICS LSB	Left shoulder	Medium	Harsh	Crescendo decrescendo, midsystolic	Rare, pathologic
Regurgitation							
Mitral	Often loud	Mitral	Left axilla	High	Blowing	Pansystolic	Common, pulmonary edema, arrhythmia, CHF
Tricuspid	Variable	Tricuspid	Right of sternum, left MCL	High	Blowing	Pansystolic	Always pathologic
Diastolic							
Stenosis							
Mitral	Variable	Mitral	Little	Low	Rumbling	Begins after short pause after S_2, decrescendo, crescendo	Rare, pulmonary edema, atrial fibrillation
Regurgitation							
Aortic	Often faint	Aortic	Down LSB	High	Blowing	Decrescendo, early systole	LVH, dilation of left ventricle

HYPERTENSION

Description
- The following discussion is based primarily on the Seventh Report of the Joint National Committee on Prevention, Detection, Evaluation, and Treatment of High Blood Pressure (JNC VII), 2003 (JNC VIII is anticipated in 2010)
- Systolic blood pressure (SBP) ≥ 140 mm Hg and/or diastolic blood pressure (DBP) ≥ 90 mm Hg
- Hypertension is classified by severity; see Table 9–5

Table 9-5. Classification of Blood Pressure

Classification of Blood Pressure for Adults Aged 18 Years and Older*

Category	Blood Pressure, mm Hg	
	Systolic	Diastolic
Normal	< 120 and	< 80
Prehypertension	120 to 139 or	80 to 89
Stage 1 hypertension	140 to 159 or	90 to 99
Stage 2 hypertension	> 160	> 100

Based on the average of 2 or more readings taken at 2 or more visits after an initial screening.

- Hypertension is classified as either primary (essential) or secondary
  - Primary hypertension constitutes 95% of hypertension cases
    - Isolated systolic hypertension: a subset of primary hypertension
    - More common in older adults
    - Defined as systolic > 140 with DBP < 90
    - Stronger cardiovascular risk factor than elevated DBP in older adults
  - Secondary hypertension: 5% of all hypertension cases, less common in older adults
    - Sudden onset of hypertension in the older adult is often from secondary cause

Etiology
- Primary hypertension: no known cause
- Isolated systolic hypertension: elevated pulse pressure (SBP and DBP) due to reduced vascular compliance
- Secondary hypertension
  - Renal parenchymal disease
  - Renal vascular disease
  - Cushing disease
  - Pheochromocytoma
  - Hyperaldosteronism
  - Coarctation of the aorta
  - Sleep apnea
  - Thyroid/parathyroid disease
- Pharmacologic
  - Oral corticosteroids
  - Cocaine
  - NSAIDs
  - Sympathomimetics: decongestants
  - Estrogens
  - Alcohol
  - Cyclosporine
  - Amphetamines
  - Erythropoietin
  - MAO inhibitors

Incidence and Demographics
- 64% of patients over age 60
- Males > females

- NHANES III study of Americans age 60 and older: elevated BP found in 60% non-Hispanic Whites, 71% non-Hispanic Blacks, 61% Mexican Americans
- Diastolic pressure tends to stabilize after age 60, but rising SBP increases rapidly after age 55

Risk Factors
- Smoking
- Dyslipidemia
- Diabetes mellitus
- Age older than 60 years
- Gender (men and postmenopausal women)
- Family history of cardiovascular disease: women under age 65 or men under age 55
- African American
- Obesity (BMI $\geq$ 30 kg/m^2)
- Stress
- Excessive dietary intake of sodium

Prevention and Screening
- Annual blood pressure screening

Assessment
- Identify severity of hypertension (see Table 9–5)
- Signs and symptoms of secondary hypertension
  - Renal parenchymal disease: urinalysis for proteinuria; elevated serum creatinine
  - Renal vascular disease: renal bruits, symptoms variable or absent depending on whether infarction occurred
  - Cushing disease: fatigue, weakness, bruising, osteoporosis, truncal obesity, hyperglycemia
  - Pheochromocytoma: episodes of flushing, palpitations, pallor, tremor, profuse perspiration, angina, diaphoresis
  - Hyperaldosteronism: muscle weakness, cramps, paresthesia, decreased serum potassium and magnesium, increased urine potassium and serum sodium
  - Coarctation of the aorta: weak peripheral pulses, chest x-ray
- Target organ damage (TOD)
- Heart
  - Left ventricular hypertrophy: point of maximum impulse displaced to the left, S_4 gallop
  - Angina/history of MI
  - Prior coronary revascularization
  - Chronic heart failure: S_3, bilateral basilar rales (crackles), peripheral edema
- Brain
  - Stroke or transient ischemic attack: abnormal neurological exam
- Chronic kidney disease
  - Peripheral arterial disease: decreased pedal pulses
- Retinopathy: Scheie classification
  - Grade 1: slight generalized attenuation of retinal arterioles
  - Grade 2: obvious arteriolar narrowing with focal areas of attenuation
  - Grade 3: grade 2 plus retinal exudates, cotton-wool spots, and hemorrhages
  - Grade 4: grade 3 plus optic nerve edema

History
- Known duration and levels of elevated BP
- Symptoms of cardiovascular disease, heart failure, cerebrovascular disease, peripheral vascular disease, renal disease, diabetes mellitus, dyslipidemia, other comorbid conditions, gout, or sexual dysfunction
- Family history of high blood pressure, premature cardiovascular disease, stroke, diabetes, dyslipidemia, or renal disease
- Symptoms suggesting causes of hypertension
- History of recent changes in weight, leisure time physical activity, and smoking or other tobacco use
- Dietary assessment including intake of sodium, alcohol, saturated fat, and caffeine
- History of all prescribed and OTC medications, herbal remedies, and illicit drugs
- Results and adverse effects of previous antihypertensive therapy
- Psychosocial and environmental factors that may influence hypertension control

Physical
- Two or more blood pressure measurements
- Verification in the contralateral arm
- Height, weight, and waist circumference
- Funduscopic examination for hypertensive retinopathy: arteriolar narrowing, focal arteriolar constrictions, arteriovenous crossing changes, hemorrhages and exudates, disc edema
- Neck carotid bruits, distended veins, or an enlarged thyroid gland
- Heart rate rhythm, increased size, precordial heave, clicks, murmurs, and third and fourth heart sounds
- Lungs rales and evidence for bronchospasm
- Abdomen bruits, enlarged kidneys, masses, or abnormal aortic pulsation
- Extremities for diminished or absent peripheral arterial pulsations, bruits, and edema
- Neurological assessment

Table 9-6. Essential Criteria for Measuring Blood Pressure

Criterion	Process
Have patient rest for 5 minutes	Two or more readings taken at each of 2 or more visits after an initial screening
Patient sitting in chair with arm supported	If BP is stage 3, take 3 times at 1 visit and start management at that visit
Use correct size cuff	Readings 2 minutes apart
Use mercury sphygmomanometer or recently calibrated aneroid	Patient refrain from smoking or caffeine 30 prior to reading
Patient not acutely ill	

Diagnostic Studies
- General
  - Blood chemistry: potassium, sodium, creatinine, fasting glucose
  - Lipids: total cholesterol and HDL
  - 12-lead electrocardiogram
  - CBC
  - Urinalysis

- Additional optional testing per JNC VII
  - Creatinine clearance, microalbuminuria, 24-hour urinary protein, blood calcium, uric acid, fasting triglycerides, LDL, glycosylated hemoglobin, TSH, and echocardiography
  - Renal disease suspected: renal and abdominal vascular ultrasound and renal arteriogram if indicated

Differential Diagnosis
- See Etiology

Management
- Goal is lower than 140/90 for most patients but 130/80 for those with diabetes or renal disease

Nonpharmacologic Treatment
- See Box 9–1
- Lifestyle changes are recommended for patients with prehypertension and for *all* patients with hypertension

Pharmacologic Treatment
- Because clinical studies have shown the benefit of diuretics in blood pressure reduction, the JNC VII recommends starting with a diuretic unless patient has compelling indication or comorbid condition affecting choice of medication
- Diuretics and ACE inhibitors are appropriate for initial treatment of hypertension in older adults
- Many older adults have compelling indications to start with another drug
- Individualized treatment plan should be implemented considering the patient's risk factors compelling indications, and concomitant disease
- Most patients will need two or more medications to achieve control
  Diuretic: thiazide type
  ACEI: angiotensin-converting enzyme inhibitor
  ARB: angiotensin-receptor blocker
  BB: beta blocker
  CCB: calcium-channel blocker

Box 9–1. Lifestyle Modifications for Prevention and Management of Hypertension

Smoking cessation

Lose weight if overweight, and reduce intake of dietary saturated fat and cholesterol

Limit alcohol intake to no more than 1 oz (30 mL) ethanol (e.g., 24 oz [720 mL] beer, 10 oz [300 mL] wine, or 2 oz [60 mL] 100-proof whiskey) per day or 0.5 oz (15 mL) ethanol per day for women and lighter weight people

Increase physical activity (30 to 45 minutes most days of the week)

Reduce sodium intake to no more than 100 mmol per day (2.4 g sodium, 6 g sodium chloride, or 1 teaspoon)

Maintain adequate intake of dietary potassium (approximately 90 mmol or 2 g per day), calcium, and magnesium

---

Adapted from "Seventh report of the Joint National Committee on Prevention, Detection, Evaluation, and Treatment of High Blood Pressure" by A. V. Chobanian, G. L. Bakris, H. R. Black, W. C. Cushman, L. A. Green, J. L. Izzo, Jr., et al., 2003, *Hypertension, 42*(6), pp. 1206–1252.

Table 9-7. Pharmacological Treatment for Hypertension

BP Classification	Without Compelling Indication	With Compelling Indication
Prehypertension 130–139/85–89	Lifestyle modification	Drugs for compelling indication
Stage 1 140–159/90–99	Diuretic for most; may consider ACEI, ARB, BB, CCB, or combination	Drug(s) for the compelling indications; other antihypertensive drugs (diuretics, ACEI, ARB, BB, CCB as needed)
Stage 2 160 or more/100 or more	Two drug combination for most (usually diuretic and ACEI or ARB or BB or CCB)	

Adapted from "Seventh report of the Joint National Committee on Prevention, Detection, Evaluation, and Treatment of High Blood Pressure" by A. V. Chobanian, G. L. Bakris, H. R. Black, W. C. Cushman, L. A. Green, J. L. Izzo, Jr., et al., 2003, *Hypertension, 42*(6), pp. 1206–1252.

Figure 9-2. Algorithm for Treatment of Hypertension

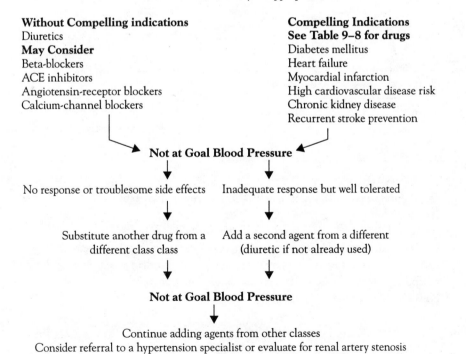

Begin or Continue Lifestyle Modifications

↓

Not at Goal Blood Pressure (<140/90 mm Hg)
130/80 mm Hg for patients with diabetes or chronic kidney disease

↓

Initial Drug Choices
Start with a low dose of a long-acting once-daily drug, and titrate dose
Low-dose combinations may be appropriate

Without Compelling indications
Diuretics
May Consider
Beta-blockers
ACE inhibitors
Angiotensin-receptor blockers
Calcium-channel blockers

Compelling Indications
See Table 9–8 for drugs
Diabetes mellitus
Heart failure
Myocardial infarction
High cardiovascular disease risk
Chronic kidney disease
Recurrent stroke prevention

Not at Goal Blood Pressure

No response or troublesome side effects   Inadequate response but well tolerated

↓   ↓

Substitute another drug from a   Add a second agent from a different
different class class   (diuretic if not already used)

↓   ↓

Not at Goal Blood Pressure

↓

Continue adding agents from other classes
Consider referral to a hypertension specialist or evaluate for renal artery stenosis

Adapted from "Seventh report of the Joint National Committee on Prevention, Detection, Evaluation, and Treatment of High Blood Pressure" by A. V. Chobanian, G. L. Bakris, H. R. Black, W. C. Cushman, L. A. Green, J. L. Izzo, Jr., et al., 2003, *Hypertension, 42*(6), pp. 1206–1252.

Table 9-8. Drug Choices for Compelling Indications

Compelling Indication	Diuretic	BB	ACEI	ARB	CCB	Aldo Ant
Heart Failure	x	x	x	x		x
Post-MI		x	x			x
High CVD risk	x	x	x		x	
Diabetes	x	x	x	x	x	
Chronic kidney disease			x	x		
Recurrent stroke prevention	x		x			

Adapted from "Seventh report of the Joint National Committee on Prevention, Detection, Evaluation, and Treatment of High Blood Pressure" by A. V. Chobanian, G. L. Bakris, H. R. Black, W. C. Cushman, L. A. Green, J. L. Izzo, Jr., et al., 2003, *Hypertension, 42*(6), pp. 1206–1252.

Note. Aldo Ant: aldosterone antagonist diuretic, spironolactone

Diuretics

- Target groups: those with heart failure, older patients, African Americans, smokers
- Avoid: history of gout, DM (high dose), hyperparathyroidism, and dyslipidemia
- Thiazide-type diuretics are first-line therapy
- In general, hydrochlorothiazide is preferred over chlorthalidone in older adults because it has a shorter half-life and may have less risk for adverse effects
- Furosemide (Lasix) is used in patients with renal insufficiency
- Spironolactone is potassium-sparing diuretic often used for heart failure

Table 9-9. Examples of Recommended Diuretic Therapy

Drug	Dose Range	Side Effects
Hydrochlorothiazide (HCTZ)	12.5 to 50 mg every morning	Anorexia, nausea, vomiting, cramping, dehydration, hypokalemia, hypercalcemia, hyperlipidemia, hyperglycemia
Chlorthalidone	6.25 to 25 mg q.d.	
Furosemide (Lasix)	20 to 80 mg q.d.	
Spironolactone	12.5 to 50 q.d.	Hyperkalemia, hyponatremia, gynecomastia, GI disturbances, drowsiness

Beta Blockers (BB)

- Target groups: post-MI, angina, arrhythmias, tremor, hyperthyroid
- First-line therapy
- Avoid asthma, conduction disorders, bradycardia, heart block
- Use with caution in diabetes mellitus (masks symptoms of hypoglycemia)
- Cardioselective beta blockers have greater effect on cardiac receptors than lung receptors at lower doses and are recommended in older adults
- Heart failure: carvedilol (Coreg)

Table 9-10. Examples of Recommended Beta Blocker Therapy

Drug	Dosage	Side Effects
Metoprolol (Lopressor)	50 to 100 mg q.d. or b.i.d.	Bradycardia, depression, fatigue, exercise intolerance, asthma, sexual dysfunction
Atenolol (Tenormin)	25 to 100 mg q.d.	

Angiotensin-Converting Enzyme Inhibitors (ACE)
- Target groups: DM, CHF, post-MI
- Well tolerated; do not cause hyperlipidemia or hyperglycemia
- Avoid use in renal stenosis, elevated creatinine
- Captopril seldom used because of increased incidence of cough, frequency of dosing

Table 9–11. Examples of Recommended Ace Inhibitor Therapy

Drug	Dosage	Side Effects
Lisinopril (Prinivil, Zestril)	2.5 to 40 mg q.d.	Hyperkalemia, angioedema, headache, dizziness, fatigue
Ramipril (Altace)	1.25 to 20 mg q.d.	

Angiotensin-Receptor Blockers (ARB)
- Target groups: identical to those for ACE inhibitors, with inability to tolerate ACE inhibitors because of cough
- Avoid in renovascular disease

Table 9–12. Examples of Recommended Angiotensin Receptor Blockers

Drug	Dosage	Side Effects
Losartan (Cozaar)	25 to 100 mg q.d.	Rare side effects: dizziness, insomnia, muscle cramps, leg pain, hyperkalemia
Valsartan (Diovan)	40 to 320 mg q.d.	

Calcium-Channel Blockers (CCB)
- Target groups: angina, CAD, Blacks, migraine, isolated systolic in older adults, arrhythmia (non-dihydropyridine)
- Contraindicated in conduction disorders
- Three types of calcium-channel blockers
- Dihydropyridine calcium-channel blockers: prototype nifedipine, now many others including amlodipine
  – Do not affect cardiac conduction system
- Non-dihydropyridine calcium-channel blockers
  – Verapamil: affects cardiac conduction system
  – Cardizem: has characteristics of both verapamil and dihydropyridine calcium-channel blockers
- Avoid beta blocker and non-dihydropyridine calcium-channel blocker combination
- Research has shown that short-acting nifedipine increases cardiac morbidity

Table 9–13. Examples of Recommended Calcium Channel Blocker Therapy

Drug	Dosage	Side Effects
Dihydropyridines Nifedipine (Procardia XL) Amlodipine (Norvasc)	30 to 90 mg p.o. q.d. 2.5 to 10 mg q.d.	Edema, fatigue, palpitations, dizziness, GI upset, flushing abdominal pain, drowsiness
Verapamil (Calan SR)	120 to 480 mg q.d.	Constipation, edema, bradycardia, headache constipation, fatigue, heart failure, AV block
Diltiazem (Cardizem LA)	120 to 360 mg q.d.	Edema, headache, bradycardia, fatigue, AV block, flushing, nausea, heart failure, liver abnormalities

Special Considerations
- Monitor for side effects of medications, particularly orthostatic hypotension and dehydration in frail older adults and those with comorbid disease and polypharmacy

When to Consult, Refer, Hospitalize
- Refer as needed for secondary causes of hypertension
- Consult physician when no response to first-line therapy
- Hypertension emergencies
- Refer for target organ damage/clinical cardiovascular disease

Follow-up
- Follow up 4 to 6 weeks until BP is controlled, every 3 to 6 months depending on clinical situation
- Routine visits every 3 to 6 months depending on patient clinical situation
- SBP > 180 or DBP > 110 and follow-up in 48 to 72 hours

Complications
- Stroke, CAD, heart failure, target organ damage, aortic dissection

HYPERLIPIDEMIA

Description
- A laboratory measurement of blood lipids showing elevation of cholesterol and/or triglycerides
- Lipids are carried in lipoproteins, which are classified by density
- High-density lipoproteins facilitate the transfer of cholesterol from the periphery to the liver
- Low-density lipoproteins facilitate transfer of cholesterol from the liver to the periphery
- This discussion is based on the *Third Report of the National Cholesterol Education Program (NCEP) Expert Panel on Detection, Evaluation, and Treatment of High Blood Cholesterol in Adults* (Adult Treatment Panel III); see References, available at www.nhlbi.nih.gov/guidelines/cholesterol; ATP IV is anticipated in 2010
- The third report emphasizes importance of LDL, with recommendations to further decreasing LDL levels, and recognizes diabetes and peripheral arterial disease as well as clinical CAD as high-risk equivalents for coronary heart disease
- While the NCEP panel emphasizes LDL, triglycerides are known to be an independent risk factor for CVD

Etiology
- Genetic hyperlipidemia
- Diet: excessive carbohydrate intake, weight gain; increased saturated fat or alcohol intake
- Diseases: diabetes mellitus, hypothyroidism, pancreatitis, renal disease, liver disease
- Medications: oral contraceptives, diuretics, beta blockers, corticosteroids

Incidence and Demographics
- See CVD, metabolic syndrome
- Total cholesterol levels increase and achieve plateau in middle age and decline slightly after age 70

Risk Factors
- Hyperlipidemia is a major risk factor for cardiovascular disease
- See Assessment

Prevention and Screening
- Low-fat diet
- Annual screening for hyperlipidemia indicated up to age 65
- Meta-analyses have not found cholesterol to be a risk factor for CVD for persons over age 75
- Consider general health, comorbidities, and life expectancy when counseling regarding screening and treatment of cholesterol over age 75, remembering that statins seem to confer protective qualities beyond lowering LDL

Assessment
- Determine the patient's overall risk status for CVD
  - LDL level
  - Presence of CVD
  - Determine whether patient has CVD risk equivalent:
    - Presence of clinical forms of atherosclerotic disease
    - Type 2 diabetes
    - Multiple risk factors that confer a 10-year risk for CVD greater than 20% (use Framingham calculation found online at http://hp2010.nhlbihin.net/atpiii/calculator.asp?usertype=prof)
  - Count number of risk factors:
    - Age: male age 45 or older, or female age 55 or older
    - Family history of premature CVD: CVD in male first-degree relative less than 55 years *or* CVD in female first-degree relative less than 65 years
    - Current cigarette smoking
    - Hypertension: blood pressure greater than or equal to 140/90 *or* patient is taking antihypertensive medication
    - Low HDL cholesterol (less than 40)
    - Negative risk factor: high HDL, greater than 60

History
- CVD risk factors
- Comorbid disease
- Medications
- Family history

Physical
- Xanthomas
- Obesity
- Funduscopic exam
- Look for signs of comorbid disease, complications of hyperlipidemia

Diagnostic Studies
- Complete fasting lipid profile: total cholesterol, HDL, LDL, triglycerides
- Liver function tests
- Routine blood chemistries
- Urinalysis

Table 9-14. Classification of LDL, Total, and HDL Cholesterol

LDL Cholesterol	< 100	Optimal
	100 to 129	Near optimal
	130 to 159	Borderline high
	160 to 189	High
	190+	Very high
Total Cholesterol	< 200	Desirable
	200 to 239	Borderline high
	240+	High
HDL Cholesterol	< 40	Low
	60+	High
Triglycerides	< 200	Normal
	200 to 400	Borderline high
	400 to 1000	High
	1000+	Very high

Differential Diagnosis
- See Etiology

Management
- Intensity of treatment depends on the patient's overall risk status for CVD

Table 9-15. Treatment Decisions Based on Risk Category: LDL-C

Risk Category	Initiate Lifestyle Changes	Initiate Drug Therapy	LDL goal
High risk	≥ 100	≥ 100	< 100
Moderately high risk	≥ 130	≥ 130	< 130
Moderate risk	≥ 130	≥ 160	< 130
Low risk	≥ 160	≥ 190	< 160

Nonpharmacologic Treatment
- Diet: all patients with hyperlipidemia should be started on a therapeutic lifestyle diet
  - Caloric restriction
  - Increased dietary fiber: oatmeal, oat bran, raw fruits and vegetables
  - Weight loss in overweight patients
- Exercise
  - All patients should be started on an appropriate exercise program: 30 minutes of aerobic activity 5 to 7 days/week

Pharmacologic Treatment

Table 9–16. Effect of Medications on Lipids

Drug Type	LDL	HDL	Triglycerides
HMG CoA reductase inhibitors ("statins")	–20% to –50%	+5% to 15%	–10% to –25%
Fibric acids	–10% to –25%	+10% to +15%	–20% to –50%
Bile acid sequestrants	–15% to –30%	+3% to 5%	+5% to –30%
Niacin	–10% to –25%	+15% to +35%	–20% to –50%
Selective cholesterol absorption inhibitor	–15% to –20%	+2% to 4%	–4% to –6%

- HMG CoA reductase inhibitors ("statins")
  - Generally well tolerated
  - Contraindication: liver disease
  - Most are metabolized by cytochrome P450 (CYP) 3A4, except pravastatin (Pravachol)
    - Drug interaction with cyclosporine, erythromycin, itraconazole, ketoconazole
    - Use caution in combination with fibric acid, increased risk for rhabdomyolysis
  - Monitor for adverse reactions
    - Muscle pain and elevated creatine phosphokinase (CPK) may indicate rhabdomyolysis, which may lead to renal dysfunction
    - Elevated liver function tests (LFT): monitor liver function tests prior to initiation of therapy, then every 6 to12 weeks for a year, then periodically
- Fibric acids
  - Generally well tolerated
  - Adverse reactions: hepatotoxicity, cholelithiasis, dizziness, dyspepsia, bloating, diarrhea, myalgia
  - Contraindicated in renal or hepatic dysfunction
- Bile acid sequestrants
  - Not absorbed systemically
  - May safely be used in combination other lipid-lowering medications
  - Interfere with absorption of other drugs and fat-soluble vitamins: take 1 hour before other medication/vitamin or 4 hours after
  - Few able to tolerate because of unpalatability
  - Side effects: constipation, flatulence, nausea, bloating abdominal cramps, malabsorption
- Nicotinic acid
  - Use with caution in DM, heart failure, peptic ulcer, gout; monitor for liver toxicity.
  - Liver function tests, blood glucose, uric acid prior to initiation
  - Low dose; titrate slowly to avoid flushing; pre-treat with aspirin ½ hr prior to dose
  - Long-acting form has less flushing but more liver toxicity
  - Side effects: flushing, pruritus, impaired glucose tolerance, hyperuricemia, nausea, abdominal pain, diarrhea hypotension, nausea

Table 9–17. Recommended Lipid Drug Therapy

Drug	Dose
HMG CoA Inhibitor (Statin)	
Atorvastatin (Lipitor)	10 to 80 mg p.o. daily
Rosuvastatin (Crestor)	5 to 40 mg p.o. daily
Fluvastatin (Lescol)	20 to 40 mg p.o. daily
Lovastatin (Mevacor)	10 to 80 mg p.o. daily
Pravastatin (Pravachol)	20 to 40 mg p.o. daily
Simvastatin (Zocor)	5 to 80 mg p.o. daily
Bile Acid Sequestrant	
Cholestyramine (Questran)	4 g b.i.d. to 24 g divided
Colestipol (Colestid)	5 g b.i.d. to 30 g divided
Fibric Acid	
Gemfibrozil (Lopid)	600 mg q.d. to 1200 mg divided
Fenofibrate (Tricor)	48 mg to 145 mg p.o. daily
Nicotinic Acid Derivative	
Niacin	100 mg q.d. to 3.0 g divided
Nicotinic Acid (Niaspan) extended release	500 mg q.d. to 2.0 g
Selective Cholesterol Absorption Inhibitor	
Ezetimibe (Zetia)	10 mg p.o. daily

When to Consult, Refer, Hospitalize
- Patients with the following conditions may require physician consultation and/or referral: diabetes mellitus (especially if poorly controlled); existing CVD, poorly controlled hypertension, chronic renal insufficiency
- Dietitian: poor dietary compliance

Follow-up
- Assessment of adverse reactions to medication, diet assessment, compliance with exercise routine, 24-hour recall of diet
- Monitor CPK and LFT as described above
- Visits: 8 weeks initially, until lipid control is achieved; then every 6 months

Expected Course
- Dependent on etiology, CAD

Complications
- CAD progression
- Stroke

ARRHYTHMIAS
Atrial Fibrillation
Description
- Acute or chronic arrhythmia that is characterized by a non-synchronized irregular atrial and ventricular activity; untreated rates vary from atrial rate of 200 to 600 beats per minute with ventricular rate of 80 to 180 beats per minute; this is an irregularly irregular rhythm in which conduction varies from the atrial to the ventricular

- Pulse deficit is the difference between apical rate and radial pulse rate
- Can be life-threatening in older adults because of risk for embolism (stroke) and inability to tolerate tachycardia (increases risk for heart failure)
- Often starts as acute episodes, later becomes chronic
- Associated with increase in mortality in otherwise healthy patients; thus, should never be considered as a benign condition even though no organic heart disease may be found

Etiology
- Rheumatic heart disease
- Cardiomyopathy
- Hypertension
- Acute myocardial infarction
- Pulmonary embolus (PE)
- Chronic heart failure
- Pericarditis
- Hyperthyroidism
- Idiopathic

Incidence and Demographics
- The most common chronic arrhythmia
- Increases with age, steep increase after age 70
- Male preponderance
- High reoccurrence of episodes
- Approximately 4% of people over 60 have sustained atrial fibrillation

Risk Factors
- Patients with atrial fibrillation are at increased risk for stroke
- Profile for those most at risk of stroke includes:
  - Age over 65 years
  - Previous TIA or stroke
  - High blood pressure
  - Heart failure
  - Thyrotoxicosis
  - Clinical coronary disease
  - Mitral stenosis
  - Prosthetic heart valve
  - Diabetes

Prevention and Screening
- Avoid excessive alcohol, caffeine, and nicotine
- Treat comorbid conditions
- Assess and aggressively respond to triggers that comprise hemodynamic stability

Assessment
Evaluate for hemodynamic stability
- Shock, severe hypotension, pulmonary edema, myocardial ischemia

History
- Variable symptoms from asymptomatic to severe
- Palpitations

- Angina
- Fatigue
- Decline in activity level
- Marked dyspnea
- Dizziness
- Syncope

Physical
- Tachycardia
- Irregular pulse: marked deficit between apical rate and radial pulse rate
- Pallor
- Orthostatic blood pressure
- Assess comorbid conditions
- Peripheral edema
- Jugular venous distension
- Tachypnea
- Thyromegaly
- CNS disturbance: decreased mental acuity

Diagnostic Studies
- Serum electrolytes
- ECG: confirmatory with absent p waves, irregular ventricular rate, and rhythm 100 to 160 beats
- Cardiac event monitor
- Echocardiogram
- Thyroid function tests
- NT pro BNP (elevated in AF, decreases after cardioversion)
- Ventilation perfusion scan/angio CT: rule out pulmonary embolus

Differential Diagnosis
- Atrial flutter
- Sinus tachycardia

Management
- Initial treatment directed toward slowing ventricular response to 60 to 100 beats/minute; restoring sinus rhythm when feasible; and decreasing risk of stroke from embolism
- Chronic treatment goal is rate control and prevention of stroke from embolism

Nonpharmacologic Treatment
- Treat underlying disorders (such as pneumonia)
- Invasive therapy for refractory cases
- Cardioversion to normal sinus rhythm
- Surgical or catheter ablation
- Pacing
- Internal atrial defibrillator
- Patients on warfarin require extensive patient education regarding diet, signs and symptoms of bleeding, and monitoring and dosing

Pharmacologic Treatment
- Acute
  - Managed in hospital setting under care of cardiologist

  - Rate control managed with esmolol, metoprolol, propranolol, diltiazem, or verapamil
  - Pharmacologic conversion with dofetilide, flecainide, ibutilide, propafenone, or amiodarone; less effective drugs include disopyramide, procainamide and quinidine; digoxin and sotalol are not recommended.
- Chronic
  - Rate control and antithrombotic therapy
  - Antiarrhythmic agent if needed
- Antithromboembolic therapy
  - Antithrombotic therapy to prevent thromboembolism is recommended for all patients with AF, except those with contraindications.
  - The selection of the antithrombotic agent should be based upon the absolute risks of stroke and bleeding and the relative risk and benefit for a given patient
  - Anticoagulation with a vitamin K antagonist is recommended for patients with more than 1 moderate risk factor; such factors include age 75 years or older, hypertension, heart failure, impaired LV systolic function (ejection fraction 35% or less or fractional shortening less than 25%), and diabetes mellitus
  - INR should be determined at least weekly during initiation of therapy and monthly when anticoagulation is stable
  - Aspirin, 81 to 325 mg daily, is recommended as an alternative to vitamin K antagonists in low-risk patients or in those with contraindications to oral anticoagulation
  - Antithrombotic therapy is recommended for patients with atrial flutter as for those with AF

Table 9-18. Antithrombotic Therapy and Risk

No risk factors	ASA 81 to 325 mg/day
One moderate risk factor	ASA 81 to 325 mg/day or warfarin (INR 2.0 to 3.0)
Any high-risk factor	Warfarin (INR 2.0 to 3.0)

Table 9-19. Risk Factors

Less Validated or Weaker Risk Factors	Moderate Risk Factors	High Risk Factors
Female gender	Age greater than or equal to 75 years	Previous stroke, TIA, or embolism
Age 65 to 74 years	Hypertension	Mitral stenosis
Coronary artery disease	Heart failure	Prosthetic heart valve
Thyrotoxicosis	LV ejection fraction 35% or less Diabetes mellitus	

How Long to Treat
- Anticoagulation therapy is indefinite unless situations arise that would contraindicate therapy

Special Considerations
- To take warfarin safely, the patient must keep regular office appointments, have blood work done regularly, and be reliable in taking his or her medication correctly

- For frail and demented older adults and patients unable or unwilling to take warfarin, consider ASA 325 mg q.d.

Follow-up
Expected Course
- Prognosis dependent on heart disease
- Exercise and activity levels may be limited

Complications
- Heart failure
- Stroke
- Peripheral arterial embolism
- Pharmacologic: bradycardia, torsade de pointes
- Warfarin therapy confers increased risk for intracranial hemorrhage

Heart Failure (HF)
Description
- A common clinical syndrome that arises from impairment of the heart's ability to effectively meet the metabolic demands of the body; formerly called congestive heart failure (CHF). The use of the acronym CHF now refers to chronic heart failure.
- Can result from any structural or functional cardiac disorder that impairs the ability of the ventricle to fill with or eject blood; the cardinal manifestations of HF are dyspnea and fatigue, which may limit exercise tolerance, and fluid retention, which may lead to pulmonary congestion and peripheral edema
- Syndrome may be chronic with episodic exacerbations or acute with mild, moderate, or severe symptoms
- Major complication of heart disease with serious life-threatening outcomes that need aggressive management
- The prevalence of HF rises from 2% to 3% at age 65 to more than 80% in persons over 80 years of age
- Life expectancy: 5-year survival rate is 50%

Etiology
- Basic causes are from:
  - Myocardial damage due to ischemic heart disease, myocarditis, or cardiomyopathy
  - Ventricular overload due to:
    - Pressure overload as in hypertension, coarctation of aorta, aortic stenosis, or pulmonary stenosis
    - Volume overload as from mitral regurgitation, aortic regurgitation, ventral septal defect (VSD), atrial septal defect, patent ductus arteriosus
  - Restriction and obstruction to ventricular filling
    - Mitral stenosis, cardiac tamponade, constrictive pericarditis, restrictive cardiomyopathies, atrial myxoma
  - Cor pulmonale and other problems such as AV fistula, thyrotoxicosis, or myxedema

Incidence and Demographics
- Common syndrome, increasing in incidence
- Most common in older adult patients
- Male preponderance until age 75, then equal occurrence
- Frequent hospital admitting diagnosis

Risk Factors
- Factors precipitating HF in patients with underlying heart disease include:
  - Progression or complications of basic causes
  - Patient noncompliance with medications
  - Excess salt intake
  - Stress
  - Obesity
  - Arrhythmias
  - Cardiac muscle damage
  - Blood problems
  - Increased volume
  - Decreased volume
  - Anemia
  - Electrolyte imbalance
  - Drugs
    - NSAIDs
    - Beta blockers
    - Steroids
    - Digitalis toxicity
    - Alcohol

Prevention and Screening
- Treat underlying cause if possible
- Monitor for and treat risk factors

Assessment
- Usually begins with left-sided failure, which causes pulmonary signs, then right-sided failure, which causes systemic signs
- Both left-sided and right-sided failure are usually present

History
- General: diminished exercise capacity, weakness, fatigue, anorexia, nocturia
- Respiratory: cough, at first nonproductive at night, progressing to frequent cough productive of pink, frothy sputum
- Dyspnea on exertion (DOE), orthopnea, paroxysmal nocturnal dyspnea (PND)

Physical
- General: cyanosis, hypotension/hypertension
- Respiratory: basilar rales, frothy pink sputum
- Cardiac: S_3 gallop rhythm, elevated jugular venous pressure (JVD), cardiac enlargement
- Extremities: dependent edema
- Abdomen: hepatomegaly
- CNS: delirium

Diagnostic Studies
- Chest x-ray: pleural effusions, pulmonary edema, cardiomegaly, and to rule out pneumonia
- Electrolytes, CBC, TSH
- NT-proBNP (for patients < 75 years, > 125 pg/mL; > 75 years, > 450 pg/mL
- Urinalysis
- ECG: possible left-ventricular strain

- Echocardiogram: ejection fraction (EF) determines severity and diagnoses failure as systolic or diastolic, which determines appropriate treatment

Table 9-20. New York Heart Association Functional Classification of HF

Class	Activities That Are Tolerated
Functional class 1	Ordinary physical exertion does not limit activity
Functional class 2	Ordinary physical activity presents slight limitations Patient experiences fatigue, dyspnea, angina
Functional class 3	Comfortable at rest; physical activity presents marked limitations
Functional class 4	Symptoms at rest; any physical activity presents marked limitations

Table 9-21. American Heart Association Stages and Recommendations for Treatment of HF

Stage	Treatment Goals	Drugs/Treatment
Stage A: Patients at high risk for developing HF	Treat HTN Smoking cessation Treat lipid disorder Encourage regular exercise Discourage alcohol, illicit drugs Control metabolic disorder	ACEI/ARB if indicated (as in cases of HTN, DM)
Stage B: Patients with cardiac structural abnormalities or remodeling who have not developed HF symptoms	All measures in Stage A	ACEI/ARB BB (if indicated)
Stage C: Patients with current or prior symptoms of HF	All measures in A and B Dietary salt restriction	Diuretics for fluid retention ACEI BB For selected patients: aldosterone antagonist, ARB, digoxin, hydrazaline, nitrates Biventricular pacing Implantable defibrillator
Stage D: Patients with refractory end-stage HF	All measures in A, B, C Appropriate level of care	Compassionate end-of-life care/hospice Extraordinary measures: Heart transplant Chronic inotropes Permanent mechanical support Experimental drugs/surgery

Differential Diagnosis

- Chronic obstructive pulmonary disease
- Cirrhosis
- Pulmonary emboli
- Acute MI
- Pneumonia
- Asthma
- Chronic venous insufficiency
- Nephrotic syndrome

Table 9–22. Drug Treatment in Heart Failure

Drugs	Treatment Regimen	Common Side Effects
Diuretics		
Loop diuretics:		Electrolyte disturbances, orthostatic hypotension, dizziness, weakness, GI upset
Furosemide	20 to 40 mg once or twice a day (max: 600 mg/day)	
Bumetanide	0.5 to 1.0 mg once or twice a day (max: 10 mg/day)	
Torsemide	10 to 20 mg/day (max: 200 mg/day)	
Thiazide diuretics:		Anorexia, nausea, vomiting, cramping
Chlorothiazide	250 to 500 mg once or twice (max: 1000 mg/day)	
Chlorthalidone	12.5 to 25 mg once (max: 100 mg/day)	
Hydrochlorothiazide	25 mg once or twice (max: 200 mg/day)	
Indapamide	2.5 mg once/day (max: 5 mg/day)	
Metolazone	2.5 mg once/day (max: 20 mg/day)	
Potassium-sparing diuretics:		Hyperkalemia
Amiloride	5 mg once/day (max: 20 mg/day)	
Spironolactone	12.5 to 25 mg/day (max: 50 mg/day)	
Triamterene	50 to 75 mg/day (max: 200/day)	
Sequential nephron blockade:		
Metolazone	2.5 to 10 mg once/day plus loop diuretic	
Hydorchlorothiazide	25 to 100 mg once or twice a day plus loop diuretic	
Chlorothiazide (IV)	500 to 100 mg/day plus loop diuretic	

continued

Table 9-22. Drug Treatment in Heart Failure (cont.)

Drugs	Treatment Regimen	Common Side Effects
Angiotensin-Converting Enzyme Inhibitors (ACE)		
Lisinopril	2.5 once a day, titrate up to 20 mg once a day	Renal impairment, angioedema, hypotension
Enalapril	2.5 mg twice a day (max: 20 mg/day)	Cough (common), dizziness, weakness
Quinapril	5 mg twice a day (max: 20 mg/day)	Hyperkalemia—use with caution in renal impairment
Fosinopril	5 to 10 mg once/day (max: 40 mg/day)	
Perindopril	2 mg once (8 to 16 mg/day)	
Ramipril	1.25 to 2.5 mg once (10 mg/day)	
Trandolapril	1 mg once (4 mg/day)	
Angiotensin-Receptor Blockers (ARB)		
Losartan	25 to 50 mg/day (max:100 mg/day)	Rare side effects: dizziness, insomnia, muscle cramps, leg pain, hyperkalemia
Valsartan	20 to 40 mg/day (max: 160 mg/day)	
Candasartan	4 to 8 mg/day (max: 32 mg/day)	
Beta Blockers (BB)		
Carvedilol	3.125 mg twice/day (max: 25 to 50 mg/day)	Bradycardia, depression, fatigue
Metoprolol XL	12.5 to 25 mg/day (max 200 mg/day)	
Bisoprolol	1.25 mg/day (max: 10 mg/day)	

Management
Nonpharmacologic Treatment
- Identify and treat underlying disease
- Control precipitating factors
- Control leg edema with elastic pressure stockings and elevation of legs
- Exercise
- Sodium and fluid restriction (Stage C and D)
- Daily weights
- Patient education: goal identification to balance activity with metabolic restriction
- Importance of medication and diet compliance
- Other options (surgical): valve replacement and cardiac transplant

Pharmacologic Treatment
- Patient frequently needs a 3- to 4-drug regimen to control symptoms
- Diuretics: reduce preload and left-ventricular filling
- ACEI is cornerstone therapy; prevents progression of left ventricular dysfunction

- ARB is used if patient is unable to tolerate ACEI
- Beta blockers: improve ventricular function and reduce post-infarction mortality
- Cardiac glycoside (digoxin): improves contractility in systolic failure
- Vasodilators: reduce afterload; used if patient is unable to tolerate ACEI or ARB
- Anticoagulants: prevent thrombus formation

How Long to Treat
- Acute episodes: until resolution and stabilization of symptoms
- Chronic condition: indefinite

When to Consult, Refer, Hospitalize
- Physician consult for initial assessment and management
- Hospitalize if acute pulmonary edema
- In chronic disease: refer if exacerbation is not responsive to treatment
- Consider referral for:
  - Arterial bypass graft (ABG)
  - Cardiac catheterization: important for determining primary etiology
  - Endomyocardial biopsy: only useful with myocarditis or infiltrative disease

Follow-up
Expected Course
- Patient usually experiences a steady decline after diagnosis
- Acute: generally responsive to initial treatment
- Chronic: EF good indicator of morbidity and mortality
- Poor prognosis if EF less than 20%

Complications
- Electrolyte disturbances
- Adverse reactions to medications
- Arrhythmias, especially atrial fibrillation
- Death

PERIPHERAL VASCULAR DISORDERS
Peripheral Arterial Disease (PAD)
Description
- Obstruction or narrowing of the major arteries, usually in the lower extremities, that may be acute or chronic and is frequently a result of atherosclerosis
- Intermittent claudication is the most common symptom of peripheral arterial disease

Etiology
- Acute thrombus leading to embolus
- Chronic atherosclerotic lesions
- Inflammatory component: thromboangiitis obliterans (Buerger's disease), giant cell arteritis

Incidence and Demographics
- Elderly
- Male preponderance

Risk Factors
- Age greater than 40
- Tobacco use
- Hyperlipidemia
- Diabetes mellitus
- Hypertension

Prevention and Screening
- Lifestyle modification—stop smoking
- Identification and treatment of comorbid conditions

Assessment
History
- Acute: pain, paresthesia, paralysis, pallor, pulselessness
- Chronic: intermittent claudication—lower-extremity aching, fatigue, and tiredness occurring with activity and relieved by cessation of activity
- Aorta: back or abdominal pain
- Femoral: hip, buttock, calf pain
- Peripheral vascular disease progresses from silent, asymptomatic disease to intermittent claudication to rest pain, then to ulceration or gangrene

Physical
- Pallor, pulseless extremity
- Severity determined by amount of time required for venous filling and return of color
- Cool extremity, dependent rubor
- Absent or decreased hair on extremity
- Femoral artery bruit

Diagnostic Studies
- Doppler ultrasound
- Angiography for acute or surgical candidates

Differential Diagnosis
- Musculoskeletal strains
- Osteoarthritis
- Acute arterial spasm
- Acute deep vein thrombus

Management
Nonpharmacologic Treatment
- Acute arterial occlusion: avoid elevating affected extremity; protect extremity and refer for heparin therapy immediately
- In chronic disease, smoking cessation counseling and/or program is crucial
- Control comorbid diseases such as hyperlipidemia, diabetes mellitus, hypertension
- Initiate prescribed exercise program
- Education patient about signs and symptoms that require medical attention, care of feet

Pharmacologic Treatment
- Acute: heparin 5000 units IV
  - Embolectomy, thrombolytic therapy

- Chronic
  - Indicated for intermittent claudication
    - Cilostazol (Pletal) 100 mg b.i.d.; antiplatelet/vasodilator, contraindicated in CHF
    - Pentoxifylline (Trental) 400 mg t.i.d.
  - Antiplatelet therapy
    - Aspirin 325 mg
    - Clopidogrel (Plavix) 75 mg q.d.

When to Consult, Refer, Hospitalize
- Acute arterial occlusion
- Arteriosclerosis obliterans
- Recurrent thromboembolism
- New onset, severe symptoms: possible vascular surgery

Follow-up
Expected Course
- Chronic: symptoms differ, with slow progression to rapid deterioration

Complications
- Gangrene
- Amputation

VENOUS DISORDERS
Superficial and Deep Venous Thrombosis
Description
- Deep venous thrombosis (DVT): acute formation of blood clot(s) in the deep venous system of the lower extremities or pelvic veins
- Superficial: acute inflammation and clot formation with associated redness and tenderness along superficial veins

Etiology
- DVT: three primary predisposing factors
  - Venous stasis: obesity, CHF, prolonged immobility, arrhythmias (especially atrial fibrillation)
  - Hypercoagulability: postoperative state, some malignancies, dehydration, acute or chronic inflammation, abrupt discontinuation of anticoagulants, inherited coagulation deficits, estrogen usage
  - Injury to venous wall intima: PVD, varicose veins, trauma (especially hip fractures)
  - Effect of predisposing factors increased by advanced age and prior history of DVT
- Superficial
  - IV therapy
  - Trauma
  - Bacterial infection

Incidence and Demographics
- Common, approximately 1 to 2 million cases per year
- Female preponderance
- High incidence with total hip replacement

Risk Factors
- DVT
  - Orthopedic surgery
  - Immobility
  - Carcinoma
  - Venous catheters
  - Rheumatoid disease—lupus
  - High altitude elevation
  - Coagulation defects
  - Polycythemia vera
- Superficial
  - Aseptic procedures

Prevention and Screening
- Administration of short-term low-molecular-weight heparin, such as enoxaparin (Lovenox), after hip surgery
- Post-surgical mechanical leg compression

Assessment
History
- DVT
  - Frequently asymptomatic
  - Possible unilateral leg pain or tenderness and swelling
  - Pain specific to limb or calf
- Superficial
  - Saphenous vein frequently involved
  - Acute episode with defined time frame
  - Local redness, tender cord
  - Swelling
  - Dull pain over inflamed vein
  - Fever

Physical
- DVT
  - Signs unreliable
  - Reproducible tenderness with calf compression
  - Positive Homan's sign: pain in calf with dorsiflexion of foot; note that a negative Homan's sign does not conclusively rule out DVT
  - Leg circumference greater than that of uninvolved leg
  - Swelling of calf or thigh
  - Cool extremity with weak distal pulses
- Superficial
  - No significant swelling of extremity
  - Isolated induration, redness, and tenderness along vein

Diagnostic Studies
- Laboratory
  - Anticoagulation therapy baseline: platelets, prothrombin time (PT), activated partial thromboplastin time (aPTT), hemoglobin, LFT, occult blood; monitor platelets daily with heparin

- Referral for testing
  - B-mode ultrasound combined with Doppler flow detection: highly sensitive
- Contrast venography: most sensitive and specific; superficial
  - Culture and sensitivity if superficial vein appears infected

Differential Diagnosis
- Cellulitis
- Musculoskeletal strain
- Lymphedema
- Acute arterial occlusion
- Ruptured Baker cyst

Management
Nonpharmacologic Treatment
- DVT
  - Initially hospitalize with bed rest, anticoagulation; after stabilization prompt mobilization
  - Intermittent pneumatic compression followed graded pressure stockings
  - Filtering devices: umbrella in vena cava traps emboli, useful if anticoagulants are contraindicated and for recurrent emboli
  - Following hospitalization
    - Leg exercises
    - Avoidance of leg crossing
    - Elevation of legs in bed
    - Educate patient regarding signs and symptoms
- Calf DVT: outpatient management
  - Superficial
    - Leg elevation when patient is sitting
    - Local heat
    - If septic, hospitalization often required

Pharmacologic Treatment
- DVT
  - Anticoagulation therapy: acute treatment and prophylaxis
    - Baseline laboratory tests—platelets, aPTT, PT, INR, LFT, fecal occult blood, hemoglobin
    - Heparin IV on inpatient basis
      - Does not dissolve thrombi; stops propagation, allows natural fibrinolysis
      - Heparin side effects: thrombocytopenia, bleeding; use caution with liver disease
      - Heparin and warfarin concurrent with heparin starting day 3; keep INR at 2.0–3.0
    - Low-molecular-weight heparin effective treatment for uncomplicated DVT
    - Thrombolytic agents may be given in ER
    - Aspirin not beneficial
- Superficial
  - Aseptic: NSAIDs
  - Septic: appropriate antibiotic for 6 weeks, sometimes excision of vein

How Long to Treat
- DVT
  - Single episode: 3 to 6 months
  - Indefinite: CHF, recurrent embolism, DVT, or PE
- Superficial
  - Aseptic inflammation subsides in 1 to 2 weeks

When to Consult, Refer, Hospitalize
- Refer acute DVT
- Refer recurrences or complications

Follow-up
- See regularly to get blood work and management of warfarin dosage

Expected Course
- Good once danger of PE has passed
- Superficial: untreated condition may become septic, which increases mortality

Complications
- DVT
  - Pulmonary embolism
  - Chronic venous insufficiency
- Superficial
  - Septic thrombophlebitis, osteomyelitis

Venous Insufficiency
Description
- Venous valve incompetence with venous engorgement and edema of the lower leg that is often chronic but noninflammatory

Etiology
- Leg trauma
- Incompetent venous valves
- High venous pressure

Incidence and Demographics
- Female predominance
- Onset late adulthood

Risk Factors
- Prior history of pregnancy, deep vein thrombosis
- Prolonged immobility, particularly standing
- Family tendency
- Age
- Obesity

Prevention and Screening
- Early aggressive treatment of thrombophlebitis
- Moisturizers to areas of xerosis with avoidance of scratching
- Avoidance of prolonged standing and immobility

- Elastic compression stockings with ambulation
- Weight loss if appropriate
- Avoidance of restrictive lower-extremity garments

Assessment
History
- Fatigue, aching, heaviness in lower extremities
- Lower-extremity edema worsens with prolonged standing
- Mild pruritus of lower extremity, scratching

Physical
- Hyperpigmentation of distal extremity: brown, brawny thickened skin, red
- Ulceration, if present, distal often medial aspect
- Edema of lower extremities
- Eczema
- Varicosities may be present
- Recurrent stasis ulcers, weeping, crust formation

Differential Diagnosis
- Cellulitis
- Chronic renal disease
- Lymphedema
- Acute phlebitis
- Fungal infection
- Atopic dermatitis
- Severe contact dermatitis
- Neurodermatitis

Management
Nonpharmacologic Treatment
- Elastic stockings prior to ambulation
- Elevation of foot of bed
- Avoidance of prolonged positions or inactivity
- Ulcers: see Chapter 6, Dermatologic Disorders

Pharmacologic Treatment
- Diuretic therapy: generally not recommended unless edema is causing ulcers
- Steroid creams: hydrocortisone cream, triamcinolone 1%, or betamethasone topical (Valisone)
- Cordran tape
- Zinc oxide ointment with ichthammol

How Long to Treat
- Chronic condition
- Treat exacerbations until resolution

When to Consult, Refer, Hospitalize
- Refractory conditions, ulcers that will not heal

Follow-up

Expected Course
- Chronic, recurrent with frequent exacerbation and poor compliance with preventive measures

Complications
- Bacterial infection
- Thrombophlebitis
- DVT
- Stasis ulcers

CASE STUDIES

Case 1. A 68-year-old male is following up after consultation with an orthopedist for a recent fractured thumb. Orthopedist noted that the patient had a blood pressure of 166/104.

PMH: Chart shows that the patient had, at the last office visit, BP 144/92. Laboratory work was ordered. Review of chart shows labile blood pressure readings for the previous 2 years, which decreased after weight loss undertaken to treat hyperlipidemia. States he follows low-salt, low-fat diet and exercises 2 to 3 times a week. Nonsmoker.

Medications: Atorvastatin (Lipitor) 10 mg daily; ibuprofen (Motrin) 400 mg p.o. 3 times daily

FH: Diabetes type 2 and CAD

1. What cardiac risk factors does he have?

Lab findings on previous visits:
BUN 22
Creatinine 0.8
Na+ 136
K+ 4.0
Glucose 162
   Cholesterol 230
   Triglycerides 250
   LDL 148
   HDL 32

2. What additional problem does this lab identify? Is this a significant coronary risk factor?
3. Is his hyperlipidemia well controlled?

Physical: Vital signs current visit: BP 160/102; pulse 98; resp 16; weight 205 lbs; height 5'9"
Cardiac: RRR, no murmur, no carotid bruits or pedal edema, no renal bruits
Resp: vesicular sounds throughout all lung fields
Funduscopic: clear disc, obvious arteriolar narrowing with focal areas of attenuation
UA: trace glucose and protein
ECG sinus rhythm

4. What is the significance of these findings?
5. What stage hypertension does he have?
6. How would you manage this patient's hypertension? List steps.

Case 2. A 73-year-old White female complains of increasing shortness of breath and cough productive of frothy sputum over the last 24 hours. She has had trouble sleeping because of a cough she attributes to allergies, and has felt tired for the past 3 months. Two days ago she celebrated her 73rd birthday.

PMH: Two years ago she had an episode of weakness and dizziness. At that time, her EKG showed changes indicative of a mild MI. She was placed on atenolol (Tenormin) 100 mg and has remained stable. Has mild hypertension, hyperlipidemia; menopause 10 years ago. Smoking history ½ pack a day for 20 years; quit 5 years ago.

Lab: Chest x-ray showing mild cardiomegaly, otherwise unremarkable. An echocardiogram showing EF 40%, moderate left-ventricular dysfunction.

1. What is the most likely diagnosis?
2. What factor(s) most likely to have precipitated this?
3. What is the most likely the basic cause(s)?
4. What over-the-counter drugs should you specifically ask about?

Exam: BP 142/94, pulse 88; resp 22; temp 98.8° F; weight: 180 lbs
Ht: 5'4"; general appearance: appears mildly short of breath
Resp: tachypnea, occasional nonproductive cough, bibasilar rales (crackles)
Extremities: 2+ edema extending halfway up lower legs

5. What other physical exam do you need to do and what would you look for?

Medications: Atenolol (Tenormin) 100 mg p.o. daily, lovastatin (Mevacor) 20 mg daily, aspirin 81 mg daily

6. What medications would you start today?
7. What lab work would you need to check before starting these medications?
8. What adverse reactions would you monitor for?

Case 3. A 70-year-old White female presents for routine follow-up of lipids.
PMH: Her last visit she was started on a low-saturated-fat diet. Medical history significant for osteoporosis and hypercholesteremia. Ex-smoker with 15 pack-years, quit 7 years ago. Occasional ETOH with glass of wine once a week.
Medications: Fosamax 10 mg q.d.; calcium and vitamin D supplements
Exam: general appearance: alert, oriented, NAD; weight 130 lbs; Height 5'5"
BP 138/82
Cardiac: RRR, no murmurs; no edema, peripheral pulses present
Resp: vesicular breath sounds throughout all lung fields
Abdomen: soft, no hepatosplenomegaly or masses

Labs:	Last Visit	This Visit
Cholesterol, total	275	230
Triglycerides	118	104
HDL	62	56
LDL	189	140

Basic metabolic panel, CBC, and LFT unremarkable

1. What is your assessment?
2. What cardiac risk factors does this patient have?
3. What other risk factors should you assess?
4. What is your plan?

REFERENCES

Ahmed, A. (2003). American College of Cardiology/American Heart Association chronic heart failure evaluation and management guidelines: Relevance to the geriatric practice. *Journal of the American Geriatric Society, 51,* 123–126.

ALLHAT Collaborative Research Group. (2002). Major outcomes in high-risk hypertensive patients randomized to angiotensin converting enzyme inhibitor or calcium channel blocker vs diuretic. The antihypertensive and lipid lowering treatment to prevent heart attack trial. *Journal of the American Medical Association, 288,* 2981–2997.

American College of Cardiology/American Heart Association. (2004). Guidelines for the management of ST-elevation MI. Retrieved from http://circ.ahajournals.org/cgi/reprint/110/9/e82

American College of Cardiology/American Heart Association. (2005). 2005 Update to the guidelines for the evaluation and management of chronic heart failure. *Circulation, 112,* e154–e235.

American College of Cardiology/American Heart Association. (2006). Guidelines for the management of atrial fibrillation. *Circulation, 114,* 257–354.

American College of Cardiology/American Heart Association. (2007). 2007 guidelines for the management of patients with unstable angina//non ST elevation myocardial infarction: Executive summary. *Circulation, 116,* 803–877.

American Heart Association. (2007). Universal definition of myocardial infarction. *Circulation, 116,* 2634–2653.

Antman, E. M., Hand, M., Armstrong, P. W., Bates, C. R., Green, H. A., Halasyamani, L. K., et al. (2008). 2007 focused update of the ACC/AHA 2004 guidelines for the management of patients with ST elevation myocardial infarction. *Circulation, 117,* 296–329.

Appel, I. J. (2002). The verdict from ALLHAT: Thiazide diuretics are the preferred initial therapy for hypertension. *Journal of the American Medical Association, 288,* 3039–3042.

Chobanian, A. V., Bakris, G. L., Black, H. R., Cushman, W. C., Green, L. A., Izzo, J. L., Jr., et al. (2003). Seventh report of the Joint National Committee on Prevention, Detection, Evaluation, and Treatment of High Blood Pressure. *Hypertension, 42*(6), 1206–1252.

Expert Panel on Detection, Evaluation and Treatment of High Blood Cholesterol. (2001). Executive summary of the Third Report of the NCEP Expert Panel in adults. *JAMA, 285*(10), 2486.

Falk, R. H. (2001). Atrial fibrillation. *New England Journal of Medicine, 344,* 1067–1078.

Fraker, T. D., & Fihn, S. D. (2007). 2007 chronic angina focused update of the ACC/AHA 2002 guidelines for the management of patients with chronic stable angina. *Circulation, 116,* 2762–2772.

Gibbons, R. J., Abrams, J., Chatterjee, K., Daley, J., Deedwania, P. C., Douglas, J. S., et al. (2002). Guideline update for the management of patients with chronic stable angina: A Report of the American College of Cardiology/American Heart Association Task Force of Practice Guidelines. *Journal of the American College of Cardiology, 41,* 159–168.

Go, A. S., Hylek, E. M., Chang, Y., Phillips, K. A., Henault, L. E. Capra, A. M., et al. (2003). Anticoagulation therapy for stroke prevention in atrial fibrillation: How well do randomized trials translate into clinical practice? *Journal of the American Medical Association, 290,* 2685–2692.

Levy, P. J. (2002). Epidemiology and pathophysiology of peripheral arterial disease. *Clinical Cornerstone, 4,* 1–15.

National Cholesterol Education Program. (2001). *Third report of the Expert Panel on Detection, Evaluation, and Treatment of High Blood Cholesterol in Adults* (Adult Treatment Panel III). Bethesda, MD: Author.

National Cholesterol Education Program. (2004). *Adult Treatment Panel Update. Implications of recent trials for ATP III guidelines*. Bethesda, MD: Author.

National Heart, Lung, and Blood Institute. (2003). *Seventh report of the Joint National Committee on Prevention, Detection, Evaluation, and Treatment of High Blood Pressure* (JNC 7) Express. (NIH Publication No. 5233). Bethesda, MD: National Institutes of Health.

Redfield, M. M., Jacobsen, S. J., Burnett, J. C., Jr., Mahoney, D. W., Bailey, K. R., & Rodeheffer, R. J. (2003). Burden of systolic and diastolic ventricular dysfunction in the community. Appreciating the scope of the heart failure epidemic. *Journal of the American Medical Association, 289*, 194–202.

Sander, G. E. (2002). High blood pressure in the geriatric population: Treatment considerations. *American Journal of Geriatric Cardiology, 11*, 223–232.

Shocken, D. D., Benjamin, E. J., Fonarrow, G. C., Karumholz, H. H., Levy, D., Mensah, G. A., et al. (2008). Prevention of heart failure. *Circulation, 117*, 2544-2565.

Snow, V., Barry, P., Fihn, S. D., Gibbons, R. J., Owens, D. K., Williams, S. V., et al. (2004). Primary care management of chronic stable angina and asymptomatic suspected or known coronary artery disease: A clinical practice guideline from the American College of Physicians. *Annals Internal Medicine, 141*(7), 562–567.

Snow, V., Barry, P., Fihn, S. D., Gibbons, R. J., Owens, D. K., Williams, S. V., et al. (2004). Evaluation of primary care patients with chronic stable angina: Guidelines from the American College of Physicians. *Annals of Internal Medicine, 141*(1), 57–64.

Sonnenblick, E. H. (2000). Detecting and treating heart failure: An update on strategies. *Consultant, 40*(1), 170–176.

Theyus, J., & Francis, J. (2009). N-terminal pro-brain naturetic peptide and atrial fibrillation. *Indian Pacing Electrophysiology Journal, 9*, 1–4.

Tsikouris, J. P., & Cox, C. D. (2001). A review of class III antiarrhythmic agents for atrial fibrillation: Maintenance of normal sinus rhythm. *Pharmacotherapy, 21*, 1514–1529.

U.S. Preventive Services Task Force. (2002) Aspirin for the primary prevention of cardiovascular events: Recommendation and rationale. *Annals of Internal Medicine, 136*, 157–160.

Wald, D. S., Law, M., & Morris, J. K. (2002). Homocysteine and cardiovascular disease: Evidence on causality from a meta-analysis. *British Medical Journal, 325*, 1202–1206

White, H. D. (2003). Should all patients with coronary disease receive angiotensin converting enzyme inhibitors? *Lancet, 362*, 755–757.

Wing, L. M., Reid, C. M., Ryan, P., Beilin, L. J., Brown, M. A., Jennings, G. L., et al. (2003). A comparison of outcomes with angiotensin converting enzyme inhibitors and diuretics for hypertension in the elderly. *New England Journal of Medicine, 348*, 583–592.

Yusuf, S., Sleight, P., Pogue, J., Bosch, J., Davies, R., & Dagenais, G. (2000). Effects of an angiotensin converting enzyme inhibitor, ramipril, on cardiovascular events in high risk patients: The Heart Outcomes Prevention Evaluation (HOPE) Study Investigators. *New England Journal of Medicine, 342*,145–153.

Zepf, B. (2001). Diagnosis and treatment of venous stasis ulcers. *American Family Physician, 64*, 1452.

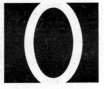

Gastrointestinal Disorders

Katherine Tardiff, MSN, GNP-BC, ACHPN

GENERAL APPROACH

Normal Changes of Aging

- Age-related changes often begin before age 50 and continue gradually throughout life
- Most clinically important changes:
  - Changes in the mouth, including fewer taste buds, decline in sense of taste, decreased saliva secretion
  - Decreased esophageal, gastric, and intestinal motility
  - Decreased hydrochloric acid in the stomach
  - Decreased intestinal absorption, motility, and blood flow
  - Decreased liver size and blood flow
- Effect of aging GI system on absorption and metabolism of medications:
  - Dry mouth and reduced secretions results in difficulty swallowing medications
  - Decreased motility and absorption of some medications in the GI tract
  - Decreased activity of the cytochrome P450 system in the liver
    - Decreased metabolism of some drugs; increased frequency of drug interactions and drug toxicity
- Decreased immune function in GI tract leads to increased susceptibility to infection
  - Decreased production of antibodies and other specialized immune cells in the intestinal wall as well as decreased cytokine activity
  - Increased risk for GI infectious diseases (especially food-borne illnesses) and for all infections
- See Table 10–1 for specific changes

Table 10-1. Summary of Physiologic Aging Effects on GI Tract

Part of System	Effect of Aging	Implications	Contributing Factors
Oropharynx	Impaired neuromuscular coordination	Dysphagia Choking Aspiration	Neuromuscular diseases such as stroke
Esophagus	Decreased Motility	Increased risk of indigestion & GERD	Concurrent medications, obesity, hiatal hernia, DM
Stomach	Decreased lower esophageal sphincter of stomach (LES) function No change in baseline gastric acid secretion Decreased response to acid Blood flow decreased	Delayed emptying Impaired gastric mucosal protection, decreased response to injury Increased risk of GERD & PUD	DM, alcohol, medications, tobacco CHF, atherosclerosis Decreased blood flow
Liver	Decreased liver size, blood flow, and perfusion Increased susceptibility to stress	Altered drug metabolism, increased risk of drug interactions	Alcohol, medication use, herbal remedies
Pancreas	Decreased exocrine reserve	Usually not a problem, increased risk of DM	DM
Gallbladder/ biliary tree	Less complete emptying due to decreased contractility	Increased risk of cholelithiasis	Obesity, multiparity
Small bowel	No significant changes	Decreased nutrient absorption	Vascular disease
Colon	Decreased mucosal cell growth, increased transit time	Increased susceptibility to carcinogens, constipation	Colon cancer, diverticulosis, and altered bowel habits
Anal sphincter	Decreased resting and maximum squeeze pressures in the anal canal	Fecal incontinence	Dementia, neurologic diseases

Clinical Implications

History
- Older adults less likely to feel pain with abdominal conditions
- Older adults are more likely to present with nonspecific complaints

Physical
- Tend to have a less acute presentation
- Weight loss an important sign

Assessment
- Stool for occult blood:

- False positives can be caused by ingestion of iron, aspirin, cimetidine, iodine, or large portions of rare red meat, raw broccoli, turnips, radishes, parsnips, or cauliflower
- False negatives can occur from vitamin C ingestion and intermittent bleeding (sensitivity is only 50%)

Treatment

- All patients with positive stool guaiac test require GI referral
- Diet is often an important part of management of GI problems
  - For acute problems, fluid replacement to keep up with fluid loss
  - Start with ice chips and clear liquids such as Pedialyte, Gatorade, tea, ginger ale
  - Gradually progress to soups, crackers, and other bland foods as tolerated
  - For management of many chronic problems, older adults often need to increase the amount of fiber in their food and increase their fluid intake

Drugs Used for a Multitude of GI Problems

- Antacids
  - Liquid more effective than tablet form
  - Antacids can decrease absorption of other medications (such as fluoroquinolones, tetracycline, ferrous sulfate); separate dosing by 2 hours
  - Various preparations are available over the counter:
    - Maalox and Mylanta (antacids) or Gaviscon (antacid with alginic acid) 15 to 30 mL 4 times daily, taken 1 hour after meals and before bed as needed
    - Calcium carbonate can cause constipation; milk-alkali syndrome
    - Sodium bicarbonate causes elevated sodium levels; fluid retention
    - Aluminum products cause constipation; CNS adverse effects
    - Magnesium hydroxide causes diarrhea; hypermagnesemia
    - Bismuth subsalicylate (Pepto-Bismol) for nausea and diarrhea: 524 mg (tablets or liquid) Q 30 to 60 minutes up to 8 doses in 24 hours or q.i.d. with meals and HS for traveler's diarrhea
    - Will cause black stool
    - Radiopaque
- H2-receptor antagonists: suppress gastric acid secretion (some available OTC at reduced doses)
  - Ranitidine (Zantac) 75 to 150 mg q.d.–b.i.d.; 300 mg q.d.
  - Famotidine (Pepcid) 10 to 40mg q.d.–b.i.d.
  - Nizatidine (Axid) 150 to 300 mg p.o. q.d.–b.i.d.
- Proton-pump inhibitors (PPI): suppress gastric acid secretion to a greater degree than H2 blockers
  - Omeprazole (Prilosec) 20 mg q.d.
  - Lansoprazole (Prevacid) 15 to 30 mg q.d.
  - Pantoprazole (Protonix) 20 to 40 mg p.o. q.d.
  - Rabeprazole (Aciphex) 20 mg p.o. q.d.
  - Esomeprazole (Nexium) 20 to 40 mg p.o. q.d.
- Prokinetic agents: increase lower esophageal sphincter (LES) tone and promote gastric emptying
  - Metoclopramide (Reglan) 5 to 10 mg q.i.d.; used less frequently because of potential for central nervous system side effects such as drowsiness, confusion, depression, extrapyramidal reactions

RED FLAGS

- Acute abdominal pain
- Upper GI bleeding (hematemesis, coffee-ground emesis)
- Lower GI bleeding (maroon stools or frank red blood per rectum, melena)
- Intractable nausea or vomiting
- Intractable diarrhea
- Change in bowel patterns, anorexia, weight loss

ACUTE ABDOMEN

Description
- Acute onset of severe pain; requires emergency management
- May be difficult to differentiate between cardiac pain and abdominal pain
  - Cardiac pain can extend from jaw to epigastric area

Etiology
- Acute abdomen: five groups of symptoms and signs
  - Pain
    - Capsular distension of the outer membrane that often surrounds an organ such as the liver
    - Rebound tenderness cased by peritoneal irritation
  - Shock: tachycardia, decreased blood pressure, decreased or increased temperature, pallor, diaphoresis
    - Often indicates pancreatitis, hemorrhage, vascular insufficiency
  - Vomiting often indicates obstruction of bowel or biliary duct
  - Muscular rigidity often indicates visceral perforation, mucosal ulceration
  - Abdominal distension often indicates obstruction of large bowel

Incidence and Demographics
- Extremely common; often related to other medical conditions
- Approximately 25% of patients who present to the emergency department with acute abdominal pain are older than 50 years
- Biliary disease is the leading cause for acute abdominal surgery among older adults
- Pancreatitis is the most common nonsurgical cause of abdominal pain in older adults

Risk Factors
- History of abdominal surgery
- Use of certain medications, including NSAIDs
- Chronic constipation
- Infection
- Alcohol or drug use

Assessment
History
- Onset, duration, progression, migration, character, intensity, and localization
  - Monitor over time
  - Associated symptoms such as anorexia, nausea, vomiting, diarrhea, constipation, urinary symptoms

- Determine whether pain interferes with sleep
- Factors that precipitate or relieve the pain; relationship of pain to meals, specific foods, urination, defecation, exertion, and inspiration
- Any self-treatments
- Presence of blood in the stool, urine, or emesis
- Social history including alcohol and intravenous drug use
- Gynecological history: evaluate for vaginal bleeding, HRT use (particularly unopposed estrogen), hysterectomy or oophorectomy
- Any new medications or medications that can cause constipation
- Previous abdominal surgery

Physical
- General appearance and evaluation of volume status
  - Vital signs may be normal despite pathology
  - Assess for restlessness and body positioning
- Abdominal exam, perform with knees flexed
  - Observe for distension or any surgical scars indicating history of abdominal surgery
  - Bowel sounds:
    - High-pitched tinkling sounds suggest a dilated bowel with air and fluid under tension
    - Rushes of high-pitched sounds indicate intestinal obstruction
    - Absent bowel sounds indicate an ileus or peritonitis
  - Palpate for localized tenderness, rigidity, guarding, and rebound tenderness (an indication of peritonitis)
    - Check for CVA tenderness
    - Evaluate for hepatosplenomegaly and fluid wave (ascites)
- Rectal exam: rectal wall pain can be an indication of appendicitis or abscess
- Pelvic exam: if no obvious GI explanation and a GYN cause is suspected in a postmenopausal woman

Diagnostic Studies
- Laboratory studies
  - CBC with differential; may show leukocytosis or anemia
  - Serum electrolytes, glucose, BUN, and creatinine
  - Liver function tests (AST, ALT, alkaline phosphatase, bilirubin, PT, PTT)
  - Amylase and lipase
  - Urinalysis to rule out urinary tract infection and hematuria
  - Stool for occult blood
- Imaging
  - Flat plate and upright abdominal film to evaluate for bowel obstruction, paralytic ileus, perforation (free air in peritoneal cavity), and biliary or renal stones
  - Ultrasound for suspected biliary and pelvic diseases, to rule out AAA
  - Computerized tomography (CT) to diagnose perforation, AAA, appendicitis, mesenteric venous thrombosis
  - Angiography is the gold standard for diagnosis of acute mesenteric ischemia
  - Consider ECG to rule out referred pain from cardiac etiology
  - Consider chest x-ray to evaluate for heart, lung, and mediastinal disease

Differential Diagnosis

Diffuse Pain

- Generalized peritonitis
- Gastroenteritis
- Metabolic disturbances
- Psychogenic illness

Right Upper Quadrant

- Cholecystitis
- Cholelithiasis
- Hepatitis
- Hepatic abscess
- Right lower lobe pneumonia
- Subphrenic abscess

Right Lower Quadrant

- Appendicitis
- Cecal diverticulitis
- Ureteral calculi
- Ovarian cyst/torsion

Left Upper Quadrant

- Splenic enlargement/hematoma
- Left lower lobe pneumonia
- Pancreatitis
- Cardiac disease

Left Lower Quadrant

- Diverticulitis
- Ureteral calculi
- Ovarian cyst/torsion

Epigastric or Midline

- Gastritis
- Cardiac disease
- Peptic ulcer disease
- Pancreatitis
- Abdominal aortic aneurysm

Management

- Varies depending on etiology

Special Considerations

- Signs and symptoms in older adults may be more subtle, as they often do not have a classic presentation
- Morbidity and mortality among patients with abdominal pain are high

When to Consult, Refer, Hospitalize

- Refer for immediate surgical evaluation in cases of acute abdominal symptoms and signs
- Refer to gastroenterologist if less acute

COMMON GASTROINTESTINAL DISORDERS

Constipation

Description

- Decrease in frequency of stools to less than 3 per week; patients may describe constipation as straining, hard stools, or feeling of incomplete evacuation
- The Rome III Diagnostic Criteria
  - Presence of the following for at least 3 months, with symptom onset at least 6 months prior to diagnosis
  - Must include two or more of the following:
    - Straining during at least 25% of defecations
    - Lumpy or hard stools in at least 25% of defecations
    - Sensation of incomplete evacuation for at least 25% of defecations
    - Sensation of anorectal obstruction/blockage for at least 25% of evacuations
    - Manual evacuation or assistance to facilitate at least 25% of defecations (e.g., digital evacuation, support of pelvic floor)
    - Fewer than 3 defecations per week
  - Loose stools are rarely present without the use of laxatives
  - Insufficient criteria for irritable bowel syndrome

Etiology

- Mechanical obstruction (partial or complete): colon cancer, strictures, anal stenosis
- Neurologic dysfunction causing a change in colonic motility, as in diabetes, spinal cord injury, stroke, multiple sclerosis, and Parkinson's disease
- Metabolic disorders: hypothyroidism, hyperparathyroidism, hypokalemia, hypercalcemia, and uremia
- Psychogenic causes
- Medications: opiate analgesics, calcium-channel blockers, anticholinergics, diuretics, aluminum-based antacids, calcium and iron supplements, NSAIDs, antihistamines, antipsychotic and antiparkinson agents, laxative abuse
- Other causes include: decreased colonic motility due to aging, poor dietary intake of fiber and fluids, decreased mobility

Incidence and Demographics

- 25% of older adults have constipation; upwards of 45% of frail older adults have constipation
- More common in women, most likely because of increased self-reporting
- More common in long-term care than in assisted living or the community

Risk Factors

- Immobility
- Lack of fiber and fluids in diet
- Increasing age
- Comorbidities and medications

Prevention and Screening

- Regular physical activity; increase daily fiber and fluid intake
- Avoid all unnecessary medications that may predispose to constipation
- Do not ignore the urge to defecate

Assessment

History
- Nature and duration of constipation
- Change in pattern, character, and color of stool; fecal and urinary incontinence; anorexia; abdominal or rectal pain; rectal bleeding; hemorrhoids; weight loss; and laxative use
- Medications, diet, fluid intake

Physical Exam
- Distension, abdominal tenderness, palpable stool in the colon, and decreased bowel sounds may be present; check for obstruction
- Digital rectal exam to assess for sphincter tone, masses, impacted stool, stool for guaiac, hemorrhoids, fissures, abscesses, rectal prolapse, rectocele
- In frail older adults, physical exam may reveal fever, delirium, abdominal distension, urinary retention, decreased bowel sounds, arrhythmias, tachypnea, weight loss

Diagnostic Studies
- Stool for occult blood
- CBC to check for leukocytosis and anemia
- Electrolytes, calcium, BUN, creatinine and glucose
- Thyroid function tests to rule out hypothyroidism
- Flat plate and upright abdominal films to evaluate for obstruction
- Colonoscopy or sigmoidoscopy may be indicated

Differential Diagnosis
- See Etiology

Management
- Must be individualized; start with mild, increase dose, add another medication as needed

Nonpharmacologic
- Fiber: 15 grams/day: e.g., 2 tbsp bran powder b.i.d. mixed with fluids or sprinkled over food
- Ensure adequate fluid intake with fiber or will worsen constipation
- Fluid: 1.5 to 2 liters/day
- Physical exercise
- Bowel training program
- Avoid medications that precipitate constipation, especially opioids

Pharmacologic
Initial treatment of mild constipation
- Hydrophilic colloids or bulk-forming agents
  - Take daily to increase fiber intake; must take adequate fluids or obstruction may occur
  - Psyllium (Metamucil, Fiberall) 3 to 4 grams 1 to 3 times daily; methylcellulose (Citrucel) 2 grams 1 to 3 times daily; polycarbophil 1 gram 1 to 4 times daily
- Surfactants: stool softener; not a stimulant, no dependency
  - Take daily, should produce soft stool in 1 to 3 days
  - Useful instead of hydrophilic agents if patient has low fluid intake
  - Few side effects, but less effective than laxatives

– Docusate sodium (Colace) 50 to 200 mg daily

More severe constipation

- Osmotic laxatives; sorbitol is as effective and less expensive than lactulose
  – Lactulose 15 to 30 mL (10 to 20 grams) p.o. q.d.–b.i.d.
  – Sorbitol 15 to 30 mL (70% solution) p.o. q.d.–b.i.d.
  – Polyethylene glycol 8.5 to 34 g in 240 mL liquids once daily; effective in 2 to 4 days
  – Lactulose and sorbitol effective in 24 to 48 hours
  – May cause bloating and hypernatremia
- Stimulant laxatives
  – Used for acute constipation and chronic laxative-dependent patients
  – Should result in a bowel movement in 0.5 to 3 hours when given rectally, 6 to 8 hours when given orally
    - Senna 1 to 2 of 187-mg tablets at HS or 1 of 652-mg suppository at HS
    - Bisacodyl 5 mg tablet at HS or 10 mg suppository
  – May cause dependency; many older adults have become stimulant dependent; patients on opioids are usually dependent on a stimulant laxative
  – Do not use if obstruction is a possibility, may cause rupture
- Enemas may be necessary; use instead of stimulant for rectal outlet delay or if obstruction/impaction is a possibility
  – Results in 2 to 30 minutes
  – Sodium phosphate (Fleets) prepared in a 4.5-oz. squeeze bottle
    - May cause fluid retention and hyperphosphatemia
    - Use with caution in those with renal failure and underlying bowel disease
  – Warm tap water 750 to 1000 cc for suspected high impaction
    - May cause water toxicity and hypervolemia
- Many older adults require long-term routine medication plus a p.r.n. medication

Special Considerations
- Any older adult reporting constipation should have depression considered as a diagnosis

When to Consult, Refer, Hospitalize
- Emergently hospitalize for signs and symptoms of acute abdomen or obstruction
- Refer to gastroenterologist
  – Treatment failure
  – Stool positive for occult blood
  – Weight loss
  – Unexplained change in bowel pattern

Follow-up
Expected Outcomes
- With treatment, resolves in several days if no significant underlying problem
- Older adults frequently need chronic management of constipation

Complications
- Bowel obstruction, fecal impaction, chronic constipation, rectal prolapse, abdominal pain, painful bowel movements
- Delirium, verbal and physical aggression

Diarrhea

Description

- Acute diarrhea: sudden onset, lasting ≤ 14 days
  - Inflammatory—invades mucosa
  - Noninflammatory
- Persistent diarrhea: > 14 days duration
- Chronic diarrhea: > 30 days duration

Etiology

- Acute diarrhea: medications (including laxatives and antibiotics), viral, bacterial, or protozoal/parasitic infections; also can be caused by the presence of a small bowel obstruction
- Chronic diarrhea: can have many causes, including medications, osmosis, secretion, inflammation, malabsorption, motility disorder, and infection

Incidence and Demographics

- Common, almost universal experience
- C. *difficile* is the cause of approximately 25% of all cases of antibiotic-associated diarrhea
  - Mostly occurs in hospital or long-term-care facility

Risk Factors

- Foreign travel
- Ingesting contaminated food or water
- Institutional living or living in close approximation to others having infectious gastroenteritis
- Recent course of antibiotics
- Lactose intolerance
- Medications: antibiotics, laxatives, or antacid use
- GI surgery
- Medical conditions such as hyperthyroidism

Prevention and Screening

- Careful food preparation (such as proper cleaning of fresh fruits/vegetables), good hand-washing, drinking bottled water when traveling to foreign countries
- C. *difficile*–associated diarrhea (CDAD)
  - Decrease environmental contamination
  - Spores of C. *difficile* are resistant to alcohol hand gels and foams
  - Vinyl glove use for all patients with CDAD followed by hand-washing with soap and water
  - Cleanse and disinfect surfaces with detergent and unbuffered 1:10 hypochlorite solution (bleach)
  - Reduce or limit the use and overuse of certain types of antibiotics (clindamycin, third-generation cephalosporins, and fluoroquinolones)

Assessment

History

Sudden onset, acute symptoms of diarrhea

- Food history, particularly unpasteurized dairy products and raw or undercooked meat or fish and timing of symptoms in relation to exposure

- Recent antibiotic use
- Description of the diarrhea and any associated symptoms including GI symptoms, fever, malaise
  - Noninflammatory diarrhea: watery stool, periumbilical cramping, bloating, nausea, and vomiting
  - Inflammatory diarrhea: bloody stool, fever, left lower-quadrant pain, cramping, urgency, and tenesmus
- Possible exposure to pathogens via residential or occupational exposure, recent and remote travel, pets, and hobbies

Chronic diarrhea symptoms
- Obtain description of long-term bowel pattern, contributing factors such as certain foods or stress, family history, and stool characteristics (bloody, watery, presence of mucus)

Physical Exam
- Fever, weight loss may be present
- Observe for signs of dehydration: tachycardia, orthostatic hypotension, altered mental status, poor skin turgor, dry mucous membranes, decreased urine output
- Abdominal exam: hyperactive bowel sounds and generalized tenderness
- Signs of peritonitis may be seen with severe inflammatory diarrhea
- Rectal exam: stool guaiac may be positive

Diagnostic Studies
- None indicated for diarrhea lasting < 48 hours without systemic signs and symptoms
- Stool cultures, ova, and parasites, *Clostridium difficile* (C. diff) toxin
- Stool for fecal leukocytes: present in inflammatory diarrhea
- Stool for occult blood
- CBC to look for anemia, leukocytosis, and eosinophilia, which may be present in parasitic infections and inflammatory bowel disease
- Electrolytes; evaluate for dehydration and electrolyte abnormalities
- BUN and creatinine; elevations may be indicative of dehydration
- Abdominal x-ray to evaluate for small bowel obstruction or fecal impaction

Chronic diarrhea:
- Sigmoidoscopy or colonoscopy with mucosal biopsy to diagnose colitis
- Vitamin B_{12}, folate, vitamin D, albumin, cholesterol, iron, iron binding capacity, prothrombin time to evaluate for malabsorption
- 24 hour fecal fat collection to diagnose steatorrhea

Differential Diagnosis
- Infectious agents (viral, bacterial, parasitic)
- Gastrointestinal disease
- Fecal impaction
- Ileus
- Bowel obstruction
- Malabsorption
- Celiac sprue
- Inflammatory bowel disease
- Lactose intolerance
- Irritable bowel syndrome
- Ischemia secondary to mesenteric atherosclerosis

- Acute appendicitis
- Cholecystitis

Systemic disease
- Diabetic neuropathy
- Hyperthyroidism

Neoplasia
- Obstruction
- Secretory tumors

Management

Nonpharmacologic
- Diet changes: avoid high-fiber foods, milk products, fats, alcohol, and caffeine
- Hydration (oral or IV)

Pharmacologic Treatment
- Antidiarrheal agent use is controversial
  - Causative pathogen needs to be eliminated from the body
  - Never use in patients with high fever, bloody diarrhea, or leukocytosis; retained stool may lead to systemic toxicity
  - Antidiarrheal agents can be used in mild to moderate diarrheal illness if it is necessary to control the diarrhea for a short time for a specific purpose
    - Loperamide (Imodium): initially, 4 mg, followed by 2 mg after each loose stool for a maximum of 16 mg in 24 hrs, use for 2 days only
    - Bismuth subsalicylate (Pepto-Bismol): 2 tablets or 30 mL 4 times daily, maximum 8 doses/day

Inflammatory Diarrhea
- Empirical antibiotic treatment while awaiting stool culture results for patients with moderate to severe fever, bloody stools, tenesmus, or the presence of fecal leukocytes; fluoroquinolones are the drug of choice because they provide good coverage for most invasive bacterial pathogens.
  - Ciprofloxacin 500 mg b.i.d. for 5 to 7 days
  - Levofloxacin 500 mg daily for 5 to 7 days
  - Alternate treatment: doxycycline 100 mg b.i.d.
  - Macrolides and penicillins are no longer recommended because of resistance

If *Giardia* organisms or *C. difficile* is suspected
- Metronidazole (Flagyl) 500 mg p.o. t.i.d. or 250 mg q.i.d. for 10 to 14 days; patients should avoid alcohol use during treatment and for 48 hours after treatment
- Vancomycin 125 mg p.o. q.i.d. for 10 to 14 days
- Antiemetics if vomiting and nausea preclude adequate fluid intake
  - Antiemetics listed below belong to the phenothiazine class, which are anticholinergics and have the standard anticholinergic precautions and adverse reactions
    - Promethazine (Phenergan): p.o. or by rectal suppository
    - Prochlorperazine (Compazine) p.o. or by rectal suppository

Special Considerations
- Consideration of risk versus benefit of antimicrobial therapy must be carefully weighed prior to initiation

When to Consult, Refer, Hospitalize
- Any patient with bloody diarrhea, fever, acute abdominal pain, and leukocytosis should be referred and evaluated immediately in an acute care setting
- Anyone who has not had resolution of diarrhea within 3 weeks needs to be referred to a gastroenterologist for evaluation
- Hospitalize older adults unable to take adequate fluids

Follow-up
Expected Outcomes
- Acute diarrhea should resolve in 24 to 48 hours
- Inflammation of the bowel because of a drug reaction may last for several weeks
- Acute diarrhea may be prolonged if patient does not adhere to GI diet
- Complications
- Dehydration, electrolyte imbalance, sepsis, shock, malnutrition, anal fissures, and hemorrhoids

Dysphagia
Description
- Difficulty in swallowing (oropharyngeal dysphagia) and passing food from the mouth down the esophagus to the stomach (esophageal dysphagia)

Etiology
- As many as 50 pairs of muscles in the head and neck are responsible for swallowing
- Oropharyngeal: common in older adults
  - Neurologic disorders: brainstem CVA, dementia, mass lesion, Parkinson's disease, MS, myasthenia gravis
  - Muscular disorders: myopathies, polymyositis, hypothyroidism
  - Motility disorders: upper esophageal sphincter dysfunction
  - Structural defects: diverticulum, malignancy; defects related to surgery or radiation
- Esophageal dysphagia
  - Mechanical obstruction
    - Esophageal stricture (from GERD)
    - Carcinoma
  - Motility disorder
    - Achalasia: syndrome in which there is a lack of lower esophageal peristalsis
    - Esophageal spasm (spastic motor disorders of the esophagus); normal peristalsis interrupted by simultaneous nonperistaltic contractions; underlying cause not known
    - Scleroderma
  - Esophagitis
    - Most commonly medication-induced (alendronate, risedronate, tetracycline, quinidine, potassium chloride, and ferrous sulfate)

Incidence and Demographics
- Extremely common; 14% of community-dwelling older adults report symptoms consistent with dysphagia
- Neurologic disorders may cause dysphagia in 300,000 to 600,000 Americans annually

Risk Factors
- Comorbid medical and surgical conditions that increase with age
- Frailty or advanced disease
- Radiation of the neck
- Medication use, particularly potassium chloride, alendronate, ferrous sulfate, quinidine, ascorbic acid, tetracycline, aspirin and NSAIDs

Assessment
History
- Oropharyngeal
  - Coughing, choking, and regurgitation that occurs immediately upon initiating swallowing
  - Liquids are more difficult to swallow than soft foods
  - May have neurologic signs and symptoms such as dysphonia, dysarthria
- Esophageal dysphagia
  - Mechanical dysphagia
    - Primarily for solids; recurrent, predictable, may worsen as lumen narrows
    - Patient may have sensation of food sticking after swallowed
  - Motility disorders
    - Dysphagia for both solids and liquids; episodic, unpredictable, and nonprogressive
    - May have chest pain
- Assess alcohol and tobacco use, weight loss, malnutrition, bleeding
- Medical history for diseases that may cause dysphagia

Physical Exam
- Comprehensive exam in all patients with dysphagia, include weight
- Examination of oral cavity, head, neck, and supraclavicular region
- Observe patient swallowing
- Neurological exam: check for gag reflex, tongue movement, and upper palate mobility

Diagnostic Studies
- CBC, liver function tests, BUN, albumin, thyroid function tests
- Stool guaiac
- Referral to specialist for more extensive diagnostic testing
  - Endoscopy: standard test for the diagnosis and management of esophageal diseases because it allows for biopsy and a definitive tissue diagnosis; done first if mechanical obstruction suspected
  - Barium swallow or upper GI series; done first if a motility problem is suspected.

Differential Diagnosis
- See Etiology

Management
- Depends on underlying cause

Nonpharmacologic
- Speech therapy evaluation and treatment
- Swallowing rehabilitation
- Dietary modifications
- Endoscopy with dilation for patients with stricture

Special Considerations
- Dysphagia is an independent predictor of mortality

When to Consult, Refer, Hospitalize
- Always refer patients with new symptoms of dysphagia to a gastroenterologist
- Refer to speech therapy for evaluation and management

Follow-up
Expected Outcomes
- Treatment aimed at managing symptoms and reducing risk for complications
- Dysphagia related to advancing cognitive impairment is progressive

Complications
- Aspiration pneumonia

Gastroesophageal Reflux Disease (GERD)
Description
- Reflux of gastric contents into the esophagus producing a variety of symptoms that affect quality of life
- Classification of patients with GERD:
  - Individuals with uninvestigated GERD symptoms
  - Individuals with erosive esophagitis on endoscopy
  - Individuals with nonerosive reflux disease on endoscopy

Etiology
- Lower esophageal sphincter (LES) dysfunction: The LES works in combination with the diaphragm to maintain a physiological barrier against gastric contents entering the esophagus; transient, spontaneous relaxation in LES tone allows reflux to occur
- Acidic reflux then causes irritation of the esophageal mucosa because of decreased esophageal mucosal resistance to acid
- Ineffective esophageal clearance of reflux caused by decreased saliva production and esophageal peristalsis occurs typically during sleep
- Delayed gastric emptying: gastroparesis (common in diabetics)
- Sliding hiatal hernia (protrusion of the stomach through the diaphragm into the esophagus): may predispose patients to GERD

Incidence and Demographics
- Affects approximately 25% of the U.S. adult population
- Common in older adults

Risk Factors
- Agents that decrease LES tone: anticholinergics, meperidine, morphine, theophylline, calcium-channel blockers, nitrates, diazepam, barbiturates, nicotine, alcohol, caffeine, mints, chocolate, citrus, spicy foods, and foods high in fat
- Obesity
- Anxiety
- Smoking
- Hiatal hernia
- Diabetes
- Gastric outlet obstruction caused by scar tissue, ulceration, or a tumor

- Delayed gastric emptying
- Connective tissue disorders (e.g., scleroderma)

Prevention and Screening
- Lifestyle changes: losing weight, stopping smoking, avoiding alcohol and certain foods

Assessment
History
- Typical symptoms:
  - Heartburn (pyrosis): burning retrosternal discomfort radiating upward toward the neck and occurring 30 to 60 minutes after meals
  - Regurgitation: flow of gastric contents into the mouth or throat; a sour or bitter taste in the mouth is common
- Symptoms exacerbated by lying supine or bending over, improved by sitting up or taking antacids
- Less common symptoms include: dysphagia, odynophagia (painful swallowing), chest pain, hoarseness, cough, sore throat, nausea, and asthma

Physical Exam
- Abdominal exam may have mild epigastric tenderness, otherwise abdominal exam is normal
- Stool negative for occult blood

Diagnostic Studies
- Not indicated if typical symptoms of heartburn and regurgitation are present and symptoms are relieved by treatment
- Endoscopy: best study to document GERD and diagnose complications; consider whether patient presenting with complicated disease, risk for Barrett esophagus

Differential Diagnosis
- Esophageal motility disorders
- Peptic ulcer disease
- Esophageal tumor
- Cholelithiasis
- Angina pectoris
- Pill and radiation-induced esophagitis
- Infectious esophagitis

Management
- Goals are to relieve symptoms, heal esophagitis, and prevent complications

Nonpharmacologic
- Lifestyle modification is the key component to management
- Elevate head of bed on 6 inch blocks or use wedge under mattress
- Avoid eating 2 to 3 hours before lying down and eat smaller, more frequent meals
- Lose weight if overweight
- Avoid tight-fitting clothing
- Avoid substances that cause symptom, including foods high in fat, citrus and spicy foods, mints, chocolate, caffeine, and alcohol; stop smoking

- If appropriate consider changing medications that decrease LES tone
- Surgical intervention for severe disease

Pharmacologic
- Antacids neutralize gastric acid
  - First-line treatment of mild intermittent symptoms
  - Taken after meals and at bedtime
- H2-receptor antagonists: suppress gastric acid secretion; symptomatic improvement occurs in approximately 80% of cases within 6 weeks
  - First-line treatment of mild-to-moderate symptoms and second-line treatment of mild, intermittent symptoms that are not relieved by lifestyle modification or antacids within 2–3 weeks
  - Reevaluate after 2 weeks; if effective, reevaluate at 6 weeks; continue for 8 to 12 weeks
- Proton-pump inhibitors (PPI): suppress gastric acid secretion to a greater degree than H2 blockers
  - First-line treatment of severe symptoms; erosive esophagitis confirmed by endoscopy and second-line treatment of moderate symptoms if H2 blocker not effective within 6 weeks
  - Reconsider diagnosis if no response to PPI after 8 weeks
  - Treat erosive esophagitis with PPI for 12 weeks
- Prokinetic agents: increase LES tone and promote gastric emptying
  - Second- to third-line treatment of mild-to-moderate symptoms often requires combination therapy with PPI
  - Use with caution because of potential for CNS side effects; should not be used long term

Special Considerations
- If patient has a good response to therapy, gradually withdraw medications while continuing lifestyle modifications
- Lifestyle modification should continue throughout treatment and indefinitely to prevent relapse
- Maintenance therapy with H2 blockers should be considered to prevent relapse that occurs in 80% of cases within 6 months

When to Consult, Refer, Hospitalize
- Consult with or refer to gastroenterologist when the patient does not respond to treatment or has symptoms of dysphagia, evidence of blood loss, iron deficiency anemia, or significant weight loss

Follow-up
Expected Outcomes
- Often a chronic, relapsing condition; however, the majority of patients with GERD respond well to medical therapy without developing complications or requiring surgery

Complications
- Older adults have increased incidence of respiratory complications, including aspiration pneumonitis, asthma, laryngeal granulomas, and subglottic stenosis
- Hemorrhage, esophageal stricture, Barrett esophagus, adenocarcinoma

Peptic Ulcer Disease

Description
- Symptomatic ulceration in the gastric or duodenal mucosa secondary to pepsin and gastric acid secretion that extends through the muscularis mucosa

Etiology
- Two major factors: nonsteroidal antiinflammatory drug (NSAID) use and chronic *H. pylori* infection
- NSAIDs and *H. pylori* are about equal in frequency of causing PUD; hypersecretory states are rare
- Acid hypersecretory states (e.g., Zollinger-Ellison syndrome, caused by a gastrin-secreting tumor)

Incidence and Demographics
- In the United States, there are approximately 500,000 new cases and 4 million reoccurrences per year
- The incidence of PUD in NSAID users is about 36%
- The incidence of PUD in *H. pylori*–infected patients is about 42%
- Duodenal ulcers are 5 times more common than gastric ulcers
- Benign gastric ulcers occur more often in older adults
- Ulcers occur more often in males than in females
- About 5% of gastric ulcers are malignant at time of presentation

Risk Factors
- Aging: decrease in gastric mucosal protective mechanisms
- Chronic NSAID use (increased risk of gastric ulcers)
- Prior history of ulceration
- Corticosteroid use
- Smoking
- Stress

Prevention and Screening
- Smoking cessation
- Stress management

Assessment
History
- Classic symptoms:
  - Epigastric pain (dyspepsia): gnawing or dull ache that fluctuates throughout the day
  - Pain often occurs 2 to 5 hours after meals or on an empty stomach
  - Nocturnal pain relieved by food intake, antacids, or antisecretory agents
- Nausea, anorexia, and weight loss may be present, more often with gastric ulcer
- Ask about medications

Physical Exam
- Abdominal exam is unreliable; may reveal mild, localized epigastric tenderness to deep palpation
- Stool may be positive for occult blood

Diagnostic Studies
- Blood tests are not reliable in predicting the presence of PUD
  - CBC to exclude anemia from GI blood loss and leukocytosis due to ulcer perforation
  - Blood chemistries, including liver function testing and serum calcium, are often obtained
  - Amylase in patients with significant epigastric pain to exclude ulcer penetration into the pancreas
- Noninvasive testing for the diagnosis of H. pylori:
  - Urea breath test (H. pylori generates urease): diagnoses active H. pylori infection; useful in evaluating symptomatic patients who have been previously treated for H. pylori; if breath test positive, indicates unsuccessful eradication
  - H. pylori serum antibodies (do not imply active infection; patient may remain positive as long as 18 months); PPI should be held for 7 days prior to test because they may cause a false-negative result; inaccurate results more likely in older adults
  - Fecal antigen assay: positive result indicates active infection and may cost less than the urea breath test
- Upper endoscopy: best test to diagnose peptic ulcer disease; allows for biopsy to detect malignancy (gastric ulcer) and H. pylori infection (through rapid urease test or histology)

Differential Diagnosis
- Gastroesophageal reflux
- Cholecystitis
- Pancreatitis
- Biliary tract disease
- Gastric carcinoma
- Cardiovascular disease

Management
Nonpharmacologic
- Stop NSAIDs, cigarettes, and excess alcohol (modest alcohol consumption may promote ulcer healing)
- Avoid foods that precipitate dyspepsia
- Surgery for refractory ulcers is rarely performed
  - Duodenal ulcer; selective vagotomy
  - Gastric ulcer; ulcer removal with antrectomy or hemigastrectomy without vagotomy

Pharmacologic
- Eradicate H. pylori in infected individuals
  - PPI for 7 to 14 days *and*
  - Clarithromycin 500 mg p.o. b.i.d. for 7 to 14 days *and*
  - Amoxicillin 1 g b.i.d. for 7 to 14 days (metronidazole 500 mg b.i.d. can be substituted in penicillin-allergic individuals)
  - After H. pylori treatment regimen completed, continue treatment with PPI in patients with a complicated duodenal ulcer or if the ulcer was extremely large or high risk
  - Ulcers not due to H. Pylori:
  - PPI or H2-receptor antagonists generally effective
  - Treatment for NSAID-associated ulcer
  - Discontinue offending agent if possible

How Long to Treat
- Gastric ulcer: 4 weeks
- Duodenal ulcer: 8 weeks
- Maintenance therapy is indicated in the following: older adults for 1 to 2 years; patients who are H. pylori negative with recurrent ulcer; patients who have failed therapy to eradicate H. pylori; those with a history of peptic ulcer complications
  - H2-receptor antagonists may be used every night when going to sleep

When to Consult, Refer, Hospitalize
- Refer to a gastroenterologist for endoscopic evaluation (esophagogastroduodenoscopy [EGD]) in patients with symptoms of GI bleeding (iron deficiency anemia, hematemesis, or melena), persistent vomiting, and weight loss; severe epigastric pain that may suggest ulcer penetration or perforation; persistent symptoms after several weeks of treatment; for recurrent symptoms after finishing treatment; all gastric ulcers

Special Considerations
- Concurrent use of a PPI, antibiotics, or bismuth will cause false-negative results on endoscopic urease tests, culture, histology for H. pylori density, and stool antigen and breath tests
- Silent ulcerations common in older adults and may present with massive hemorrhage or perforation
- Lack of symptoms can be due to diminished perception and regular NSAID use that can mask pain

Follow-up
Expected Outcomes
- Evaluate effectiveness of therapy 2 weeks after initiation, and again after completion (between 4 and 12 weeks)
- Using a urea breath test or fecal antigen test, confirm eradication of H. pylori in patients that continue to have symptoms or relapse; these patients may require retreatment with a different antibiotic regimen
  - PPIs reduce sensitivity; stop 7 to 14 days before test
- Successful H. pylori eradication decreases peptic ulcer recurrence to 20% per year
- All gastric ulcers should be reevaluated by endoscopy with biopsy after treatment to document resolution and exclude malignancy

Complications
- Hemorrhage, ulcer perforation or penetration, gastric outlet obstruction, death

Gastric Cancer
Description
- Cancer of the stomach

Etiology
- Gastric cancer generally takes the form of gastric adenocarcinoma (95%)
- Other kinds of gastric cancer include primary gastrointestinal lymphoma, stromal tumors, or other rare tumors

Incidence and Demographics
- More common in men

- Generally does not occur before age 60
- Decreasing incidence in the United States; this may be attributed to improved diets and eradication of *H. pylori* infection
- High incidence of gastric cancer in South America and Japan
- Native Americans, Hispanic Americans, and Blacks are twice as likely as Whites to have gastric cancer

Risk Factors
- *H. pylori* infection
- Epstein-Barr virus
- Chronic atrophic gastritis
- Diet high in salt, fried food, processed meat, fish, and alcohol and low in vegetables, fruits, milk, and vitamin A
- Smoking
- History of gastric surgery

Prevention and Screening
- Value of mass screening is controversial
- Periodic upper endoscopy can be offered to patients considered to be high risk
- Treatment of *H. pylori* infection
- Diets high in fresh fruits and vegetables

Assessment
History
- 80% are asymptomatic during early stages of disease
- Weight loss and abdominal (commonly epigastric) pain are the most common symptoms at initial diagnosis
- Dysphagia, nausea, early satiety, and evidence of occult GI bleeding may be reported

Physical Exam
- Weight loss
- Rare hematemesis and melena
- Rare palpation of a gastric mass
- Left supraclavicular lymph node enlargement is a sign of metastatic spread

Diagnostic Studies
- CBC/diff: assess for iron deficiency anemia
- Stool for occult blood is often positive
- Liver function tests may be elevated indicating metastatic disease
- Upper endoscopy with biopsy
- Abdominal CT after diagnosis to evaluate extent of disease

Differential Diagnosis
- Gastric ulcer
- Gastritis
- GERD

Management
- Depends on staging of disease; the staging schema of the American Joint Committee on Cancer/International Union Against Cancer is based on tumor (T), node (N), and metastasis (M) classifications

- Surgical resection: total gastrectomy, esophagogastrectomy for tumors of the cardia and gastroesophageal junction, or subtotal gastrectomy for tumors of the distal stomach
  - Extent of lymph node dissection is controversial
  - For curative resection, 5-year survival rates are 60% to 90% (stage I), 30% to 50% (stage II), 10% to 25% (stage III)
  - Adjuvant (postoperative) and neoadjuvant (preoperative) treatment strategies incorporating chemotherapy and radiation therapy (RT) may be trialed

Special Considerations
- Pernicious anemia is often caused by chronic atrophic gastritis in older adults; patients with pernicious anemia may be at a greater risk for developing gastric cancer

When to Consult, Refer, Hospitalize
- Any older adult with new onset of dyspeptic symptoms especially associated with weight loss, iron deficiency anemia, and occult blood in the stool should be referred to a gastroenterologist
- Most patients will require palliative care at some point in their disease

Follow-up
Expected Outcomes
- Most patients will have a recurrence

Complications
- Early postoperative complications: anastomotic failure, bleeding, ileus, transit failure at the anastomosis, cholecystitis, pancreatitis, pulmonary infections, and thromboembolism
- Late postoperative complications: dumping syndrome, vitamin B_{12} deficiency, reflux esophagitis, and bone disorders, especially osteoporosis

Cholelithiasis/Cholecystitis
Description
- Cholelithiasis is presence of gallstones in the gallbladder
  - Gallstones consist predominantly of either cholesterol or calcium
- Cholecystitis is inflammation of the gallbladder

Etiology
- Over 90% of cases are due to cystic duct obstruction by an impacted stone
- Carcinoma or other tumor that compresses the gallbladder or bile ducts

Incidence and Demographics
- Over 10% of men and 20% of women have gallstones by age 65
- Higher incidence of cholelithiasis in western Europeans and people of western European ancestry, Hispanic, and Native American populations; lower incidence in eastern European, Black, and Japanese populations
- Cholecystitis is the most common indication for abdominal surgery in patients over age 55

Risk Factors
- Age-related changes in the biliary tract
- Genetic predisposition

- Obesity, rapid weight loss
- Diabetes mellitus
- Crohn disease
- Cirrhosis
- Hyperlipidemia
- Medications that cause cholesterol saturation such as estrogen and gemfibrozil (Lopid)

Prevention and Screening
- Low-fat, low-carbohydrate, high-fiber diet and physical activity
- Using ursodiol (Actigall) during rapid weight loss may prevent stone formation

Assessment
- Older adults generally have an atypical presentation; are less likely to present as acute cholecystitis

History
Cholelithiasis
- Frequently asymptomatic
- May have nausea and vomiting, right upper quadrant pain
- Pain is usually precipitated by a large or fatty meal

Cholecystitis
- May present with colicky epigastric or right upper quadrant pain, nausea, vomiting, and fever
  - More than half of older adults with acute cholecystitis have no nausea, vomiting, or fever
- Pain may radiate to the right shoulder, scapula, or between the shoulder blades if there is irritation of the phrenic nerve

Physical Exam
- Murphy's sign: increased pain on inspiration during palpation of the right upper quadrant under the costal margin, present in approximately half of older adults
- Jaundice may be present if there is biliary obstruction
- Guarding and rebound tenderness may be present

Diagnostic Studies
Cholelithiasis
- Abdominal ultrasound
- Flat plate and upright abdominal films may show gallstones

Cholecystitis
- Leukocytosis; elevated ALT, AST, GGT, and alkaline phosphatase usually present
- Elevated bilirubin may be seen with or without obstruction
- Serum amylase may also be elevated especially if a biliary duct obstruction has occurred at or near the pancreatic duct, causing concomitant pancreatitis
- Abdominal ultrasound to detect the presence of stones
- Hepatobiliary iminodiacetic acid (HIDA) scan in cases with negative findings on ultrasonography, combined with a high clinical suspicion for cholecystitis

Differential Diagnosis
- Appendicitis
- Bowel obstruction
- Pancreatitis

- Hepatitis
- Peptic ulcer disease
- Gastroesophageal reflux disease (GERD)
- Carcinoma of the gallbladder or bile ducts
- Irritable bowel syndrome
- Pneumonia
- Thoracic disease
- Angina

Management
Nonpharmacologic
- Cholelithiasis:
  - Low-fat diet
- Cholecystitis:
  - Supportive care including bowel rest and IV hydration, nasogastric tube placement if vomiting

Pharmacologic
- Cholelithiasis:
  - Asymptomatic gallstones that are discovered incidentally on imaging should not be treated
- Cholecystitis:
  - Selection of treatment depends on the severity of symptoms
  - Pain management may include the use of opioids or NSAIDs
  - Empiric coverage of Gram-negative and anaerobic organisms should be considered
  - Cholecystectomy
  - Ursodiol (Actigall): a naturally occurring bile acid that inhibits intestinal absorption of cholesterol; 8 to 10 mg/kg/day p.o. in divided b.i.d./t.i.d. doses in patients who refuse or cannot tolerate surgery

Special Considerations
- Older adults have an increased likelihood of acalculous cholecystitis
- Delayed surgical intervention is associated with increased morbidity and mortality

When to Consult, Refer, Hospitalize
- Cholelithiasis requires surgical consult
- Cholecystitis requires hospitalization with surgical evaluation

Follow-up
Expected Course
- Uncomplicated cholecystectomy usually followed by complete resolution of symptoms
- Mortality of an episode of cholecystitis approaches 10% in high-risk patients or in those who have developed complications

Complications
- Occur in more than 50% of patients over age 65
- In obese, diabetic, older adult, or immunosuppressed patients, may have severe complications with minimal symptoms
- Gangrene, necrosis, pancreatitis, perforation and peritonitis, liver abscess, suppurative cholangitis, and other complications of surgery

- Mortality rate is markedly increased in older adults who have an open cholecystectomy for acute cholecystitis

Irritable Bowel Syndrome (IBS)

Description
- Chronic, recurrent functional disorder of the GI tract characterized by abdominal pain and altered bowel habits in the absence of organic disease
- Four subtypes of IBS:
  - IBS with constipation: hard or lumpy stools on ≥ 25% of bowel movements and loose or watery stools on < 25% of bowel movements
  - IBS with diarrhea: loose or watery stools on ≥ 25% of bowel movements and hard or lumpy stools on < 5% of bowel movements
  - Mixed IBS: hard or lumpy stools on ≥ 25% of bowel movements and loose or watery stools on ≥ 25% of bowel movements
  - Unsubtyped IBS: insufficient abnormality of stool consistency to meet the above subtypes
- Presence of symptoms for at least 12 weeks in the preceding 12 months

Etiology
- Unknown, but may be related to the following
- Abnormal intestinal motility, described as excessive spastic contractions causing constipation, or decreased contractions (replaced by infrequent propulsive movements) causing diarrhea
- Decreased pain threshold in response to abdominal distension from flatulence
- Specific food intolerances (lactose, high-fat, citrus, or spicy foods; dietetic sweeteners; and gas-producing foods such as beans, cabbage, and raw onions)
- Malabsorption of bile acids
- Psychological problems are present in approximately three-fourths of patients (anxiety, depression, somatization, personality disorders, etc.)

Incidence and Demographics
- Common; estimated that 10% to 20% of the older adult population is affected
- More common in women than in men
- More common in Whites than in Blacks

Risk Factors
- Familial history
- Emotional and physical stress, manifested as anxiety, excessive worry, major loss, improper diet, overwork, decreased sleep, and poor physical fitness, can exacerbate symptoms

Prevention and Screening
- Stress reduction
- Maintain healthy lifestyle by eating a well-balanced, high-fiber, low-fat diet; exercising regularly; and getting adequate sleep
- Avoid foods or other substances that exacerbate symptoms (see specific foods listed above)
- Avoid caffeine, tobacco, and alcohol

Assessment

History

- Pain: intermittent, crampy, lower abdominal pain that may radiate to the upper abdomen or chest
- Altered bowel habits: may report diarrhea, constipation, alternating diarrhea and constipation, or normal bowel habits alternating with either diarrhea or constipation
  - Constipation, a more common symptom in older adults, is described as small, infrequent, hard stools or straining to defecate
  - Diarrhea (usually 4 to 6 stools day) described as watery, ribbon-like, with clear mucus in the stool; should not wake patient from sleep; symptoms of incomplete evacuation and urgency may also be present
- Other symptoms may include: increased flatulence and bloating, gastroesophageal reflux, dysphagia, early satiety, intermittent dyspepsia, nausea
- Symptoms typically exacerbated by meals and stress, relieved by defecation
- History of increased emotional or physical stress, depression, or preoccupation with bowel habits
- Older adults more likely to report increased urinary frequency, urgency, nocturia, and bladder instability

Physical Exam

- Usually normal, may have mild weight loss
- Abdominal exam: lower abdominal tenderness may be present, not pronounced; tender cord may be palpated over the sigmoid colon (left lower quadrant), indicates presence of stool; abdominal tympany if air trapping present; mildly hyperactive bowel sounds may be present
- Digital rectal exam normal

Diagnostic Studies

- Limited diagnostic evaluation (including laboratory evaluation, stool samples, and colonoscopy as described below) is appropriate in patients without alarm symptoms and rules out organic disease in 95% of patients
  - Laboratory evaluation
  - CBC with differential, erythrocyte sedimentation rate (ESR), and thyroid function tests are normal
  - Stool test for occult blood negative
  - In patients with diarrhea, 3 separate stool studies are negative (culture, ova and parasite, and C. *difficile*)
- Diagnostic tests
  - Colonoscopy recommended for all patients over the age of 50
  - Mucosal biopsies in patients with persistent and continuous diarrhea
- It is reasonable to consider additional diagnostic studies in patients who do not respond to treatment

Differential Diagnosis

- Inflammatory bowel disease
- Infectious diarrhea
- Thyroid disease
- Diverticulitis
- Colon cancer
- Lactose intolerance

Management
Nonpharmacologic
- Patients should keep a diary in which foods, symptoms, and daily events are recorded to identify possible exacerbating factors
- Dietary changes include: lactose-free diet trial for 2 weeks to exclude lactose intolerance; avoidance of gas-producing foods (beans, onions, celery, carrots, raisins, bananas, apricots, prunes, brussels sprouts, wheat germ, pretzels, and bagels)
- High-fiber diet (20 to 30 g/day) is recommended; may cause bloating and flatulence initially but should resolve in few weeks (increase gradually); use 1 teaspoon bran powder 2 to 3 times a day added to food or in 8 ounces of liquid
- Management of stress through relaxation techniques and behavior modification

Pharmacologic
- Depends on the nature of the symptoms
- Bulk-forming agents may be better tolerated than bran
  - Psyllium (Metamucil) 1 tablespoon in 8 ounces of fluid up to 3 times a day
  - Methylcellulose (Citrucel) 5 to 20 mL in 8 ounces of fluid up to 3 times a day
- Anticholinergic agents: relieve spasm and abdominal pain; to be used on a p.r.n. basis
  - Dicyclomine hydrochloride (Bentyl) 10 to 20 mg q.i.d. p.r.n.
  - Hyoscyamine sulfate (Levsin) 0.125 mg 1 to 2 (tabs or teaspoons) q.i.d. orally or sublingually p.r.n.
  - May increase constipation and increase risk for disorientation in frail older adults
- Antidiarrheal agents: used on an as-needed basis
- Laxatives used intermittently as needed
- Antidepressants: tricyclic or SSRI in patients with chronic, unremitting abdominal pain
- Other anxiolytics and opioids should not be used chronically in these patients because of the risk for habituation, drug interactions, and increased constipation with opioids

How Long to Treat
- High-fiber diet and avoidance of exacerbating agents should be continued indefinitely
- Use other agents as needed for symptomatic management

Special Considerations
- Reassurance and explanation about the disease is helpful in relieving the patient's anxiety and facilitating coping abilities

When to Consult, Refer, Hospitalize
- Refer to or consult with a physician or gastroenterologist for initial evaluation or for severe disease, nocturnal diarrhea, fever, and weight loss
- Refer to a psychologist for counseling and stress management if appropriate

Follow-up
Expected Outcomes
- Most respond well to treatment during the initial 12-month period; however, irritable bowel syndrome is a chronic, relapsing condition that may require prolonged therapy
- Symptoms usually decrease with age

Complications
- Generally none

Diverticulosis/Diverticulitis

Description
- Diverticulosis is the presence of diverticula, sac-like outpouchings in the wall of the colon
- Diverticulitis is an inflammation of diverticula that can vary from subclinical inflammation to peritonitis
  - Size of the diverticula can vary from small to large; number can be one to several dozen
  - Diverticula are more common in the sigmoid colon than in the proximal colon
  - Uncomplicated diverticulitis: 75% of cases; most respond to medical therapy
  - Complicated diverticulitis: 25% of cases; presence of perforation, obstruction, abscess, or fistula; nearly all require surgery

Etiology
- Environmental and lifestyle factors are thought to play an important role in the development of diverticula:
  - Poor dietary fiber intake over many years results in hypertrophy, thickening, and fibrosis of the bowel wall from movement of hard stool under increased intraluminal pressures
- Diverticulitis thought to be caused by erosion of the diverticular wall by increased intraluminal pressure or dried food particles; this results in inflammation, focal necrosis, and ultimately perforation
  - Small perforations are walled off by pericolic fat and mesentery, and may result in formation of an abscess, fistula, or obstruction

Incidence and Demographics
- Diverticulosis: 30% at age 60; more than 50% over age 80
- Approximately 20% of patients with diverticula will develop diverticulitis or bleeding episodes
- More predominant in females over age 70
- Most common cause of lower GI bleeding in older adults

Risk Factors
- Diet low in fiber and high in red meats and fat
- Sedentary lifestyle
- Obesity
- Increased age

Prevention and Screening
- High-fiber diet
- Active lifestyle

Assessment
History
- Classic presentation such as fever, leukocytosis, or significant abdominal pain may be decreased in older adults
- Clinical presentation depends on the presence or absence of complications
Diverticulosis
- Usually no complaints

- May have chronic constipation, cramping abdominal pain, bloating, flatulence, or fluctuating bowel habits
- May have painless rectal bleeding with intermittent passage of maroon stools or bright red blood

Diverticulitis
- Complaints may vary according to severity of the inflammation and infection
- Crampy left-lower or mid-abdominal pain that may radiate to the back, or acute pain that is localized to the left-lower quadrant
  - Pain usually exacerbated after meals and improved with bowel movement or passage of flatus
- Fever, constipation, loose stool or nausea and vomiting may be present

Physical Exam
Diverticulosis
- Usually normal but may have mild left-lower quadrant tenderness with a palpable mass

Diverticulitis
- Abdomen is often distended and tympanitic to percussion with diminished bowel sounds
- Rebound tenderness may also be present and may be suggestive of a perforated diverticula
- Rectal exam may reveal a palpable mass indicating a pelvic abscess

Diagnostic Studies
Diverticulosis
- Laboratory evaluation is normal

Diverticulitis
- CBC may show a mild-to-moderate leukocytosis
- Flat plate and upright abdominal film is obtained to look for free air (sign of perforation), ileus, and small or large bowel obstruction
  - Air in the bladder may indicate a fistula
- CT scan of the abdomen is the diagnostic test of choice in patients suspected of having acute diverticulitis

Differential Diagnosis
Diverticulosis
- Irritable bowel syndrome
- Constipation

Diverticulitis
- See Acute Abdomen

Management
Nonpharmacologic
- Dietary management:
  - During acute phase, clear liquids only for 2 to 3 days, after which diet may be advanced as tolerated
  - If hospitalized, clear liquids or NPO with IV hydration
  - High-fiber diet
  - Avoidance of whole pieces of fiber (seeds, corn, and nuts) is not necessary
- Surgical management required for abscess or perforation; laparoscopic surgery preferred

Pharmacologic
- Uncomplicated diverticulitis
  - Ciprofloxacin 500 mg p.o. b.i.d. plus metronidazole 500 mg p.o. t.i.d.
    - Amoxicillin-clavulanate 875/125 mg p.o. b.i.d. is an alternative to metronidazole
    - Treat for 7 to 10 days
  - For patients requiring hospitalization and IV hydration and antibiotics:
    - Metronidazole is the antibiotic of choice for anaerobic coverage
    - Gram-negative coverage with ceftriaxone 1 to 2 g daily or cefoxatime 1 to 2 g every 6 hours or ciprofloxacin 400 mg IV every 12 hours or levofloxacin 500 mg IV daily
- Complicated diverticulitis: should be managed in the acute care setting with IV fluids, broad-spectrum antibiotics, and emergency exploration

Special Considerations
- Diverticular bleeding occurs in 15% of patients with diverticulosis; it is more common in the older adult

When to Consult, Refer, Hospitalize
- Hospitalization with surgical consultation should be obtained in all patients with severe diverticulitis (fever, elevated WBC, rebound tenderness, vomiting, rectal pain) and for failure to improve after 72 hours of medical management

Follow-up
Expected Outcomes
- Response to antibiotics should occur in 3 days
- Following successful medical management for a first attack of diverticulitis, approximately one-third of patients will remain asymptomatic, one-third will have episodic symptoms, and one-third will have a second attack of diverticulitis
- Colon requires full evaluation after resolution of acute diverticulitis to assess extent of diverticular disease
  - Colonoscopy or combination of barium enema plus flexible sigmoidoscopy 2 to 6 weeks after resolution

Complications
- Perforation, peritonitis, hemorrhage, fistula, bowel obstruction, abscess, septicemia

Colorectal Cancer
Description
- Cancer of the large intestine including the rectum

Etiology
- Most colon cancers are adenocarcinomas that begin as adenomatous polyps (benign epithelial growths)

Incidence and Demographics
- Third most common cancer in both men and women and third leading cause of death due to malignancy in the United States
- Estimated new cases and deaths for 2008:
  - New cases: 108,070 (colon); 40,740 (rectal)
  - Deaths: 49,960 (colon and rectal combined)

- Increased prevalence in developed countries, urban areas, and advantaged socioeconomic groups
- Incidence increases after age 40 with 90% of new cases occurring over age 50
- Higher incidence in people of German, Irish, Czech/Slovak, and French descent

Risk Factors
- Age
- Familial adenomatous polyposis (FAP)
- Hereditary nonpolyposis colorectal cancer (HNPCC)
- Personal or family history of sporadic cancers or adenomatous polyps
- Inflammatory bowel disease
- Diabetes mellitus and insulin resistance
- Cholecystectomy
- Alcohol consumption
- Obesity

Prevention and Screening
- Protective effects have been associated with:
  - Diet high in fruits and vegetables, calcium, and folic acid, and low in red meat, animal fat, and cholesterol
  - Physical activity
  - NSAIDs and a daily aspirin

Screening
- Average risk: patients who lack signs or symptoms of colorectal cancer, are without a personal or family history of colorectal cancer or adenomatous polyps, and are without associated diseases that could increase risk
  - Screening should begin at age 50:
    - Fecal occult blood testing (FOBT) by guaiac method, performed annually; 2 to 3 stool samples collected at home (single stool sample obtained on digital exam is not an acceptable stool test)
    - Colonoscopy every 10 years *or* flexible sigmoidoscopy every 5 years *or* double-contrast barium enema every 5 years *or* computed tomography colonography every 5 years
- Increased risk: family history of adenomatous polyps in a first-degree relative under age 60
  - Screening should begin at age 40 or 10 years before the earliest case in a first-degree relative
  - May require more frequent surveillance colonoscopy
- Most guidelines recommend that screening for colorectal cancer stop when the patient's life expectancy is less than 10 years

Assessment
History
- Often reaches advanced stages without symptoms, with approximately 20% of patients having distant metastases at time of presentation
  - Common sites of metastasis are regional lymph nodes, liver, lungs, and peritoneum
  - May present with signs or symptoms related to metastatic disease
- Most patients present with bright red blood per rectum or melena, abdominal pain, and a change in bowel habits

- Left-sided colon cancers more commonly cause rectal bleeding and altered bowel habits; obstructive symptoms may occur; pencil-thin stools and occasional diarrhea may occur
- Right-sided colon cancers rarely present with obstructive symptoms; bleeding is slow and not visible in the stool; therefore, anemia is the most common presenting symptom

Physical
- A mass may be palpated in the abdomen
- Rectal mass may be palpated on digital exam
- The liver should be evaluated for enlargement suggesting metastatic disease

Diagnostic Studies
- Stool for occult blood
- CBC to evaluate for iron deficiency anemia
- Carcinoembryonic antigen (CEA): normally secreted in the GI tract; useful for monitoring colorectal cancer, especially metastatic disease; may also be elevated with any mucosal damage to the GI tract such as inflammatory bowel disease; also secreted by tumors of the lung, pancreas, and liver; highest levels are with metastatic disease to the liver
- Elevated liver function tests raise concern for possible liver metastasis
- Colonoscopy with biopsy confirms diagnosis; also used in screening high-risk patients
- Abdominal CT used to evaluate for metastatic disease in patients with colorectal cancer

Differential Diagnosis
- Rectal polyps
- Hemorrhoids
- Rectal fissures
- Colorectal strictures
- Diverticulosis
- Colorectal infections
- Inflammatory lesions
- Other neoplasms
- Inflammatory bowel disease
- Arteriovenous malformations
- Masses outside bowel wall

Management
- Depends on cancer stage (tumor size and extent of bowel wall invasion, lymph node involvement, and presence of metastasis) and type of tumor

Nonpharmacologic
- Surgery is the treatment of choice and is the only curative modality for localized colon cancer
- Adjuvant radiation therapy may be beneficial in some patients

Pharmacologic
- Adjuvant chemotherapy for patients who have undergone potentially curative surgery
- Palliative chemotherapy for patients with metastatic colorectal cancer who cannot undergo surgical resection of their disease

Special Considerations
- Prognosis in older adults is comparable to that of younger patients

When to Consult, Refer, Hospitalize
- If colon cancer is diagnosed or suspected refer to a surgeon
- Symptoms or signs of colorectal cancer (anemia, iron deficiency, blood in stool, change in bowel habits, unexplained abdominal pain, weight loss) should be referred for colonoscopy
- Patients with high risk should be followed regularly by a gastroenterologist

Follow-up
- CEA is a marker for treatment response in patients who have been diagnosed with colorectal cancer; if treatment response occurs, CEA level should decrease

Expected Course
- Depends on the stage of the cancer and type of tumor

Complications
- Complications associated with surgery, chemotherapy, and radiation; metastasis, death

Hernias
Description
- A defect in the abdominal wall that allows intra-abdominal contents to protrude
  - Types of hernias, based on their location, are inguinal, femoral, umbilical, epigastric, and incisional
  - Inguinal hernias are further subdivided into direct (through the inguinal floor) and indirect (through the internal inguinal ring)
- Clinically, all hernias can be described as:
  - Reducible: contents can be pushed back into the abdominal cavity
  - Nonreducible (incarcerated): contents cannot be pushed back into the abdominal cavity
  - Strangulated: an incarcerated hernia, in which the blood supply of the hernial contents is compromised

Etiology
- Congenital or acquired defect in the abdominal wall
- Situations or conditions that raise intra-abdominal pressure (e.g., Valsalva maneuver, ascites, obesity)

Incidence and Demographics
- Common in middle-aged and older adults
- Up to 40% of hernia repairs are performed for incarceration or bowel obstruction in patients over age 65

Risk Factors
- Constipation
- Prostatic hypertrophy (outflow obstruction causes straining during micturition)
- Chronic cough
- Ascites
- Obesity

Prevention and Screening
- Avoid excessive straining
- Weight loss

Assessment
History
- Bulging mass exacerbated by standing or straining; may be asymptomatic or described as dull ache or burning discomfort; dragging sensation may occur with large hernia that extends into scrotum
- Strangulated hernias present with severe pain, fever, nausea and vomiting, abdominal distension, and constipation

Physical Exam
- Inspection and palpation in both the supine and standing positions, while the patient performs a Valsalva maneuver; abdominal exam to evaluate tenderness, masses, hepatomegaly, and ascites; digital rectal exam to exclude enlarged prostate
- Inguinal: with the index finger, invaginate the scrotum following the spermatic cord to the opening of the external inguinal ring and, if possible, follow the inguinal canal up to the internal inguinal ring; have the patient Valsalva while your index finger is at the external inguinal ring or in the inguinal canal
  - Indirect hernia occurs near the internal inguinal ring and often extends into the scrotum
  - Direct hernia occurs near the external inguinal ring
- Femoral: palpate medial to the femoral vessels and inferior to the inguinal canal
- Umbilical: palpate the umbilical region in the supine position while the patient raises his head and performs a Valsalva maneuver
- Epigastric: usually a small mass located midline between the umbilicus and xiphoid cartilage
- Incisional: presents as a bulge through a surgical incision

Diagnostic Studies
- Mostly a clinical dianosis
- CBC may show leukocytosis if strangulation is present
- Ultrasound may be helpful for diagnosing a hernia in patients who report symptoms but have no palpable mass; can differentiate an incarcerated hernia from an enlarged lymph node or other cause

Differential Diagnosis
- Muscle strain
- Arthritis
- Lipoma
- Lymphadenopathy
- Groin abscess
- Hydrocele
- Varicocele
- Testicular tumor
- Undescended testicle

Management
Nonpharmacologic
- Patients with symptomatic, reducible inguinal hernias who have relative contraindications to surgery, may wear a truss (which keeps hernia reduced); however, this is not always effective and only should be rarely recommended
- Patients with evidence indicating a strangulated hernia must undergo emergent surgery
- Elective herniorrhaphy (hernia repair) is indicated for all abdominal hernias before incarceration and strangulation occur
- Uncomplicated hernia repair is often done under local or spinal anesthesia as outpatient surgery and can be tolerated by most older adults

Pharmacologic
- None indicated

Special Considerations
- Hernias are most likely to incarcerate shortly after initial development

When to Consult, Refer, Hospitalize
- Refer to a surgeon for evaluation
- Emergent referral for surgery within 4 to 6 hours to prevent loss of bowel from a strangulated hernia

Follow-up
Expected Outcomes
- Risk of reoccurrence after hernia repair

Complications
- Ischemic bowel with a strangulated hernia; bowel obstruction

Hemorrhoids
Description
- Hemorrhoids are venous varicosities of the hemorrhoidal venous plexus that are classified as either internal (above pectinate line) or external (below pectinate line)
- Internal hemorrhoids may prolapse and strangulate causing thrombosis, an extremely painful condition

Etiology
- May be caused by straining that occurs while lifting or having a bowel movement
- Increased portal venous pressure may contribute

Incidence and Demographics
- Occurs in 50% of adults over age 50; incidence peaks between ages of 45 and 65 and declines thereafter
- Men = women

Risk Factors
- Many risk factors have been suggested, though little evidence exists to support them
- Constipation
- Straining
- Prolonged sitting or standing

Prevention and Screening

- Consume a high-fiber diet
- Avoiding constipation and straining to defecate
- Avoid straining while lifting
- Avoid prolonged periods of sitting or standing, change position frequently
- Weight loss if overweight

Assessment

History

- Rectal bleeding (usually painless and bright red)
- Rectal discomfort, itching, burning
- Constipation or straining
- Previous management including surgery
- Acutely painful mass at the rectum if external hemorrhoid is thrombosed

Physical Exam

- Preferred position for the digital rectal examination is the left lateral decubitus with the patient's knees flexed toward the chest
- Rectal exam:
  - External hemorrhoids: inspection reveals a soft and painless mass exterior to the anal verge
  - Internal hemorrhoids: palpated by digital rectal exam or visualized by anoscopy
  - If thrombosed, hemorrhoids are bluish in color, firm, and tender to palpation

Diagnostic Studies

- CBC to rule out anemia
- Sigmoidoscopy or colonoscopy may be done to rule out other causes of rectal bleeding

Differential Diagnosis

- Anal skin tags
- Anal fissure
- Abscess
- Hypertrophied anal papilla
- Prolapse of rectal mucosa
- Rectal polyps
- Rectal or anal carcinoma

Management

Nonpharmacologic

- Eliminate risk factors when possible
- Warm sitz baths 2 to 3 times daily for 20 minutes
- High fiber diet (20 to 30 g/day) and increased fluid intake (six to eight 8-ounce glasses/day, recommend increasing fluids with caution in those with CHF or hyponatremia)
- Witch hazel compresses (Tucks) t.i.d.-q.i.d. p.r.n.
- Minimally invasive procedures: rubber band ligation (most commonly used); bipolar, infrared, and laser coagulation; sclerotherapy; cryosurgery
- Surgery: hemorrhoidectomy

Pharmacologic

- Bulk-forming laxatives to soften stool and prevent constipation
- Stool softeners to reduce straining during defecation

- Topical hydrocortisone preparations: relieve pain, itching, and inflammation; cream, foam, and suppositories are available
  - Pramoxine HCL 1%, zinc oxide 12.5%, mineral oil (Anusol); and Anusol-HC with hydrocortisone 25 mg p.r.n. up to 6 times a day
  - ProctoFoam-HC, hydrocortisone cream 1%–2.5%
- Local analgesic spray, suppository, or cream: provides pain relief
  - Benzocaine (Hurricane), pramoxine (Anusol), or dibucaine (Nupercainal)

How Long to Treat
- Use topical analgesics and hydrocortisone preparations for a maximum of 1 week because of risk for adverse effects such as contact dermatitis with analgesic creams or mucosal atrophy with steroid creams
- Stool softeners and bulk-forming laxatives may be used indefinitely to prevent recurrence

Special Considerations
- Topical anesthetics (20% benzocaine or 5% lidocaine ointment) may reduce discomfort caused by examination

When to Consult, Refer, Hospitalize
- Refer to a colorectal surgeon when symptoms do not respond to conservative treatment within 3 to 4 weeks
- Refer to a gastroenterologist if patient has severe pain, rectal bleeding, strangulation, ulceration, perianal infection, rectal prolapse, or recurrent symptomatic hemorrhoids

Follow-up
Expected Outcomes
- Patients should follow up for further evaluation if no improvement in symptoms within 2 weeks of initiating treatment, if rectal bleeding is excessive or persists, or if constipation continues

Complications
- Bleeding, thrombosis, strangulation, secondary infection, ulceration, and anemia
- Complications of surgery including pain, thrombosis, infection, abscess

Abnormal Liver Function Tests
Description
- Serum liver chemistries useful in evaluating liver function:
  - Alanine aminotransferase (ALT) and aspartate aminotransferase (AST) evaluate hepatic cellular integrity
  - Bilirubin (direct and indirect), alkaline phosphatase (ALP), and gamma-glutamyl transpeptidase (GGT) assess hepatic excretion
  - Prothrombin time (PT) and serum albumin evaluate hepatic protein synthesis

Etiology
- Elevated aminotransferases (ALT and AST) are typically caused by acute hepatocellular injury
  - Enzymes are found in multiple tissues and released into the plasma in response to cellular injury

- AST: predominantly in the liver; more specific than ALT for evaluating hepatocellular damage
- ALT: found in liver, cardiac, skeletal, kidney, and brain tissue; elevated levels alone may indicate tissue damage in any of those organ systems (e.g., myocardial ischemia or musculoskeletal injury)
- ALT and AST do not indicate the severity of liver injury, as they may be normal in severe disease
- Highest levels of ALT and AST (usually > 500 u/liter): severe viral hepatitis, drug-induced liver injury (e.g., acetaminophen, phenytoin, rifampin), or ischemic hepatitis
- Moderate elevations (usually < 300 u/liter): mild acute viral hepatitis, chronic active hepatitis, cirrhosis, and liver metastases
- Mild elevations: biliary obstruction, with higher levels suggesting the development of cholangitis (causing hepatic cell necrosis)
- In alcoholic liver disease, the AST/ALT ratio may be > 2:1
- Bilirubin: degradation product of heme; elevated level should be fractionated to determine if it is predominantly conjugated (direct, processed by the liver) or unconjugated (indirect, not processed by the liver)
  - Elevations in direct bilirubin are usually caused by impaired excretion of bilirubin from the liver due to hepatocellular disease (above), biliary tract obstruction, drugs, or sepsis
  - Indirect bilirubin elevation is caused by hemolysis or ineffective erythropoiesis (increased bilirubin production); Gilbert or Crigler-Najjar syndromes (impaired bilirubin conjugation because of enzyme deficiency); or when hepatic bilirubin uptake is decreased because of hepatotoxic drugs, heart failure, or portosystemic shunting
- ALP is an enzyme found in various tissues including the liver, bone, intestine, and placenta (more than 80% from liver and bone)
  - Elevated ALP levels, in the absence of bone disease, usually represent impaired biliary tract function
  - Fractionation of an elevated serum ALP can be done to determine the source; however, elevation of other liver function tests is helpful in establishing a hepatic cause
  - Mild to moderate increases (usually 1 to 2 times normal) occur with hepatocellular disorders such as hepatitis or cirrhosis
  - High serum elevations (up to 10 times normal or greater) can occur with extrahepatic biliary tract obstruction (usually a gallstone blocking the common bile duct) or intrahepatic cholestasis (bile retention in the liver) as seen with drug-induced cholestasis and biliary cirrhosis
  - Usually mildly elevated in incomplete biliary tract obstruction and in metastatic and infiltrative liver disease (e.g. leukemia, lymphoma, and sarcoid)
  - Also present in nonhepatic disorders, with the most common being bone disease (Paget disease and bone metastases)
- GGT is useful in differentiating the origin of an elevated ALP (hepatic vs. bone), as both ALP and GGT tend to increase in similar hepatic diseases
  - Also a highly sensitive indicator of acute alcohol ingestion and of other agents that stimulate the hepatic microsomal oxidase system, such as barbiturates and phenytoin
  - GGT enzyme also present in the pancreas, kidney, heart, and brain, and elevations may occur in disorders involving those organ systems

- PT: A prolonged PT is caused by impaired hepatic synthesis of coagulation factors seen in significant liver disease or with vitamin K deficiency that may occur with malnutrition, malabsorption (e.g., cholestasis, steatorrhea, pancreatic insufficiency), and warfarin use; if administration of vitamin K corrects the PT, then a deficiency was present
- Albumin: primary protein synthesized by the liver
  - Decreased levels may be caused by chronic liver disease or by other nonhepatic factors such as malnutrition, hormonal factors, or excessive protein loss (nephrotic syndrome or protein-losing enteropathy)
  - Inadequate hepatic protein synthesis may lead to a decreased serum albumin; however, because of its long half-life (14 to 20 days), albumin stores are often adequate
  - In liver disease, it is often an indicator of a chronic process

Incidence and Demographics
- Frequently detected in asymptomatic patients because of the large number of screening tests that incorporate LFT
- Chronic liver disease is the 12th leading cause of death in the United States

Risk Factors
- Alcoholism
- Obesity
- Diabetes
- Hyperlipidemia
- Hepatitis B and C infection
- Medication use: e.g., oral corticosteroids, amiodarone, tamoxifen, methotrexate

Prevention and Screening
- Abstinence from alcohol
- Reduce exposure to hepatotoxic drugs (including over-the-counter medications/supplements)
- Low-fat diet

Assessment
History
- Exposure to chemicals or medications (prescription, over-the-counter medications, and herbal therapies)
- Generalized symptoms of fever, anorexia, malaise, weight loss, and pruritus may be present
- Gastrointestinal symptoms: nausea, vomiting, abdominal pain, dark urine, and pale stools
- Additional history is aimed at identifying potential risk factors:
  - History of hepatitis exposure, transfusions, medications, alcohol and IV and intranasal drug use, sexual practices, tattoos, occupational exposure, and travel history

Physical Exam
- Skin exam: jaundice (include sclera), spider angiomas, palmar erythema, and ecchymosis

- Abdominal exam: ascites, tenderness (usually right upper quadrant), enlarged gallbladder, hepatomegaly, and splenomegaly
  - Liver may be smaller than normal in advanced liver disease
- Extremities: asterixis and peripheral edema

Table 10-2. Interpreting Liver Function Tests

Liver Function Test	Enzyme Found In	Cause of Elevation	Seen in the Following Conditions	Comments
Direct bilirubin (conjugated, processed by liver)		Impaired excretion of bilirubin from the liver	Hepatocellular disease, biliary tract obstruction, hepatotoxic drugs	
Indirect bilirubin (unconjugated, not processed by the liver)		Hepatic bilirubin uptake is decreased	Hemolysis, defects in hepatic uptake or conjugation of bilirubin (Gilbert's syndrome), heart failure	
Alkaline phosphatase	Bone, liver	Impaired biliary tract function (cholestasis) or infiltrative liver disease, hepatic excretion	**Mild:** hepatitis or cirrhosis, early cancer **High:** biliary tract obstruction, cholestasis	Increases with age, women > men Also elevated in bone disease
GGT	Liver, pancreas, kidney, heart brain	Hepatic excretion	Sensitive for acute alcohol ingestion	Differentiates the origin of an elevated ALP between bone and liver
Transaminases	Many tissues	Acute hepatocellular injury from necrosis or inflammation	**Mild:** biliary obstruction; mild viral chronic or active and alcoholic hepatitis; cirrhosis; and liver metastases **High:** viral hepatitis, drug-induced liver injury	Do not indicate severity of liver injury; most common cause of elevation is alcoholic hepatitis
ALT	Predominantly liver, more specific test	Celiac disease		
AST	Liver, cardiac, skeletal, kidney, brain			AST twice as high as ALT typical of alcoholic liver injury

continued

Table 10–2. Interpreting Liver Function Tests (cont.)

Liver Function Test	Enzyme Found In	Cause of Elevation	Seen in the Following Conditions	Comments
Prothrombin time		Impaired hepatic synthesis of coagulation factors	Significant liver disease	
Albumin	Blood serum	Impaired hepatic protein synthesis, excess protein loss	Chronic liver disease, malnutrition	May decrease with age

Diagnostic Studies
- If the patient is asymptomatic, repeat liver function tests first; if normal, repeat testing in 3 to 6 months
  - If repeat is abnormal, obtain hepatitis serologies to exclude viral hepatitis A, B, and C (see section on viral hepatitis)
- If the patient is symptomatic, further tests are guided by history and physical; consider:
  - Hepatitis B surface antigen, surface antibody, and core antibody
  - Hepatitis C antibody
  - Monospot and CMV; IgG, IgM titers
  - Abdominal ultrasound: best screening test to evaluate for gallstones; it can also detect biliary tree dilation, biliary obstruction, cholecystitis, and liver parenchymal disease
  - Computed tomography (CT) scan (with IV contrast): best test for evaluating liver parenchymal disease and space-occupying lesions (tumor or abscess); can also assess biliary tree dilation and identify obstructing lesion
  - Magnetic resonance imaging (MRI): similar to CT scan but can better visualize vessels without the use of IV contrast
  - Endoscopic retrograde cholangiopancreatography (ERCP) and percutaneous transhepatic cholangiography (PTC): usually done after screening with ultrasound, CT, or MRI to further assess cause, location, and extent of biliary tree abnormalities
  - Liver biopsy: definitive study to determine the cause and extent of hepatocellular and infiltrative liver disease; biopsy may be guided using ultrasound or CT

Management
- Aimed at correcting underlying cause

Nonpharmacologic
- Discontinue hepatotoxic drugs and avoid drugs and other agents that are hepatotoxic
- Management will vary depending on etiology

Special Considerations
- Higher incidence of neoplasm in older adults

When to Consult, Refer, Hospitalize
- Consult with, or refer to, a physician or specialist when significantly abnormal liver function tests persist without an identifiable cause, or for symptomatic patients in need of specialized diagnostic tests and management

Follow-up
- Depends on etiology

Viral Hepatitis

Description
- Inflammation of the liver caused by a viral infection that may be acute (< 6 months duration) or chronic (> 6 months duration)
- Five types of viral hepatitis have been identified: hepatitis A virus (HAV); hepatitis B virus (HBV); hepatitis C virus (HCV); hepatitis D virus (HDV), which requires coexisting HBV infection; and hepatitis E virus (HEV)
  - Hepatitis G virus (HGV) may be pathogenic in humans, though this is unclear

Etiology

Table 10-3. Etiology of Viral Hepatitis

Type	Causative Virus	Transmission	Incubation Days	Comments
HAV	RNA	Fecal-oral route; contaminated food and water, food handlers, crowding, poor sanitary conditions	15 to 45	Rare complications, not chronic
HBV	DNA with an inner core protein and outer surface coat component	Infected blood, blood products, via body fluids (semen, vaginal mucus, saliva, tears)	40 to 150	Less acute onset, chronic infection common
HCV	RNA, six major genotypes	Infected blood or blood products, body fluids	15 to 160	Usually mild, can become chronic
HDV	RNA	Occurs only in persons with HBV; parenteral/sexual transmission	30 to 180	Only in HBV
HEV	RNA	Fecal-oral route; contaminated food and water, poor sanitary conditions	14 to 60	Rare in USA
HGV		Transmission similar to HCV	Unknown	Rarely causes hepatitis; questionable pathogenicity in humans

Incidence and Demographics
- HAV is the most common cause of acute hepatitis; HCV is the most common cause of chronic hepatitis
- After 60 years of age there is a decreased incidence of HAV because of decreased exposure and increased immunity
- Sexual activity is thought to account for 50% of HBV cases in the United States; IV drug use accounts for 20% of cases

- Rates of HCV have declined in the United States because of a reduction in cases of transfusion-associated hepatitis

Risk Factors
- Persons receiving blood transfusions or blood products
- IV drug use
- Risky sexual behaviors
- Eating contaminated foods
- Patients on hemodialysis
- Foreign travel to endemic areas
- Exposure to infected individuals

Prevention and Screening
- Universal precautions
- Vaccination against hepatitis A and B

Assessment
- Older adults tend to have more severe symptoms, including jaundice, mental changes, and prolonged course

Table 10–4. Serologic Tests for Viral Hepatitis

Lab tests	Name	Indicates	Use
HAV			
IgM anti-HAV	IgM antibody to HAV	Acute disease, resolves in 3 to 6 months	Diagnostic for HAV
IgG anti-HAV	IgG antibody to HAV	Early infection, peaks after 1 month	When persists, indicates previous exposure, noninfectivity, and immunity to HAV
HBV			
HBsAg	Hepatitis B surface antigen	Appears first, persists through clinical illness; remains positive in chronic hepatitis and asymptomatic carriers	First evidence of HBV; establishes infection, indicates infectivity
Anti-HBs	Antibody to hepatitis B surface antigen	Appears after HBsAg disappears, present after HBV vaccination	Indicates recovery from HBV infection, not infective and immunity
Anti-HBc	IgM and IgG antibody to hepatitis B core antigen	Appears after HBsAg is detected; IgM anti-HBc may persist for 3-6 months and reappear with flares of chronic HBV; IgG anti-HBc is positive during acute HBV and may persist indefinitely despite recovery	Indicates acute HBV infection; may be negative in chronic infection; may be the only indicator of infection when there is a delay between the disappearance of HBsAg and appearance of anti-HBs (the window period)

continued

Table 10–4. Serologic Tests for Viral Hepatitis (cont.)

Lab tests	Name	Indicates	Use
HBeAg	Hepatitis B core antigen	Appears during incubation period shortly after the detection of HBsAg	Indicates active viral replication and increased infectivity; if persists for 3 months after acute infection suggests increased risk for developing chronic HBV infection
Anti-HBeAg	Antibody to HBeAg	Appears when HBeAg disappears	Indicates decreased viral replication and infectivity
HBV DNA		Parallels presence of HBeAg	More sensitive than HBeAg in detecting viral replication and infectivity
HCV			
Anti-HCV	Antibodies to HCV	Initial screening test; confirm with RIBA test	Indicates acute or chronic HCV infection, not protective
RIBA	Recombinant immunoblot assay	Positive in HCV confirmed with HCV RNA	Indicates current or past infection
HCV RNA	Hepatitis C RNA	Ongoing viremia; detects viral load	Most sensitive test to detect infection
HDV			
Anti-HDV	Antibody to HDV	Detects hepatitis D infection	In persons with HBV
HEV & HGV	Serologic markers not widely available	Acute: IgM anti-HAV, HBsAg, IgM anti HBc, and anti-HCV Chronic: HBsAg and anti HCV	

History

- Symptoms appear after the incubation period; presentation varies according to the type of virus involved
- Symptoms of viral hepatitis are similar; however, the severity of symptoms may vary among types, ranging from asymptomatic infection without jaundice to fulminant hepatitis (severe form of acute hepatitis indicated by encephalopathy, hypoglycemia, bleeding, and prolonged prothrombin time)
- Symptoms are categorized into three phases:
  - Prodromal phase: flu-like symptoms described as low-grade fever, chills, general malaise, fatigue, anorexia, myalgias, and arthralgias; nausea and vomiting usually occur; mild but constant abdominal pain in the right upper quadrant is present (occasionally more severe); pruritus, constipation, diarrhea, dark urine, and clay-colored stools may occur; most infectious in the 2 weeks before the icteric stage
  - Icteric phase: if clinical jaundice occurs, it usually presents 5 to 10 days after the onset of symptoms; prodromal symptoms begin to improve; may have enlarged liver, pruritus, abdominal pain, anorexia

– Convalescent/recovery phase: symptoms continue to improve; jaundice and abdominal pain resolve

Physical Exam
- General toxicity varies with disease severity
- Jaundice of the skin, sclera, and mucous membranes
- Lymphadenopathy usually presents in the cervical and epitrochlear areas
- Abdominal exam: liver tenderness with hepatomegaly in 70%
- Dark urine or clay-colored stools

Diagnostic Studies
Laboratory evaluation
- ALT and AST are elevated; levels peak (400-several thousand u/L) during the icteric phase, then progressively decrease during the convalescent phase
- Serum bilirubin normal to markedly elevated; clinical jaundice evident at levels > 2.5
- Alkaline phosphatase may be normal or mildly elevated
- Prothrombin time: if prolonged may indicate serious disease
- CBC may reveal an increased number of atypical-appearing lymphocytes
- Glucose and electrolytes should be normal
- Urinalysis may be positive for protein and bilirubin

LIVER BIOPSY
- Performed if the diagnosis is uncertain
- Gold standard for assessing severity and activity of chronic hepatitis

Differential Diagnosis
- Acute cholecystitis
- Common bile duct stone
- Cirrhosis
- Hepatotoxic agents such as acetaminophen
- Alcoholic hepatitis
- Ischemic hepatitis
- CMV, herpes simplex
- Coxsackie virus
- Toxoplasmosis
- *Candida, Mycobacteria* infection
- *Pneumocystis* infection
- *Leptospira* infection

Management
Nonpharmacologic
- Activity as tolerated, avoid overexertion
- Normal-caloric, high-protein diet
- Hydration
- Avoid hepatotoxic agents (acetaminophen and alcohol)
- Colloid baths and lotions to decrease pruritus if present
- Antiemetics for nausea and vomiting if needed

Pharmacologic
- For acute, uncomplicated hepatitis, no pharmacologic treatment is indicated
- Vitamin K IM is indicated if the PT is prolonged, greater than 1½ times normal

- Avoid sedatives, as they can cause hepatic encephalopathy
- Both chronic hepatitis B and C are treated with recombinant human interferon alfa or nucleoside analogs
- HAV
  - Pre-exposure: hepatitis A vaccine (Havrix or Vaqta) with a second dose given at 6 to 12 months; recommended for persons at high risk and persons with chronic liver disease (including HBV and HCV)
  - Postexposure: immune globulin, given within 2 weeks of exposure, prevents illness in 80% to 90%
- HBV:
  - Pre-exposure: hepatitis B vaccine (Recombivax or Engerix-B) IM given in 3 doses at 0, 1, and 6 months; recommended for persons at increased risk and persons with chronic liver disease (including HCV)
  - Postexposure: immune globulin (HBIG) given as soon as possible (within 7 days of exposure), followed by initiation of the HBV vaccination series (above), prevents illness in approximately 75%; recommended after direct transmucosal or parenteral exposure with HBsAg-infected blood or body fluids
  - Treatment options for some patients with chronic HBV include: interferon alfa, lamivudine, adefovir dipivoxil, entecavir, telbivudine
- HCV:
  - Interferon alfa-2b, interferon alfa-2a, consensus interferon, and ribavirin (used in combination with interferon)
  - Interferon: treat for 6 months, approximately 50% respond; after stopping drug, 30% to 50% of those treated do not relapse
  - Prolonged treatment (12 to 18 months) is recommended
  - Ribavirin taken in combination with interferon results in higher sustained response rates

Special Considerations
- Report hepatitis A to health department
- Monitor patients on interferon closely for depression, suicidal ideation
- Protect skin while on interferon, which can cause photosensitivity

When to Consult, Refer, Hospitalize
- Refer all patients with hepatitis B, C, or D
- Hospitalization should be considered for patients over 60 because of severity of illness

Follow-up
Expected Outcomes
- Most patients recover from acute viral hepatitis without any sequelae
- Older adults are more likely to have a prolonged course and increased mortality
- Main cause of death is fulminant hepatitis, which is more common with HBV
- Patients over age 50 with acute HCV more likely to progress to chronic hepatitis and cirrhosis
- Chronic carriers of HBsAg and HCV RNA have an increased risk of developing hepatocellular carcinoma

Complications
- Hepatic necrosis, chronic active or chronic hepatitis, cirrhosis, hepatic failure, hepatocellular carcinoma (HBV and HCV)

CASE STUDIES

Case 1. A 68-year-old male presents to your clinic with complaints of burning epigastric pain after meals associated with nausea, especially when he lies down after eating. He has lost 15 lb over the past month, which he attributes to poor appetite.

HPI: The patient is a recovering alcoholic. He stopped drinking 8 months ago and has been going to AA meetings on a regular basis. The patient is also a heavy smoker and has frequent episodes of bronchitis. He continues to smoke but has cut back significantly. His past medical history includes treatment for a gastric ulcer 1 year ago. He is not taking any medication.

1. What other questions would you ask this patient?

Exam: Vital signs are stable. No lymphadenopathy. Heart and lung exams are normal. Abdomen is soft, nontender, normal bowel sounds, no hepatosplenomegaly, no masses, no abdominal bruits. Rectal exam is normal with guaiac negative stools.

2. What laboratory tests would you order?
3. What other studies would you order?
4. What treatment would you provide?

Case 2. A 72-year-old male with HTN is in your office for a follow-up visit. He complains of being constipated.

HPI: The patient states that he's always had a regular bowel movement every morning. For the past month, bowel movements occur every 4 to 5 days only after he uses a laxative. Medications include a calcium-channel blocker and one aspirin a day.

1. Is a new onset of constipation in a 72-year-old concerning? Or is this a normal change related to the aging process?
2. What other history would you obtain?

Exam: The patient is alert and oriented × 3. Blood pressure and other vital signs are normal. His abdomen is mildly distended but nontender. Bowel sounds are present in all quadrants. No enlarged liver or spleen. No bruises. Rectal exam is normal, no impacted stool. The remainder of his examination is normal.

3. What laboratory tests would you order?
4. What other studies would you order?
5. What treatment would you provide?

Case 3. A 62-year-old obese White female presents with right upper quadrant pain, nausea, and vomiting. The onset of pain was sudden and occurred after eating at a restaurant. She has had similar episodes in the past but not as severe.

1. What additional history would you like?

Exam: Temp is 99.5° F, with remaining vital signs normal. Abdomen is soft. Right upper quadrant pain increases when palpating the right upper quadrant during inspiration and there is localized guarding. There is no rebound tenderness. Bowel sounds are normal. No hepatosplenomegaly. There are no abdominal bruits. Rectal exam is normal. The remainder of her exam is normal.

2. What diagnostic tests would you order?
3. What is the most likely differential?
4. How would you treat her?

REFERENCES

Chait, M. (2007). Lower gastrointestinal bleeding in the elderly. *Annals of Long-Term Care, 15*(4), 40–44.

Chait, M. M. (2008). The new era of *C. difficile*-associated diarrhea. *Annals of Long-Term Care, 16*(7), 25–31.

Chey, W. D., & Wong, B. C. Y. (2007). American College of Gastroenterology guideline on the management of *Helicobacter pylori* infection. *American Journal of Gastroenterology, 102*(8), 1808–1825.

Dienstag, J. L. (2008). Hepatitis B virus infection. *New England Journal of Medicine, 359*(14), 1486–1500.

Ehrenpreis, E. D. (2005). Irritable bowel syndrome. *Geriatrics, 60*(1), 25–28.

Freston, J. W. (2004). Therapeutic choices in reflux disease: Defining the criteria for selecting a proton pump inhibitor. *American Journal Medicine, 117*(Suppl 5A), 14S–22S.

Lacy, B. E., & Cole, M. S. (2004). Constipation in the older adult. *Clinical Geriatrics, 12*(11), 44–54.

Lyon, C., & Clark, D. C. (2006). Diagnosis of acute abdominal pain in older patients. *American Family Physician, 74*(9), 1537–1544.

Minocha, A. (2005). Irritable bowel syndrome in the older patient. *Clinical Geriatrics, 13*(4), 19–24.

Palmer, J. L., & Metheny, N. A. (2008). Preventing aspiration in older adults with dysphagia. *American Journal of Nursing, 108*(2), 40–48.

Peppas, G., Bliziotis, I. A., Oikonomaki, D., & Falagas, M. E. (2007). Outcomes after medical and surgical treatment of diverticulitis: A systematic review of the available evidence. *Journal of Gastroenterology and Hepatology, 22*(9), 1360–1368.

Ramakrishnan, K., & Salinas, R. C. (2007). Peptic ulcer disease. *American Family Physician, 76*(7), 1005–1012.

Sharma, S., Habib, S., & Agrawal, P. (2008). Hepatitis C virus infection in the elderly population. *Clinical Geriatrics, 16*(5), 38–48.

Silverblatt, A., & Eisen, G. (2007). Current status of screening for colon cancer in older adults. *Clinical Geriatrics, 15*(1), 33–37.

Tabloski, P. A. (2006). *Gerontological nursing.* Upper Saddle River, NJ: Pearson Education.

Tarik, S. H. (2008). Constipation in long-term care. *Annals of Long-Term Care, 16*(12), Supplement.

Tazkarji, M. B. (2008). Abdominal pain among older adults. *Geriatrics and Aging, 11*(7), 410–415.

van Zanten, S. V. (2008). Diagnosis and management of gastroesophageal reflux disease and dyspepsia among older adults. *Geriatrics and Aging, 11*(6), 363–367.

Wolf, D. C. (2008). *Viral hepatitis.* Retrieved from http://emedicine.medscape.com/article/185463-overview

Renal and Urologic Disorders

MJ Henderson, MS, RN, GNP-BC

GERIATRIC APPROACH

Normal Changes of Aging

Prerenal Changes

- Impaired thirst perception predisposes patient to dehydration

Renal Changes (see Table 11-1)

- Renal blood flow decreased because of sclerosis of pre- and postglomerular arterioles
  - Decrease in renal blood flow of 50% by age 80
  - The kidneys compensate with increased arteriolar resistance to maintain filtration; however, stress can cause the compensatory mechanism to fail
- Glomerular filtration rate (GFR) decreased because of increased number of sclerotic and nonfunctioning glomeruli
  - After age 40, GFR declines; most people have a decrease of *more than* 30% by age 70
  - However, one-third of older persons who are free of renal and cardiovascular disease—have well-preserved kidney function
  - Reduced GFR leads to reduced clearance of toxins, some electrolytes, and medications

Postrenal Changes in Older Adults Predisposed to Renal Damage

- Females commonly experience mucosal atrophy, increasing risk for incontinence and infection
- In males, enlargement of the prostate may cause urethral obstruction

Table 11-1. Age-Related Changes in the Renal System Due to Decreased Renal Blood Flow and GFR

Function	Age Related Change Noted by the 8th Decade	Consequences
Maximum concentration of urine	20% to 30% decrease	Increased risk of volume loss
Dilutional capacity	Decreased	May predispose to overhydration and hyponatremia after vigorous fluid administration, causing pulmonary or cerebral edema
Sodium handling	Impaired	Increased risk of volume, acidosis, and either hypernatremia or hyponatremia
Formation of NH_4^+ (ammonia)	Decreased 20%	Impaired ability to correct acidosis
Synthesis of renin	Decreased	Serum abnormalities such as hyperkalemia, hypocalcemia, and elevated parathyroid activity
Renin response to volume loss	Decreased	Inability to autoregulate in effort to maintain acceptable perfusion when renal blood flow decreases

Clinical Implications

History
- Chronic medical conditions such as diabetes or hypertension that affect renal function
- Medications for hypertension and other nephrotoxins to which they have been exposed
- Genitourinary symptoms
- Symptoms that are affected by renal function, such as cardiovascular, respiratory, neurologic, and hematologic changes
- Fatigue, edema, weight changes, and change in mental or functional status
- Allergies, especially antibiotics and dyes

Physical
- Complete physical exam
- Detection of prerenal problems, such as dehydration with skin turgor changes, condition of mucous membranes, weight changes
- Detection of postrenal problems, such as BPH mucosal atrophy

Assessment

Table 11-2. Possible Implications of Renal Symptoms

Symptom	Possible Implications
Pain or urgency in lower urinary tract	Acute inflammatory process (can occur even when very small quantities of urine are in bladder)
Pain in upper urinary tract	Usually secondary to distension of a hollow viscus, such as obstruction in a ureter or the urethra, or the capsule of an organ (as in pyelonephritis or nephrolithiasis).
Constant pain	Usually an infection
Colicky pain	Obstruction secondary to kidney or ureteral stones
Urinary frequency	Excess fluid intake, caffeine, diuretics, hyperglycemia Lesions of bladder or urethra Detrusor overactivity Infection
Suprapubic ache	Bladder distension
Perineal pain	Prostate pain is often perineal and may radiate to the lumbosacral spine or to the groin Women—prolapsed uterus
Weight loss and malaise	May be associated with malignancy (pain is usually a late sign of malignancy)
Urgency	Occurs secondary to trigonal or posterior urethral irritation produced by inflammation, stones, or tumor; most commonly occurs with cystitis, urinary incontinence
Dysuria	Infection or inflammation
Frequency, hesitancy, urgency and strangury (slow, painful urination)	Commonly associated with micturition disorders
Hematuria	Should be considered an indication of malignancy until proven otherwise Could also be stones, hemorrhagic cystitis, or prostate disease

- Assessment principles
  - Identification of risk for renal insufficiency in older adults prior to any surgical procedure is crucial, as mortality is as high as 60%
  - Evaluate renal function prior to procedures or surgery because of increased risk of postoperative renal failure
  - Diagnostic tests requiring contrast dyes are used with caution because of potential for adverse reactions

Treatment
- Careful administration of most pharmacologic agents because of decreased renal clearance and narrowed therapeutic index; older adults are also at increased risk for adverse drug reactions because of altered volume of distribution and impaired renal clearance of medications

- Avoid administration of nephrotoxic drugs or drugs cleared by the kidneys (digoxin, some calcium-channel blockers, NSAIDs, aminoglycosides) that can accelerate or cause side effects

ASYMPTOMATIC BACTERIURIA

Description
- Significant bacterial count in urine of a patient who has no symptoms; i.e., > 100,000 bacteria/mL urine

Etiology
- Most commonly caused by *E. coli*
- Other Gram-negative bacteria include *Proteus mirabilis*, *Klebsiella pneumoniae*, and *Staphylococcus saprophyticus*

Incidence and Demographics
- Asymptomatic bacteriuria common in older adults (for example, in 15% to 50% of institutionalized older adults)

Risk Factors
- Female gender
- Aging
- Incontinence
- Structural abnormalities in urinary tract
- Prostatic hypertrophy
- Asymptomatic calculi
- Indwelling urinary catheters

Prevention and Screening
- Hygiene
- Hydration
- Encourage complete voiding
- Avoid use of catheters, even condom catheters

Assessment
History
- No symptoms

Physical
- Usually no findings

Diagnostic studies
- Urinalysis reveals bacteria without WBC
- Urine culture may be positive

Differential Diagnosis
- Contaminated specimen
- UTI

Management
Nonpharmacologic Treatment
- Increase fluids to flush urinary tract
- Empty bladder fully and frequently to avoid stasis

Pharmacologic Treatment
- None
- Consider antibiotic therapy if patient is immunosuppressed, as in AIDS or has a malignancy

When to Consult, Refer, Hospitalize
- Usually not required

Follow-up
Expected Course
- Uneventful

Complications
- UTI, sepsis

URINARY TRACT INFECTION

Description
- Infection of one or more of the structures of the lower urinary tract
- May involve the ureter(s), bladder, or urethra

Etiology
- Most commonly caused by *E. coli*; many strains now resistant to many drugs
- Other Gram-negative bacteria from gastrointestinal tract such as *P. mirabilis*, *K. pneumoniae*, *Enterobacter* species, and *Staphylococcus* organisms
- In institutionalized older adults, staff may inadvertently transfer organisms that colonize perineum as a result of inadequate infection control measures

Incidence and Demographics
- Most frequent bacterial infection and most common reason for antibiotic use in older adults
- Prevalence reported to be 15% to 30% of females and 5% to 15% of males; prevalence may rise to 50% in institutionalized older adults
- When indwelling catheters are used, biofilm collects on the foreign body and creates medium for bacterial growth

Risk Factors
- Female gender
- History of prior UTI
- Diabetes mellitus or other immunocompromised state
- Structural urinary tract abnormalities (strictures, stones, tumors, neuropathic bladder)
- Procedures: catheterization, recent surgery
- Relaxation of pelvic supporting structures
- BPH or prostatitis
- Incontinence of urine/stool
- Cognitive impairment

- Altered barriers: use of catheters, age-related changes in genital and urethral mucosa
- Underlying neurologic conditions (such as stroke)

Prevention and Screening
- Meticulous perineal care
- Avoidance of long-term indwelling catheters in all older adults and condom catheters in males whenever possible; in patients who must have indwelling catheters, maintain closed systems
- Drinking cranberry juice/taking cranberry capsules may reduce pyuria and bacilluria
- In postmenopausal women, systemic or topical estrogen therapy markedly reduces the incidence of recurrent UTI
- For those who can void spontaneously, encourage complete voiding

Assessment
History
- Burning or pain during voiding, nocturia, frequent small voids, urgency, hematuria or cloudy urine, suprapubic/lower abdominal or low back pain
- Fever, chills
- Nonspecific complaints: fatigue, malaise, weakness, or confusion
- New or worsening incontinence of urine (especially in patients with underlying neurologic impairment or cognitive function)

Physical
- Fever, suprapubic tenderness to palpation
- CVA tenderness if upper-tract infection
- Mental status changes may be the only sign
- Males should have careful GU exam with rectal exam to evaluate prostate

Diagnostic Studies
- Bacteria and WBC in adequate clean-caught urine, or in-and-out catheter specimen
- Urine culture shows more than 100,000 bacteria/mL urine
- Consider re-culture after antibiotics completed
- Repeat or refractory infections: urine culture, renal/bladder ultrasound, or IVP
- Other tests if indicated
  - CBC with differential
  - Serum electrolytes
  - Serum BUN and creatinine
  - Blood cultures in septic-appearing patients
- If bladder outlet obstruction suspected, do in-and-out catheter specimen to determine post-void residual
- Suspicion of obstruction with an upper-tract infection requires emergent ultrasound

Differential Diagnosis
- Urethritis
- Diabetes
- Pyelonephritis
- Renal calculi
- Vaginitis
- Female urethral syndrome
- Chemical vaginitis

- Prostatitis
- Meatal stenosis

Management
Nonpharmacologic Treatment
- Hygiene measures
- Hydration
- Remove bladder catheters as soon as possible
- In patients with indwelling catheters, change catheter prior to initiating antibiotic therapy
- Surgical correction of known anatomic abnormalities
- If no contraindications, may encourage use of cranberry juice or tablets to acidify urine

Pharmacologic Treatment
- If symptoms mild, consider waiting to treat until culture results are available
- Treat moderate symptoms with empiric therapy until culture is available
- For dysuria (some with involuntarily retention), consider phenazopyridine (Pyridium)
- Antibiotics
    - Quinolones such as ciprofloxacin 250 to 500 mg b.i.d., norfloxacin 400 mg b.i.d., or ofloxacin 200 to 400 mg b.i.d.
    - Trimethoprim/sulfamethoxazole (TMP/SMZ) DS (160/800mg) b.i.d.
    - Nitrofurantoin 100 mg b.i.d. for 10 days
    - Cephalosporins such as cephalexin or cefaclor 500 mg q.i.d.; cefadroxil 1g/day or b.i.d.

How Long to Treat
- Uncomplicated first UTI in women 3 days; men usually receive 10- to 14-day courses
- In recurrent infection, longer courses of antibiotics are necessary
- Patients with indwelling catheters treated only until asymptomatic (usually 5 to 7 days), as it is impossible to sterilize their urine; prolonged antibiotic use promotes resistance

Special Considerations
- Uncomplicated cystitis is rare in men; men require further investigation of symptoms to rule out other pathological process
- Vaginal estrogen in postmenopausal women may decrease frequency of UTI

When to Consult, Refer, Hospitalize
- Consult for recurrent infections if anatomic abnormality is suspected
- Refer men to urologist for likelihood of concomitant prostatic involvement
- Hemodynamically unstable patients, or those in whom urosepsis is a potential concern, may require hospitalization or intravenous antibiotics
- Patients with signs/symptoms of fever, nausea, vomiting, confusion, or increased WBC generally require admission for IV antibiotics and close observation

Follow-up
- Check urine culture to determine susceptibility of bacteria to antibiotic

Expected Course
- If using correct antibiotic (per culture and sensitivity) signs and symptoms should dissipate at 72 hours
- Bacterial cure rates of 7% to 80% are expected for ambulatory elderly

- Patient may have asymptomatic bacteriuria
- Reculture those with atypical course
- Indwelling catheters increase morbidity and UTI

Complications
- Pyelonephritis, recurrent or relapse of infection, renal abscess, urosepsis

PYELONEPHRITIS

Description
- Infection of renal parenchyma or other portion of upper urinary tract

Etiology
- 75% of cases caused by *E. coli* organism
- 10% to 15% caused by other Gram-negative species (*P. mirabilis, K. pneumoniae, Enterobacter* organisms); 10% to 15% caused by *S. aureus* or *S. saprophyticus*
- Most common route of infections is ascension from bladder

Incidence and Demographics
- Estimated at 10 to 15 hospitalizations for acute pyelonephritis per 10,000 persons over 70

Risk Factors
- Urinary tract structural abnormalities
- Instrumentation
- Stones
- Catheters
- Diabetes or other immunocompromised states
- BPH
- Fecal incontinence

Prevention and Screening
- Hygiene
- Hydration
- Avoid catheters when possible
- May require prophylactic antibiotics if patient has frequent UTI

Assessment
History
- Fever, shaking chills, flank pain, CVA tenderness, myalgias, abdominal pain, hematuria, pyuria, dysuria, frequency, urgency, nausea, and vomiting

Physical
- Classic: acutely ill, shaking chills, high fever with CVA tenderness
- Subacute: low grade fever, low back pain

Diagnostic Studies
- Urinalysis: bacteria, WBC, + leukocyte esterase on dipstick, also present in UTI
- Urinalysis: proteinuria, casts indicate renal involvement
- Leukocytosis on CBC indicates systemic involvement
- Urine culture and sensitivity
- Urologist may order x-rays, renal ultrasound

Differential Diagnosis
- Stones in renal pelvis or proximal ureter
- Prostatitis
- TB
- Tumors
- Lower urinary tract infection
- Lower-lobe pneumonia
- Any acute abdominal infection (diverticulitis, cholecystitis, appendicitis, pancreatitis)

Management
- Acute: refer immediately for probable hospitalization
- Subacute: may be treated at home

Nonpharmacologic Treatment
- Fluids
- Nonpharmacologic relief measures for symptoms: sitz baths, warm packs, or heating pads

Pharmacologic Treatment
- Antibiotics (check creatinine clearance first for accurate dosing)
- Oral regimens for outpatient treatment
  - Ciprofloxacin 500 mg every 12 hours or other fluoroquinolone for 7 days
  - Amoxicillin/clavulanate 875/125 mg b.i.d. or 500/125 mg t.i.d. for 14 days

How Long to Treat
- Oral regimens treat 7 to 21 days, depending on severity of illness
- Chronic pyelonephritis: therapy required for 3 to 6 months
- If obstruction cannot be eliminated and recurrent UTI is common, long-term therapy is useful

Special Considerations
- Rule out renal mass/lesion if no improvement in 3 days

When to Consult, Refer, Hospitalize
- Inpatient management required if patient appears toxic or is hemodynamically unstable
- Outpatient management if patient is able to tolerate oral therapy, has adequate renal reserve and reliable supervision
- Immediate access to health care provider if condition worsens.
- Refer for urologic consultation

Follow-up
- Repeat culture 2 weeks after completion of therapy and again at 12 weeks

Expected Course
- Symptoms should resolve within 72 hours of initiation of appropriate therapy
- Advanced age may lead to less favorable outcome
- Recurrence rates as high as 15%

Complications
- Sepsis, chronic renal insufficiency, chronic pyelonephritis

URINARY INCONTINENCE

Description
- Involuntary, accidental loss of urine on a regular basis
- Not a disease state, but a clinical symptom of an underlying disease process

Etiology
- Multiple disorders interact to cause UI
- Age-related changes contribute
- *Drugs:* sedatives, hypnotics, diuretics, opioids, anticholinergics (antidepressants, antihistamines, psychotropics) and cardiac medications (calcium-channel blockers, alpha-adrenergic blockers/agonists, ACE inhibitors, beta-adrenergic agonists)
- *Acute incontinence:* sudden onset, related to an acute process or iatrogenic problem, resolves with resolution of problem
- **D**—delirium, anything that can cause delirium, depression
- **R**—restricted mobility, retention (acute)
- **I**—infection, inflammation (atrophic vaginitis or urethritis), impaction (stool)
- **P**—pharmaceuticals, polyuria (hyperglycemia, excess fluid intake, volume overload due to venous insufficiency or CHF)
- *Persistent Incontinence*
  - Stress incontinence: estrogen deficiency in women combined with pelvic floor muscle weakness, urethral hypermobility, and bladder outlet or urethral sphincter weakness
  - Urge incontinence: due to detrusor instability with or without local genitourinary conditions; CNS disorders such as stroke, dementia, parkinsonism, spinal cord injury; acute or chronic UTI; irradiation of bladder
  - Overflow incontinence: due to anatomic obstruction from prostatic enlargement, stricture, cystocele, acontractile bladder from diabetes mellitus, or spinal cord injury; neurogenic bladder from MS and other spinal cord conditions and from anticholinergic medications
  - Functional incontinence: due to physical (immobility) or cognitive disability, environmental barriers

Incidence and Demographics
- Occurs in 30% of older women and 15% of older men in community setting
- Affects 60% to 80% of nursing home residents
- Overall affects 12 million adults
- Over 10 billion dollars per year in the United States are spent on the management of incontinence
- Underreported because many consider it an inevitable consequence of aging

Risk Factors
- Depends on type of incontinence
- Dementia

Prevention and Screening
- Kegel exercises for women, regular pelvic examination to detect pathology early
- Monitor prostate for BPH and initiate therapy before symptom presents
- Initiate estrogen cream for older women

Assessment
- Confirm urinary incontinence, identify type, and identify factors that might contribute to or exacerbate problem

Table 11-3. Assessment of the Four Types of Persistent Incontinence

Type of Incontinence	History	Physical	Test
Stress	Leakage of small amounts precipitated by increased intra-abdominal pressure, as in cough	Leaks when upright, not supine, cough test when standing—loose urine, atrophic vaginitis	Normal urodynamic studies, minimal post-void residual if needed to rule out mixed incontinence
Urge	Urgency with loss of large amount of urine; inability to delay voiding; unrelated to activity or position	Prolapse, atrophic vaginitis	Urodynamic testing shows detrusor instability
Overflow	Leak small amounts of urine, a persistent dribbling, no precipitating factor	Suprapubic dullness to percussion, tenderness; may find prolapse in women, enlarged prostate in men	Post-void residual > 100 mL
Functional	Urinary accidents because of inability to toilet	Dementia, immobility	None

History
- Requires specific questions such as, "Do you have trouble with urine leaking?"
- Urgency, leaking, dribbling, burning, hesitancy, nocturia, hematuria
- Assess current medications and other provoking factors such as caffeinated drinks or alcohol
- Bladder habit pattern/record; fluid intake pattern
- GYN history

Physical
- Complete physical
- Mental status exam
- Exam of abdomen for masses, suprapubic tenderness, or fullness
- Observe voiding to detect problems with hesitancy, dribbling, or interrupted stream
- Pelvic exam to assess perineal skin, cystocele, uterine prolapse, pelvic mass, perivaginal muscle tone, atrophic vaginitis
- Estimate post-void residual by abdominal palpation and percussion or bimanual exam
- Rectal exam for perineal sensation, resting and active sphincter tone, rectal mass and fecal impaction; assess consistency and contour of prostate
- Neurological exam with deep tendon reflex, sensation; normal sphincter tone indicates intact neurological system to the bladder
- Musculoskeletal exam for secondary causes such as weakness, ambulation problems

Diagnostic Studies
- Urinalysis and culture to rule out UTI, glycosuria
- Serum BUN and creatinine may reveal decreased renal function
- Serum glucose to rule out diabetes
- Measure post-void residual urine (less than 100 mL is adequate)
- Additional tests may include
  - Urodynamic testing, such as bladder ultrasound after voiding
  - Pelvic ultrasound may reveal source of obstruction
- Other tests as indicated by suspected etiology

Differential Diagnosis
- Type of incontinence
- Urinary tract infection
- Urinary retention/obstruction
- Diabetes mellitus
- Neurologic disease

Management
- Good hygiene, frequent voiding, complete voiding, and Kegel exercises

Table 11–4. Treatment for Specific Causes of Incontinence

Type of Incontinence	Treatments, in Order of Preference
Stress	Pelvic floor muscle training (Kegels)
	Bladder training
	Estrogen cream
	Vaginal cones
	Biofeedback
	Alpha-adrenergic agonists
	Surgery
Urge	Bladder relaxants
	Estrogen cream
	Bladder training
	Pelvic floor muscle training (Kegels)
Overflow	Surgical removal of obstruction
	Bladder retraining
	Intermittent catheterization
	Indwelling catheter
Functional	Behavioral interventions
	Environmental changes
	Incontinence undergarments

Nonpharmacologic Treatment
- Increase access to toilet or commode
- Limit use of diuretics
- Dietary modifications (avoid caffeine and alcohol)
- Condom catheters in males (only as last resort)
- Incontinence pads (minimize use)

Table 11-5. Pharmacologic Treatment for Urge or Mixed Incontinence

Class	Drug	Dosage
Anticholinergic and smooth muscle relaxant	Oxybutynin (Ditropan, Ditropan XL, Oxytrol)	2.5 to 5.0 mg t.i.d./q.i.d. 5 to 20 mg p.o. q.d. 3.9 mg/day (apply patch 2x/wk)
	Tolterodine (Detrol, Detrol LA)	2 mg p.o. b.i.d. or for LA use 4 mg p.o. q.d.
Estradiol	Estradiol vaginal cream (Estrace) 1%; see Chapter 12, Gynecologic Disorders	0.5 to 2 g intravaginally/day for 2 weeks then 0.5 to 1 g 1 to 3 times per week
Muscarinic receptor antagonist	Trospium (Sanctura)	20 mg q.d. on empty stomach Dose q.d. at HS on patients > 75 years, and those with Cr Cl (creatinine clearance) < 30 mL
	Darifenacin (Enablex)	7.5 to 15 mg/day
	Solifenacin (Vesicare)	5 to 10 mg/day

Table 11-6. Pharmacologic Treatment for Stress Incontinence

Class	Drug	Dosage
Estradiol; see Chapter 12, Gynecologic Disorders	Estradiol vaginal cream (Estrace); see Chapter 12, Gynecologic Disorders	0.5 to 2 g intravaginally per day for 2 weeks, then 1 to 3 times per week

How Long to Treat
- Indefinitely or until surgical correction

When to Consult, Refer, Hospitalize
- Consult specialist for patients with stress and urge incontinence who fail to respond to behavioral therapy and initial drug treatment
- Refer atrophic vaginitis with prolapse to gynecologist
- Refer overflow incontinence, suspected BPH to urologist
- Refer neurologic abnormalities to neurologist

Follow-up
- Weekly visits until symptom controlled

Expected Course
- Prognosis is poor

Complications
- Physical: recurrent UTI, falls, skin breakdown
- Psychological: depression, social isolation, leads to nursing home placement
- Economic costs

HEMATURIA

Description
- The presence of red blood cells (RBC) in the urine
- May be microscopic (greater than 3 RBC/high-power field) or gross (visible to naked eye)

Etiology
- Infection is a frequent cause, and can be renal, bladder, or urethral
- Neoplasms anywhere in tract—blood in the urine necessitates a diagnostic study for GU cancer
- Glomerulonephritis
- Kidney stones
- Benign prostatic hypertrophy, prostatitis, epididymitis
- Tuberculosis
- Connective tissue diseases (systemic lupus erythematosus)
- Medications (anticoagulants—heparin, warfarin, aspirin, NSAIDs)

Incidence and Demographics
- Dependent on etiology
- Hematuria due to UTI is common in women

Risk Factors
- Depends on etiology

Prevention and Screening
- Prevention of infections

Assessment
History
- Determine onset and appearance
- Associated systemic symptoms: fever, chills, myalgias, weight loss or gain
- Local symptoms dysuria, nocturia, discharge

Physical
- Vital signs: hypertension may indicate renal disease; fever may indicate infectious etiology
- Genitourinary exam: lesions, tenderness, discharge
- Rectal exam: prostate enlargement, bogginess
- Abdominal exam: note tenderness, organomegaly, masses, bruits; percuss for CVA tenderness
- Extremities: lesions, rashes, edema

Diagnostic Studies
- Urinalysis, urine culture, microscopic exam of urinary sediment
- Renal function studies: BUN, creatinine
- CBC/differential, ESR: rule out infection, inflammation
- Additional testing may be ordered by GU: IVP, renal ultrasound, or cystourethrogram

Differential Diagnosis
- See Etiology

Management
- Dependent on etiology

When to Consult, Refer, Hospitalize
- Unexplained hematuria for invasive testing

Follow-up
- Depends on etiology

EVALUATING RENAL FUNCTION

Table 11–7. Interpretation of Renal Function Studies

Test	Normal	Renal Insufficiency	Renal Failure	Uremic Syndrome (End-Stage Renal Disease)	Nephrotic Syndrome
BUN	7 to 22	Increases after 50% loss of renal function	Increases by 10 to 20 mg/dL	60 to 100	Normal
Creatinine	Less than 1.0 for women; less than 1.2 for men	1.5 to 3	Above 3	5 to 6	Normal
24-hour urine for protein	Less than 200 mg/24 hr	Greater than 200 mg/24 hr		Over 3 g/24 hr	Over 3.5 g/24 hr
For creatinine clearance	Men 85 to 125 mL/min; women 75 to 115 mL/min	50 to 90 mL/min	10 to 50 mL/min	< 10 mL/min	
Change in GFR	Men 100 to 140 mL/min; women 85 to 115 mL/min	30 to 50 50% of normal	Less than 30 29% of normal	Less than 15 mL/min 10% to 15% of normal	

- GFR is the standard measure of renal function
  - It is best measured by creatinine clearance, from a 24-hour urine
  - Creatinine clearance is not sensitive to early disease
  - It can also be estimated from serum creatinine concentration, a blood test
  - It can be calculated by the following formula:
    - [(140 – patients's age) × body weight in kilograms] divided by (72 × serum) creatinine concentration
    - Take the sum above and multiply it by 0.85 for women

Elevated BUN/Creatinine
- Azotemia: increased urea (nitrogen compounds) in the blood measured by BUN (blood urea nitrogen)
- Prerenal azotemia: high BUN not caused by kidney disease but by CHF or volume depletion, as in dehydration; the most common cause of acute renal failure

- Uremia: increased urea in the urine, an older term for azotemia/elevated BUN
- Uremic syndrome: a term for advanced renal failure (end-stage renal disease), when patient has large amounts of urea in the urine; an older term, from when urea in urine was an important lab test; we now rely on serum BUN and creatinine to assess renal function
- Urea and creatinine are end products of protein metabolism; both are used as measures of kidney function; creatinine is more accurate because it is less affected by other factors
- Serum creatinine tends to remain stable despite decreased GFR because of decreased muscle mass in the older adult
- BUN/creatinine ratio is used to help decide if the problem is extrarenal (pre- or post-) or from intrinsic renal disease; the ratio decreases when the disease is in the kidney because creatinine rises more than the BUN; for example, when the patient is dehydrated, mainly the BUN rises. The creatinine rises only slightly but in renal disease the creatinine goes up along with the BUN prerenal failure BUN:creatinine ratio is > 20:1; in intrinsic renal disease less than 15:1

Proteinuria

- The presence of proteinuria means the kidney is leaking protein, usually from glomerular disease but also some nonrenal causes
- Nephrotic syndrome is proteinuria of more than 3.5 g of protein in 24-hour urine, with casts in urine; has a variety of causes
- Sediment/casts
  - Sediment is what is in the bottom of the test tube after urine has been spun in a centrifuge
  - The two important constituents of sediment are:
    - Casts: gel-like substances that form in the renal tubules and collecting ducts; they are an indication of serious renal disease
    - Crystals: not usually important in renal disease

GLOMERULAR DISEASE

Description

- Immune complex–mediated damage to glomeruli that produces thickening of the glomerular basement membrane and an associated decrease in glomerular surface area, which decreases glomerular filtration rate
- Characterized by diffuse inflammatory changes in the glomeruli and clinically by the nephrotic syndrome
- The nephrotic syndrome is the abrupt onset of hematuria, RBC casts, and proteinuria in association with hypoalbuminemia, hypercholesterolemia, and peripheral edema

Etiology

- Postinfection: after streptococcal infection or infections in surgical implants, (especially salmonella), endocarditis, hepatitis B and C
- Renal vasculitis
- Multisystem disorders: SLE; lymphoma; amyloidosis; carcinoma of lung, bladder, prostate
- Drug reactions: allopurinol, hydralazine, rifampin, captopril, lithium, probenecid, NSAIDs

Incidence and Demographics

- Unknown

Risk Factors
- Unknown

Prevention and Screening
- Early and aggressive treatment of underlying cause

Assessment
History
- Edema
- Malaise, fatigue
- Hematuria, oliguria, or anuria

Physical
- Edema, hypertension

Diagnostic Studies
- Urinalysis will demonstrate proteinuria, hematuria
- Serum creatinine, albumin, and cholesterol
- 24-hour urine to measure proteinuria and creatinine clearance
- Serum protein electrophoresis and immunophoresis
- Total serum complement
- Renal biopsy with ultrasonographic guidance

Differential Diagnosis
- Acute renal failure
- Chronic renal failure
- Cancer

Management
- Refer to nephrologist for renal biopsy and management

When to Consult, Refer, Hospitalize
- Refer to nephrologist

Follow-up
Complications
- Hypertensive encephalopathy or retinopathy
- Rapidly progressive glomerulonephritis, acute renal failure, CHF

ACUTE RENAL FAILURE (ARF)

Description
- Rapid reduction of renal function associated with elevated BUN (azotemia)
- Classified by etiology as prerenal, intrarenal, or postrenal
- Commonly but not exclusively associated with oliguria (decreased/absent urine)

Etiology
Prerenal: amount of blood flow to kidneys decreased, most common cause of ARF
- Hypovolemia from fluid loss due to diarrhea, vomiting, hemorrhage, diuretics, inappropriate fluid restriction
- CHF-decreased cardiac output

Renal: intrinsic ARF
- Acute glomerulonephritis
- Collagen vascular diseases affecting kidney (systemic lupus erythematosus [SLE]) scleroderma, Wegener granulomatosis, polyarteritis nodosa)
- Drugs such as ACE inhibitors, allopurinol, ampicillin, trimethoprim and sulfamethoxazole, cimetidine, phenytoin, methicillin, thiazides, NSAIDs, aminoglycosides
- Infection: acute pyelonephritis, others
- Infiltrative conditions: leukemia, lymphoma, sarcoidosis
- Hypercalcemia
- Vascular obstructions: clots, aneurysms, atheroembolic disease

Postrenal: obstructive ARF
- Ureteral and urethral obstruction due to prostatic hypertrophy, renal stones, urethral stricture

Incidence and Demographics
- Three times as prevalent in older adult as in the overall adult population

Risk Factors
- See Etiology

Prevention and Screening
- Early treatment of above-mentioned conditions
- ACE inhibitors have been demonstrated to decrease progression to renal failure in both diabetic and nondiabetic patients; can also precipitate ARF in dehydrated patients and may cause elevated potassium
- Blood pressure control is crucial
- Avoid dehydration

Assessment
History
- Patients may remain asymptomatic until GFR is less than 10% of normal
- Early manifestations may include only nocturia because of inability to concentrate urine
- Later: anorexia, fatigue, weakness, edema, pruritus, nausea, vomiting, constipation or diarrhea, shortness of breath, lethargy

Physical
- General: delirium, dehydration
- Vital signs: hypertension, tachycardia, tachypnea
- Skin: ecchymosis, petechiae, rash
- Lungs: crackles
- Look for evidence of infection
- Kidneys may be tender to palpation
- Bladder may be enlarged

Diagnostic Studies
- Daily increase in creatinine
- Urinalysis for sediment (casts) and protein—normal in pre- and postrenal failure
- Urine osmolarity

- Elevated BUN and creatinine
- Prerenal failure BUN/creatinine ratio greater than 20:1; in intrinsic renal disease less than 15:1
- Renal ultrasound

Differential Diagnosis
- Glomerulonephritis
- Systemic vasculitis
- Urinary tract obstruction
- Pyelonephritis

Management
Nonpharmacologic Treatment
- Refer to nephrology for care, often with dialysis

Special Considerations
- Avoid urinary catheters when feasible as they dramatically increase risk of infection

When to Consult, Refer, Hospitalize
- Refer to nephrologist or, if patient wishes, hospice

Follow-up
Expected Course
- If cause corrected promptly, failure can be reversed or progression arrested

Complications
- Pulmonary edema
- Hypertensive crisis
- Hyperkalemia
- Chronic kidney disease
- Death

CHRONIC KIDNEY DISEASE (CKD)

Description
- Decrease in GFR associated with progressive, irreversible damage to both kidneys

Etiology
- Acute renal failure untreated leads to CKD
- Most common causes of CKD
  - Diabetic nephropathy
  - Hypertensive disease
  - Glomerulonephritis
  - Atherosclerotic renovascular disease

Incidence and Demographics
- Incidence increases with age
- Older adults over 65 comprise more than one third of the dialysis population
- Males > females
- Increased incidence in non-Whites

Risk Factors
- Older adults with chronic disease
- Family history

Prevention and Screening
- Control diabetes and blood pressure
- Avoid use of NSAIDs in older adults
- Keep patients adequately hydrated
- Avoid/monitor use of contrast dyes for diagnostic testing

Assessment
History
- Symptoms are same as ARF but present less acutely

Physical
- Hypertension
- Peripheral neuropathies with sensory and motor deficits
- In late stages
  - Confusion
  - Breathlessness
  - Intractable hiccups
  - Yellow-brown skin

Diagnostic Studies
- Significant proteinuria and urinary casts
- Decreased creatinine clearance
- Plasma sodium concentrations may be normal or slightly reduced
- Metabolic acidosis with CO_2 level between 15 and 20 mmol/L
- Low levels of serum calcium and phosphorus are common
- Potassium may be elevated
- Normochromic normocytic anemia
- Reduced kidney size on ultrasound

Differential Diagnosis
- Urinary tract obstruction
- Vasculitis
- Pyelonephritis

Management
Nonpharmacologic Treatment
- Dietary restrictions required to maintain appropriate fluid and electrolyte balance
- Protein restricted to 20 to 25 g per day of balanced amino acid protein source
- Potassium restriction to 2 g per day may be required
- Phosphate should be limited (eggs, dairy, meat)

  DIALYSIS
  - Hemodialysis is the mode of choice; is equivalent to 10% to 15% of normal renal function
  - Peritoneal dialysis may be better tolerated by those with unstable cardiovascular status; in these individuals, sudden volume or electrolyte shifts can cause hypotension, ischemia, or arrhythmias

TRANSPLANTATION
- In recent years, more older adults have been deemed eligible for transplantation, as there have been demonstrated benefits; the major complications are infection, rejection, and cardiovascular disease

Pharmacologic Treatment
- To remove excess free water if kidneys lose the ability to regulate sodium, diuretics (such as furosemide) can be used; usually not problematic until late in course
- Acidosis may require treatment with sodium bicarbonate if symptomatic (fatigue, tachypnea, lethargy)
- Hyperphosphatemia may require phosphate binders such as oral calcium acetate or calcium carbonate to prevent development of renal osteodystrophy
- Anemia may require erythropoietin
- Bleeding: fresh-frozen plasma may be used to correct bleeding times; conjugated estrogens have been used for bleeding as well
- Aldosterone resistance may require fludrocortisone (Florinef) and potassium-binding resins

How Long to Treat
- Indefinitely

Special Considerations
- Impairments due to renal failure
- Water balance
  - Loss of ability to dilute urine leads to fluid retention and decreased sodium
- Acid-base balance
  - Dietary protein metabolism produces hydrogen ion (H^+), causing metabolic acidosis
  - The body compensates with respiratory alkalosis and by taking calcium from bones
- Altered calcium and phosphate
  - Decreased phosphate excretion leads to increased calcium release from bones, which leads to osteoporosis
- Sodium
  - Reduced ability to maintain sodium homeostasis
  - Inability to eliminate extra sodium leads to fluid retention, hypertension, and edema
  - Too little sodium leads to hypovolemia and decreased renal blood flow
- Potassium: becomes a problem later in CKD
  - Kidney loses ability to excrete K^+, which leads to elevated potassium level
- Lipid disorders
  - Kidney participates in clearing fat from bloodstream
- Anemia
  - Reduction in production of erythropoietin leads to anemia

When to Consult, Refer, Hospitalize
- Refer to nephrologist when renal failure is suspected
- Patient may require dialysis or transplantation
- Refer to urologist if obstruction or other surgically correctable conditions are suspected
- Refer to hospice if transplantation and dialysis are not options or if patient refuses treatment

Follow-up

Expected Course

- If untreated and creatinine rises to > 10, death is imminent within 3 to 5 months
- Patients asking to be taken off dialysis because of poor quality of life is the leading cause of death in dialysis patients older than 70 years

Complications

- Anemia
- Malnutrition
- CHF
- Infection
- Bleeding
- Death

CASE STUDIES

Case 1. A 94-year-old female patient with dementia returned home from the hospital for hip surgery with a Foley catheter. She complains of hip pain but not low back pain or suprapubic tenderness. She has been incontinent of bowel and bladder for many years. She requires total care. Patient is afebrile.

1. What lab tests would you order?

Lab: Her creatinine is 1.2 and her BUN is 36. Urinalysis shows many bacteria, no WBC.

2. How do you interpret this lab work?
3. What are your initial interventions?

Lab: The nurse obtains a urine culture and C&S without your order. It shows 10,000 colonies each of 3 microorganisms, which are sensitive to ciprofloxin, sulfamethoxazole/trimethoprim, and levofloxacin (Levaquin).

4. Would you treat the patient with an antibiotic?
5. What would the urinalysis show if the patient did have a UTI?
6. What are the possible complications of a UTI in this patient?

Case 2. While talking to a 74-year-old female patient, you discover that she has stopped going downstairs for meals in her senior apartment building. She has also stopped going on trips and does not have enough groceries. She denies any pain or fatigue. Seems reluctant to talk about it. Admits to urinary frequency.
History: Upon questioning, patient is afraid she might not make it to the bathroom in time, so has restricted her activities. Urinates every 1 to 2 hours so she won't be incontinent. Still has an occasional accident, in which she loses a large amount of urine.

1. What is the significance of loss of a large amount of urine?
2. What risk factors would you inquire about?
3. What medications can contribute to incontinence?
4. What treatment is effective for her type of incontinence?
5. What medications would you consider?

Case 3. An 83-year-old man has been taking ibuprofen for 20 years for degenerative joint disease. He also has hypertension, for which he takes hydrochlorothiazide. His blood pressure today is 160/94. He states that is what it usually is and that is fine with him. Routine screening lab shows BUN of 64 and creatinine of 1.8.

1. What is your initial assessment?
2. What other lab tests would you order? What would you look for?
3. Which diuretic is most effective in patients with renal insufficiency?
4. What complications should you monitor for?

REFERENCES

Alexander, I. M., & Knight, K. A. (2005). *100 questions & answers about menopause.* Sudbury, MA: Jones & Bartlett.

Barry, M. J., Fowler, F. J., Jr., O'Leary, M. P., Bruskewitz, R. C., Holtgrewe, H. L., Mebust, W. K., et al. (1992). The American Urological Association symptoms index for benign prostatic hyperplasia. *Journal of Urology, 148,* 1549–1557.

Brown, J. S., Vittinghoff, E., Wyman, J. F., Stone, K. L., Nevitt, M. C., Ensrud, K. E., et al. (2000). Urinary incontinence: Does it increase risk for falls and fractures? *Journal of the American Geriatrics Association, 48,* 721–725.

Burgio, K. L., Goode, P. S., Locher, J. L., Umlauf, M. G., Roth, D. L., Richter, H. E., et al. (2002). Behavioral training with and without biofeedback in the treatment of urge incontinence in older women. *JAMA, 288*(18), 2293–2299.

Ellerkmann, R. M., & McBride, A. (2003). Management of obstructive voiding dysfunction. *Drugs Today, 39*(7), 513–540.

Grodstein, F., Fretts, R., Lifford, K., Resnick, N., & Curhan, G. (2003). Association of age, race, and obstetric history with urinary symptoms among women in the Nurses' Health Study. *American Journal of Obstetrics & Gynecology, 189,* 428–434.

Liu, C. C., Wang, C. J., Huang, S. P., Chou, Y. H., Wu, W. J., & Huang, C. H. (2004). Relationships between American Urological Association symptom index, prostate volume, and disease-specific quality of life question in patients with benign prostatic hyperplasia. *Kaohsiung Journal of Medical Science, 20*(6), 273–278.

Miller, L. G., & Tang, A. W. (2004). Treatment of uncomplicated urinary tract infections in an era of increasing antimicrobial resistance. *Mayo Clinic Proceedings, 79*(8), 1048–1053.

Ouslander, J. G., Maloney, C., Grasela, T. H., Rogers, L., & Walawander, C. A. (2001). Implementation of a nursing home urinary incontinence management program with and without tolterodine. *Journal of the American Medical Directors Association, 2,* 207–214.

Reuben, D. B. (Ed.) (2009). *Geriatrics at your fingertips 2008–2009* (10th ed.). New York: American Geriatrics Society.

Srulevich, M., & Chopra, A. (2008). Voiding disorders in long term care. *Annals of Long-Term Care and Aging, 16*(12;suppl 1), 39–45.

Tan, T. L. (2003). Urinary incontinence in older persons. A simple approach to a complex problem. *Annals Academy Medicine Singapore, 32*(6), 731–739.

Yoshimura, N., & Chancellor, M. B. (2002). Current and future pharmacological treatment for overactive bladder. *Journal of Urology, 168,* 1897–1913.

Gynecologic Disorders

Vaunette Fay, PhD, RN, FNP-BC, GNP-BC

GERIATRIC APPROACH

Normal Changes of Aging

- For women, menopause is a normal change of aging
  - Loss of bone mass puts patient at increased risk for osteopenia or osteoporosis and fractures
  - Breast: involution of glandular structures after menopause; breast density decreases with age; glandular breast tissue replaced by fat, with increased risk for breast cancer
  - Urogenital atrophy: thinning and shrinkage of vulva; thinning of vagina wall and loss of rugae, leading to thin, friable tissue; increased pH, less acidic environment; decreased lubrication; cervix atrophy
  - Atrophy of the urethra and bladder mucosal thinning, sphincter weakening, decrease in bladder capacity, all of which contribute to urinary frequency and stress incontinence
  - Body composition changes, with the percentage of body fat increasing and muscle mass decreasing

Clinical Implications

History

- Many women accept gynecologic symptoms as inevitable and are reluctant to seek help
- Susceptible to recurrent urinary tract infections because of decreased estrogen levels and increased pH in vagina
- Often feel pelvic exams and Papanicolau tests are no longer needed
- Often feel that a hysterectomy has eliminated any risk of gynecologic cancer, although they are still at risk for ovarian, vulvar, and vaginal cancer

- Sexual activity should be a part of the history

Physical
- Many patients will have arthritis, with stiff joints and pain that will make the lithotomy position difficult or impossible; they may only be able tolerate the position for a short amount of time
- If unable to get into the lithotomy positions, a limited exam can be done with patient on her back or side with one leg raised and supported; a speculum exam may not be possible, but the external genitalia will be accessible to exam
- Delicate, friable tissue will make insertion of speculum difficult and likely to cause bleeding, which will then be difficult to differentiate from abnormal vaginal bleeding
- Use smaller speculum; Pederson and pediatric specula available
- Breast exam: may do initial exam with patient in sitting position

Assessment
- Carefully evaluate the risks of the expected conditions and their treatment vs. the benefits of treatment or nontreatment before embarking on an extensive diagnostic study in the geriatric patient; include the patient in the decision-making process.
- Dementia may lead to an inability to tolerate the gynecologic exam; for example, older women may interpret an exam as rape and have a catastrophic reaction
- While less common in older adults, sexually transmitted infections (STI) should remain in your differential
- Up to 20% of HIV-positive individuals are now older adults

Treatment
- In general, age alone should not determine whether or not a patient receives optimal therapy for a gynecologic cancer; many older adults can tolerate and benefit from full treatment; a well-informed patient can choose her plan of care

MENOPAUSE

Description
- Perimenopause defined as the time during which age-related biologic reduction in ovarian function results in gradual end of fertility and absence of menstrual periods
- Menopause defined as the point at which menstrual function stops because of loss of ovarian activity; only identified in retrospect, after cessation of menses for 1 year
- Many gynecologic disorders in older adults are due to hormonal changes of menopause

Etiology
- Estrogen and progestin production wanes, reducing inhibition of hypothalamic pituitary axis, which results in gradual rise in follicle-stimulating hormone (FSH)
- Perimenopause confirmed when FSH levels reach > 20 IU/L despite continued menses
- Estrogen production in the postmenopausal ovary is minimal; most is produced by the adrenal glands; the postmenopausal ovary continues to produce androgens
- Fluctuation in estrogen level is responsible for perimenopausal symptoms

Incidence and Demographics
- Average age at perimenopause is 47 years; duration of perimenopause is approximately 3.5 years
- Average age of biological menopause is 51, typical age range 45 to 55

- About 10% of women have abrupt cessation of menses; 90% have menstrual changes prior to menstrual cessation
- About 1% of women experience menopause before age 40 (premature ovarian failure)
- Artificial menopause can occur any time that the ovaries are removed or irradiated, before biologic failure occurs

Risk Factors
- Normal change of aging
- Hysterectomy
- Family history of early or late menopause

Assessment
History
- Symptoms vary in individuals because of nonovarian production of estrogen, as in obesity
- Menstrual cycle irregularity, hot flushes, and sweats (vasomotor instability); sleep disturbances, fatigue; irritability, mood changes; vaginal dryness, urinary complaints
- Hot flushes, also called hot flashes, are the predominant complaint
  - Sudden, transient sensation of heat that spreads through body, especially chest, face, and head
  - Accompanied by increased heart rate and profuse sweating
  - Frequently occur during night, causing increase in nighttime awakenings and fatigue during day
- Many women have other symptoms such as decreased libido and depression; these are not a direct effect of menopause but are due to the above changes
- Obtain history of hormone use including hormone replacement therapy (HRT) and oral contraceptives

Physical
- Cardiac exam: for cardiovascular disease
- Musculoskeletal exam: for osteoporosis
- Breast exam: increased risk for breast cancer after menopause
- Pelvic exam
  - Lighter pink vagina; thin with fewer rugae; smaller labia; dry to little thin, watery discharge
  - Vaginal pH 5.5 to 7 (a rise over premenopausal levels of approximately 4.0)
  - Cervix is atrophied
  - Uterus and ovaries smaller
  - Leiomyomata or adenomyosis reduced

Diagnostic Studies
- Labs: not generally required
- Fluctuation of FSH, luteinizing hormone (LH), and estradiol levels common until menopause
- Within 1 year of cessation of menses, 3- to 4-fold increase in FSH and 3-fold increase in LH (confirm ovarian failure) with estradiol levels below 20 pg/mL
- Papanicolau test, wet prep, maturational index: more parabasal cells and fewer intermediate and superficial cells (changes consistent with reduced estrogen)
- Vaginal atrophy
  - Abnormal amount of WBC (greater than 10 per high-power field) on wet prep

- Reduced or absent of lactobacilli: reflects increase in vaginal pH > 5
- Abnormal flora, including pathogenic bacteria, may be present
- Any vaginal specimen with blood should prompt a work-up for cervical or uterine bleeding sources; minimal trauma during the examination should not cause vaginal bleeding (except the use of a Cytobrush, which often causes slight spotting)
- Endometrial biopsy recommended if:
  - Cessation of menses for more than 6 months, then vaginal bleeding
  - Bleeding more often than every 3 weeks
  - Bleeding longer than 8 days
  - Increased amount of bleeding with clots

Consequences of Menopause

- Urogenital atrophy
  - Thinning of vulva and vagina lead to thin, friable tissue; increased vaginal pH; less acidic environment; decreased secretions lead to increased risk for infection and dyspareunia
  - Atrophy of the urethra and bladder trigone may lead to urinary frequency, urgency, and urge incontinence (may occur months to years later)
- Osteoporosis (also see section in Chapter 14, Musculosketelal Disorders)
  - Increased bone resorption and decreased bone formation
  - Postmenopausal women who smoke have lower bone density, putting them at an increased risk for hip fracture

Differential Diagnosis

- Depression
- Thyroid and other endocrine disorders
- Hot flushes
- Pheochromocytoma
- Cancer
- Leukemia
- Thyroid tumors
- Pancreatic tumors

Vaginal atrophy

- Infectious vaginitis (trichomoniasis, yeast)
- Bacterial vaginosis
- Vulvar or vaginal cancer
- Diabetes

Management

- Management goals: symptom relief, prevention of long-term complications

Nonpharmacologic Treatment

- Hot flushes: eliminate precipitating factors such as hot drinks, alcohol, caffeine, warm environment, stress, tobacco
- Vitamin B complex, vitamin E may be helpful
- Many women try natural remedies such as soy; none have been proven effective
  - Kegel exercises to prevent urinary incontinence
  - Vaginal lubricants such as KY jelly for coitus;
    - Petroleum jelly and other oil-based lubricants increase the risk of bacterial growth
  - Vaginal atrophy
    - Limit use of perfumed products that can cause genital area irritation; use cotton undergarments (synthetic materials may cause irritation)

- For patients with dysuria, adding cranberry juice to diet may help urinary symptoms
- Water-soluble lubricants before coitus

Pharmacologic Treatment
- Perimenopause may be managed with low-dose oral contraceptives
  - These include the brands Alesse, Ortho Tri-Cyclen, Desogen, Loestrin
  - Estrogen dose in oral contraceptives is about 4 times greater than menopausal therapy estrogens
  - Prevents inadvertent pregnancy
  - Low androgenic progestin recommended
  - Progestin alone if estrogen contraindicated
  - Transdermal clonidine 0.1 mg/day patch once a week for hot flashes and other symptoms

  ### HORMONE REPLACEMENT THERAPY (HRT)
  - The Women's Health Initiative study has changed what the medical profession thinks about HRT
    - Long-term estrogen and estrogen plus progestin increase the risk for breast cancer
    - HRT is not recommended for the primary indication of protecting women against coronary heart disease (CHD); may reduce risk for CHD when started in early menopause
    - HRT may increase the risk for CHD among women who are farther into menopause when therapy is started, especially during the first year after the initiation of hormone use
    - HRT increases the risk for thromboembolic events and stroke
  - Other research suggests HRT may increase risk for dementia
  - Many formulations of estrogen and progestin for HRT are available
    - North American Menopause Society (NAMS) recommends lowest effective dose of estrogen that meets the treatment goals
  - See Table 12–1 for some of the more common products

  ### CURRENT RECOMMENDATIONS
  - The U.S. Preventive Services Task Force concluded that the harmful effects of combined HRT exceed the benefits in most women
  - In those individuals who desire to have or continue HRT, treatment regimen should be individualized
    - Begin HRT at time of menopause
    - Give the lowest dose of estrogen needed to alleviate vasomotor instability and other symptoms
    - Women who still have a uterus must take progesterone in addition to estrogen to prevent endometrial cancer; estrogen alone is adequate in women without a uterus
  - Use for a limited number of years
  - HRT usually given orally as either continuous or cyclic therapy
    - Usually begin with cyclic therapy, as it reduces the risk for withdrawal bleeding
    - Usually change to continuous therapy after about a year
      » More convenient regime

» Less breakthrough bleeding
» Many have better relief of vaginal atrophy with combination HRT

BENEFICIAL EFFECTS OF HRT
- Vasomotor stability and sleep patterns improve
- Urogenital atrophy is diminished
    - Vaginal estrogen best for prevention or alleviation of symptoms of atrophy
        » May be used in addition to oral HRT
- Osteoporosis
    - HRT will stabilize osteoporosis and prevent further deterioration
    - HRT will not stimulate new bone growth
    - Adequate calcium and exercise are also required
- Colon cancer: HRT decreases the risk for colon cancer

ADVERSE EFFECTS OF HRT
- Estrogen alone greatly increases risk for endometrial cancer; also increases risk for breast cancer
- Possible increased risk of CHD; increased risk for thromboembolic events and stroke, dementia
- Common estrogen therapy side effects include nausea, breast tenderness, mood swings, migraines (like menstrual migraines)
- Common progestin side effects include nausea, acne, headaches
- Progestin may also cause PMS-type symptoms (irritability) and breast tenderness until cessation of menses is complete
- Common androgenic side effects of progestin include acne and hirsutism

ABSOLUTE CONTRAINDICATIONS TO ESTROGEN THERAPY
- Current or history of ovarian or breast cancer, undiagnosed breast mass
- Thromboembolia, unexplained genital bleeding, endometrial cancer (unopposed estrogen)

PRECAUTIONS TO USE OF ESTROGENS OR "RELATIVE CONTRAINDICATIONS"
- Seizure disorder, hypertension, familial hyperlipidemia, migraines, gallbladder disease, past history of thrombosis, high risk for breast cancer

TRANSDERMAL OR VAGINAL ROUTE PREFERRED OVER ORAL ESTROGENS IN THE FOLLOWING
- Chronic impaired liver function, significant liver disease/liver tumors (increased growth of benign vascular tumors in 1950s studies) because it misses the first-pass effect through the liver and allows for lower doses
- Migraines (risk for stroke, increased migraines due to estrogen use in one-third of patients)
- Active or history of thrombophlebitis or thromboembolic disorders
- Vaginal cream used for atrophic vaginitis; can help reverse genitourinary changes, may have some systemic effect; initial rapid absorption can cause breast tenderness; overall systemic estrogen absorption during local therapy is negligible

How Long to Treat
- Treat perimenopause with low-dose oral contraceptives for about 1 year, then switch to HRT

- Recommendation: limit use of HRT to 5 to 7 years, as risk for adverse effects rises with duration of use
- Discontinue treatment if patient develops contraindications to use or significant adverse reaction to medication

Table 12-1. Hormone Replacement Therapy Choices

Drug Class	Trade	Form	Strength	Starting Dose	Comment
Estrogens					
Conjugated equine estrogens	Premarin	Tablet	0.3, 0.625, 0.9 mg	0.625 q.d.	Continuous— no uterus
		Cream	0.625 mg/gram	0.5 to 2 g every night	Gradually taper to lowest dose to maintain vaginal mucosa
Synthetic conjugated estrogens	Cenestin	Tablet	0.625, 0.9, 1.25 mg	Cyclic: 0.625, 3 weeks on, 1 week off	Cyclic
		Vaginal cream	0.5, 1.0, 1.1, 2.0 mg	0.5 to 2 g every night	Gradually taper to lowest dose to maintain vaginal mucosa
17 beta estradiol	Estrace	Tablet	0.5, 1.0, 2.0 mg	1 mg q.d.	
	Estrace	Cream	1%	2 to 4 g q.d. × 2 weeks then 1 to 3 doses/week	Gradually taper to lowest dose to maintain vaginal health
	Estring	Vaginal ring	One ring	every 90 days	Reassess need every 3 to 6 months
	Alora, Climara, Estraderm	Patch	0.37, 0.5, 0.75, 0.1 mg	0.05 mg/day	Change 1 to 2x/week depending on brand
	Vagifem	Vaginal tab	25 mcg	q.d. for 2 weeks then 2x/week	

continued

Table 12–1. Hormone Replacement Therapy Choices (cont.)

Drug Class	Trade	Form	Strength	Starting Dose	Comment
Esterified estrogen	Menest	Tablet	0.3, 0.625, 1.25, 2.5 mg	0.625 mg q.d.	
Estropipate	Ogen, Ortho-Est	Tablet	0.625, 1.25, 2.5 mg	0.75 mg q.d.	
Ethinyl estradiol	Estinyl	Tablet	0.02, 0.05 mg	Cyclic: 0.02 mg every 1 to 2 days, 3 weeks on, 1 week off	
Progestins					
Medroxyprogesterone acetate	Amen, Cycrin, Provera	Tablet	2.5, 5, 10 mg	Cyclic: 5 to 10 mg for 10 to 14 days; continuous: 2.5 to 5 mg q.d.	
Norethindrone acetate	Aygestin	Tablet	5 mg	2.5 to 5 mg q.d.	
Micronized progesterone	Prometrium	Tablet	100 mg	200 to 400 mg q.d. for 10 to 14 days	
	Crinone	Vaginal gel	4% (45 mg/dose); 8% (90 mg/dose)	45 mg q.o.d. × 6 doses	
Combination					
Conjugated estrogen (Medroxyprogesterone acetate: MPA)	Prempro	Tablet	03/1.5 mg 0.45/1.5 mg 0.625/2.5 mg 0.625/5 mg	1 tab q.d. in EZ dial dispensers	
	Premphase	Tablet	0.625 estrogen days 1 to 14; 5 mg MPA added days 15 to 28	1 tab q.d. in EZ dial dispensers	
Esterified estrogen (methyl-testosterone)	Estratest, Estratest HS	Tablet	1.25 mg/2.5 mg 0.625/1.25 mg	Cyclic: 0.625/1.25 3 weeks on, 1 week off	

continued

Table 12-1. Hormone Replacement Therapy Choices (cont.)

Drug Class	Trade	Form	Strength	Starting Dose	Comment
Estradiol, norethindrone	Activelle	Tablet	1 mg/0.5 mg	1 q.d.	Continuous, intact uterus
17 beta-estradiol, norethindrone acetate	CombiPatch	Patch	0.05/0.14 0.05/0.25	0.05/0.14 q.d.	
Ethinyl estradiol, norethindrone	FemHRT	Tabs	5 mcg/1 mg	1 q.d.	

Special Considerations
- Include patient's preferences and needs when selecting HRT

When to Consult, Refer, Hospitalize
- If patient has absolute or relative contraindications for HRT
- Adverse reaction to HRT
- Usual HRT not satisfactory to patient, usually because of breakthrough bleeding

Follow-up
Complications
- Adverse effects of HRT
- Adverse effects of menopause
- Vaginal atrophy
  - Pelvic prolapse
  - Urinary incontinence
- Osteoporosis
  - Kyphosis
  - Fractures
  - Disability

POSTMENOPAUSAL VAGINAL BLEEDING

Description
- Vaginal bleeding that occurs 6 months or more following menopause
- Not due to hormone replacement therapy

Etiology
- Atrophic endometrium, vaginitis
- Endometrial proliferation
- Hyperplasia
- Endometrial or cervical cancer
- Administration of estrogens without added progestin
- Anticoagulant administration

Incidence and Demographics
- Common

Risk Factors
- Endometrial hyperplasia and endometrial carcinoma

- Genitourinary problems
- Thyroid disease
- Thrombocytopenia
- Blood dyscrasia

Prevention and Screening
- Always combine estrogen therapy with progestin in patients who still have a uterus
- Periodic pelvic exams to assess uterus size

Assessment
- Any postmenopausal bleeding must be evaluated thoroughly because of risk for cancer

History
- Timing, duration, amount
- Usually painless
- May report single episode of spotting or profuse bleeding for days or months
- Vaginal discharge, pain, heat/cold intolerance, bleeding or bruising, weight changes
- Associated activity
- Bowel or bladder symptoms
- Anticoagulants, NSAIDs, aspirin

Physical
- Thyroid nodules, enlargement, tenderness
- Hepatomegaly, abdominal pain, guarding, rebound pain
- Pelvic: vulvar or vaginal bleeding, lesions, or neoplasms
- Rectal blood, hemorrhoids

Diagnostic Studies
- Cytologic smear of the cervix and vaginal pool
- CBC, TSH
- Transvaginal sonogram of uterus to rule out vaginal wall thickening (< 5mm virtually excludes malignancy)
- Endometrial biopsy

Differential Diagnosis
- Endometrial polyps
- Hyper-/hypothyroidism
- Urinary tract infection
- Atrophic vaginitis
- Cancer
- Endometriosis
- Fibroids
- Thrombocytopenia
- Coagulopathy
- Blood dyscrasia

Management
- Treat any causes identified as indicated

Nonpharmacologic Treatment
- Dilation and curettage (D&C) should be offered to all postmenopausal women with vaginal bleeding
- Hysterectomy if endometrial hyperplasia with atypical cells or carcinoma is found

Pharmacologic Treatment
- Simple endometrial hyperplasia: cyclic progestin therapy for 21 days of each month for 3 months with repeat D&C

When to Consult, Refer, Hospitalize
- Refer all cases to gynecologist
- Consider admission for acute management of heavy bleeding

Follow-up
Expected Course
- Dependent on etiology

Complications
- Dependent on etiology

PELVIC PROLAPSE

Description
- Loss of normal pelvic support, allows descent and herniation of these organs
- Symptomology depends upon degree and location of the pelvic prolapse
- May present as
  - Uterine/vaginal prolapse
  - Cystocele: bulge of bladder into vagina
  - Rectocele: bulge of rectum into vagina
  - Enterocele: bulge of small intestine into vagina

Etiology
- Multiparous with vaginal delivery
- Menopause: lack of estrogen
- Aging process: decreased tissue turgor
- Hysterectomy

Incidence and Demographics
- Incidence unknown due to underreporting
- Estimate 15% to 30% of multiparous women have some degree of pelvic prolapse

Risk Factors
- See Etiology

Prevention and Screening
- Rectocele: avoid constipation

Assessment
- Correlate symptoms to clinical findings
- Graded by severity: leading edge of prolapsing organ
  - Mild (also called a first degree): descending halfway to the vaginal introitus
  - Moderate: descent to the introitus
  - Severe (fourth degree): prolapsed beyond introitus

History
- Pelvic pressure or heaviness
- Complaint of protrusion or bulge through the vagina
- Irritation with walking or exercising secondary to a bulge felt in the vagina
- Feeling of obstruction in the vagina
- Urinary and/or bowel dysfunction

- Low back pain
- Chronic pelvic aching
- Decrease in pain or pressure when lying down
- Sexual dysfunction and painful intercourse

Physical
- Examine in lithotomy and standing positions to evaluate degree of prolapse
- Have patient strain—Q-tip test
- Bimanual exam and rectovaginal exam
- Repeat in standing position
- Bladder-function studies: for women with urinary incontinence symptoms (Cystocele)
- Pelvic floor strength tests: strength of pelvic floor and sphinter muscles; helpful in determining if patient will benefit from Kegel exercises

Diagnostic Studies
- None

Differential Diagnosis
- Urinary incontinence
- Rectocele: constipation, incontinence of stool

Management
Nonpharmacologic Treatment
- Mild to moderate prolapse
  - Avoid stress to the pelvic floor: heavy lifting, high-impact aerobics, repetitive stooping, obesity, chronic cough
  - Kegel exercises
  - Weighted vaginal cones
- Severe
  - Intravaginal pessary if patient does not want surgery, or if surgery is contraindicated
  - Teach patient correct use; remove and clean monthly
  - If patient unable to use, may have family member insert
  - Surgical repair of the specific defect

Pharmacologic Treatment
- None

How Long to Treat
- Pessary indefinitely
- Surgery curative

Special Considerations
- Patients who are fitted with a pessary occasionally become lost to follow-up and/or demented, and the pessary may remain in the patient without cleaning for long periods of time

When to Consult, Refer, Hospitalize
- Consider surgery

Follow-up
- Pessary: see weekly until comfortable with pessary
- Pessary must be removed and cleaned monthly

Expected Course
- Variable

Complications
- Prolapse: bleeding, ulceration infection, pain, organ incarceration, urinary retention
- Pessary: infection, incarceration, erosion into bladder, rectum, or abdominal cavity

BARTHOLIN GLAND CYSTS AND ABSCESSES

Description
- Infection of the Bartholin gland (unilaterally or bilaterally), which obstructs the duct and prevents drainage; pain, swelling, abscess formation results, with chronic ductal stenosis and residual distension

Etiology
- Most common pathogen is *E. coli*
- Trauma

Incidence and Demographics
- Uncommon

Risk Factors
- None known

Prevention and Screening
- None known

Assessment
History
- Previous episodes; any prior surgical treatment (incision and drainage [I&D])
- Pain on the sides of the introitus, dyspareunia, painful sitting or walking

Physical
- Physical exam may show fluctuant mass at 4 o'clock, 8 o'clock or both; if active infection, there may be pain; size can vary up to 4 cm
- Swelling on the sides of the introitus
- Tenderness indicates active infection

Diagnostic Studies
- I&D and wound cultures should be done for gonorrhea, chlamydia, *E. coli*

Differential Diagnosis
- Inclusion cysts
- Lipoma
- Fibroma
- Hematoma
- Bartholin gland cancer (rare)

Management
Nonpharmacologic Treatment
- Cyst needs no treatment if not symptomatic

- Mild—warm soaks can alleviate pain and promote spontaneous ductal opening
- Treatment is to perform I&D or refer for marsupialization to establish new ductal opening; laser incision can also be used.
- Wound catheter can be inserted at time of I&D; suture if needed or tape into place, and let drain over 4 weeks

Pharmacologic Treatment
- None

How Long to Treat
- Warm soaks for a week; if not resolved, refer

When to Consult, Refer, Hospitalize
- Refer to gynecologist if not resolved by warm soaks

Follow-up
Expected Course
- Recurrent episodes unless patient has treatment

Complications
- Stenosis of the duct outlet with distension may persist
- Reinfection causes recurrent tenderness and enlargement of the duct

ABNORMAL GROWTHS
Benign Growths
Leiomyomas
Description
- Leiomyomas are also known as uterine fibroids, myomas
- Benign uterine smooth muscle and connective tissue growth responsive to estrogens
- Discrete, firm, roundish, often multiple in various anatomic locations: intramural, submucous, subserous, intraligamentous, pedunculated, cervical
- Mostly asymptomatic and found incidentally on examination

Incidence and Demographics
- Occurs in 4% to 11% of women; increases with age (20% of women over 35 and 40% of women over 50)

Assessment
Physical
- Occasionally causes menorrhagia (with degeneration and calcification) and anemia, dysmenorrhea, pelvic pain (enlargement, encroachment on adjacent structures, torsion), bladder pressure, and back or lower pelvic pressure
- Reduces in size and symptoms after menopause
- Enlarged, firm, irregular uterus; mobile, mostly nontender, and negative for other exam findings; clinically useful to note size comparable to gestational size ("10–12 weeks size"; "umbilicus minus 1 cm") for comparative evaluation over time

Diagnostic Studies
- Labs: HCG, CBC (iron deficiency anemia), screening Papanicolau tests and other health maintenance as indicated

- Pelvic ultrasonography can identify characteristic fibroid changes (hypoechoic, no cysts, uniform structure), map number and location, measure size, and assess normalcy of adjacent structures (endometrial thickness); helpful to rule out other concerns (such as ovarian cysts)

Differential Diagnosis
- Endometriosis
- Endometrial carcinoma
- Ovarian cysts
- Uterine cancer
- Abnormal vaginal bleeding
- Adenomyosis
- Cervical cancer
- Ovarian cancer
- Leiomyosarcoma (0.5% of fibroids; more common over age 40)

Management
Pharmacologic Treatment
- No treatment needed if asymptomatic
- Iron replacement therapy if needed
- Chronic pain
  - NSAIDs work well
  - Analgesics with narcotics only if unremitting pain, needs gynecological consultation
  - Reduce size medically (medroxyprogesterone [Depo-Provera], leuprolide [Lupron]) then surgical excision or hysterectomy

When to Consult, Refer, Hospitalize
- Consult with gynecology about options to reduce bleeding (Lupron, surgical excision, hysterectomy) and if endometrial sampling is indicated

GYNECOLOGIC CANCER
Abnormal Cervical Cytology/Cervical Cancer
Description
- Hyperplasia of the intraepithelial cells of the cervix
- Malignant transformation of intraepithelial cells of the cervix
- Invasion of the surrounding tissues occurs in 2 to 10 years

Etiology
- About 85% of cervical cancer is squamous cell carcinoma
- Endocervical adenocarcinoma is more rare
- 13% of all cancers in postmenopausal women are gynecologic cancers; risk increases with age
- Optimal treatment of patients with gynecologic cancer should not be withheld because of age

Incidence and Demographics
- The Papanicolau test has moved cervical cancer from a top killer (United States in the 1940s) to a preventable disease
- Accounts for about 20% of all gynecologic cancers

- Current lifetime risk for death by cervical cancer in the United States is 0.83%
- Average age at diagnosis of precancerous lesions is the mid-30s
- Average age at onset of cervical cancer is 45 to 55
- 25% of invasive cervical cancers and 41% of deaths occur in women over age 65
- Under-screening is the # 1 reason more than 11,000 women are diagnosed with invasive cervical cancer annually; nearly 4,000 die of cervical cancer annually (American Cancer Society)
- Half of women diagnosed with invasive cervical cancer have never been screened, and another 10% have not had a Pap in 5 years
- Least likely to be screened: older, poor, African American, Hispanic, and uninsured women

Risk Factors
Abnormal Cervical Cytology
- History of early sex, with multiple partners; STI, HPV, HIV, HSV
- Tobacco: nicotine and other substances bind to cells (cancer cofactor)
- Diethylstilbestrol (DES) exposure

Cervical Cancer
- Advanced age
- Those who have not received regular screening (Black, Hispanic and Native Americans, low socioeconomic status)

Prevention and Screening
- No smoking
- Pap smear to collect cells for analysis; highest-risk area on the uterine cervix for cancer is the "transformation zone" (TZ), where stratified squamous epithelial tissue intersects with columnar epithelial tissue
- TZ appears well outside the external os in very young women and migrates into the canal as the woman ages, or as there is disruption in the cervix (childbirth, invasive procedures, cancer treatment)
- With hormonal stimulation, the TZ may be more visible (hormonal contraception, pregnancy); in DES-exposed women, the TZ may extend into the vagina
- All women who are or have been sexually active should have regular cervical cytological screening from the time they are sexually active or 18 years old
- If 3 or more normal Paps and annual examinations, screen every 3 years; because of the prevalence of HPV and the false-negative rate of Pap smears, some clinicians will opt to screen women yearly despite this recommendation
- If not screened for 10 years prior to age 66, screen every 3 years to age 75
- Women who have had a hysterectomy in which the cervix was removed do not require cytologic screening (< 10% yield on vaginal cuff smears) but should continue to have vaginal inspection annually
- Annual cytology is advised if a hysterectomy was done to treat cervical dysplasia, cervical cancer, uterine cancer
- Remember that a hysterectomy might *not* remove the cervix; it is important to view the vagina and assess for the presence of a cervix
- If a woman happens to have two cervices, be sure to collect a Pap on each one and to label the Paps appropriately (e.g., right cervix, right Pap)

Assessment

History
- Cervical cancer is asymptomatic until well advanced
- Later symptoms include pain in lower abdomen, pelvis, or back; anorexia; urinary frequency
- Irregular vaginal bleeding or any kind of vaginal bleeding
- Assess the history of cervical cancer screening and management of any abnormalities
- Note any colposcopy, biopsy, and any past ablative or surgical therapy

Physical
- On pelvic exam, the cervix may appear normal or may have small, ulcerated lesion
- Late signs include weight loss
- If frank cervicitis noted, collect appropriate cultures or screens for common etiologies (trichomoniasis, gonorrhea, chlamydia, mycoplasma, ureaplasma, herpes simplex, syphilis)
- Collect cervical cytology specimens after treatment of cervicitis, wait at least 4 to 6 weeks
- If frank cervicitis is not cleared up, make note of this finding on the cytology lab form and strongly consider colposcopy and biopsy regardless of the cytologic results

Common complaints that suggest a cervical process
- Altered vaginal discharge (without odor or itch)
  - Unusual color or amount: suggests change in cervical mucus production or an inflammatory process that has secondary discharge
  - The most ominous etiology is advanced cervical cancer
- Vaginal bleeding
  - Vaginal bleeding of purely cervical origin is most commonly caused by cervical polyps, which can cause postdouching or postcoital bleeding (but are mostly asymptomatic)
  - Infectious diseases often cause postcoital spotting but also cause bleeding from the endometrium
  - Advanced cervical cancer can also cause frank bleeding

Diagnostic Studies
- Paramount lab test is the Pap smear
- If Pap smear is abnormal, colposcopy (examination of the cervix using a magnifying lens) and a biopsy (the collection and examination of tissue)
- Late laboratory abnormalities include hematuria, anemia
- Recall that false negatives occur from sampling error and from detection error

Reasons for inaccurate conventional cytology (Pap)
- Laboratory error (detection error): 1/3 of errors: false negatives 5%, false positives 3% to 10%
- Poor specimen collection technique (sampling error): estimated 2/3 of errors; even with excellent technique, can miss endocervical cells (ECC) in up to 10%; false negatives are more common in specimens without ECC

Thin prep
- Cervical specimen is placed directly into preservative vial
- Increases number of cells sampled by removing confounding mucus, blood, and debris
- Reduces inadequate specimens or sampling error by 50%
- Increases detection of low-grade intraepithelial lesions by 65% (screening) but only 6% in high-risk samples

Conventional Papanicolaou screening
- Pap cytology is most accurate and very specific for carcinoma or invasive cancer and high-grade lesions
- Not very specific for low grade lesions, and these are often overdiagnosed

When to Consult, Refer, Hospitalize
- Refer all abnormal Pap findings to gynecologist
- Refer cervical cancer to gynecologic oncologist for management

Follow-up
- If undetected or untreated, 15%–20% cervical lesions progress while the rest either stay stable or regress
- With appropriate management, future cancer risk is less than 5%. Many clinicians use automated cytology procedures if the patient has had therapy
- After ablative treatment, screening cytology should be repeated at accelerated intervals, commonly every 3–4 months for the first year, then every 6 months for the next year, then annually once a pattern of normal readings have been established
- Most treatment failures show up within 1–2 years post-procedure
- Any recurrent abnormals need colposcopic follow-up and repeat endocervical curettage and biopsy
- After invasion has occurred, death usually occurs in 3–5 years without treatment, or in unresponsive cancers

Expected Course
- Invasion pattern moves from the cervix to the uterus then the pelvis, internal lymphs, ureters, bladder and rectum
- Five year survival rates vary by stage from 99+% for early to 2% for advanced
- 75% of recurrences occur in first 2 years, carry a poor prognosis (less than 5%)

Complications
- Vaginal fistulas, urinary and fecal incontinence, back pain, leg edema, ureteral obstruction, and eventually renal failure, death

Endometrial Cancer
Description
- Malignant changes of endometrial stroma and glands (adenocarcinoma)

Incidence and Demographics
- The most common invasive gynecologic cancer
- Incidence 21 per 100,000; average age at onset 60; only 5% occur < 40 years old

Risk Factors
- Atypical endometrial hyperplasia
- Obesity
- Nulliparity
- Early menarche/late menopause
- Estrogen therapy without progestin
- Diabetes
- Cigarette smoking
- Tamoxifen

Prevention and Screening
- Not proven to be of much clinical value in endometrial cancer
- Annual Pap screening at vaginal cuff site (insensitive for endometrial cancer but rules out cervical changes)
- Mammography advised because of increased risk for breast cancer
- Occult blood stool screening also advised because of increased risk for metastasis to colon

Assessment
History
- 80% to 90% of patients present with painless abnormal bleeding pattern as cardinal sign
- Less common are leukorrhea, pelvic pressure, and symptoms of metastasis

Physical
- All women over age 40 with abnormal Pap finding should have referral for endometrial biopsy
- Vaginal bleeding occurring after established menopause merits diagnostic study
- Assess for tenderness, uterine or adnexal enlargement, cervical lesions, hemorrhoids

Diagnostic Studies
- Papanicolau test
- CBC
- Ultrasound of endometrial thickness (< 5 mm atrophic, > 15 mm hypertrophic)
- Endometrial biopsy
- Chest x-ray (most common metastasis site)

Differential Diagnosis
- Endometrial hyperplasia
- HRT-related breakthrough bleeding
- Cervical cancer
- Vaginal cancer
- Hemorrhoids
- Bleeding disorders
- Polyps

Management—refer to Gynecologist
Nonpharmacologic Treatment
- Treatment is total abdominal hysterectomy with bilateral salpingectomy and oophorectomy (TAH-BSO)
- Radiation therapy is for later stages

Pharmacologic Treatment
- Hormone therapy for metastatic or recurrent cancer
- Cytotoxic chemotherapy for palliation

When to Consult, Refer, Hospitalize
- Refer for endometrial biopsy (90% accuracy)

Follow-up
- Every 3 months for 2 years then, every 6 months, and annually afterwards

Complications
- Recurrence
- 5-year survival rate varies by stage of cancer from 95% for early detection to 25% for late detection
- Death

Ovarian Cancer
Description
- Cancer of the ovary; most ovarian cancers are advanced with extensive spread at the time of diagnosis; in about three-fourths of patients, it is not detected until it has spread in the abdomen.

Incidence and Demographics
- Incidence of 12.9 to 15.1 per 100,000 women; median age 61 with peak age 75 to 79
- Leading cause of death among gynecologic cancers

Risk Factors
- Inverse relationship between number of lifetime ovulatory cycles and ovarian cancer risk; conditions that suppress ovulation, such as multiparity, oral contraceptives, anovulatory disorders, are protective
- Increased risk: low parity, delayed childbearing, infertility, late menopause
- Lifetime risk 1.6% without family history, 5% if first-degree relative had ovarian cancer, 7% with 2 or more affected first-degree relatives (3% of these will be BCRA positive, with risk of developing breast cancer > 40% in these women)

Prevention and Screening
- Not shown to be effective

Assessment
- 60% to 75% present with advanced disease and metastasis

History
- Few symptoms in early stages
- Nonspecific GI symptoms such as dyspepsia, nausea, early satiety, change in bowel habits, and abdominal fullness
- Presentation is vague: mild dyspareunia, irregular vaginal bleeding, fatigue, or pelvic pressure

Physical
- Weight loss and anorexia are poor prognostic signs
- Careful abdominal, pelvic, and lymph node examinations
- A palpable ovary in a postmenopausal women requires a diagnostic study to rule out cancer
- Physical exam findings occur late in disease; palpable adnexal mass; ascites is a poor prognostic sign

Diagnostic Studies
- Transvaginal sonography and CA-125 assessment
- Pelvic ultrasonography: findings suggestive of cancer are solid, multiple septations; free fluid noted; irregular borders to lesion or papillation
- Abdominal CT with contrast

- Labs: CBC, comprehensive metabolic panel
- Serum CA-125 is often not elevated until advanced disease (> 35 units suggests cancer); false positives occur with endometriosis, leiomyoma
- Laparoscopy

Differential Diagnosis
- Gastrointestinal or other gynecologic malignancies
- Chronic pelvic pain syndromes
- Benign ovarian mass
- Endometriosis
- Irritable bowel syndrome
- Colitis
- Hepatic disease (ascites)
- Diverticulitis
- Fibroids
- Urinary tract disease
- Ovarian cyst

Management
- By oncology

Nonpharmacologic Treatment
- Treatment is TAH-BSO with lymph sampling

Pharmacologic Treatment
- Postoperative chemotherapy is indicated in most cases

When to Consult, Refer, Hospitalize
- Oncology or gynecology consult
- Any ovarian masses should have surgical evaluation

Follow-up
- Careful follow up with oncology

Expected Course
- Survival rate decreases with increased age
- 5-year survival varies from 85% for an early cancer, 36% for local spread only, 18% for an advanced cancer with metastases
- Those with metastatic disease to breast or colon usually die within 1 year

Complications
- Death

Vulvar Cancer (Bowen's Disease)
Description
- Skin cancer on the vulva

Etiology
A form of intraepidermal carcinoma; it may ultimately become an invasive squamous cell carcinoma
- Squamous cell accounts for 85%
- Melanomas account for 5%

Incidence and Demographics
- Only 5% of genital tract cancers; incidence is on the rise
- Primarily postmenopausal; mean age at diagnosis 65, most commonly reported in White people
- 30% to 50% of patients are HPV+
- In situ disease: 40s
- Invasive disease: 60s

Risk Factors
- Cervical cancer, HPV, smoking, genital warts

Assessment
History
- Symptoms mild, nonspecific
- Persistent itching or pain, raised area on vulva, poorly healing lesion, occasional bleeding, vaginal odor
- Advanced stage: rectal bleeding, urethral obstruction

Physical
- Pelvic exam including palpation of Bartholin glands
- Toluidine blue dye (1%) or dilute acetic acid may make lesion more visible
- Raised area on vulva, leukoplakia, altered skin tones; may be multifocal in nature; ulcerations
- Inguinal lymphs may be palpable, suggests advanced disease

Diagnostic Studies
- Cytologic smear should target focal lesions on vulva, vagina, and cervix (unreliable)
- Vulvar biopsy if qualified or refer to gynecologic specialist for biopsy

Differential Diagnosis
- Atrophic vulvitis (atrophy)
- Tuberculosis
- Vulvar dystrophies
- STDs (syphilis, granuloma inguinale, lymphogranuloma inguinale, herpes)
- Paget disease
- Squamous cell carcinoma

Management
- By gynecology
- Treatment is surgical excision; chemotherapy and radiation depend on staging
- Aggressive wound care is essential

When to Consult, Refer, Hospitalize
- Refer to gynecology for biopsy

Follow-up
Expected Course
- 5-year survival rate varies by stage from 90% for early to 20% for late
- Squamous cell cancer is slow growing and late to metastasize
- Melanomas grow quickly, with early metastasis

Vaginal Cancer

Description
- Malignant changes in epithelial layer (90% squamous, 10% adenocarcinoma) of the vagina

Incidence and Demographics
- Most rare of all genital tract cancers
- If lesions on cervix or on vulva, then not classified as vaginal cancer
- May be metastasis from other cancer in body
- Carcinoma in situ: mid-40s to 60s; invasive stage mid-60s to 70s

Risk Factors
- Cervical malignancy, HPV, smokers, DES exposure, multiple partners

Assessment
History
- Abnormal bleeding, dyspareunia, postcoital bleeding
- Pain is a late sign (spread)

Physical
- Exam shows gross lesion, "fungating" tumor inside vagina

When to Consult, Refer, Hospitalize
- Refer for colposcopy, biopsy, and surgical management (vaginectomy) to gynecological oncologist

BREAST MASSES

Description
- Benign mammary dysplasia also referred to as fibrocystic changes; majority not at risk for breast cancer
- Fibroadenomas are solid benign masses
- Duct ectasia is a collection of dilated terminal collecting ducts
- Abscesses represent bacterial colonization
- Most newly developed breast masses in older women are cancer
- Retraction is often a sign of malignancy, although it can also be of benign etiology
- Galactorrhea is milky nipple discharge not associated with lactation

Etiology
- Breast cancer incidence increases with age
- Fibrocystic changes are the most common benign breast condition; caused by ductal dilation usually 2 mm or less; 20% to 40% enlarge to palpable cysts (usually fluid-filled) and may increase and decrease with menstrual cycle
- Fibroadenomas are made of glandular and fibrous tissue, often located in upper quadrant, caused by an inflammatory reaction from ductal irritation, with onset late teens to early 20s
- Galactorrhea can be caused by any lesion or medication (such as phenothiazine, oral contraceptives, tricyclic antidepressants, opiates) affecting hypothalamic inhibition of dopamine; about 10% to 12% of breast cancers are associated with nipple discharge

- Physiologic etiologies for galactorrhea include stress, breast stimulation, exercise, eating, and sleep; bilateral nipple discharge can be expressed in up to 80% of asymptomatic women
- Fat necrosis of the breast may occur after substantial trauma

Incidence and Demographics
- Most common ages 30 to 50; up to 50% of women affected
- Cysts and fibroadenomas most common benign breast changes, followed by duct ectasia
- Duct ectasia typically occurs in 40s and is most common cause of nipple discharge
- Fibroadenomas often occur in younger women within 10 years of menarche
- Cancer: peak age at diagnosis is 45 to 60; occurs in 1 of 8 women

Risk Factors
- Fibrocystic disease: caffeine intake, chocolate, smoking, family history
- Mastitis: usually seen in lactating women, but its presence in a nonlactating woman should prompt evaluation for an inflammatory carcinoma
- Cancer: risk increased with early menarche, late menopause, first pregnancy after age 35, obesity, android fat distribution

Prevention and Screening
- Monthly breast self-exam and periodic clinical breast exam
- Mammography on routine screening schedule unless focal area of concern (dominant mass of different texture, new mass); women > 40 should have screening mammography every 1 to 2 years

Assessment
History
- Achy, tender, or painless lumpy breasts
- More tender with menses
- Vision problems, headaches
- Any nipple discharge—may be seen in galactocele or ductal ectasia, papilloma, or cancer
- Cold intolerance, weight gain, fatigue

Physical
- Benign multiple breast masses, fluctuating size with menses (cystic, adenosis, fibrosis, ductal hyperplasia), occasionally with unilateral or bilateral nipple discharge
- Fibroadenomas: unilateral mass, often solitary; well defined, round, rubbery, mobile masses
- Fibrocystic disease: multiple masses, tender with menses, fluctuating size, rare nipple discharge
- Nipple discharge typically green to yellow to black in color if physiologic; coming from multiple ducts versus spontaneous, unilateral, and bloody, which is more likely associated with cancer
- Nipple discharge often associated with duct ectasia; often thick and cheesy
- Cancer: solitary, hard mass; nonmovable, nontender mass without well-defined margins; skin dimpling, nipple retraction, discharge
- Axillary, supraclavicular, and infraclavicular lymph node exam for suspicious nodes
- Abscess (mastitis): sudden onset; unilateral, tender, fluctuant; erythema; edema; induration; fever

- Visual field defects

Diagnostic Studies
- Breast ultrasonography can identify cystic structures vs. solid mass
- Mammograms more useful for older women with less dense breast tissue
- Fine-needle aspiration or biopsy any suspicious area; if bloody fluid obtained or no fluid or persistent mass, refer for excision
- TSH, prolactin, and MRI of sella turcica as needed

Differential Diagnosis
- Breast cancer
- Fibroadenoma
- Breast abscess
- Galactocele
- Fat necrosis
- Benign cyst
- Prolactinoma

Management
Nonpharmacologic Treatment
- Fibroadenoma: excise or aspirate
- Fibrocystic disease: vitamin E supplements, reduce caffeine and chocolate in diet, supportive brassiere
- Abscesses: warm compresses
- Monthly breast self exams encouraged
- Avoid nipple stimulation
- Evening primrose oil

Pharmacologic Treatment
- Vitamin E supplements 400 IU daily, vitamin B_6 25 to 50 mg daily, magnesium supplements
- Oral contraceptives may or may not relieve symptoms
- Antibiotics and OTC analgesics for abscess

Special Considerations
- Breast pain in postmenopausal women not on HRT should be examined for cancer
- Despite limitations of mammography for women with implants, such as reduced sensitivity, these women should continue to be radiographically screened as appropriate for their age and risk factors

When to Consult, Refer, Hospitalize
- Refer to a surgeon for fine-needle aspiration to confirm that cyst is fluid-filled, for excisional biopsy, or for suspicious findings as outlined above
- Refer to oncologist for suspicion of cancer

Follow-up
- Reevaluate in 1 to 2 months soon after menses to determine efficacy of therapy and if further study is required

Complications
- Usually none if benign process

BREAST CANCER

Description
- Malignant neoplasm of the breast

Etiology
- Precise etiology unknown
- Noninvasive: intraductal tumors including ductal carcinoma in situ (DCIS) or lobular carcinoma in situ (LCIS)
- Invasive: tumor no longer contained within basement membrane
  - Invasive ductal carcinoma originates from epithelial cells lining mammary ducts; subtypes include medullary, papillary, tubular, and colloid
  - Invasive lobular carcinoma arises from mammary lobules

Incidence and Demographics
- 1 in 8 women (lifetime risk)
- Peak age at diagnosis 45 to 65, with > 75% occurring over age 50
- About 70% are invasive; invasive ductal more common than lobular (96% to 97% vs. 3% to 4%)
- Most common site is upper outer quadrant (49%)

Risk Factors
- Risks include early menarche, late menopause (after 53), nulliparity, first pregnancy after age 35 (1.5x risk), prior breast cancer (5 to 10x risk), obesity (may be linked to hyperinsulinemia or fat cell production of androgens converted to estrogens), android fat distribution, excess alcohol use, tobacco use; data are mixed on whether estrogen use increases risk
- 20% family history (autosomal dominant with maternal linkage); relative risk (RR) 2.2 with first degree relatives; 10.5 RR with bilateral disease in premenopausal relatives; 5.5 RR with bilateral disease in postmenopausal relatives
- 90% of women with breast cancer have *no* family history
- People with mutations in the BRCA1 or BRCA2 tumor suppressor genes have greater risk for breast and ovarian cancers, usually early onset

Prevention and Screening
- Protection may be conferred by exercise, dietary soy, weight control especially in postmenopausal years
- Tamoxifen as prophylaxis in high-risk women (watch for endometrial abnormalities)

Screening for Breast Cancer
- 40 and over: monthly BSE and annual clinical breast examination and mammography every year (reduces cancer mortality by 30% to 50% in women ages 50 to 69; over age 70 the data are conflicting; no evidence to benefit women over age 75; the American Geriatric Society recommends screenings stop at age 85
- False-negative rate of 10% to 15% and a false-positive rate of 15% to 20% for screening mammogram
- Clinical breast examination to find changes that may indicate a malignancy soon enough for timely intervention and to teach or to reinforce breast self examination
- Yearly mammogram for women who have had breast cancer—for women at high risk, a screening MRI is recommended along with the yearly mammogram.

- Genetic testing for breast cancer: testing for mutations in the BRCA genes; not generally recommended except for those at elevated risk for breast cancer

Assessment
History and Physical
- 55% palpable nontender mass; 35% abnormal mammogram without palpable mass
- Persistent nipple itching or burning suggests Paget disease; may present with minimal skin changes and no mass palpable; may have erosion or ulceration
- Exam shows solitary, nontender, firm-to-hard mass without well-defined margins; often fixed position
- Ominous signs are enlarged or tender lymph nodes, skin color changes, skin erosion, peau d'orange (pitted skin surface with edema), dimpling, nipple retraction, pain, breast enlargement

Diagnostic Studies
- Fine-needle aspiration: occasionally may not yield enough tissue to make a diagnosis, or may miss the cancer entirely
- Mammography
- Ultrasound (US): most current is ultrasound computed tomography
- CBC, liver function tests, chest x-ray, estrogen and progesterone receptor determination (usually ordered once biopsy done), bone scan, CT or US to assess lymph node involvement and metastasis

Differential Diagnosis
- Fibrocystic changes
- Fibroadenoma
- Intraductal papilloma
- Lipoma
- Fat necrosis

Management
- Decision making
  - Risk/benefit analysis
  - Consider life expectancy, comorbidities, treatment risks, patient values, quality of life
  - Older women generally tolerate surgery and radiation well; comorbidity influences surgical morbidity
  - Postmenopausal women tend to have a better prognosis than younger women
- Local therapy
  - Breast conserving therapy (BCT) or mastectomy: treatment patterns influenced by age, patient preferences
  - Modified radical mastectomy for multifocal disease, diffuse suspicious micro-calcifications, or prior breast irradiation
  - Sentinel node evaluation of axilla (less risk for lymphedema)
  - Local radiation following BCT: benefit less certain in older women
  - Radiation after mastectomy in high-risk women (large tumors, positive lymph nodes) and after partial mastectomy
  - All mastectomy specimens should be tested for hormone receptors, proliferation rates, and HER-2/neu antigens
  - Genomic profiles may help to identify patients who benefit from adjuvant chemotherapy and those who would not

- Systemic therapy (adjuvant)
  - Tamoxifen for 5 years after surgery: beneficial for estrogen receptor (ER) positive tumors
    - Reduces risk for recurrence and improves survival
    - Reduces risk for new primary breast cancer
    - Marked benefit in women over 70
  - Tamoxifen first-line therapy in women unable to tolerate surgery
  - Consider chemotherapy if high risk for recurrence
  - Decreasing benefit of chemotherapy with increasing age (chemotherapy may be less effective and more toxic in older adults)
    - Consider toxicities, comorbidities, preferences in women over 70
    - Benefits negligible with major comorbidities especially dementia

Special Considerations

- Tamoxifen may be given for prevention to women at high risk for breast cancer
- Delayed diagnosis and inadequate treatment associated with poor social support, transportation problems, impaired cognition
- Risk for undertreatment with advanced age, even controlling for comorbidity, functional status, cognitive disorders

When to Consult, Refer, Hospitalize

- Breast mass or abnormal calcifications on mammogram
- Eczema of nipple, new-onset nipple or breast retraction, persistent nipple discharge

Follow-up

- Periodic physical examinations (every 3 to 4 months for 3 years, every 6 months for the next 2 to 3 years, then yearly)
- Yearly mammogram after BCT
- Routine screening for other cancers such as colorectal, uterine
- Periodic lab tests: CBC, liver function tests
- Intensive follow-up to detect recurrence after primary therapy is not indicated in asymptomatic persons

Expected Course

- Stage of breast cancer is the most reliable indicator of prognosis
- Localized cancer cure rate is 75% to 90%
- When axillary lymph nodes are involved with tumor, survival is 4% to 50% at 5 years and about 25% at 10 years

Complications

- Increased risk for endometrial cancer, thromboemboli, stroke in postmenopausal women on tamoxifen
- Exacerbation of postmenopausal symptoms may occur with tamoxifen (hot flushes, vaginal dryness, cognitive changes)

CASE STUDIES

Case 1. A 69-year-old female comes to your office for her annual physical exam. On exam, you note a lump in the upper outer aspect of the right breast. The lump is about 1 cm, mobile, firm, with regular borders. There is no dimpling, retraction, or other breast or chest wall lesions. There is no tenderness. There is no adenopathy. The remainder of the physical exam is normal. She was not aware of this lump or other changes in her breasts. However, she does not perform regular breast self exam. Her last mammogram was 3 years ago and last Papanicolau test was 1 year ago.

Breast History: The patient has no prior history of breast cancer or breast biopsies. Menarche: age 9. The patient is gravida 1, para 1, miscarriages/abortions 0. Age at first full-term pregnancy: 36. Age at menopause: 54. Hormones: HRT (Prempro): 10 yr.

Past Medical History: Hypercholesterolemia, osteopenia

Medications: Conjugated estrogens/medroxyprogesterone (Prempro), atorvastatin (Lipitor) 20 mg, multivitamin, calcium

Habits: Diet: generally follows low-fat diet; exercise: walks 3 times a week for ½ hour; alcohol: 3 to 4 drinks/week; tobacco: none

1. Based on the history and physical, what is your recommendation regarding diagnostic evaluation of the breast lump?
2. The mammogram shows a small mass in the upper outer quadrant of the right breast. The sonogram shows a cystic lesion with a small solid component in the area of the palpable mass. What would be your next recommendation for follow-up of this mass?
3. What aspects of the patient's history would be considered risk factors in assessing her risk for breast cancer?

Case 2. A 70-year-old female comes to the clinic because she thinks she is shrinking. She is 5'2", weighs 98 pounds, has smoked for 30 years, and has COPD. Upon questioning, admits to having difficulty holding her urine due to frequency and urgency. She wears pads when she goes out, but she doesn't go out much because she is embarrassed.

1. What consequences of menopause does she have?
2. What other consequence would you evaluate her for?
3. What physical exam is indicated?
4. What diagnostic tests would you order?
5. What is the single most important thing she can do to improve her health?
6. The pelvic exam shows moderate vaginal atrophy. How would you manage the vaginal atrophy?

Case 3. A 78-year-old healthy female has a routine Pap results of CIN II.

1. What does the CIN II mean?
2. What counseling would you give when you told her about the results?
3. What would your actions be?
4. What would her life expectancy be if she were not treated?
5. What follow-up would the patient need?

REFERENCES

Anderson, G. L., Judd, H. L., Kaunitz, A. M., Barad, D. H., Beresford, S. A., Pettinger, M., et al. (2003). Effects of estrogen plus progestin on gynecologic cancers and associated diagnostic procedures: The Women's Health Initiative randomized trial. *JAMA, 290*(13), 1739–1748.

Anderson, G. L., Limacher, M., Assaf, A. R., Bassford, T., Beresford, S. A., Black, H., et al. (2004). Effects of conjugated equine estrogen in postmenopausal women with hysterectomy: The Women's Health Initiative randomized controlled trial. *JAMA, 291*(14), 1701–1712.

Basil, B., & Horowitz, I. R. (2001). Cervical carcinoma: contemporary management. *Obstetrics and Gynecology Clinics of North America, 28,* 727–742.

Cauley, J. A., Robbins, J., Chen, Z., Cummings, S. R., Jackson, R. D., LaCroix, A. Z., et al. (2003). Effects of estrogen plus progestin on risk of fracture and bone mineral density: The Women's Health Initiative randomized trial. *JAMA, 290*(13), 1729–1738.

Cauley, J. A., Zmuda, J. M., Lui, L., Hillier, T. A., Ness, R. B., Stone, K. L., et al. (2003). Lipid-lowering drug use and breast cancer in older women: A prospective study. *Journal of Women's Health, 23*(9), 749–756.

Centers for Disease Control and Prevention. (2006). *Preventive Services Task Force mammography screening guidelines.* Retrieved from http://www.cdc.gov/cancer/breast/basic_info/screening. htm

Chlebowski, R. T., Hendrix, S. L., Langer, R. D., Stefanick, M. L., Gass, M., Lane, D., et al. (2003). Influence of estrogen plus progestin on breast cancer and mammography in healthy postmenopausal women: The Women's Health Initiative randomized trial. *JAMA, 289*(24), 3243–3253.

Chlebowski, R. T., Wactawski-Wende, J., Ritenbaugh, C., Hubbell, F. A., Ascensao, J., Rodabough, R. J., et al. (2004). Estrogen plus progestin and colorectal cancer in postmenopausal women. *New England Journal of Medicine, 350*(10), 991–1004.

Gull, B., Carlsson, S., Karlsson, B., Ylostalo, P., Milsom, I., & Granberg, S. (2000). Transvaginal ultrasonography of the endometrium in women with postmenopausal bleeding: Is it always necessary to perform an endometrial biopsy? *American Journal of Obstetrics and Gynecology, 185,* 509.

Harris, J. M., Lippman, M., Morrow, M., & Osborne, C. (Eds.) (2000). *Diseases of the breast.* Philadelphia: Lippincott Williams & Wilkins.

Kimmick, G. G., & Balducci, L. (2000). Breast cancer and aging. *Hematology/Oncology Clinics of North America, 14*(1), 213–234.

Loose, D. S., & Stancel, G. M. (2006). Estrogen and progestin. In L. Burnton (Ed.), *Goodman & Gilman's the pharmacologic basis for therapeutics* (11th ed.). New York: McGraw Hill. Available at http://www.accessmedicine.com/content.aspx?aID=953504

Mailhot, T., & Richard, A. (2006). *Uterine prolapse.* Retrieved from http://emedicine.medscape.com/ article/797295-overview

Mandelblatt, J. S., Hadley, J., Kerner, J. F., Schulman, K. A., Gold, K., Dunmore-Griffith, J., et al. (2000). Patterns of breast carcinoma treatment in older women. *Cancer, 89*(3), 561–572.

Manson, J. E. (2003). Estrogen plus progestin and the risk of coronary heart disease. *New England Journal of Medicine, 349,* 523–534.

North American Menopause Society. (2004). Treatment of menopause associated vasomotor symptoms: Position statement of The North American Menopause Society. *Menopause, 11*(1), 11–33.

North American Menopause Society. (2007). The role of local vaginal estrogen for treatment of vaginal atrophy in postmenopausal women: 2007 position statement of The North American Menopause Society. *Menopause, 14*(3), 168–182.

North American Menopause Society. (2008). Estrogen and progestogen use in postmenmopausal women: July 2008 position statement of the North American Menopause Society. *Menopause, 15*(4), 584–602.

Randolph, W. M., Goodwin, J. S., Mahnken, J. D., & Freeman, J. L. (2002). Regular mammography use is associated with elimination of age related disparities in size and stage of breast cancer at diagnosis. *Annals of Internal Medicine, 137,* 783–790.

Rossouw, J. E., Anderson, G. L., Prentice, R. L., LaCroix, A. Z., Kooperberg, C., Stefanick, M. L., et al. (2002). Risks and benefits of estrogen plus progestin in healthy postmenopausal women: Principal results from the Women's Health Initiative randomized controlled trial. *JAMA, 288,* 321–333.

Sawaya, G. F. (2003). Risk of cervical cancer associated with extending the interval between cervical cancer screenings. *New England Journal of Medicine, 349,* 1501–1509.

Shumaker, S. A., Legault, C., Rapp, S. R., Thal, L., Wallace, R. B., Ockene, J. K., et al. (2003). Estrogen plus progestin and the incidence of dementia and mild cognitive impairment in postmenopausal women: The Women's Health Initiative Memory Study: A randomized controlled trial. *JAMA, 289,* 2651–2662.

Speroff, L., Glass, R. H., & Kase, N. G. (1999). *Clinical gynecologic endocrinology and infertility* (6th ed.). Philadelphia: Lippincott Williams & Wilkins.

Tabor, A., Watt, H. C., & Wald, N. J. (2002). Endometrial thickness as a test for endometrial cancer in women with postmenopausal vaginal bleeding. *Obstetrics & Gynecology, 99,* 663–670.

U.S. Preventive Services Task Force. (2002). Postmenopausal hormone replacement therapy for primary prevention of chronic conditions: Recommendations and rationale. *Annals of Internal Medicine, 137,* 834–839.

Warren, M. P. (2004). A comparative review of the risks and benefits of hormone replacement therapy regimens. *American Journal of Obstetrics and Gynecology, 190,* 1141–1167.

Wassertheil-Smoller, S., Hendrix, S. L., Limacher, M., Heiss, G., Kooperberg, C., Baird, A., et al. (2003). Effect of estrogen plus progestin on stroke in postmenopausal women: The Women's Health Initiative: A randomized trial. *JAMA, 289,* 2673–2684.

Wysocki, S. (2008). Etiology, consequences, and management of vaginal atrophy. *American Journal for Nurse Practitioners, 12*(11/12), 36–38, 44–46.

Male Reproductive System Disorders

Vaunette Fay, PhD, RN, FNP-BC, GNP-BC

GERIATRIC APPROACH

Normal Changes of Aging

Male Reproductive System
- Decreased testosterone level leads to increased estrogen-to-androgen ratio
- Testicular atrophy
- Decreased sperm motility; fertility reduced but extant
- Increased incidence of gynecomastia

Sexual Function
- Slowed arousal—increased time to achieve erection
- Erection less firm, shorter lasting
- Delayed ejaculation and decreased forcefulness at ejaculation
- Longer interval to achieving subsequent erection

Prostate
- By fourth decade of life, stromal fibrous elements and glandular tissue hypertrophy, stimulated by dihydrotestosterone (DHT, the active androgen within the prostate); hyperplastic nodules enlarge in size, ultimately leading to urethral obstruction

Clinical Implications
History
- Many men are overly sensitive about complaints of the male genitourinary system; men are often not inclined to initiate discussion, seek help; important to take active role in screening with an approach that is open, trustworthy, and nonjudgmental
- Sexual function remains important to many men, even at ages over 80
- Lack of an available partner, poor health, erectile dysfunction, medication adverse effects, and lack of desire are the main reasons men do not continue to have sex
- Acute and chronic alcohol use can lead to impotence in men
- Nocturia is reported in 66% of patients over 65
  - Due to impaired ability to concentrate urine, reduced in bladder capacity or BPH
  - Frequent cause of insomnia

Physical
- Digital rectal exam (DRE) is almost universally dreaded by men; provide privacy, allow for dignity

Assessment
- In men diagnosed with benign prostatic hyperplasia (BPH), periodic evaluation for prostate cancer must continue

Treatment
- A man may not want treatment for BPH because of fear of erectile dysfunction

PROSTATE GLAND DISORDERS
Prostatitis
Description
- Acute or chronic inflammation of the prostate gland secondary to bacterial or nonbacterial causes

Etiology
- Various causes: allergic, autoimmune response; infectious, related to instrumentation, UTIs, prostatic abscess, or stone
- Acute infection: generally Gram-negative bacilli; primarily *E. coli*; may also be *Enterobacter* organisms, *Klebsiella* organisms, *Proteus* organisms, *Staphylococcus aureus*
- Infectious causes usually occur by direct invasion from the urethra, typically UTI

Incidence and Demographics
- Chronic bacterial prostatitis occurs primarily in older men
- Acute bacterial prostatitis is uncommon

Risk Factors
- Age over 50
- Instrumentation of urinary tract
- Abscess elsewhere in the body
- Recurrent UTIs

Prevention and Screening
- Avoidance of unnecessary procedures

Assessment (see Table 13–1)

History

- Symptoms of dysuria due to compression of the urethra by the inflamed prostate
- Chronic bacterial prostatitis characterized by remissions and exacerbations with recurrent UTIs
- Acute bacterial prostatitis characterized by acute onset with systemic symptoms and pattern of pain and dysuria
- Current medications (such as anticholinergics), other medical illness, and sexual history to assess risk of infection

Physical

- Abdominal exam: check for tenderness or distended bladder from urinary retention
- Genitalia: urethral discharge
- CVA tenderness to assess kidneys
- Rectal exam
- *Warning regarding prostate examinations:* examining the prostate is a part of this exam; however, because of exquisite tenderness and risk for bacteremia, it is to be done very gently or, in the case of suspected acute prostatitis, perhaps not at all until treatment has been initiated
- In the nonacute patient, prostatic massage *is* indicated for carrying out the three-step urinalysis and culture for evaluation of prostatic secretions, and as part of therapeutic treatment

Table 13–1. Clinical Presentation of Prostatitis

Assess	Acute Bacterial	Chronic Bacterial
Symptoms	Chills, fever, malaise Dysuria Urgency Burning Frequency Hematuria Pain: pelvis, perineum, lower back, scrotum, with defecation, with intercourse	+/– low grade fever Dysuria Hesitancy Hematuria Hematospermia Pain mild: perineal, scrotal, abdominal, with ejaculation
Physical Findings	Fever Prostate very tender, boggy, warm Urethral discharge	No systemic findings Prostate may be normal, indurated, mildly tender, boggy, or irregular +/–Prostatic stones Scrotum +/– edema, erythema, and tenderness

Diagnostic Studies

- Urinalysis and culture/sensitivity: If pyuria on initial clean-catch wet prep and positive urine culture, adequate diagnosis for acute bacterial prostatitis
- If initial clean-catch wet prep is negative for bacteria, proceed to prostatic massage and collect postmassage urine for wet prep and culture
- If prostatic massage wet prep has at least 10 to 15 WBC, culture will usually yield gram-negative organisms indicative of chronic prostatitis

- Negative culture with WBC indicates nonbacterial prostatitis; if no WBC and negative culture, suspect prostatodynia and refer
- Chronic prostatitis is additionally evaluated with CBC, serum BUN and creatinine, and possible IV pyelogram and/or transrectal ultrasound
- Bladder cancer screening via urine cytology

Differential Diagnosis
- BPH
- Prostatodynia
- Urethral stricture
- Nonbacterial prostatitis
- Cancer of the bladder or prostate
- Renal colic
- Other infections: abscess, epididymitis, cystitis, urethritis

Management
Nonpharmacologic Treatment
- Avoidance of known irritants: caffeine, alcohol, OTC antihistamine or decongestants
- Hydration maintenance (force fluids)
- Rest and sitz baths 20 minutes 2 to 3 times a day for pain as needed

Pharmacologic Treatment
- Prostate gland difficult to penetrate with antibiotics; first-line treatment with trimethoprim-sulfamethoxazole (Bactrim) or fluoroquinolones
- NSAIDs recommended for both anti-inflammatory effects and pain relief; choice of medications may be limited because of intolerance/side effects of NSAIDs.
- Stool softeners as needed

Table 13–2. Antibiotic Management of Infections—Based on Gram Stain and Culture

Treatment	Acute Bacterial	Chronic Bacterial
Antibiotics	Ciprofloxacin 500 mg PO b.i.d. Levofloxacin 500 qd Trimethoprim/ sulfamethoxazole (Bactrim) DS b.i.d. Ofloxacin 400 mg p.o. once, then 300 mg every 12 hours for 10 days Other antibiotic appropriate to the organism	Cipro 500 mg PO b.i.d. Trimethoprim/ sulfamethoxazole (Bactrim) DS b.i.d. Ofloxacin 200 mg every12 hours for 3 months
How long to treat	2 to 6 weeks	1 to 4 months

When to Consult, Refer, Hospitalize
- Hospitalization indicated for all patients with systemic involvement for IV antibiotics, treatment of possible septicemia
- Refer to a urologist if no improvement within 48 hours of treatment
- Refer to a urologist older patients (> 50) who are symptomatic, have recurrent prostatitis, or have acute bacterial prostatitis, as BPH may be a compounding problem

Follow-up
Expected Course
- Chronic prostatitis: follow-up appointments with urinalysis, culture and sensitivity every 30 days; sooner as indicated based on response to treatment and changes in symptoms
- Acute prostatitis: reevaluation in 48 to 72 hours, then 2 to 4 weeks later for urinalysis, urine and prostatic secretion cultures to monitor treatment effectiveness and assess for complications; repeat one month after completion of antibiotic course

Complications
- Potential for serious sequelae including development of prostatic abscess, stones, ascending or recurrent UTIs, epididymitis, urinary retention, renal infection

Benign Prostatic Hyperplasia
Description
- Benign, gradual enlargement of the periurethral prostate gland in which the enlargement mechanically obstructs urination by compressing the urethra
- Differentiate between BPH and prostate cancer

Etiology
- Combination of hormonal changes, growth factors—stromal and epithelial cell hyperplasia
- Begins in the periuretheral zone of prostate
- Medications known to increase symptoms: alpha-adrenergic agonists, anticholinergics, antihistamines, opioids, tricyclics, sedative hypnotics, alcohol

Incidence and Demographics
- Approximately half of 50-year-old men, 70% of 70-year-olds, 90% of those 85+
- Initially asymptomatic, many develop urinary symptoms by age 60

Risk Factors
- Age
- Presence of androgens

Prevention and Screening
- Most organizations recommend annual DRE examination after the age of 40
- Use of the PSA for screening remains controversial; PSA should be drawn prior to doing the DRE
- Early screening starting in the 40s may allow for earlier treatment, slowing of the progression of hyperplasia, and possible reduction of symptoms

Assessment
History
- Assess degree of impairment using the American Urological Association BPH Symptom Index
  - Not emptying bladder completely, urinary frequency, repeated stopping and starting, urgency, weak stream, pushing or straining to begin urination, nocturia
- Obstructive symptoms: difficulty starting/stopping stream, hesitancy, dribbling, weakening force/size of stream, sensation of full bladder after voiding, urinary retention
- Irritative symptoms: urgency, frequency, nocturia, urge incontinence, dysuria, suprapubic discomfort

- Medications: anticholinergics (decongestants, antihistamines, tricyclic antidepressants, tranquilizers) impair bladder contractility; sympathomimetics increase outflow resistance
- Past medical history: explore for other conditions that may be associated with these symptoms—surgery, diabetes, neuromuscular disease (multiple sclerosis), psychogenic disorder, cardiovascular disease (CHF), and hypercalcemia
- General: fever, malaise, back pain, hematuria, and pain with voiding indicate possible complication of BPH

Physical
- Abdomen: possible distended bladder on percussion or palpation; costovertebral angle tenderness if renal sequelae
- Neurologic: screening exam to note nonprostate etiology for symptoms of neurogenic or myogenic etiology, detrusor muscle impairment, compression of nerves
- Digital rectal exam (DRE): intact anal sphincter tone; prostate nontender, firm, smooth, and rubbery consistency with blunting or obliteration of midline median sulcus
- Enlargement may be symmetric, nodular or asymmetric; any nodules should be considered possibly malignant

Diagnostic Studies
- Urinalysis: hematuria, glycosuria, or infection
- Urine culture and sensitivity if evidence of infection
- Serum creatinine to assess renal function: may be abnormal if urinary retention or obstruction has affected upper urinary tract, as well as with underlying renal disease
- Urine culture and sensitivity if evidence of infection
- Prostate specific antigen (PSA): controversial if patient is asymptomatic, normal is 4 to 7 ng/mL for the older adult; > 10 ng/mL may indicate cancer or prostatitis
- Urinary flowmetry studies (flow rate), postresidual urine, and urodynamic studies, transrectal ultrasound (to guide needle biopsy), and abdominal ultrasound done by urologist

Differential Diagnosis
- Prostate cancer
- Prostatitis
- Urethral stricture
- Urinary tract infection
- Bladder neck contracture or cancer
- Infectious or inflammatory disease (prostatitis, cystitis, urethritis)
- Diseases associated with increased urination (CHF, DM, hypercalcemia)
- Neurologic disease

Management
Nonpharmacologic Treatment

MILD SYMPTOMS
- Watchful waiting, monitoring of symptoms
- Avoidance of bladder irritants: coffee, alcohol, medications listed in Etiology
- Limit intake of fluids in the evening, avoid large quantities in short time

MODERATE
- Treatment initiated when symptoms interfere with quality of life (such as frequent nocturia disrupting sleep, incontinence) or recurrent UTI

SEVERE
- Treatment required if patient has refractory retention, recurrent urinary tract infections, recurrent or persistent gross hematuria, bladder stones, or renal insufficiency due to BPH
- Surgical options include transurethral resection of prostate (TURP), transurethral incision of prostate (TUIP), and open prostatectomy via abdominal incision (rarely used)
- Laser surgery and coagulation necrosis techniques performed under ultrasound guidance are newer techniques that are minimally invasive

Pharmacologic Treatment
- Aggravating medications should be discontinued when feasible

MILD TO MODERATE
- Two classes of medications are available (see Table 13–3)
- Alpha-adrenergic blockers: reduce muscle tone through effect on alpha-adrenergic nerves in both bladder neck and prostatic urethra, so there is decreased resistance to urine flow
- 5-alpha-reductase inhibitors block conversion of testosterone to DHT, decreasing hormonal (androgen) effect on prostate, shrinking prostate size and symptoms, resulting in increased peak urinary flow rate
- Less commonly used drugs include GnRH agonists, progestational antiandrogens, flutamide, and testolactone
- Saw palmetto is an alternative therapy that is controversial but commonly used
- Treat UTI if present

How Long to Treat
- Depends on type and severity of symptoms and impact on daily functioning
- Medications may be prescribed until symptoms are no longer manageable and nonpharmacologic treatment may be needed

Table 13-3. Pharmacologic Management of BPH

Drugs	Dosage	Comment
α_1–Adrenergic Blockers		
Terazosin (Hytrin)	Always begin with 1mg PO QHS, may increase to 2 mg, then 5 mg up to 10 mg/day to achieve symptom relief or desired flow rate	Drugs of choice for smaller prostate and acute irritative symptoms Improvement dose dependent; 4 to 6 weeks for maximal therapeutic effect May cause postural hypotension, dizziness, palpitations, or syncope First-dose syncope requires first pill be taken while patient is in bed May be beneficial for those with concomitant BPH and HTN, can reduce number of medications needed
Doxazosin (Cardura)	1 mg q.d. HS, may double every 1 to 2 weeks to max of 8 mg/day	
Prazosin (Minipress)	1 mg q.d. HS or every 12 hours with a max of 20 mg/day	
Alfuzosin (Uroxatral)	10-mg extended-release tablet taken at the same time daily after a meal	

continued

Table 13-3. Pharmacologic Management of BPH (cont.)

Drugs	Dosage	Comment
Tamsulosin HCL (Flomax) α-1A blocker	0.4 mg q.d. 30 min before meal at same time each day. May increase to 0.8 mg after 2 to 4 weeks	No cardiovascular side effects; postural hypotension not common May cause dizziness, abnormal ejaculation, rhinitis
5 α-Reductase Inhibitor		
Finasteride (Proscar)	5 mg q.d. no titration needed	Drug of choice for large prostate and those with contraindications or failed treatment with α-adrenergics
Dutasteride (Avodart)	0.5 mg/day	Improvement not noted for up to 6 to 12 months Must be used indefinitely to sustain effect Decreases PSA by up to 50%, blocking effectiveness of PSA as screening tool for CA

Special Considerations
- In presence of concomitant diseases (diabetes mellitus; CV or neurologic disease), care should be coordinated with regard to medications, ability for self care, and recommendations for procedural or surgical treatment
- Must always rule out prostate cancer

When to Consult, Refer, Hospitalize
- Referral to a urologist is indicated for AUA index score of 8 or more, symptoms not responsive to medications, infections (epididymitis, repeat UTIs), obstruction or acute urinary retention, renal disease, or suspicion of malignancy
- Refer if surgical procedure may be indicated

Follow-up
- Annual evaluation with DRE indicated for asymptomatic or minor symptoms, sooner if symptoms warrant

Expected Course
- Without intervention, prostate gland will continue to increase in size, ultimately causing symptoms of obstruction
- Depending on response to medication, may have prolonged course of milder symptoms, slowing of hyperplasia
- Follow up initially every 2 to 4 weeks until stable
- Individuals on finasteride need follow-up in 6 months

Complications
- Recurrent UTI/sepsis
- Obstruction of urinary flow with urinary retention
- Incontinence
- Azotemia
- Chronic renal failure

Prostate Cancer
Description
- Malignant neoplasm of the prostate gland

Etiology
- Unknown

Incidence and Demographics
- 190,000 new cases per year
- Second most common cause of cancer deaths in men
- One in five men develop prostate cancer; average age at diagnosis is 72 years
- About 85% of all clinically diagnosed cases of prostate cancer are men > age 65
- 40% greater incidence in Black men; at all ages, Black men are diagnosed with prostate cancer at later stages and are 2.5 times more likely to die of the disease than White men

Risk Factors
- Age
- Exposure to chemical carcinogens, history of STIs
- Family history
- Possibly related to prior vasectomy
- Diet high in fat and meat or low intake of fruit
- More common in Blacks
- Low vitamin D levels
- Sun exposure
- History of agricultural work

Prevention and Screening
- Annual digital rectal exam (DRE) beginning between age 40 and 50
- Annual PSA test from age 50 is recommended for screening and early detection by some groups; U.S. Preventive Health Services Task Force suggests research does not support this practice because of high number of both false positives and false negatives
- Avoid use of androgen supplements

Assessment
History
- Asymptomatic initially
- May include any or all BPH symptoms described above
- With enlargement, frequency, nocturia, and dribbling develop
- Bone pain in hips, pelvis, or back occurs with advanced metastatic cancer

Physical
- Depending upon stage of the cancer, the prostate on DRE may be normal on the palpable lateral and posterior portion of the gland or may be asymmetrical, and generally firmer with hard induration, localized nodules, and obliterated median sulcus
- Hematuria may be present
- Examine back for spinous process tenderness and lower extremities for neurological abnormalities if metastatic disease is suspected

Diagnostic Studies
- PSA level > 4 ng/mL indicates possible cancer
- Normal PSA in 40% of patients with cancer; PSA discredited as good screening examination
- CBC, urinalysis, urine C&S for study of urinary symptoms
- Acid phosphatase increased with late stage (metastatic) disease in bone

Differential Diagnosis
- BPH
- Prostatitis
- UTI
- Proximal urethral stone
- Bladder or renal cancer
- Urethral stricture

Management by the Urologist
- Treatment choice based on stage of disease

Nonpharmacologic Treatment
- Asymptomatic with life expectancy < 10 years, watchful waiting is option
- If localized, treatment options include watchful waiting, radical prostatectomy and external beam radiation therapy, brachytherapy (radioactive seed implant)
- Disseminated disease treated with surgical or chemical castration (hormonal therapy) or chemotherapy

Pharmacologic Treatment
- LHRH agonist: leuprolide (Lupron) monthly injection
- Antiestrogen: flutamide 250 mg t.i.d.

How Long to Treat
- Follow-up exam and PSA every 3 months first year, then every 6 months for 1 year
- Chest x-ray and bone scan every 6 months for 1 year then as indicated by changes in PSA
- Early stage may be cured with no further treatment needed if localized and surgically removed
- Hormonal treatment is maintained throughout the course of the advanced stages
- Radiation, chemotherapy treatments vary depending upon staging

When to Consult, Refer, Hospitalize
- All patients with PSA > 10, sudden increase in serial PSA even if still within normal limits, abnormalities on DRE, or symptomatic are referred to urologist

Follow-up
Expected Course
- PSA should be undetectable after prostatectomy, negligible after radiation
- Rise in PSA after treatment indicates recurrence
- Concurrent with treatment of the cancer is the need to address the effects of the diagnosis, sequelae of the disease, and side effects of treatments
  - Coping with a chronic or terminal illness
  - Loss of self-image or self-esteem
  - Transient or permanent incontinence (2% to 5%)
  - Loss of libido and impotence

Complications
- Incontinence, erectile dysfunction, pain, pathologic fractures related to bone metastases to regional lymph nodes and bone (axial skeleton most common site), death

- Impotence occurs in 40% postoperatively and 25% to 35% postradiation; hormonal treatment may additionally result in gynecomastia, cardiovascular complications, or hot flashes

PENILE DISORDERS

Phimosis

Description
- Inability to retract the foreskin of uncircumcised penis that had formerly been retractable

Etiology
- Occurs when orifice of the prepuce is too small to allow retraction of the foreskin
- Acquired from trauma, prior infection, or poor hygiene (retained smegma and dirt) that results in inflammation and development of adhesions
- Geriatric patients may develop phimosis with use of condom catheters

Incidence and Demographics
- Elderly at increased risk because of inability to care for self

Risk Factors
- Poor hygiene
- In diabetics, levels of glucose in the urine are higher than normal—increased risk of bacteria infection
- Trauma

Prevention and Screening
- Hygiene of the genitalia with retraction of the foreskin during washing
- Make sure to replace foreskin after washing.

Assessment
History
- May be asymptomatic, with phimosis discovered on examination
- When related to an infectious or inflamed process, patients complain of irritation and tenderness of the glans, discomfort with voiding, or pain on erection
- If severe enough, outflow of urine may be compromised by an opening that is too small, presenting as a **urological emergency**

Physical
- Glans nonretractable, prepuce pallid, striated, and thickened
- If actively infected: erythema, smegma, and/or exudate and tenderness

Differential Diagnosis
- Penile lymphedema associated with trauma, allergic reaction, insect bite

Management
Nonpharmacologic Treatment
- Treatment of the underlying cause such as infection or inflammation with good hygiene, sitz baths, and warm compresses
- Surgical release or circumcision

Pharmacologic Treatment
- If concurrent infection or inflammation, treatment with topical antifungals or steroids may be sufficient to allow for retraction

How Long to Treat
- Topical treatment for underlying infection or inflammation for 1 to 2 weeks

When to Consult, Refer, Hospitalize
- Refer to urologist for surgical release or circumcision if nonresponsive to topical treatment and hygiene, urinary flow compromised, or asymptomatic phimosis remains

Follow-up
Expected Course
- Resolves with treatment

Complications
- Inflamed prepuce
- Meatal stenosis
- UTI
- Premalignant changes

Erectile Dysfunction
Description
- Inability to achieve or maintain a satisfactory erection more than 25% to 50% of the time
- May be defined by patients as loss of orgasm, premature ejaculation, or loss of emission, libido, or erections

Etiology
- Classified as either psychological or organic
- Psychological origin is likely with loss of orgasm when libido and erection are intact and with premature ejaculation concurrent with anxiety, depression, relationship problems, new partner, or emotional disorders
- If patient has nocturnal erections, problem is probably psychological, not organic
- Gradual loss of erections over time is indicative of organic causes
- Libido problems more associated with low testosterone level
- Medications such as anabolic steroids, digoxin (Lanoxin), antihypertensives, especially centrally acting (reserpine, clonidine, methyldopa); beta-blockers; and spironolactone (loss of libido); anti-depressants (MAOI, tricyclics, SSRI)
- Lifestyle issues of alcohol, drug, and cigarette (or other nicotine) use
- Hormonal and endocrine disorders of the thyroid, kidney, pituitary gland; or testicular function, Addison's disease and Cushing syndrome
- Vascular disorders such as arterial insufficiency, venous disease, atherosclerosis
- Neurologic disorders: cortical, brainstem, and spinal cord disorders; peripheral neuropathies; Parkinson's disease
- Posttreatment of prostate disorders
- Diabetes mellitus, increased with poor glucose control
- Renal failure
- Pain
- Arthritis

Incidence and Demographics

- Widely unreported; estimated that 10% of the male population and 35% of men over 60 affected
- 20 to 30 million men in the United States; increases with age

Risk Factors

- See Etiology

Prevention and Screening

- Maintaining a healthy relationship, seeking support or counseling
- Avoidance of known stressors that affect sexual relationships
- Close management of chronic diseases, especially diabetes

Assessment

History

- Determine the patient's perception or definition of erectile dysfunction to clarify the problem and symptoms, as well as the timing, circumstances, frequency of occurrence
- Complaints include any of the following: reduced size and strength of erection, lack of ability to achieve or maintain erections adequate for intercourse, rapid loss of erection with penetration, or lack of libido
- Determine nature of patient's relationship, sexual partners, lifestyle, and stress
- Inquire about nocturnal or morning erections: presence reflects intact blood supply, nervous system, and sexual apparatus; reduced likelihood of organic cause
- Associated symptoms indicative of underlying disease: decreased body hair; gynecomastia; neuropathies; anxiety; headaches; vision changes; decreased circulation; excessive skin dryness or skin changes; changes in testicles' size, consistency, or shape; and changes in penis such as rash, discharge, or phimosis
- Review past medical history for other diseases, testicular infections or insults, medications (prescription, OTC, and herbal), and history of smoking, drug, alcohol use

Physical

- Complete screening physical noting general appearance, generalized anxiety or hyperactivity, vital signs for postural hypotension, dry hair, loss of secondary sex characteristics, spider angiomas, hyperpigmentation, palmar erythema, or goiter
- Chest, abdomen, and extremities for cardiac abnormalities, gynecomastia, aortic or femoral bruits, peripheral vascular deficits
- Genital examination for penile circulation, discharge, fibrosis, or lesions; testicles for size, masses, varicoceles, or atrophy; DRE for prostate abnormalities, sphincter tone
- Neurologic screening for cortical, brainstem, spinal, or peripheral neuropathies, noting especially bulbocavernosi reflex, cremasteric reflex, pinprick, or light touch to genital and perianal area, focal tenderness of spine

Diagnostic Studies

- Key studies to screen for underlying etiology begin with plasma glucose, prolactin, and free testosterone, CBC, UA, and lipid profile
- Ultrasound to check for blood flow to penis
- Other tests dependent on findings of history/physical and results of preliminary tests
- For libido problems check total testosterone, luteinizing hormone, TSH, prolactin

- Urologist may include nocturnal penile tumescence and rigidity testing, duplex ultrasonography, penile angiography, nerve conduction studies, or a trial injection of prostaglandin E_1, phentolamine, and papaverine intracorporeally to assess vascular integrity, noting penile response

Differential Diagnosis
- See Etiology

Management
Nonpharmacologic Treatment
- Modify lifestyle: stress reduction techniques; stop alcohol, drugs, and cigarettes
- Use of a vacuum constriction device for those with venous disorders of the penis or nonresponsiveness to vasoactive injections
- Surgical treatment—penile implants

Pharmacologic Treatment
- Substitute or discontinue medications known to cause erectile dysfunction
- Some antihypertensives that are less likely to cause ED are calcium-channel blockers (nifedipine), angiotensin-converting enzyme blockers (lisinopril), selective beta-blockers (atenolol)
- Alternative antidepressants instead of SSRI (fluoxetine [Prozac], sertraline [Zoloft], paroxetine [Paxil], citalopram [Celexa])
- Some antidepressants less likely to cause ED are bupropion (Wellbutrin) and venlafaxine (Effexor)
- Treat hormonal abnormalities as follows
  - Insufficient testosterone treated with a 3-month testosterone trial (if indicated by androgen deficiency, without prostatic cancer) using testosterone injections 200 mg IM every 3 weeks or topical patches of 2.5 to 6 mg/day
  - Hyperprolactinemia treated with bromocriptine initially 2.5 mg b.i.d., up to 40 mg/d
- Phosphodiesterase type 5 inhibitor—do not give if patient on nitroglycerin
  - Sildenafil (Viagra) 25 to 50 mg 1 hour prior to desired erection (works within 30 min to 4 hours)
  - Tadalafil (Cialis) 2 to 20 mg
  - Vardenafil (Levitra) 2.5 to 20 mg
- Controversial oral agents include yohimbine, trazodone, and ginkgo biloba
- Penile injections such as alprostadil (Caverject), first dose in office setting, 1.25 to 2.5 mcg with repeat dose after 1 hour if no response; patient to remain in office until detumescence completed; partial response may have second injection within 24 hours
- Use of injections or oral agents requires thorough patient teaching on proper use, frequency of use, side effects and risk of priapism, and when to seek medical help, such as erection lasting more than 6 hours
- Alternatives to alprostadil are papaverine or phentolamine
- Urethral suppository of alprostadil (Muse) in various strength pellets

How Long to Treat
- Variable depending upon treatment methods

Special Considerations
- Age 70+: rarely seek help; most likely have physical problems

When to Consult, Refer, Hospitalize
- Psychotherapist for individual or couples therapy, sex therapy
- Urologist, endocrinologist, cardiologist, neurologist referrals as indicated by diagnosis and requirements for further evaluation or advanced treatment

Follow-up
- Follow-up is varied depending upon diagnosis, underlying etiology, response to treatment, and need for therapy; patients should be seen initially at shorter intervals to adjust and monitor responsiveness to treatment, then every 3 months

Expected Course
- Improvement in many patients with oral medications, vacuum devices, suppository and penile implants; 15% spontaneously improve
- 20% failure rate with vacuum device; 10% to 30% dissatisfaction with penile implant
- Alprostadil injections have an 85% to 90% response rate, while the urethral pellet method rates are 40% to 60%
- Phosphodiesterase type 5 inhibitors are effective for 70% of patients at maximal dose

Complications
- Variable depending upon underlying etiology and treatment method side effects
- Phosphodiesterase type 5 inhibitors cause hypotension, headache, flushing, nausea, nasal congestion, abnormal vision, cardiovascular events, priapism, prolonged erections

CASE STUDIES

Case 1. An 83-year-old man complains of urinary hesitancy, dribbling, urinary frequency of small amounts, nocturia 4x/night. This has been gradually getting worse of past few months.

1. What is the most likely diagnosis?
2. What physical exam is required?
3. If the symptoms are not troublesome, what is the usual approach?
4. What symptoms would require referral for treatment?
5. What nonpharmacologic treatment may be helpful?
6. Which medications would you consider starting the patient on? What are their main disadvantages?

Case 2. A 78-year-old Black man comes to you feeling poorly. He complains of fatigue and low back pain, which has been gradually increasing for the past few months. He has had urinary symptoms, which he attributed to BPH for the past 6 years, gradually worsening so that he is now having hesitancy, dribbling, and a feeling of not emptying his bladder completely. He has never sought treatment for the BPH symptoms because he thought it was an inevitable consequence of aging.
PMH: 50 pack/year smoking, COPD, osteoarthritis, hypertension, and hyperlipidemia.
Medications: ipratropium/albuterol (Combivent) inhaler, acetaminophen (Tylenol) p.r.n. pain, hydrochlorothiazide 25 mg p.o. q.d., atorvastatin (Lipitor) 40 mg p.o. q.d.

1. What do his urinary symptoms indicate?
2. What are the most likely possibilities for a differential diagnosis?
3. What lab work would you order?
4. Which would be most useful for deciding between the differential?
5. What risk factors does he have?
6. What would you do?
7. What follow-up is required?

Case 3. A 68-year-old man comes to your office with the complaint of insomnia. Says he is having some problems with his wife. She is not too happy with him. Patient seems reluctant to say what is really bothering him

1. How would you approach this situation?
2. What normal changes of aging affect sexual function?

History: Patient tells you he has a gradual loss of the ability to maintain an erection for the past year or so. His wife is upset about this and has been nagging him to do something about it. The problem became worse recently, after an argument with his wife.

3. Is this ED psychological or organic?

PMH: Patient has hypertension, diabetes, lipid disorder, osteoarthritis

4. How do these diseases affect ED?
5. What would be your initial approach?

REFERENCES

Barry, M. J., Fowler, F. J., O'Leary, M. P., Bruskewitz, R. C., Holtgrewe, H. L., & Mebust, W. K. (1992). Correlation of the American Urological Association symptom index with self-administered versions of the Madsen-Iverson, Boyarsky and Maine Medical Assessment Program Symptoms Indexes. *Journal of Urology, 148*, 1558–1563.

Carson, C. C. (2004). Erectile dysfunction: Evaluation and new treatment options. *Psychosomatic Medicine, 55*, 664–671.

Chapple, C. R. (2004). Pharmacological therapy of benign prostatic hyperplasia/lower urinary tract symptoms: An overview for the practicing clinician. *British Journal Urology International, 94*(5), 738–744.

Dambro, M. R. (2004). *The 5-minute clinical consult.* Philadelphia: Lippincott, Williams & Wilkins.

DeLuca, G. (2001). Prostatitis. *American Journal for Nurse Practitioners, 5*(3), 45–54.

Edmunds, M. W., & Mayhew, M. S. (2004). *Pharmacology for the primary care provider* (2nd ed.). St. Louis, MO: Mosby.

Ellsworth, P., & Kirshenbaum, E. M. (2008). Current concepts in the evaluation and management of erectile dysfunction. *Urologic Nursing, 28*(5), 357–369.

Ferri, F. F. (2003). *Ferri's clinical advisor* (6th ed.). St. Louis, MO: Mosby.

Gambert, S. R. (2001). Prostate cancer: When to offer screening in the primary care setting. *Geriatrics, 56*(1), 22–31.

Islam, J., & Cass, A. R. (2007). In R. J. Ham, P. D. Sloane, G. A. Warshaw, M. A. Bernard, & E. Flaherty (Eds.), *Primary care geriatrics: A case-based approach* (5th ed., pp. 575–590). New York: Mosby Elsevier

Lovejoy, B. (2001). Diagnosis and management of chronic prostatitis by primary care providers. *Journal of the American Academy of Nurse Practitioners, 13*(7), 317–321.

Meredith, P. V., & Horan, N. M. (2000). *Adult primary care.* Philadelphia: WB Saunders.

Raja, S. G., & Nayak, S. H. (2004). Sildenafil: Emerging cardiovascular indications. *Annals of Thoracic Surgery, 78*(4), 1496–1506.

Reuben, D. B., Herr, K. A., Pacala, J. T., Pollock, B. G., Potter, J. F., & Semla, T. P. (2007). *Geriatrics at your fingertips* (9th ed.). New York: American Geriatric Society.

Spalding, M. C., & Sebesta, S. C. (2008). Geriatric screening and preventive care. *American Family Physician, 78*(2), 206–215.

Tierney, L. M., McPhee, S. J., & Papadakis, A. (2005). *Current medical diagnosis and treatment* (44th ed.). Stamford, CT: Appleton & Lange.

Wagenlehner, F. M., & Naber, K. G. (2003) Antimicrobial treatment of prostatitis. *Expert Review of Anti-Infective Therapy, 1*(2), 275–282.

Musculoskeletal Disorders

MJ Henderson, MS, RN, GNP-BC

GERIATRIC APPROACH

Normal Changes of Aging

- Body composition: fat mass increases; bone and muscle mass and strength decrease
- Decreased water content leads to stiffness in tendons, ligaments, and cartilage
- Endocrine changes affecting bones and muscle
  - Adrenopause—reduced dehydroepiandrosterone (DHEA) levels may play part in increased adiposity and decreased lean muscle mass
  - Andropause
    - Reduction of total and free testosterone in men
    - Decreased testosterone in postmenopausal women has been associated with increased fracture risk
  - Menopause increases bone resorption, increasing the risk of osteopenia and osteoporosis
  - Growth hormone (GH) and insulin-like growth factor I (IGF-I) levels decrease; lower levels may assist in increasing adiposity, decreasing lean muscle mass and strength
  - Parathyroid hormone (PTH)—PTH levels increase; higher levels associated with increased bone resorption, increased osteoblast activity

Clinical Implications

History

- Family history of autoimmune disease, previous/current occupation, military service, athletics
- Onset of problem (Insidious or sudden? Progression of symptoms?)

- Timing: When does pain occur? Worse at night? With rest? With activity? With weather?
- Mechanism of injury (such as fall, twisting motion—how much force was involved?)
- Symptoms associated with pain: certain movements, positions, activities—any locking, catching, or giving way of a joint?
- Does the pain or symptoms interfere with function (activities of daily living [ADL], instrumental activities of daily living)?
- Previous pain, injury, or surgery in same area?
- Previous treatment? Self-treated or another provider? Include any medications, OTCs, herbs
- Concomitant medical problems, medications

Physical
- Assess for inflammation, swelling around joints, shape of joints, systemic disease
- Compare sides to assess for abnormalities
- Inspection: note signs of underlying pathology (such as vascular changes of skin, poor healing of wounds, presence of deformity, or malalignment, gait)
- Movements: check unaffected side first; first active, then passive range of motion (ROM, painful movements last); check ADL/transfer, ambulation/gait
- Tenderness to palpation, with active/passive movement (normal ROM may be decreased)
- Palpate for crepitus, grinding, catching of joints
- Manual muscle testing against resistance to assess strength; rate on scale of 1/5 to 5/5
- Provocative tests specific to area

Assessment
- Intra-articular processes will produce decreased range of motion, swelling, and inflammation
- Involvement of small joints (elbows, wrist, metacarpal, phalangeal joints and ankles) may indicate an inflammatory joint process rather than mechanical problem
- False-positive rheumatoid factor and elevated sedimentation rates are common; order these tests to make a specific diagnosis based on history and physical exam
- Consider deconditioning when evaluating a musculoskeletal problem
  - Immobility, for any reason, causes a rapid decrease in muscle strength very quickly; any decrease in activity will cause a corresponding decrease in strength
  - Reduced muscle mass and strength is associated with increased risk of physical frailty, falls, fractures, decreased function
  - Exercise can improve functional performance in older adults and increase muscle strength
  - Consider depression in the patient with chronic pain

Treatment
- Normal changes of aging may delay healing of musculoskeletal injuries
- Physical modalities of rest, ice, heat, compression, elevation, massage, and exercise may need to be modified because of changes in muscle mass, bone density, visual disturbances, or decreased sensory acuity, but are essential to management of musculoskeletal conditions in the older adult

- Medications
  - Acetaminophen is usually first-line pain medication for most musculoskeletal pain or injuries
    - Acetaminophen at 3,000 to 4,000 mg per day divided on regular basis
    - Maximum dose of acetaminophen is 4,000 mg in 24-hour period
    - Use with caution in presence of liver disease and alcohol use
  - Nonselective NSAIDs
    - Useful for short-term relief of pain in chronic arthritis, acute injury
    - Adverse effects more common in the older adult
    - Side effects include GI bleed, renal failure, liver failure, CHF, edema, confusion, and elevated blood pressure; use with extra caution in patients with these conditions
    - Patients with history of peptic ulcer disease or GI bleed have 10 times greater risk of GI bleed
    - When used long term, use lowest dose, monitor for;
      - Symptoms of blood loss/GI bleed, heart and renal failure
      - CBC for anemia and renal failure every 3 to 6 months
    - Ibuprofen: 400 to 800 mg with food t.i.d.-q.i.d.
    - Nabumetone (Relafen): 1,000 to 1,500 mg, may be give q.d. or divided b.i.d. with food
  - Selective COX-2 inhibitors
    - COX-2 inhibitors pose less risk of GI side effects and GI bleeding in those with risk
    - Celecoxib (Celebrex) 100 to 200 mg q.d.-b.i.d.; sulfa allergy a relative contraindication
    - Do not use for patients with concurrent cardiac disease or for those on warfarin
  - Narcotics may be safely used for noncancer pain not amenable to other treatment; use lowest effective doses; use with extreme caution regarding confusion, drowsiness, and constipation
    - Oxycodone generally fairly well tolerated; start at low doses and frequency, 5mg at HS; may give b.i.d.-q.i.d.; use for shortest possible duration
    - Propoxyphene has increased risk of delirium in older adults; use with caution in situations involving antidepressants or anxiolytics, excessive alcohol use, addiction risk, or suicidal ideation
    - Monitor use of OTC medications particularly with regard to prescribed medications and dosages of acetaminophen, NSAIDs, or aspirin
    - Other adverse effects include respiratory and cardiac depression, dizziness, nausea, vomiting, diaphoresis
    - Narcotics almost always cause constipation; start bowel regime (see GI, constipation), try stool softener with osmotic agent or stimulant; avoid hydrophilic colloid or bulk-forming agents particularly if inadequate fluid intake is an issue
    - Encourage fluids, increased dietary fiber, and mobility for all older adults on narcotics
    - Ultram (tramadol) 50 mg every 4 to 6 hours p.r.n. not to exceed 300 mg/day; a non-narcotic used for pain control
  - Use muscle relaxants (cyclobenzaprine, methocarbamol, metaxalone) with caution, **if at all,** as they may cause dizziness and falls

– Alternative treatments for pain: behavioral interventions
  • Try heat/ice to affected areas
  • Consider physical therapy and physical activity/movement to decrease pain

ARTHRITIS AND OTHER DISEASES

Osteoporosis

Description
• Osteoporosis: bone resorption occurs faster than bone formation, causing increased bone porosity in the trabecular bone (larger marrow spaces) and thinning of cortical bone
• Bone mineral density (BMD) at least 2.5 standard deviations (SD) below peak bone density (30-year-old control); represented as T-score of –2.5 or lower
• Osteopenia: BMD T score of –1 to –2.4

Etiology
• Hormone deficiency: estrogen, androgen
• Cushing syndrome or steroid use
• Malignancy (multiple myeloma, leukemia)
• Chronic hyperthyroidism, hyperparathyroidism
• Rheumatoid arthritis
• Vitamin D deficiency, vitamin A excess
• Chronic heparin use

Incidence and Demographics
• Approximately 11 million people in the United States have osteoporoisis of the hip
• 4/10 women and 1/10 men > 50 years of age will have a fracture of the hip, spine, or wrist
• Primarily affects postmenopausal women (over 50) and men over 70
• 21% of postmenopausal women have osteoporosis
• About 40% of women over 50 have had a fracture due to osteoporosis
• It costs 18 billion dollars per year to treat osteoporotic fractures

Risk Factors
• Menopause, early menopause < 45 years (natural or surgical)
• Inadequate calcium intake; premenopausal intake important
• Fracture in 1st-degree relative
• Petite frame, low weight (less that 127 pounds)
• Tall, thin women and men
• Dementia
• Recurrent falls
• Depression
• Frailty
• Decreased physical activity; immobilization
• Reduced vision
• Smoking
• Excessive alcohol intake, > 2 drinks/day
• Any fracture after age 50

Prevention and Screening
- Nutritional diet with adequate intake of calcium and vitamin D
- Regular weight-bearing exercise/resistance exercise
- Smoking cessation
- Avoiding high alcohol intake
- Bone densitometry or dual-energy x-ray absorptiometry (DXA) scan of axial skeleton for screening and diagnosis recommended for all women 65 and older and for women 60 and older with increased risk, such as those who have lost height or had a fracture after age 50

Assessment
History
- Any fracture after age 50 especially spine, hip, wrist
- Loss of height
- Back pain (from vertebral fracture)
- Diet, exercise, medications
- Articular stiffness, developing into pain with motion; pain relieved by rest

Physical
- Usually no finding specific to osteoporosis, especially early
- Kyphosis with bulging abdomen is common in more advanced osteoporosis
- Fracture is the most common presenting sign
- Documented decrease in height over time

Diagnostic Studies
- Bone densitometry
- Osteoporosis shows on regular x-rays after more than 30% of bone is lost
- To rule out secondary causes of osteoporosis, check TSH, free T4, PTH, CA, 25-hydroxy vitamin D, phosphate, albumin, alkaline phosphatase, kidney and liver tests, electrolytes, protein electrophoresis, CBC, UA, and bioavailable testosterone in men

Differential Diagnosis
- Osteoarthritis
- Paget disease
- Metastatic bone disease
- Rheumatic disease
- Fibromyalgia
- Gout
- Multiple myeloma
- Acute injury

Management
Nonpharmacologic Treatment
- Regular weight-bearing exercise (20 to 30 minutes/day, 6 to 7 days/week)
- Fall-prevention management and education
- Smoking cessation
- No more than 1 to 2 alcoholic drinks per day

Pharmacologic Treatment
- Calcium supplementation (1,200 to 1,500 mg/day) or adequate dietary intake; calcium citrate better for those taking PPI and those with achlorhydria

- Adequate vitamin D intake 800 IU/day (some recommend up to 4,000 mg per day)
- All pharmacological treatments for osteoporosis require optimal calcium and vitamin D intake to be effective
- Bisphosphonates: alendronate (Fosamax) 70 mg per week or 150 mg per month, or risedronate (Actonel) 35 mg p.o. once weekly or 75 mg on 2 consecutive days per month, or ibandronate (Boniva) 150 mg p.o. per month, or 3 mg IV every 3 months; must take on empty stomach in the morning and remain sitting or standing for 30 minutes (60 minutes for ibandronate) before eating or it will not be absorbed or will cause severe esophagitis; *or*
- Zoledronic acid (Reclast) 5 mg IV once a year; *or*
- Parathyroid hormone teriparatide (Forteo) 20 mcg SC q.d. for a maximum of 2 years; is more effective than bisphosphonates but must be given SC daily
- Selective estrogen receptor modulators (SERM): raloxifene (Evista) 60 mg/day p.o. for postmenopausal women may help with vertebral fracture pain
- Calcitonin nasal spray (Miacalcin) 200 units/day intranasal, alternating nostrils; for patients unable to take bisphosphonates because of GI distress; not as effective as bisphsphonates; also used as analgesic for compression fractures

How Long to Treat
- Indefinitely or until treatment is contraindicated by patient's condition

When to Consult, Refer, Hospitalize
- Refer to rheumatologist or endocrinologist if patient does not respond to treatment
- Refer to orthopedist for suspected fracture; hospitalize for any hip fracture

Follow-up
Expected Course
- Improvement or maintenance of bone density evident by DXA every 2 years after initiation of therapy
- Benefit continues to be seen after 10 years of treatment with no new adverse effects
- Follow-up monitoring (DXA) may improve adherence to treatment plan
- Monitor height changes

Complications
- Major cause of morbidity in the older adult
- Fracture (vertebral most common, associated with chronic pain; hip most disabling and has greatest mortality); see section on fractures for more information
- Impaired gait
- Chronic pain syndrome
- Inability to perform basic activities of daily living, has major impact on quality of life

Arthritis

Table 14-1. Characteristics of Osteoarthritis and Rheumatoid Arthritis

Characteristics	Osteoarthritis	Rheumatoid Arthritis
Radiographic appearance	Joint space narrowing, osteophytes, subchondral bone sclerosis, subchondral cysts	Evidence of osteoporosis with/without subchondral bone destruction (bone and cartilage involvement in later stages), joint deformities
Morning stiffness	Lasts < 30 minutes	Lasts > 1 hour
Joint involvement	Usually weight-bearing (spine, hips, knees), or distal finger joints (DIP)	Multiple small joints, symmetric joint involvement (esp. of hands); rare in spine
Laboratory findings	ESR < 20 to 40 mm/hr; RF negative	Serum RF abnormal (usually elevated) ESR usually elevated (not definitive diagnosis) anti-CCP elevated, as is CRP
Clinical findings that may be present	Joint pain, bony tenderness and hypertrophy, crepitus, may have some deformity; no palpable warmth, occasional fluid in joint.	Joint deformity, soft tissue swelling or fluid; muscle atrophy, extra-articular soft tissue nodules (rheumatoid nodules) acute—red, warm, swollen, & tender

Osteoarthritis

Description
- Degenerative disorder of the movable joints characterized by destruction of cartilage and bone hypertrophy, and formation of osteophytes and subchondral cysts; there is no systemic involvement
- Hypertrophy of bone at the articular margins
- Inflammation absent or minimal

Etiology
- May be a combination of mechanical and genetic factors
- May be secondary to injury or repetitive use

Incidence and Demographics
- Most common form of arthritis; affects more than 20 million people in the United States
- Up to 90% of U.S. population older than 40 years has radiographic evidence of osteoarthritis
- Incidence increases with advancing age
- Asians, Pacific Islanders have lower prevalence than other races
- Native Americans have greatest prevalence

Risk Factors
- Advancing age
- Repetitive joint use
- Trauma

- Obesity
- Family history

Prevention and Screening
- Moderate physical activity
- Maintain ideal body weight, avoid obesity

Assessment
History
- Gradual onset of joint pain and stiffness that often worsens with activity and is relieved by rest
- Morning stiffness common but usually lasts less than 30 minutes
- Weather changes may affect symptoms
- More advanced symptoms include:
  - More joints involved
  - Joint instability, especially with osteoarthritis of knees
  - Coarse crepitus felt in joint
  - Bony enlargement of joint with decreased range of motion
  - May have decreased sensation

Physical
- Localized to affected joints, not a systemic disease
- Bony hypertrophy of joint, tenderness at joint line; limited range of motion
  - Distal interphalangeal (DIP) joint swelling: Heberden's node
  - Proximal interphalangeal (PIP) joint swelling: Bouchard's node
- Soft tissue swelling may be present; decreased ROM
- Crepitus with movement
- Joint effusion, if present, usually mild

Diagnostic Studies
- Plain radiographs: presence of osteophytes, asymmetric joint space (narrowing), subchondral bone, sclerosis and, cysts
- Presence of radiographic changes does not correlate with presence or severity of symptoms
- Laboratory findings: ESR almost always normal; primary use is ruling out inflammatory condition; no specific laboratory tests for osteoarthritis

Differential Diagnosis
- Gout
- Fibromyalgia
- Osteoporosis
- Multiple myeloma
- Acute injury
- Rheumatoid arthritis
- Polymyalgia rheumatica
- Trauma

Management
- Goals are to relieve symptoms, maintain/improve function, avoid adverse effects of medication

Nonpharmacologic Treatment
- Physical activity/therapy is the cornerstone of treatment
- Occupational therapy
- Heat/cold to affected joint
- Non–weight-bearing exercise; arthritis self-help and water aquatics courses
- Ambulation aids (canes, braces, walkers) or assistive devices to facilitate function
- Weight loss programs if appropriate

Pharmacologic Treatment (see Clinical Implications)
- Acetaminophen up to 4000 mg/day in divided doses is first-line therapy for pain
- Topical analgesic creams such as diclofenac sodium/Voltaren 1% gel; lidocaine 5% patches
- NSAIDs can be very effective, especially in those with severe disease who have inflammatory response, but GI risks may outweigh benefits. May use COX-2 inhibitor celecoxib (Celebrex) cautiously in those at no risk for cardiac disease; again, risks may outweigh benefits.
- Intra-articular corticosteroid or hyaluronic acid injections may be helpful

Surgical Treatment
- Consider joint replacement when other modalities are not sufficient to manage pain and facilitate function

When to Consult, Refer, Hospitalize
- Patients with functional impairment, or need for intra-articular injections or moderate to severe pain should be referred to rheumatologist or orthopedic surgeon

Follow-up
Expected Course
- Gradual progressive worsening
- Limitation of activity, difficulty with ADL

Complications
- Decreased quality of life
- Chronic pain
- Adverse effects of pain medications
- Injury to specific joints: cervical and lumbar radiculopathy, rotator cuff tears, meniscus and quadriceps rupture, and impingement syndromes

Rheumatoid Arthritis (RA)
Description
- Chronic, inflammatory, systemic disease with symmetric bone erosions, small joint destruction of hands and feet, and progressive limitation in function

Etiology
- Probably autoimmune, but no specific inciting factor or infectious agent yet identified
- Genetic, environmental factors affect progression and extent of disease

Incidence and Demographics
- Prevalence in general population is 1% to 2%
- Prevalence about 2.5 times greater in females

- Usual age of onset is commonly between the fourth and fifth decade with peak age of onset between 35 and 50 years of age, but may begin at any age
- Some American Indian populations have a higher prevalence of RA, > 5%
- Persists and progresses in old age

Risk Factors
- Susceptibility is genetically determined
- Smoking

Assessment
History
- Usually insidious, gradual onset over several weeks, diagnosed after symptoms have been present for 6 weeks
- May have acute flares superimposed over chronic progressive course

  SYSTEMIC SYMPTOMS
  - Prodromal symptoms of malaise, fatigue, weight loss, low-grade fever, anorexia, and weakness, may persist indefinitely

  JOINT INVOLVEMENT
  - Stiffness and pain in smaller joints
  - Hands: proximal interphalangeal (PIP), metacarpophalangeal (MCP), and wrist joints
  - Elbow, ankle, and metatarsophalangeal (MTP) joints of foot
  - Rheumatoid nodules
  - Involvement usually symmetrical, in 3 or more joints simultaneously
  - Morning stiffness lasts longer than 1 hour

Physical
- Acute inflammation of joint with redness, heat, swelling, and tenderness to palpation may occur
- Often less acute presentation with symmetric joint swelling with stiffness
- Stiffness in the morning, after inactivity, and after strenuous activity is a good measure of activity of the disease
- Subcutaneous rheumatoid nodules are seen over the ulna, olecranon, olecranon bursa, fingers, and Achilles tendon and are usually mobile and nontender
- As disease progresses, damage to joints progresses and joint deformities become more pronounced

Diagnostic Studies
- No single test is adequate to make diagnosis
- Elevated serum rheumatoid factor (RF) in about 85% of cases (also found in infection, other autoimmune diseases)
- CBC frequently shows anemia of chronic disease; elevated platelet count may be present in severe disease
- ESR (erythrocyte sedimentation rate) correlates with degree of synovial inflammation
- C-reactive protein (CRP) may also be used to monitor inflammation
- Antibodies to cyclic citrullinated peptide (CCP antibodies) more specific to RA than other tests and found earlier in the disease
- Elevated alkaline phosphatase is seen sporadically
- Synovial fluid shows sterile leukocytosis

- Gammaglobulinemia: elevated IgM and IgG
- X-ray will show joint erosions and narrowing of joint spaces

Differential Diagnosis
- Systemic lupus erythematosus (SLE)
- Rheumatic fever
- Septic joint
- Psoriatic arthritis
- Ankylosing spondylitis
- Osteoarthritis
- Gout

Management
- Goals are early diagnosis and early treatment to prevent or limit irreversible joint damage, maximize mobility, and limit pain and depression
- Course of therapy depends on disease severity; early consultation with or referral to rheumatologist is recommended

Nonpharmacologic Treatment
- Patient education (Arthritis Foundation self-help courses)
- Physical and occupational therapy to strengthen muscles, improve joint ROM and function, protect joint(s)
- Regular exercise program, except rest during flares
- Assistive devices (canes, splints) to facilitate function

Pharmacologic Treatment
- NSAIDs are used first, while diagnosis is being confirmed. Weigh risks versus benefits for older adults.
  - Have not been shown to alter disease course but may offer symptom relief
  - Biologic agents (disease-modifying anti-rheumatic drugs [DMARD]) such as sulfasalazine, hydroxychloroquine, or methotrexate are options to start
  - Methotrexate (MTX) is considered by many to be treatment of choice
  - Beneficial effect in 2 to 6 weeks
  - Common adverse effect is gastric irritation, folic acid depletion
  - Serious adverse effects are interstitial pneumonitis, hepatotoxicity, and bone marrow suppression
  - Patients should not drink alcohol while on MTX
  - Need folic acid replacement
  - Corticosteroids
  - Prednisone PO or methylprednisolone IM
  - For acute flares; failure to respond to other medications
  - Does not alter course of disease
  - Use lowest dose for shortest period of time to avoid long-term side effects
  - Leflunomide (Arava) also used but not for consumers of alcohol; patient needs folic acid replacement
- Antimalarials: hydroxychloroquine (Plaquenil)
  - Good for mild disease, 25% to 50% will respond; takes 3 to 6 months to have effect
  - Comparative low toxicity: one adverse effect is pigmentary retinitis, which requires ophthalmology exams
  - Also may cause neuropathies, myopathies

- Anti–tumor necrosis factor (anti-TNF) blockers are new drugs that may replace methotrexate as first line therapy; examples include etanercept (Enbrel), infliximab (Remicade), adalimumab (Humira), and rituximab (Rituxan)
- Abatacept (Orencia), a soluble fusion protein, can be used if the anti-TNF agents fail; not for use with anti-TNF agents
  - All of the above may cause hypersensitivity reaction, severe infections or sepsis, and autoimmunity (lupus-type syndrome)
  - Work faster than methotrexate; good response in 60%
  - Are extremely expensive; insurance coverage is variable

How Long to Treat
- Lifelong therapy is indicated

When to Consult, Refer, Hospitalize
- Refer to rheumatologist for management; patients in long-term-care facilities are referred when symptoms are not controlled
- Physical therapy

Follow-up
- Frequent follow-ups are indicated until symptoms are controlled; then regular evaluations at 3- to 6-month intervals
- Laboratory testing as indicated by medication side-effect profile; at least a CBC and liver tests every 8 weeks

Expected Course
- Destruction of joints begins to appear within a few months of disease onset
- Variable course with remission and exacerbations
- For some patients, the acute inflammation resolves, but patient is left with deformities of joints with severely decreased functional ability

Complications
- Severe systemic effects: pleuritis, pericarditis, vasculitis
- Musculoskeletal: muscle wasting, contractures, carpal tunnel syndrome
- Patients may sustain substantial joint damage and develop poor functional status
- Adverse effects of medications, especially GI bleed and to hepatic and renal systems
- Increased vulnerability to infection

Gout
Description
- Disease resulting from hyperuricemia in which there is deposition of uric acid or monosodium urate crystals in supersaturated extracellular fluids (particularly in and around joints and tendons)
- Three classic stages: asymptomatic hyperuricemia, acute intermittent gout, chronic tophaceous gout
- Pseudogout is calcium pyrophosphate dihydrate crystal deposition disease (CPPD)

Etiology
- Underlying pathology is hyperuricemia (serum urate > 7.0 mg/dL) due to underexcretion of urate by the kidneys in 90% of cases, and less commonly caused by overproduction
  - Overproduction: inherited enzyme defects; idiopathic, lymph, and myeloproliferative disorders; high intake of ethanol and purine-rich foods (organ meats, shellfish,

peas, lentils, beans); hemolytic disorders; obesity; malignant diseases; warfarin; and cytotoxic drugs
- Underexcretion: chronic renal failure, hypertension, dehydration, obesity, hyperparathyroidism, hypothyroidism, lead nephropathy, and drugs such as thiazide diuretics, ethanol cyclosporine, ethambutol, low-dose salicylate, cyclosporine, pyrazinamide, and levodopa

Incidence and Demographics
- Affects 2.1 million in the United States
- Higher incidence in men; occurs in postmenopausal women
- Slightly higher incidence in Black males with hypertension than in Whites
- High incidence in Pacific islanders
- Peak incidence is fifth decade

Risk Factors
- Heredity
- Obesity
- Thiazide diuretics
- Alcohol ingestion

Prevention and Screening
- Correct/control underlying etiology
- Avoid foods high in purines
- Maintain normal body weight

Assessment
History
- Classic: sudden attack of red, hot, swollen, exquisitely tender joint is common; if this occurs in first MTP joint, it's known as podagra
- More commonly: chronic joint pain, in more than one joint
- Foot, ankle, knee are most common sites; wrist, elbow, fingers also may be affected

Physical
- During acute attack, joint is red, hot, swollen, exquisitely painful; fever, chills, malaise may accompany acute attack
- Tophi (sodium urate crystals deposited in soft tissue) present in chronic tophaceous gout; usually after 2 or 3 to 10 years from onset of acute intermittent gout; may be confused with nodules from rheumatoid arthritis or osteoarthritis
- Joint swelling, restricted movement in late/chronic stages because of arthritis

Diagnostic Studies
- Joint aspiration: fluid shows presence of urate crystals on polarized light microscopy, increased WBC
- Serum uric acid > 7.0 mg/dL supports diagnosis but is not specific
- Elevated ESR in acute gout
- Excision of nodule shows gouty tophus
- X-ray: shows punched-out lesions in subchondral bone, usually first seen in first MTP joint ("Mickey Mouse" ears); tophi may be seen if at least 5 mm in diameter

Differential Diagnosis
- Septic joint
- Pseudo gout
- Acute rheumatic fever
- Rheumatoid arthritis
- Osteoarthritis

Management
Nonpharmacologic Treatment

ACUTE
- Rest
- Local application of cold; use with caution in patients with peripheral vascular disease or peripheral neuropathy

CHRONIC
- Dietary modification: avoid purines and alcohol
- Fluid intake ≥ 3 liters/day
- Weight loss in obese patients

Pharmacologic Treatment
- Asymptomatic hyperuricemia is rarely treated
- Use all gout medications with caution, especially in patients with renal insufficiency or dehydration

ACUTE
- NSAIDs or Clochicine are the treatments of choice
  - Indomethacin is not recommended for use in geriatric patients since it produces the most central nervous system side effects
  - Treat until pain resolved; COX-2 inhibitors not FDA approved for gout
- Colchicine dose is 0.6 mg p.o. every 2 hours until pain is relieved or nausea or diarrhea occurs; total dose not to exceed 8 mg/day; usually relief in 3 to 14 days
  - Nausea, diarrhea or abdominal cramping frequently occurs; bone marrow suppression and myoneuropathy may occur
  - Used for patients who are not good candidates for NSAIDs, such as individuals on anticoagulants or those with congestive heart failure, renal insufficiency
  - Drug has very narrow therapeutic index, monitor closely
- Corticosteroids p.o. or injection may be used for patients unable to take oral NSAIDs

CHRONIC
- Treat chronic gout to keep uric acid level within normal limits and minimize urate deposition in tissues
- Avoid or decrease dose of diuretics
- Colchicine 0.6 mg p.o. 1 to 2 times a day
- Allopurinol is for chronic gout only
  - 100 mg to 300 mg per day depending on creatinine clearance
  - Do not use to treat acute gout or asymptomatic hyperuricemia
  - Adverse events include fatal skin reactions, hypersensitivity reactions, and renal and hepatotoxicity

How Long to Treat
- Acute symptoms treated until symptoms are relieved
- Lifelong therapy begun if:
  - Repeated attacks of disabling gout
  - Chronic gout
  - Presence of tophi

When to Consult, Refer, Hospitalize
- Consult for any complicated presentation, renal disease, underlying metabolic pathology
- Refer to rheumatologist for joint aspiration, unclear diagnosis

Follow-up
Expected Course
- Decrease in frequency, severity of attacks with appropriate treatment

Complications
- Kidney stones, renal obstruction and infection
- Joint destruction, chronic arthritis of multiple joints with decreased mobility
- Complications frequent from medications used to treat

Polymyalgia Rheumatica
Description
- Polymyalgia rheumatica (PMR) is a syndrome characterized by aching and morning stiffness in the proximal joints (shoulder and pelvic girdles) associated with an elevated sedimentation rate
- Giant-cell arteritis (GCA) is a systemic inflammation of medium and large arteries; when it affects the temporal arteries, it is called temporal arteritis (TA) and manifests in severe temporal artery pain, scalp pain, and vision loss; TA may lead to blindness; requires immediate referral to ophthalmologist for temporal artery biopsy
- PMR, GCA, and TA appear to be related disorders; PMR responds to low-dose steroids, while GCA and TA require high-dose therapy

Etiology
- Genetic predisposition
- Cellular, immune, and humoral mechanisms involved

Incidence and Demographics
- PMR is relatively common in the older adult
- Occurs in persons aged 50 years or older
- Average age at onset is 70
- Women affected twice as often as men; Whites more than Blacks

Risk Factors
- Family history

Prevention and Screening
- None

Assessment
History
- Onset is usually gradual, but may be abrupt
- Fatigue, anorexia, and weight loss may be early symptoms
- Stiffness, malaise, aching, depression may be present
- Shoulder girdle first to be affected; may start unilaterally, then become bilateral
- Pelvic girdle often affected; patients have difficulty standing up without pushing up with arms
- Gelling (stiffening) after inactivity and early morning stiffness are prominent

Physical
- Weakness of proximal joints
- Difficulty and pain with movement of joints
- Low-grade fever may be present

Diagnostic Studies
- Sedimentation rate is essential for diagnosis; must be > 50 mm/h
- May have anemia and elevated LFT, especially alkaline phosphatase
- Not associated with rheumatoid factor, antinuclear antibodies, or other autoantibodies

Differential Diagnosis
PMR is a diagnosis of exclusion:
- Rheumatoid arthritis
- Polymyositis
- Chronic infection
- Malignancy
- Hypothyroidism
- Hyperthyroidism
- Myeloma/leukemia

Management
Nonpharmacologic Treatment
- Exercise to maintain and augment function

Pharmacologic Treatment
- High initial dose prednisone; prednisone 10 to 20 mg q.d. may be required for life
- Clinical response should be within 3 days; if no response, reevaluate diagnosis

How Long to Treat
- Continue prednisone for 6 months to 2 years
- Taper depending on ESR
- Disease flares are common as prednisone is decreased

Special Considerations
- If signs and symptoms are consistent with TA, start 60 mg prednisone immediately and refer for temporal artery biopsy; untreated TA can cause blindness
- A PMR patient on low-dose prednisone can develop TA

When to Consult, Refer, Hospitalize
- Patient should be referred to rheumatologist for confirmation of diagnosis and management

Follow-up
- Monitor ESR closely; monthly and after each change in prednisone
- Monitor for signs and symptoms indicative of temporal arteritis

Expected Course
- PMR generally resolves after about a year

Complications
- PMR can lead to TA, which can cause blindness
- Anticipate and manage side effects of prednisone, including hyperglycemia, edema, osteoporosis

INJURY/OVERUSE SYNDROMES
Neck Pain
Description
- Injury or damage to structures in the neck; may cause occipital headache or neck, trapezius, rhomboid, or parascapular pain

Etiology
- Most common causes
  - Osteoporosis or osteoarthritis
  - Trauma, especially whiplash
  - Neck strain or spasm
  - Falls
  - Significant kyphosis

Incidence and Demographics
- 50% of those over age 50 will have neck pain at some time
- 80% of those over age 55 have some evidence of degenerative disk disease on cervical spine x-rays

Risk Factors
- Age
- Previous trauma or injury, degenerative joint disease
- Osteoporosis

Assessment
History
- Identify onset or precipitating events or trauma
- Acute or chronic
- Associated neurological symptoms: paresthesia, weakness, dizziness or vertigo, drop attacks, visual or hearing impairments, particularly with neck movement
- Impact on function and sleep
- Previous attempts at pain management

Physical
- Do not test range of motion if fracture suspected (e.g., any trauma)
- Asymmetric range of motion of neck
- Distal muscle wasting
- Decreased reflexes

- Sensory impairment
- Neurological and muscular skeletal exam may reveal level of cervical lesion
  - C-5: weakness of shoulder abductors and elbow flexors
  - C-6: weakness of wrist extensors
  - C-7: weakness of finger abductors

Diagnostic Studies
- X-rays: rule out tumor; findings of degenerative changes may not correlate with severity of symptoms
- MRI to confirm positive neurological findings if herniated disk or cord compression is suspected
- Electromyogram to confirm diagnosis of radiculopathy

Differential Diagnosis
Important to rule out:
- Tumor, metastasis
- Meningitis
- Rheumatoid arthritis
- Polymyalgia rheumatica
- Compression fracture
- Torticollis
- Ankylosing spondylitis
- Cervical herniated nucleus pulposus

Management
Nonpharmacologic Treatment
- Heat
- Soft cervical collar short term for whiplash
- Exercises for neck strengthening as tolerated
- Surgery for decompression if indicated

Pharmacologic Treatment
- See Clinical Implications for pain management
- Use muscle relaxants with caution in the older adult
- Refer for consideration of injecting trigger points with local anesthetic or cortisone

Special Considerations
- Surgical decompression for myelopathy is 75% to 80% effective

When to Consult, Refer, Hospitalize
- Emergently immobilize neck and refer to ED if acute traumatic fracture is suspected
- Refer to neurosurgery for focal neurologic deficits with suspected cord or nerve root compression
- Refer for corticosteroid injection
- Physical therapy for exercises

Follow-up
Expected Course
- Most pain responds to 4 to 6 weeks of conservative treatment

Complications
- Chronic pain, limited ROM, weakness, pain, decreased function of upper extremities

Low Back Pain
Description
- Low back pain (LBP) is a symptom, not a disease; for example, aching or sharp pain in lower lumbar, lumbosacral, or sacroiliac area
- Sciatica: symptom of pain that radiates down one or both buttocks/legs; often but not always caused by herniated disk
- Herniated disk: rupture of nucleus pulposus through annulus fibrosis of intervertebral disk; compresses spinal cord or irritates associated nerve root; more often unilateral but may have central herniation
- Spinal stenosis is narrowing of the spinal canal, usually from osteoarthritis
- Cauda equina is the collection of spinal roots descending from the lower spinal cord; compression of these is a medical emergency

Etiology
- Musculoskeletal most common
- Muscle/ligament strain
- Osteoarthritis
- Degenerative disk disease
- Disk herniation
- Spinal stenosis
- Vertebral compression fracture

Incidence and Demographics
- One of the most common complaints in primary care
- Most back pain in older patients has its onset before age 65

Risk Factors
- Physical deconditioning
- Poor body mechanics
- Cigarette smoking
- Obesity
- Scoliosis
- Depression
- Degenerative joint disease
- Osteoporosis

Prevention and Screening
- Regular exercise program
- Maintain ideal body weight
- Proper body mechanics and posture (may need orthotics in shoes)

Assessment
- Key is to assess for neurological compromise from herniated disc or cauda equina

History
- Onset of back pain, any precipitating events, chronic or acute
- Impact on function, mobility, and ADL

- Stiffness usually associated with muscular injury
- Paresthesia or sciatica (burning pain in buttock and leg) is associated with herniated disk or radiculopathy
- Gait disturbance along with back pain suggests spinal stenosis
- Pain at night unrelieved by rest suggests tumor, infection, compression fracture, ankylosing spondylitis, or malignancy
- Bilateral leg weakness, saddle area anesthesia, or bladder and bowel incontinence indicate a cauda equina process from tumor, epidural abscess, or massive disk herniation

Table 14-2. Differences Between Simple LBP and LBP Due to Herniated Disk

Clinical Problem	History	Physical Examination
Simple Low Back Pain	Pain in back, buttocks, and/or thigh Onset usually after exertion No history of trauma, infection, malignancy Pain relieved by lying supine	Paravertebral tenderness, muscle spasm Loss of normal lumbar lordosis common No neurologic deficit
Low Back Pain Due to Herniated Disk	Initially, back pain severe Chronic herniation usually results in leg pain greater than back pain Often + history of trauma, forced flexion Central herniation results in bilateral leg weakness, bowel/bladder dysfunction (cauda equina syndrome)	L5-S1 (most common): pain in posterior thigh, posterior/lateral calf, heel; weak plantar flexion of foot; diminished ankle reflex L4-5: pain in lateral thigh, anterior calf, and dorsum of foot; weak dorsiflexion of foot L3-4: pain in anterior and lateral thigh, medial calf, and foot; weak quadriceps; diminished patellar reflex

Physical

- With the patient on his or her back, raise one leg with knee absolutely straight, until pain is experienced in the thigh, buttock, and calf; record angle at which pain occurs; a normal (pain-free) value would be 70° to 90°, higher in people with lax ligaments
- Then perform sciatic stretch test: dorsiflex foot at the point of discomfort; test is positive if additional pain results
- Flexing the knee will relieve the buttock pain, but this is restored by pressing on the lateral popliteal nerve
- Severe root irritation is indicated when straight raising of the leg on the unaffected side produces pain on the affected side

Diagnostic Studies

- X-ray: order when new onset and to rule out acute compression fracture, as treatment options are different; x-ray not often necessary for simple LBP but useful for identifying degenerative changes, vertebral alignment, bone tumor, disk space height
- MRI: most useful for identifying herniated nucleus pulposus and diskitis, or if considering surgery or spinal injections
- Bone scan: helpful for identifying metabolically active processes such as tumor, occult fracture, infection, abscess

- Serum studies usually not helpful but ESR elevated in infection; HLA-B27 positive in ankylosing spondylitis

Differential Diagnosis
Metabolic Disorders
- Osteoporosis with compression fractures
- Osteomalacia
- Paget's disease

Cancer
- Metastatic prostate
- Multiple myeloma
- Lymphoma

Autoimmune Connective Tissue Disorders
- Rheumatoid arthritis
- PMR
- Reiter syndrome
- Psoriatic arthritis
- Ankylosing spondylitis

Nonmusculoskeletal Origin
- Abdominal aortic aneurysm
- Peptic ulcer
- Endocarditis
- Pancreatic disease
- Renal stones
- Ovarian cysts, tumors
- Infection

Management
- Most simple LBP responds to conservative treatment
- 80% or more of patients with LBP due to herniated disk also respond to conservative treatment

Nonpharmacologic Treatment
- Relieve pain to facilitate function and maintain activity
- Avoid bed rest, which causes deconditioning
- Modified activity as tolerated; no heavy lifting; avoid activities that provoke pain
- Ice, and/or heat and massage
- Physical therapy for muscle conditioning exercises
- In certain instances, braces may reduce symptoms for vertebral compression fractures but may be uncomfortable and restrict respirations in the older adult
- Chiropractic manipulation use with caution in older adults with osteoporosis
- Resumption of normal activities with careful body mechanics, back exercises

Pharmacologic Treatment
- Short term
  - Tylenol, NSAIDs, lidocaine patch 5% (Lidoderm)
  - Use muscle relaxants with caution
- Long term (see pain management section, Chapter 4): may need to refer to pain management clinic/team for TENS units or injections

How Long to Treat
- Most episodes resolve within 4 to 6 weeks of conservative treatment; if patient in severe pain, reevaluate in 24 to 48 hours

When to Consult, Refer, Hospitalize
- Refer for vertebroplasty immediately if evidence of cauda equina syndrome, acute fractures; this is an image-guided, minimally invasive, nonsurgical therapy used to strengthen a broken vertebra by injecting an orthopedic cement mixture through a needle into the fractured bone
- Refer immediately for spinal instability, neurological deficit
- Hospitalize for suspected abscess, tumor, abdominal aneurysm, cauda equina
- Obtain consult for patients who do not respond to 6 to 8 weeks of conservative treatment
- Physical and occupational therapy

Follow-up
- Provide patient education about body mechanics, conservative therapy, use of medications and their side effects

Expected Course
- Most acute LBP resolves in 4 to 6 weeks with conservative care
- Remitting and recurring symptoms are common

Complications
- Few complications if diagnosed and treated, though recurrence is common
- Can develop a chronic pain syndrome that can be difficult to manage
- With neurologic deficit, can have permanent nerve damage if compression of nerve root not relieved in timely manner
- Depression

SPECIFIC JOINT PROBLEMS

- Older adults have many complaints of joint pain, stiffness
- Arthritis often initially presents with single joint involvement but will progress to multiple joints
- Specific joint problems may be a complication of a generalized arthritis such as RA, OA, and gout
- If the patient consistently has a specific joint problem, consider the following options:
- Bursitis, tendonitis, and muscle strain and ligament sprain will be discussed as a group
- Impingement syndromes and other problems will be discussed individually
- See Chapter 4 for discussion of fractures

Table 14-3. Common Problems of Joints, Organized by Joint and Problem

Joint	Bursitis	Tendonitis	Strain / Sprain	Entrapment Neuropathies	Other Local Conditions
Shoulder	Subacromial Subdeltoid	Rotator cuff Bicipital	Deltoid muscle strain	Impingement syndrome	Adhesive capsulitis Rotator cuff strain, tear
Wrist		De Quervain	Radiocarpal muscle strain	Carpal tunnel	Ganglion cyst
Elbow	Olecranon	Medial, lateral epicondylitis		Cubital tunnel	
Hip	Trochanteric Iliopsoas Ischial				Spontaneous fractures
Knee	Prepatellar Infrapatellar Pes anserine	Iliotibial band Patellar	Collateral ligament sprains		Meniscus tear Quadriceps rupture
Ankle	Retrocalcaneal	Achilles Posterior tibialis Peroneal	Ligaments of ankle sprain		

Bursitis

Description
- Inflammation of bursal sac, a synovial fluid-filled sac that cushions and reduces friction in joints

Etiology
- Trauma
- Infection (septic)
- Chronic overuse
- Inflammatory arthritis

Risk Factors
- Chronic pressure on bursa (kneeling, resting point of elbow on hard surface, overhead activity)
- Chronic arthritis

Prevention and Screening
- Avoidance of activities that apply pressure to bursae

Assessment
History
- Sudden or gradual onset of localized swelling, sometimes painful but swelling alone may cause patient to seek treatment

Physical
- Localized fluctuant swelling
- Sometimes red, warm, and/or painful to touch
- No loss of ROM
- If cellulitis, tissue breakdown evident in local area; consider septic bursitis

Diagnostic Studies
- Fluid aspiration analysis to evaluate for infection (elevated WBC; presence of organisms on Gram stain, culture), hemorrhage (elevated RBC), gout (presence of characteristic crystals)

Differential Diagnosis
- Septic joint
- Joint effusion
- Acute rheumatoid arthritis flare
- Osteoarthritis
- Gout

Management
Nonpharmacologic Treatment
- Temporary rest or immobilization of affected joint
- Aspiration of bursal sac

Pharmacologic Treatment
- Antibiotics if infected (*Staphylococcus aureus* most common pathogen), cephalexin 250 to 500 mg q.i.d. p.o. for 2 to 3 weeks
- NSAIDs
- Local corticosteroid injection; not performed unless infection and cellulitis is ruled out
- Retrocalcaneal injection not recommended because of risk for Achilles tendon rupture

How Long to Treat
- Antibiotics used for 7 to 14 days for infected bursa
- NSAIDs for 1 to 3 weeks until swelling subsides

When to Consult, Refer, Hospitalize
- Any local skin infection, marked cellulitis, or signs of systemic illness associated with bursitis necessitate parenteral antibiotics, possible hospitalization
- Surgical drainage may be necessary if infection does not respond to antibiotics, local aspiration
- Refer if not trained to aspirate bursa

Follow-up
- Provide patient education about need to rest joint
- To assure that there is no evidence of acute infection

Expected Course
- Symptoms usually improve within 2 to 3 days of aspirating/injecting bursa (if not infected)
- If infected, localized erythema should improve within 10 days

Complications
- Chronic bursitis

Tendonitis

Description
- Tendons are collagen fibrils, sheathed in connective tissue, which provide the elasticity and strength to transmit the forces of muscle to bone
- Overuse syndrome

Etiology
- Continued stress on tendons because of repetitive motion
- Trauma

Risk Factors
- Weak muscles
- Repetitive motion
- Increasing age

Prevention and Screening
- Strengthening of muscles

Assessment
History
- Pain initially activity-related, then continues at rest with progression of problem
- Difficulty using joint
- Numbness and tingling are *not* usually associated
- Shoulder: rotator cuff, bicipital tendonitis
  - Progressive pain with certain activities (usually overhead) that may progress to constant pain
  - Pain worse with lifting, pushing objects away
  - Difficulty lying on affected side
  - Decreased range of motion
- Elbow: medial, lateral epicondylitis
  - Lateral: pain with resisted wrist extension and power grip
  - Medial: pain with resisted wrist flexion and pronation
- Wrist: de Quervain tenosynovitis
- Insidious onset of burning, aching pain over radial aspect of wrist and base of thumb
- Pain often worse with grasping movements

Physical—All Tendonitis
- Local inflammation over the affected tendon, acute swelling
- Affected tendon is very tender to touch
- Symptoms reproduced by passive or active ROM
- Shoulder: rotator cuff, bicipital tendonitis
  - Tenderness over inflamed tendon(s)—palpated in bicipital groove
  - May have weak abduction
  - Painful arc (pain between 70 and 120 degrees of abduction)
- Elbow epicondylitis
  - Lateral (tennis elbow): swelling, tenderness just distal to and slightly anterior to lateral epicondyle
  - Medial (golfer's elbow): pain and tenderness over medial epicondyle

- Wrist: de Quervain tenosynovitis
  - Pain with passive, active thumb extension
  - May have visible thickening of tendon

Differential Diagnosis
- Fracture
- Ligament sprain
- Bursitis
- Nerve impingement
- Arthritis

Management
Nonpharmacologic Treatment
- Heat
- Physical therapy, including early passive ROM, ultrasound, stretching exercises as tolerated
- Splint affected joint: for wrist, de Quervain tendonitis, radial gutter splint for 3 weeks
- Elbow, knee band: tighten over muscle; displaces stress from tendon to muscle

Pharmacologic Treatment
- NSAIDs are mainstay of treatment
- Local corticosteroid injection may be considered
- Shoulder tendonitis symptoms should improve after 2 weeks of conservative therapy; if not, refer for physical therapy

When to Consult, Refer, Hospitalize
- Refer to orthopedist if NSAIDs not effective

Follow-up
- Provide patient education about removing underlying cause of the problem to avoid recurrence

Expected Course
- Noticeable improvement should occur within 6 weeks of treatment

Complications
- Chronic tendonitis with loss of ROM of joint
- Muscle weakness

Muscle Strain
Description
- Tearing of muscle fibers resulting in varying degrees of pain, swelling, and decreased function; graded I–III
  - Grade I: stretching, tearing of muscle fibers but fascia remains intact
  - Grade II: tearing of muscle fibers resulting in significant hemorrhage
  - Grade III: rupture of muscle, damage to fascia
- Common problem of chest wall, neck, wrist (radiocarpal), and shoulder (deltoid)

Etiology
- Excessive stress placed on any muscle (strain)

Incidence and Demographics
- Common problem, many instances self-treated
- Most common presentation to the office is chest pain due to muscles strained from coughing or unaccustomed activity

Risk Factors
- Lifting or moving objects
- Unaccustomed activity

Prevention and Screening
- Appropriate stretching, warm-up exercises prior to activity

Assessment
History
- Sudden onset of muscle pain associated with activity
- Bruising, swelling, and loss of function may occur with more severe injury
- Gradually increasing muscle pain may occur with repetitive use of specific muscle/group

Prevention and Screening
- Maintain activity, balance, coordination

Assessment
History
- Trauma: usually forced hyperextension or flexion
- Fall, twisting, or sudden pulling of a muscle
- Hearing or feeling a "pop" at joint not uncommon, followed by pain, swelling, and ecchymosis
- Pain with movement
- Decreased ROM

Physical
- Localized tenderness, swelling, ecchymosis; pain with resisted muscle contraction and passive stretching of muscle
- Assess neurovascular status
- Numbness/tingling are unusual more than a day or two after injury
- Pain with active and passive ROM
- Tenderness over joint but no point tenderness

Diagnostic Studies
- X-ray if fracture suspected (point tenderness over bony prominences or bony deformity)
- MRI may be useful to identify extent of muscle involvement but usually not necessary

Differential Diagnosis
- Tendonitis
- Fracture
- Tumor

Management
Nonpharmacologic Treatment
- Remember with the mnemonic RICE
  - **R:** rest (non-weight-bearing)
  - **I:** ice (20 minutes q.i.d. until swelling has resolved)
  - **C:** compression (elastic bandage)
  - **E:** elevation for 48 to 72 hours
- Splinting, weight bearing as tolerated; ROM and strengthening exercises
- Grade III injuries may require casting, surgery
- After 24 to 48 hours, use heat
- Physical therapy to regain strength, mobility
- Increase activity slowly and gradually to avoid reinjury

Pharmacologic Treatment
- NSAIDs are mainstay of treatment; use for 10 to 14 days; use with caution in older adults, particularly those on anticoagulant therapy

Special Considerations
- Patients should not return to full activity until they are pain free

When to Consult, Refer, Hospitalize
- Refer for any injury involving muscle weakness, neurovascular compromise, or suspected fracture

Follow-up
Expected Course
- Varies with degree of injury
- Grade I strains resolve in 2 to 3 weeks; Grade II strains require 6 to 8 weeks
- Grade III may require 8 or more weeks of treatment
- If pain does not resolve in 2 to 3 weeks, consider x-rays to rule out occult stress fractures

Complications
- Permanent deformity, loss of strength, gait disorders, falls

Ligament Sprain
Description
- Over stretching and /or partial tearing of ligaments, usually around the ankle or knee
- Standard grading indicates extent of damage:
  - Grade I: stretching but no tearing of ligaments; no joint instability
  - Grade II: partial (incomplete) tearing of ligament; some joint instability but definite end point to laxity
  - Grade III: complete ligamentous tearing; joint unstable with no definite endpoint to ligamentous stressing

Etiology
- Excessive stress placed on any ligament

Incidence and Demographics
- Common injury; often accompanies fracture

Risk Factors
- Unaccustomed activity
- Sudden forceful stretching of a joint; loss of balance

Prevention and Screening
- Appropriate stretching, warm-up exercises prior to activity
- Maintain activity, balance, coordination
- Avoidance of high-heeled shoes
- Joint-strengthening exercises

Assessment
History
- Sudden onset of pain associated with activity; bruising, swelling, and loss of function may occur with more severe injury
- Gradually increasing pain may occur with repetitive use

Assessment
History
- Fall, twisting, or sudden pulling of a joint
- Hearing or feeling a "pop" at joint not uncommon, followed by pain, swelling, and ecchymosis
- Trauma-twisting injuries; determine if inversion or eversion
- Pain with weight bearing immediately after injury suggests fracture

Physical
- Localized tenderness, swelling, ecchymosis; pain with resisted muscle contraction and passive stretching of muscle
- Rule out joint instability
- Assess neurovascular status
- Assess the assess distal and proximal joints for secondary injuries sustained in fall

Diagnostic Studies
- X-ray if fracture suspected (point tenderness over bony prominences or bony deformity)
- Ankle: x-ray if
  - Bony tenderness with palpation over medial or lateral malleolus, tarsal navicular, or base of 5th metatarsal
  - Unable to bear weight immediately after injury or during exam

Differential Diagnosis
- Tendonitis
- Fracture
- Tumor

Management
- Same as for muscle strain

Carpal Tunnel Syndrome
Description
- Entrapment neuropathy in which there is soft tissue pain because of entrapment or compression of peripheral nerves because of trauma or structural abnormalities

- Carpal tunnel syndrome of wrist: compressive neuropathy of the median nerve beneath the transverse carpal ligament
- Another entrapment neuropathy is impingement syndrome of the shoulder; see below for shoulder problems

Etiology
- Multiple causes, including any process that encroaches on peripheral nerves
  - Rheumatoid arthritis
  - Repetitive motion injury (often due to computer overuse)
  - Metabolic disorders (hypothyroidism, diabetes mellitus, acromegaly)
  - Tumors (including ganglion cyst)
  - Carpal bone osteophytes
  - Connective tissue disorders (amyloidosis, hemochromatosis)

Incidence and Demographics
- Affects approximately 2 million Americans per year
- Most common in women aged 30 to 50 years
- Women affected more often than men

Risk Factors
- Repetitive wrist flexion/extension, use of vibratory tools or machinery
- Colles fracture

Prevention and Screening
- Proper ergonomics
- Treatment of underlying problem

Assessment
History
- Initially burning or aching pain, numbness, tingling that wakes patient at night and resolves after shaking the affected hand ("wake-and-shake")
- As disorder progresses, symptoms affect thumb, index, and long fingers, may radiate into arm
- Patient may report dropping objects

Physical
- Painless thenar muscle wasting is late finding; usually no visible abnormality
- Tinel sign: positive if symptoms are reproduced by tapping the median nerve at the wrist
- Phalen sign: positive if symptoms reproduced within 60 seconds of wrist flexion

Diagnostic Studies
Electromyography/nerve conduction studies: EMG/NCS
- Mild to moderate symptoms should be present for 6 months for EMG/NCV studies to be accurate
- Electromyography/nerve conduction velocity (EMG/NCV) studies are confirmatory
- Plain x-rays if any history of trauma to rule out fracture

Differential Diagnosis
- Cervical radiculopathy (C6, C7)
- Brachial plexopathy

- Carpal navicular fracture

Management
Nonpharmacologic Treatment
- Splinting (cock-up wrist splint at night)
- Ergonomic modification of work, hobby
- Surgical release if conservative methods fail

Pharmacologic Treatment
Acetaminophen up to 4,000 mg/day p.o. in divided doses
- NSAIDs
- Corticosteroid injection into carpal tunnel (not nerve)

How Long to Treat
- Depends on severity of symptoms
- Generally, allow 6 months from onset of symptoms before obtaining EMG/NCS

When to Consult, Refer, Hospitalize
- Refer to rheumatologist or hand surgeon if patient's symptoms not improved with splinting, NSAIDs

Follow-up
Expected Course
- Mild cases usually respond to conservative measures
- Patient may require surgical release of nerve if burning, numbness, tingling persist or increase; loss of grip/pinch strength is persistent; or evidence of muscle atrophy

Complications
- Irreversible nerve damage, thenar muscle atrophy

OTHER LOCAL CONDITIONS
Shoulder—Rotator Cuff Tear, Restrictive Capsulitis
Description
- The rotator cuff is formed by four scapulohumeral muscles and their tendons that function to abduct, internally and externally rotate the humoral head; rotator cuff tendons degenerate with advancing age; tendonitis and tears are common to this region
- Restrictive capsulitis (or frozen shoulder) occurs as a result of immobility of the shoulder resulting from pain due to trauma or neuropathy (can occur within weeks)

Etiology
- Trauma; arthritic, infectious, or degenerative conditions

Incidence and Demographics
- Chronic shoulder pain and fracture due to falls are often found in older adults
- Rotator cuff tear: age usually more than 50 years
- Restrictive capsulitis: more common in women than men after age 50

Risk Factors
- Repetitive overhead activity (occupational, recreational)
- Rheumatoid arthritis

- Osteoarthritis
- Diabetics
- Previous shoulder injury

Assessment
History
- Rotator cuff tear
  - Pain in the shoulder girdle; pain may radiate into deltoid area
  - May have felt "pop" or "something give" in shoulder
  - Inability to raise arm overhead; weakness or inability to externally rotate arm
  - Inability to sleep on affected side
- Adhesive capsulitis
  - May or may not have history of trauma
  - Progressive loss of motion
  - Pain varies from minimal to severe

Physical
- Rotator cuff tear
  - Weakness or inability to externally rotate shoulder
  - Limited abduction of shoulder
  - Inability to maintain resisted abduction at 90 degrees
- Restrictive capsulitis
  - Marked restriction in active and passive ROM
  - Pain over anterior joint, rotator cuff
  - Patient often uses scapular muscles to "increase" abduction

Diagnostic Studies
- Plain x-ray: useful for evaluating fracture, deformity, presence of osteophytes, calcific tendonitis
- MRI: can show tendonitis, rotator cuff tear, ligamentous or cartilage injury, impingement syndrome

Differential Diagnosis
- Bursitis
- Tendonitis
- Fracture
- AC separation
- Septic joint
- Gout
- Chondroclavicular disease

Management
Nonpharmacologic Treatment
- Physical therapy to maintain, improve ROM, strengthen muscles
- Passive ROM exercises, progress to active, resistive exercises as healing continues
- Ice or heat for rotator cuff tear
- Surgical intervention indicated for complete rotator cuff tear, displaced fracture

Pharmacologic Treatment
- NSAIDs
- Local corticosteroid injection

When to Consult, Refer, Hospitalize
- Refer for any fracture, suspected rotator cuff tear; rheumatoid arthritis; AC separation with deformity, dislocation, or chronic instability; adhesive capsulitis; corticosteroid injection
- Consult for rotator cuff tendonitis if symptoms do not resolve within 4 to 8 weeks

Follow-up
Expected Course
- Rotator cuff: pain will gradually decrease; withhold exercise temporarily if pain reoccurs
- Restrictive capsulitis: treatment with corticosteroid injections and exercise has demonstrated quicker recovery then analgesics alone

Complications
- Permanently decreased ROM, muscular weakness, chronic pain

CASE STUDIES

Case 1. A thin, petite 75-year-old Asian woman comes to clinic for sudden onset of thoracic back pain 2 days ago when she coughed.

1. What pertinent history is it important to ask?
2. What would you expect to find on PE?
3. How would you treat this patient?
4. How soon should the pain be relieved?
5. What follow-up?

Case 2. A 68-year-old woman complains of hip and knee pain for many years. She is overweight and unable to walk more than a half block because of pain. She spends her day in a recliner eating snacks and watching television. She has become incontinent because she cannot make it to the toilet on time. Every once in a while she thinks her knee is going to give out from under her. She notes loud cracking noises when she stands up. Her knees are enlarged with decreased ROM.

1. What history would you expect?
2. Which of her symptoms are indicative of advanced disease?
3. What is the most likely diagnosis?
4. What nonpharmacologic treatment would you institute?
5. What pharmacologic treatment would you order?
6. What lab tests must be monitored if the patient is placed on a NSAID?
7. When should you refer?

Case 3. A 78-year-old man complains of low back pain (LBP) for past 5 days. Pain is in his lower lumbar area radiating into the left buttock. Pain is worse when sitting up in hard chair; he has not been able to go out to the park and play checkers with his friends.
PMH: Has had episodes of LBP for past 5 years. Patient worked as a truck driver, delivering packages before he retired. Has not been active recently due to COPD from smoking, gets SOB easily and cannot walk long distances.

1. What risk factors does he have for low back pain?
2. What symptoms would prompt an emergency referral?
3. What simple physical maneuver will be the most useful?
4. What is your most likely diagnosis?
5. If patient is compliant with therapy, how soon can he expect to have pain resolve?

REFERENCES

Arthritis Foundation. (2000). *Primer on the rheumatic diseases* (12th ed.). Atlanta: The Arthritis Foundation.

Bone, H. G., Hosking, D., Devogelaer, J. P., Tucci, J. R., Emkey, R. D., Tonino, R. P., et al. (2004). Ten years' experience with alendronate for osteoporosis in postmenopausal women. *New England Journal of Medicine, 350,* 1189–1199.

Colyar, M. (2004). Bone density testing. *Advanced Nurse Practitioner, 12*(7), 24–25.

Crowther, C. L. (2003). *Primary orthopedic care* (2nd ed.). St. Louis, MO: Mosby.

Cush, J. J., Kavanaugh, A. F., & Stein, C. M. (2005). *Rheumatology diagnosis and therapeutics* (2nd ed.). Philadelphia: Lippincott Williams and Wilkins

Diduszyn, J., Boigon, M., Glew, C., & Hofmann, M. T. (2008). Osteonecrosis of the mandible in a nursing home resident receiving bisphosphonate therapy. *Annals of Long-Term Care, 16.* Retrieved from http://www.annalsoflongtermcare.com/content/osteonecrosis-mandible-a-nursing-home-resident-receiving-bisphosphonate-therapy

Felson, D. T., Lawrence, R. C., Dieppe, P. A., Hirsch, R., Helmick, C. G., Jordan, J. M., et al. (2000). Osteoarthritis: New insights. Part I: The disease and its risk factors. *Annals of Internal Medicine, 133,* 635–646.

Hunder, G. (Ed.). (2005). *Atlas of rheumatology* (4th ed.). Philadelphia: Current Medicine LLC.

Klippel, J. H. (2001). *Primer on the rheumatic diseases* (12th ed.). Atlanta: Arthritis Foundation.

The Medical Letter. (2002). Drugs for Prevention and treatment of postmenopausal osteoporosis. Treatment Guidelines. *1*(3), 13–18.

The Medical Letter. (2008). Advertisements for TNF Inhibitors. *50*(1299), 89.

Nelson, H. D., Helfand, M., Woolf, S. H., & Allan, J. D. (2002). Screening for postmenopausal osteoporosis: A review of the evidence for the U.S. Preventive Services Task Force. *Annals of Internal Medicine, 1367,* 529–541.

NIH Consensus Development Panel on Osteoporosis Prevention, Diagnosis, and Therapy. (2001). Osteoporosis prevention, diagnosis, and therapy. *JAMA, 285,* 785–795.

Reuben, D. B., Herr, K. A., Pacala, J. T., Pollock, B. G., Potter, J. F., & Semla, T. P. (2008). *Geriatrics at your fingertips 2008–2009* (10th ed.). New York: American Geriatrics Society.

Salvarani, C., Cantini, F., Boiardi, L., & Hunder, G. G. (2002). Polymyalgia rheumatica and giant cell arteritis. *New England Journal of Medicine, 347,* 261–271.

U.S. Preventive Services Task Force. (2002). Screening for osteoporosis in postmenopausal women: Recommendations and rationale. *Annals of Internal Medicine, 334,* 1519–1525.

Neurological Disorders

Michaelene Jansen, PhD, RN, GNP-BC, NP-C

GERIATRIC APPROACH

Normal Changes of Aging

- Decreased brain weight
- 20% decrease in blood flow to the brain with changes in autoregulation
  - Contributes to risk for orthostatic hypotension and increased potential for falls
- Loss of neurons with a general decrease in dendritic connections
- Changes in neurotransmitters in specific areas
- Decrease in spinal cord motor neurons
- Increased risk for hypothermia or hyperthermia because of impaired skin vasodilatation and vasoconstriction
- Decreased thirst drive may be due to decreased endorphins or decreased response to them

Common Normal Changes of Aging Found on Physical Exam

- Decreased vibratory sensation and proprioception
- Decreased/absent Achilles reflex; other reflexes in arms and legs decreased less often
- Increased postural sway
- Gait slowed, forward flexed; and mildly unsteady; decreased arm swing
- Size of pupils unequal; pupil reaction decreased or absent
- Increased rigidity in legs

Age-Associated Memory Impairment
- Generally there is no change in thinking, behavior, or intellectual function, except decreased speed of processing
- A number of older adults experience minor changes in short-term or recent memory
- Patient notices and complains about memory loss in everyday activities
- Poor recall of specific items infrequently used, such as names of people, street addresses, vocabulary
- Items recalled later when they stop trying
- Worse under stress, then improves; not progressive or disabling

Clinical Implications
History
- Assess impact of symptoms and illness on function and ability to perform activities of daily living (ADL) and instrumental activities of daily living (IADL)
- Validate history with family member, caregiver, and medical records as appropriate

Physical
- A complete neurological examination consists of cranial nerves, motor nerves, sensory nerves, reflexes, autonomic nervous system, and a cognitive and behavioral evaluation
- Format of the neurological exam is unchanged for the older adult but may take longer
- Include functional assessment in complete history and physical of older adults and when appropriate

Assessment
- Neurological problems range from chronic to acute and fatal
- Consider cardiac or metabolic etiology or adverse medication reactions, particularly for global complaints such as syncope, weakness, or change in cognition without focal neurological symptoms
- Generalized weakness or change in cognition may also suggest a more global problem such as dementia, delirium, or depression
- Focal findings suggest a space-occupying lesion of brain or spinal cord, or a peripheral compressive neuropathy

Treatment
- Acute or sudden onset of symptoms such as headache, unilateral weakness, aphasia, visual changes, or change in level of consciousness require immediate consult, referral, or hospitalization, as do deficits resulting from head or spine trauma
- Symptoms developing over weeks or months such as headaches, memory loss, or weakness can generally be evaluated and treated in the office without patient diagnostic testing as appropriate
- Refer to neurology if unusual presentation or no response to adequate trial of standard therapy
- Dementia, delirium, and dizziness can be found in Chapter 4

STROKE AND TRANSIENT ISCHEMIC ATTACK
Description
- Strokes are ischemic or hemorrhagic
- Ischemic stroke is an interruption in blood flow to the brain causing neuronal death or infarction; further classified as thrombotic, embolic, or lacunar

- Hemorrhage accounts for less than 10% of strokes; the bleed may be intraparenchymal or subarachnoid
- Transient ischemic attack (TIA) is a temporary interruption in cerebral vascular blood flow; the deficit lasts less than 24 hours—usually 2 to 4 hours; there is no infarcted tissue or residual deficit
- Presenting signs and symptoms, management, and prognosis depend on the type and location of the stroke (see Table 15–1)

Table 15-1. Location and Signs and Symptoms of Intracranial Lesions

Location	Signs and Symptoms
Frontal lobe	Intellectual and cognitive decline Personality change Contralateral grasp reflex Expressive aphasia Focal motor seizures, contralateral weakness Loss of sense of smell (anosmia)
Temporal lobe	Seizures (may be partial without loss of consciousness) Emotional and behavioral change Auditory hallucinations Visual field cuts Receptive aphasia
Parietal lobe	Contralateral sensory loss Loss of tactile discrimination (astereognosis) Contralateral field cuts Alexia, agraphia, apraxia, acalculia Right-left confusion
Occipital	Homonymous hemianopsia Visual agnosia Cortical blindness
Cerebellum and brain stem	Ataxia and incoordination, nystagmus, vertigo Cranial nerve palsies Nausea/vomiting Motor and sensory deficits (unilateral or bilateral) Increased intracranial pressure

Etiology

Ischemic stroke
- Lack of blood flow to brain because of hypoxia, decreased cardiac output, ischemia, persistent hypertension, dyslipidemia, etc.

Thrombotic stroke
- Caused by atherosclerotic plaque leading to occlusion of an intracranial vessel
- Most common in the posterior cerebral circulation

Embolic stroke
- Caused by atherosclerotic debris from the heart, aorta, or carotids that flows into internal carotids and occludes smaller vessels of cerebral circulation

- Usually the anterior cerebral circulation

Lacunar infarcts
- Less than 5 mm, occur in internal capsule, basal ganglia, or thalamus
- Due to slow progressive occlusion of the penetrating arterioles
- TIA may be thrombotic, embolic, or lacunar in nature

Hemorrhagic stroke
- Intracerebral hemorrhage
- Spontaneous bleeding into parenchyma from microaneurysm of vessel; most commonly occurs in the basal ganglia
- Due to hypertension, hematological disorders, or anticoagulation therapy

Subarachnoid hemorrhage
- Bleeding from a ruptured aneurysm in the circle of Willis or arteriovenous malformation

Miscellaneous:
- Anemias
- Subclavian steal syndrome: occlusion of the subclavian artery proximal to the vertebral artery; blood is "stolen"; risk factors for embolization, such as atrial fibrillation, rheumatic heart disease, mitral valve disease, may be present
- More common in men
- Inflammatory arterial disorders such as giant cell arteritis, systemic lupus erythematosus

Incidence and Demographics
- Acute stroke afflicts 730,000 Americans per year
- Stroke the third leading cause of death
- Incidence is higher in men than in women
- Incidence increases in women over age 75
- Incidence doubles for each decade over age 55
- One-fourth of stroke victims die
- 50% of survivors will have some disability
- 15% to 30% will require long-term placement

Risk Factors
- Previous cerebrovascular disease, stroke, or TIA
- Risk highest in the month after TIA
- Age
- Conditions that predispose to emboli: rheumatic heart disease, atrial fibrillation, infective endocarditis, valve disease, ulcerated plaque, cardiomyopathy, coronary artery disease
- Other risk factors for vascular disease: hypertension, dyslipidemia, diabetes mellitus, smoking
- HIV/AIDS infection

Prevention and Screening

Primary Prevention

- Management of hypertension
  - Treat as directed by *Seventh Report of the Joint National Committee on Prevention, Detection, Evaluation, and Treatment of High Blood Pressure* (JNC VIII anticipated 2010)
  - Screen normotensive patients for hypertension and risk factors every 2 years
- Lipid lowering
  - Important to lower LDL levels to below 100 if arthrosclerotic disease is present, < 70 if high risk
  - HMG-CoA reductase inhibitors (statins) also contribute to plaque stabilization, reduce inflammatory markers, and have an antiplatelet effect
  - Statin therapy with intensive lipid-lowering effects is recommended for patients with atherosclerotic ischemic thrombotic stroke or TIA and without known CAD to reduce the risk for stroke and cardiovascular events
- Anticoagulation therapy
  - Warfarin for high-risk patients with atrial fibrillation or prosthetic cardiac valves
- Antiplatelet therapy
  - The combination of aspirin and extended release dipyridamole is recommended over aspirin alone
  - Antiplatelets recommended over anticoagulants to reduce the risk of recurrent stroke
- Screening for asymptomatic carotid stenosis by auscultation of carotid bruits or carotid ultrasound remains controversial, with insufficient evidence to recommend for or against
- High-risk patients over age 60 with other risk factors for vascular disease may benefit from screening and subsequent endarterectomy
- All patients will benefit from diet and exercise counseling and smoking cessation
- Educate patients and families about stokes, warning signs, and need for immediate care of stroke symptoms

Assessment

History

- Onset, duration, and progression of symptoms most important in determining etiology and management
- Resolution of symptoms in minutes to hours is a TIA
- Onset during sleep with progression suggests thrombotic
- Sudden onset with activity suggest embolic or hemorrhagic
- Detailed description of symptoms or deficits including visual changes, aphasia, motor weakness, and paresthesias may give clue to location of stroke or lesion
- Review of systems: headache, seizure, loss of consciousness, vertigo, vomiting, syncope, and cardiac symptoms
- Lack of headache excludes hemorrhagic stroke
- Loss of consciousness is associated with hemorrhage or posterior circulation thrombosis
- Vertigo usually suggests vestibular disease, but may occur with vertebrobasilar artery insufficiency
- Vomiting is most often associated with increased intracranial pressure usually due to hemorrhage, but may occur with vertebrobasilar insufficiency
- Syncope suggests arrhythmia or other cardiac etiology

- Syncope, dizziness, or vertigo alone is not indicative of a TIA
- Past medical history: cardiac disease, peripheral vascular disease, diabetes, and previous neurologic conditions such as seizure, head trauma, dementia, and brain tumors gives clues to etiology and possible differential diagnosis
- Review all medications, particularly those that can alter level of consciousness or cause bleeding

Physical

- Complete neurological exam including level of consciousness, cognitive ability (apraxia, agnosia, aphasia, amnesia), motor and sensory function (contralateral deficits), cranial nerve exam including funduscopic and visual field deficits, reflexes (hyperreflexia or Babinski on affected side)
- Cardiovascular exam including presence of hypertension, atrial fibrillation, heart murmurs, carotid bruits, abdominal aneurysm
- Symptoms of carotid TIA: weakness of contralateral arm, leg, or face, individually or in combination; numbness or paresthesia may occur alone or in combination with motor deficit; there may be dysphagia or monocular visual loss, carotid bruit; DTRs may be hyperreflexic during attack; may see atherosclerotic changes on funduscopic exam; signs and symptoms disappear as TIA resolves
- Symptoms of vertebrobasilar TIA: vertigo, ataxia, diplopia, dysarthria, dimness or blurry vision, perioral numbness, weakness, or sensory complaints on one or both sides of body or drop attacks due to bilateral leg weakness

Diagnostic Studies

- CT scan to rule out hemorrhage
- MRI if posterior circulation involved
- Lumbar puncture if CT negative for hemorrhage and SAH suspected
- Carotid duplex for evaluation of symptomatic carotid stenosis, if patient surgical candidate for endarterectomy
- Carotid studies are not indicated for evaluation of posterior circulation
- Angiography remains the "gold standard" for assessing carotid stenosis, and for identifying aneurysms, arteriovenous malformations, and vasculitis
- Electrocardiogram, chest radiograph, echocardiogram
- Holter monitor to rule paroxysmal arrhythmias
- CBC, ESR, coagulation studies, RPR, glucose
- Serum chemistries and lipids

Differential Diagnosis

- Subarachnoid or intracerebral hemorrhage
- Cerebral aneurysm or AVM
- Intracranial tumor
- Migraine with aura
- Seizure (Todd paralysis)
- Hyperventilation
- Encephalopathy
- Intoxication
- Hypoglycemia
- Syncope
- Vertigo
- Postural hypotension

Management
- Suspected hemorrhagic stroke, increased intracranial pressure, or ischemic stroke with onset of deficits of less than 3 hours must be transported by ambulance to the emergency department for immediate evaluation and management

Nonpharmacologic Treatment
- Provider should perform accurate assessment and referral for emergency care
- Educate patients and families about stroke and the need for same immediate response as heart attack
- Postacute phase: physical therapy, occupational therapy, and speech therapy should be started as soon as possible
- Emotional support of patient and family
- Referral for home health services
- Management of post-stroke complications: see Special Considerations

Pharmacologic Treatment
- Tissue plasminogen activator (TPA) must be administered in a hospital within 3 hours of onset of symptoms of ischemic stroke, after hemorrhagic stroke is excluded and qualification criteria are met.
- Patients waking with focal deficits are not appropriate for TPA because duration of deficits is unknown
- Medical management of postacute stroke as well as TIA involves anticoagulation or antiplatelet agents, and treatment of underlying heart disease, hypertension, diabetes, and hyperlipidemia
- Aspirin 50 to 325 mg monotherapy, the combination of aspirin and extended-release dipyridamole, and clopidogrel monotherapy are all acceptable options for initial therapy
- Warfarin: used for patients with symptoms who are on antiplatelet medication or those with atrial fibrillation or prosthetic heart valves; see Chapter 9, Cardiovascular Disorders, for details
  - Consider risk for falls, ability to comply with a complex medication regime, and INR monitoring when initiating warfarin therapy
- Evaluate and treat depression

How Long to Treat
- Continue antiplatelet or anticoagulation regimen for as long as such therapy is not contraindicated (increased risk for GI or intracerebral bleeding)

Special Considerations
- The nurse practitioner is an important member of the multidisciplinary team required for rehabilitation of the post-stroke patient
- Members of the team will include as needed physical therapist, occupational therapist, speech therapist, nutritionist, social worker, physician, mental health specialist
- Stroke patients have many problems depending on the location of the stroke, including immobility, impaired balance, falls, skin breakdown, incontinence of bowel and bladder, constipation, impaired vision, dysphagia, aphasia with inability to communicate, poor judgment, infections such as skin, pneumonia, UTI
- Depression is very common post–left hemisphere stroke and makes it difficult for the patient to participate in rehabilitation; aggressive treatment is necessary

When to Consult, Refer, Hospitalize
- Refer all acute stroke patients to neurology

- Emergently hospitalize all patients with focal neurological deficits of less than 3 hours for TPA if not contraindicated
- Emergently hospitalize patients with sudden, severe headache; decreasing level of consciousness, or vomiting; and focal neurological deficits
- Consult with neurologist as needed for management of TIA and postacute stroke
- Cardiology referral for management of heart disease
- Post-stroke rehabilitation may be at home or in nursing facility
- Psychiatric referral for depression if needed

Follow-up
Expected Course
- Variable; most stroke recovery occurs early; the longer deficits last the more unlikely they are to resolve, although improvement may be seen for 6 months
- Physical therapy improves functional recovery
- Older age, coma, and early acute CT changes are associated with poor prognosis
- Patients with risk for cerebrovascular disease should be monitored every 3 to 6 months for symptoms of TIA and hypertension, and counseled regarding stroke prophylaxis, diet, exercise, and smoking cessation

Complications
- Increased risk for second stroke
- Poorer prognosis and increased incidence of infection, myocardial infarction, renal failure, and delirium with advancing age
- 27% of stroke patients die within 1 year, and 53% at 5 years
- Incidence of dementia increases by 10% within a year of stroke
- TPA has a 6% increased risk of intracerebral hemorrhage but a 4% decrease in mortality at 3 months
- Antiplatelet and anticoagulation therapy has risk of intracerebral bleed or GI bleed

PARKINSON'S DISEASE

Description
- Neurodegenerative disease characterized by bradykinesia (slow movement), rigidity, and resting tremor caused by destruction of substantia nigra and nigrostriatal tract; results in damage to dopanergic neurons, leaving active unopposed acetylcholine neurons intact
- Imbalance of dopamine and acetylcholine results in loss of refinement of voluntary movement

Etiology
- Unknown, although genetics, endogenous toxins, and exogenous toxins (including manganese, carbon monoxide, and the illicit drug MPTP) have been implicated

Incidence and Demographics
- Prevalence 60 to 187 per 100,000, with 20,000 to 50,000 new cases per year
- Ethnic and gender incidence is the same
- Less prevalent in Africans and Blacks than in Asians, Europeans, and White Americans
- New onset is only 1% of those over age 65, but many patients with Parkinson's disease survive beyond age 65

Risk Factors
- Age
- Heredity
- Possible environmental factors

Prevention and Screening
- None, although older adult patients may benefit from periodic assessment of mobility, cognition, function, and fall risk

Assessment

History
- Focused detailed history of chief complaint, including time frame and progression, and aggravating and alleviating factors such as stress or rest
- Complete review of neurological symptoms including weakness, paresthesia, tremor, diplopia, aphasia, and mood and cognitive changes
- Past medical history including neurological disorders, exposure to environmental toxins, illicit drug use
- Family history of Parkinson's disease, other movement disorders, or dementia
- Medications including over-the-counter anticholinergics, antihistamines, decongestants, and cough and cold preparations
- Functional assessment: difficulty with ADL and IADL, mobility including stair climbing (patients with progressive supranuclear palsy will have difficulty descending stairs), and rising from chair
- Falls and injuries
- Review of systems for associated autonomic dysfunction, including perspiration, continence, constipation, and postural hypotension
- Assess for depression and mental status; may use Geriatric Depression Scale and Folstein Mini-Mental Status Exam or other tools
- Interview family or caregiver

Physical
- General: manner, affect, dress and hygiene; speech may be soft and monotone
- Cranial nerve exam: extraocular movements, 4th cranial nerve palsy with progressive supranuclear palsy, wide palpebral fissures, impaired swallowing
- Motor exam: no weakness; tapping over bridge of nose produces sustained blink response (Myerson sign)
- Bradykinesia: slowness of voluntary movement and difficulty initiating movement, difficulty rising from chair, shuffling gait, problems with turns and stopping movement
- Stooped, flexed posture with knees and hips flexed; hands held in front, close to body; loss of postural reflexes
- Freezing or difficulty initiating movement or changing direction
- Rigidity: cog wheeling, resistance to passive movement
- Tremor: mouth and lips; resting tremor present in one limb, limbs on one side, 4 limbs, or may be absent in 20% of patients with Parkinson's disease; see slow tremor of 4 to 6 cycles per second, most prevalent at rest
- Tremor may increase with emotional stress and decrease with voluntary activity
- "Masked faces": fixed facial expression, drooling, soft voice
- Incoordination of rapid alternating movements
- Deep tendon reflexes are unaffected, no Babinski reflex

- Seborrhea
- Orthostatic hypotension

Diagnostic Studies
- Consider head CT if diagnosis not clear and stroke or space-occupying lesion is suspected

Differential Diagnosis
- Benign essential tremor
- Progressive supranuclear palsy
- Depression
- Dementia
- Cerebrovascular disease
- Brain tumor
- Adverse effects of anticholinergic medications, particularly antipsychotics
- MPTP-induced Parkinson's disease
- Carbon monoxide poisoning
- Normal pressure hydrocephalus
- Huntington's disease
- Creutzfeldt-Jakob disease
- Shy-Drager syndrome

Management
- There is no cure for Parkinson's disease; current therapy is aimed at managing symptoms to preserve independence and mobility
- The Hoehn and Yahr Scale can be helpful for staging the disease and guiding pharmacological and supportive therapy
  - Stage I: Unilateral involvement
  - Stage II: Bilateral involvement but no postural abnormalities
  - Stage III: Bilateral involvement with mild postural instability; patient leads an independent life
  - Stage IV: Bilateral involvement with postural instability; patient requires substantial help
  - Stage V: Severe, fully developed disease; patient is restricted to bed and chair
  - Nonpharmacologic treatment
- Patient and family education regarding progressive nature of disease and complex pharmacologic treatments
- Nutritional counseling regarding low-protein diet and dietary management of constipation
- Compression stockings for postural hypotension
- Physical, occupational, and speech therapy with appropriate assistive devices for ambulation and ADL
- Fall precautions and home safety evaluation; install rails, raised toilet seats, tub chairs
- Encourage walking, social activities and interaction
- Emotional support
- Surgical intervention: pallidotomy
- Deep brain stimulation: may reduce symptoms and need for levodopa and other drugs

Pharmacologic Treatment

Table 15-2. Treatment Algorithm for Parkinson's Disease

Stage or Problem	Therapeutic Alternatives
Mild disease (Stage I and II)	Selegiline for neuro protection Anticholinergics if tremor predominant Amantadine Group support, exercise, education, nutrition
Functionally impaired (Stage III) Age ≥ 60 years	Dopamine agonist Sustained-release carbidopa/levodopa
Stage IV or V	Immediate-release carbidopa/levodopa Dopamine agonists
Poor symptom control	Increase carbidopa/levodopa dose Add or increase dopamine agonist dose Add catechol O-methyltransferase (COMT) inhibitor

Suboptimal peak response	Begin combination dopaminergic therapy
	    Add levodopa to dopamine agonist
	    Add dopamine agonist to levodopa
	Increase dose of levodopa/carbidopa or dopamine agonist
	Add COMT inhibitor as levodopa adjunct switch dopamine agonists

Wearing-off symptoms	Begin combination of dopaminergic therapy
	    Add levodopa to dopamine agonist
	    Add dopamine agonist to levodopa
	Increase frequency of levodopa dosing
	Increase dose of levodopa/carbidopa (sustained or immediate release)
	Add COMT inhibitor and decrease levodopa dose
	Change to sustained-release carbidopa/levodopa
	Add liquid levodopa/carbidopa
	Add selegiline if not already taking

On-off phenomenon	Begin combination dopaminergic therapy
	    Add levodopa to dopamine agonist
	    Add dopamine agonist to levodopa
	Add COMT inhibitor
	Modify distribution of dietary protein

Freezing	Increase or decrease carbidopa/levodopa dose Add dopamine agonist Increase or decrease dopamine agonist dose Discontinue selegiline Gait modification, assistance device
No "on" time	Manipulate time and dose of levodopa Add COMT inhibitor Avoid dietary protein Increase GI transit time

Adapted from "Antiparkinson agents," by L. R. Young, in M. W. Edmunds & M. S. Mayhew (Eds.), *Pharmacology for the Primary Care Provider* (2nd ed.), St. Louis, MO, Mosby.

DOPAMINE PRECURSOR
- Carbidopa/Levodopa
  - 25mg carbidopa/100 mg levodopa 3 times a day or 10 mg carbidopa/100 mg levodopa 3 to 4 times a day, titrate up by 1 tablet every 2 to 7 days as needed and tolerated, not to exceed 200 mg carbidopa and 8000 mg levodopa a day
  - "On-off" phenomenon occurs in 40% to 50% of patients after 2 to 3 years
  - Patients will experience inconsistent effect from the same dose
  - "Wearing-off" symptoms appear before next dose is due
  - Use lowest doses possible; consider addition of dopamine agonists

DOPAMINE AGONISTS
- Pergolide (Permax) 0.5 mg first 2 days, titrate by 0.1 to 0.15 mg/day every 3 days up to 3mg/day divided in 3 doses
- Pramipexole (Mirapex) 0.125 mg 3 times a day, titrate up to 1.5 mg 3 times a day over 7 weeks
- Ropinirole (Requip) 0.25 mg 3 times a day, titrate up weekly by 1.5 mg a day up to a total dose of 24 mg a day. Maintenance dose is 3 to 24 mg a day; discontinue slowly over 1 week

MAO-B INHIBITOR
- Selegiline (Eldepryl) 5 mg twice a day
- Rasagiline (Agilect) 1 mg daily for monotherapy; 0.5 mg daily if adjunct therapy

Anticholinergic Agents
- Benztropine (Cogentin): 1 to 2 mg a day
- Amantadine (Symmetrel): 100 mg twice a day

COMT INHIBITOR
- Tolcapone (Tasmar): 100 to 200 mg 3 times a day
  - Use with caution secondary to potential for hepatic injury
  - Do not initiate therapy in those with known liver disease or elevated LFT
  - Monitor LFT every 2 weeks for first year, then every 4 weeks for 6 months, then every 8 weeks
  - Discontinue if no improvement on tolcapone

How Long to Treat
- Medication combinations and dosages must be individualized and adjusted during the course of the disease

Special Considerations
- Prescribe Parkinson's medications with caution, particularly for those with comorbid heart, renal, or liver disease
- Avoid anticholinergics, because they tend to be poorly tolerated in those over age 60 years and have increased risk of side effects including confusion, agitation, arrhythmias, and urinary retention

When to Consult, Refer, Hospitalize
- Refer to neurologist for confirmation of diagnosis and guidance with medical management

- Neurosurgical consultation for those with severe symptoms refractory to medications, or who cannot tolerate medications; may consider deep brain stimulation to reduce symptoms

Follow-up
Expected Course
- Progressive; see Hoehn and Yahr scale for staging

Complications
- Related to immobility and falls; hip fractures are common
- Pneumonia may occur in Stage V
- Aspiration of food
- 30% have coexisting dementia with a poorer prognosis
- Depression and social isolation occur

MULTIPLE SCLEROSIS (MS)

Description
- Progressive neurodegenerative disease characterized by demyelination and inflammation of the neuronal sheath in the brain and spinal cord

Etiology
- Autoimmune disease; possible causes are genetic, viral, immunologic, or environmental

Incidence and Demographics
- Prevalence 250,000 to 300,000 in the United States
- More common in persons of Western European lineage who live in temperate zones
- Age of onset usually 15 to 55 years; 2–3:1 women to men, may be related to estrogen-progesterone levels
- Late onset of MS in the sixth or seventh decade usually severe and rapidly progressive

Risk Factors
- Familial 1% to 3% increased risk in first-degree relatives (15 times greater than in general population)
- Climate or place of residence, established by residence in the first 15 years of life
- Urban dwelling, upper socioeconomic status, Western European descent

Assessment
History
- Neurological history: paresthesias, weakness and spasticity, ataxia, fatigue, visual changes, vestibular disturbances, trigeminal neuralgia, optic neuritis, bowel and bladder dysfunction
- Time frame with exacerbations and remission
- Past medical history: systemic lupus erythematosus, Lyme disease, cerebral and spinal tumors, AIDS, seizures, peripheral neuropathy, head or spinal trauma

Physical
- Complete neurologic exam
  - Cranial nerve exam
    - Optic neuritis: decreased visual acuity, abnormal pupillary response, hyperemia-edema of optic disk

- Internuclear ophthalmoplegia: cranial nerve VI palsy or weakness of the medial rectus muscle with lateral gaze nystagmus
  - Sensorimotor exam
    - Decreased strength, increased tone, clonus, positive Babinski reflex
    - Decreased proprioception and vibratory sensation
    - Positive Romberg sign
    - Electrical sensation down the back into the legs is produced with neck flexion

Diagnostic Studies
- MRI to visualize characteristic lesions
- Cerebrospinal fluid analysis for immunoglobins and oligoclonal bands
- Visual, auditory, and sensory evoked potentials

Differential Diagnosis
- Stroke
- Cerebral or spinal tumors
- Ischemic optic neuropathy
- Systemic lupus erythematosus
- Lyme disease
- Peripheral neuropathy
- Seizure disorder
- AIDS
- Intoxication
- Amyotrophic lateral sclerosis

Management
- Aimed at delaying progress, managing chronic symptoms, and treating acute exacerbations
- Has changed recently with the advent of immune modulators

Nonpharmacologic Treatment
- Physical and occupational therapy
- Mental health services for assistance with coping strategies

Pharmacologic Treatment
- Complex; neurologist required
- Immune modulators
  - Interferon beta-1a (Avonex), interferon beta-1b (Betaseron), interferon alfa-2b (Intron), glatiramer (Copaxone), peginterferon alfa-2a (Pegasys), and interferon beta-1a (Rebif) are all available
- Acute exacerbations
  - Prednisone 60 to 80 mg/day for 1 week; taper over 2 to 3 weeks
- Spasticity
  - Baclofen: 40 to 80 mg a day in divided doses; start with 5 mg 2 to 3 times a day and titrate up every 3 days

How Long to Treat
- Use corticosteroids only for acute exacerbations, not for maintenance

When to Consult, Refer, Hospitalize
- Refer all patients with suspected MS to neurologist for confirmation of diagnosis and management
- Ophthalmology
- Continence specialist or urologist for bladder dysfunction
- Mental health referral for coping or depression

Follow-up
Expected Course
- Progressive with exacerbations and remissions
- Prognosis has changed dramatically with the advent of immune modulators

Complications
- Hydronephrosis and renal failure secondary to urinary retention
- Falls
- Depression

ESSENTIAL TREMOR

Description
- Rhythmic, involuntary movement usually of distal upper extremities; head is also frequently affected
- Usually not present at rest, occurs with sustained posture or movement

Etiology
- Unknown, familial with an autosomal dominance inheritance, although 50% have no family history

Incidence and Demographics
- May occur any time from childhood to later life
- Prevalence and severity increase with age
- Senile tremor is not a separate process

Risk Factors
- Age
- Heredity

Prevention and Screening
- None

Assessment
History
- Time of onset, duration, frequency
- Alleviating or exacerbating factors
    - Alleviating: rest, alcohol
    - Exacerbating: movement, emotional stress
- Associated neurological symptoms: weakness, paresthesias, slowed movement
- Past medical history: head trauma, stroke, Parkinson's disease, multiple sclerosis, psychiatric illness, asthma, and hypothyroidism
- Family history of tremor

- Function: problems with ADL and IADL or social life because of embarrassment
- Medications: antipsychotic, anticholinergics, theophylline, beta agonists

Physical
- Neurological exam is normal except for tremor
- Tremor may be demonstrated with rapid alternating movements
- Mild cogwheeling may be present in tense, anxious patients
- Cogwheeling is not pathognomonic for Parkinson's disease
- Normal posture and gait

Diagnostic Studies
- Usually not needed; consider electromyography if unusual presentation or difficult case
- Imaging to identify underlying pathology if abnormal neurological exam
- Thyroid function studies if hypothyroidism suspected

Differential Diagnosis
- Physiologic tremor
- Parkinson's disease
- Medication induced tremor
- Posttraumatic tremor
- Dystonia or torticollis
- Cerebellar lesions
- Demyelinating disorders

Management
Nonpharmacologic Treatment
- Reassure that disability is related only to tremor; although this can be severe and disabling, most are relieved that they do not have Parkinson's disease
- Counsel regarding genetic nature
- Refer to International Tremor Foundation
- Explain medical treatment; improvement often unpredictable
- Alcohol sometimes most effective treatment but improvement may be short
- Severe and disabling cases: contralateral thalamotomy or high-frequency unilateral thalamic stimulation

Pharmacologic Treatment
- Beta-adrenergic blockers
  - Propranolol: start with 10 to 20 mg 3 times a day, or 60 mg of sustained release each, increase each week up to 240 mg/day
  - Metoprolol (more cardio-selective for beta 1 receptors): although not approved for tremor, has been successfully used in patients with asthma and COPD
- Primidone: 50 mg a day, may gradually increase to 125 mg twice a day

How Long to Treat
- Stop medications if they are not alleviating symptoms

Special Considerations
- May be more severe and disabling in older patients
- Primidone may be poorly tolerated in older patients

When to Consult, Refer, Hospitalize
- Consider neurology consultation or referral if cause for tremor unclear
- Neurosurgical evaluation for thalamotomy or thalamic stimulation if medication not effective and tremor is disabling

Follow-up
Expected Course
- Often may require no treatment if not disabling
- May be exacerbated during predictable situations and require only intermittent medication

Complications
- Social withdrawal because of embarrassment or inability to perform ADL and IADL
- Complications secondary to medication or surgery

SEIZURES

Description
- A transient alteration in behavior, function, or consciousness that results from an abnormal electrical discharge of neurons in the brain
- Epilepsy or seizure disorder refers to chronic recurrent seizures
- Most older adults have partial seizures that may quickly generalize to tonic-clonic seizures

Etiology
- A seizure is a symptom of an underlying disorder
- Primary epilepsy cause is unknown, but is believed to be related to abnormalities of neurotransmission
- New onset of primary epilepsy is extremely rare in older adults, but patients with primary epilepsy can continue to have seizures into old age
- Secondary epilepsy is due to injury to cerebral cortex

Incidence and Demographics
- 84/100,000 persons with new-onset seizure disorder a year are older than 70 years
- In new-onset seizures after age 60, 32% are caused by stroke, 14% from brain tumors, and 25% have no identifiable cause

Risk Factors
- Trauma, use of medications that lower seizure threshold, alcohol intoxication or withdrawal, chronic illness that predisposes to metabolic abnormality, and certain triggers (flashing lights/television, emotional stress, hormonal imbalance, fever)

Prevention and Screening
- Head trauma and fall prevention, home safety counseling

Assessment
History
- Interview witness also if possible—this is the most important diagnostic information
- Detailed history of event include
  - Seizure activity (generalized or partial), loss of consciousness, incontinence

  – Prodromal symptoms such as aura, confusion, or focal neurological symptoms
  – Postictal state: antegrade amnesia, level of consciousness
- Prior seizure history including type, frequency, duration
- Triggers: stress, sleep deprivation, drug and alcohol ingestion or withdrawal
- Seizure medications: any changes, missed doses, and levels
- Medications: ciprofloxacin, metronidazole, theophylline, stimulants, antipsychotics, and bupropion can lower seizure threshold
- Diuretics, antihypertensives, and medications for diabetes can cause metabolic disturbances that can cause seizure
- Past medical history: previous intracranial lesions, trauma, stroke, migraines, diabetes, HIV, dementia, psychiatric illness
- Family history of seizure

Table 15–3. Classification of Seizures

Class	Category	Description
Partial Seizures		Only part of one cerebral hemisphere is affected
	Simple partial seizures	Focal symptoms without impaired consciousness
	Complex partial seizures	Impaired consciousness accompanies symptoms
Generalized Seizures		Affect the general cerebral cortex
	Absence (petit mal)	Impairment of consciousness
	Atypical absence	Impairment of consciousness with change in postural tone
	Myoclonic seizures	Single or multiple myoclonic jerks
	Tonic-clonic (grand mal) seizures	Sudden loss of consciousness, tonic rigid phase, followed by clonic jerking

Physical
- Assess for head trauma
- Neurological exam may be normal even with structural lesions
- Focal deficits may be worse immediately after seizure
- Evaluate cardiovascular and pulmonary status
- Blood pressure and pulse will be elevated during and immediately after a seizure

Diagnostic Studies
First-Time Seizure
- Metabolic panel, toxicology if appropriate
- CBC
- MRI
- EEG may determine seizure type and guide treatment and prognosis; does not be to be repeated
- Serologic test for syphilis

For Repeat Seizure
- Check drug level at time of seizure if possible

Differential Diagnosis

Secondary Causes for Seizure: Consider These Underlying Etiologies

NEUROLOGIC DISORDERS
- Head trauma
- Brain tumor
- Stroke
- Encephalitis

METABOLIC DISORDERS
- Electrolyte imbalance
- Hypoglycemia

OTHER
- Alcohol withdrawal
- Medications/withdrawal
- Fever

Disorders That May Appear to Be Seizures—see also Chapter 4
- Syncope
- Transient ischemic attack
- Panic attacks or psychosis
- Drug intoxication
- Migraine
- Multiple sclerosis
- Postural hypotension

Management

Nonpharmacologic Treatment
- Educate patient and family about seizure disorder and cause
- First seizures without cause do not have to be treated with anticonvulsants
- Educate family about acute seizure management; to protect patient from injury, place on left side to maintain airway if possible, do not place objects in mouth
- Patients with known recurrent seizures do not need to go to the emergency department for every seizure; only if seizure lasts more then 2 minutes or breathing is impaired (aspiration)
- Advise regarding state driving regulations
- Advise regarding swimming alone or operating dangerous equipment
- Teach about side effects and toxic effects of medications, and not to discontinue seizure medications abruptly, which may precipitate seizure
- Avoid seizure triggers: sleep deprivation, alcohol, stress, low-grade fever, and infection
- Wear medical alert bracelet

Pharmacologic Treatment
- Older adults are more responsive to antiepileptic medications than younger adults
- No one drug is better than another
- Best choice is to consider dosing, side effect profile, cost, drug interactions, low protein binding

    OLDER ANTICONVULSANTS: PHENYTOIN, PHENOBARBITAL, CARBAMAZEPINE, AND VALPROIC ACID
    - 40% to 50% of patients can be maintained seizure-free on a single agent

- Phenytoin: initially 100 mg 3 times a day; maintenance dose 300 to 600 mg/day divided
- Phenobarbital: 60 to 100 mg/day
- Carbamazepine: initially 200 mg twice a day; increase by less than 200 mg/day in divided doses 3 to 4 times a day up to 1200 mg
- Valproic acid: initially 15 mg/kg/day; increase at 1-week intervals by 5 to 10 mg/kg/day until seizures are controlled or side effects prevent further increase in dose; maximum dose 60 mg/kg/day, divide totally daily doses over 250 mg

NEWER ANTICONVULANTS: OXARBAZEPINE, TOPIRAMATE, LAMOTRIGINE, GABAPENTIN, TIAGABINE
- Oxcarbazepine (Trileptal): 600 mg twice daily
- Topiramate (Topamax): 100 mg twice daily; cognitive deficits seen with toxicity
- Lamotrigine (Lamictal): 150 mg twice daily; dizziness, tremors, ataxia with toxicity
- Gabapentin (Neurontin): 300 mg three times daily; somnolence, fatigue are side effects
- Tiagabine (Gabitril): 32 mg daily; dizziness, lethargy are side effects

Considerations
- Anticonvulsants are metabolized in the liver and involve the cytochrome P450 enzyme system; care must be used when administering these medications with multiple other medications
- Lower, less frequent doses may be needed for those with hepatic and renal dysfunction
- Anticonvulsants have small therapeutic ranges
- Some patients may do well at the lower or upper range; older adults are often controlled by subtherapeutic levels of drug
- Levels should be drawn when adjusting therapy and change in seizure frequency
- Liver enzymes must be monitored

How Long to Treat
- Consider discontinuing seizure medications in those without seizures for over 2 years
- Obtain an EEG before stopping medication
- 40% will have a recurrence, most within the first year
- Must consider risk factors of seizure recurrence and medications for each individual patient; consult with neurologist

Special Considerations
- New-onset seizures must be evaluated in those with previous history of stroke or dementia; there may be new intracranial lesions such as tumor or hematoma
- Survivors of neurosurgery or brain trauma usually do not develop epilepsy; it is common practice to administer an anticonvulsant at the time of neurosurgery or head trauma; this treatment is appropriate at the time when the brain is swollen and cerebral blood flow is compromised; however, there is no evidence that prophylactic anticonvulsant therapy prevents epilepsy; therefore, it is not necessary to maintain these patients on long-term anticonvulsants

When to Consult, Refer, Hospitalize
- Referral to neurology for first-time seizures, when considering discontinuing therapy, or for seizures refractory to adequate trials of monotherapy

- Status epilepticus is a medical emergency defined as 2 or more seizures without complete recovery or a seizure lasting over 30 minutes
- The primary care provider witnessing status epilepticus must activate 911 and be prepared to initiate emergency procedures; intravenous (IV) access and administration of IV benzodiazepines (lorazepam) should be initiated as protocols permit

Follow-up
Expected Course
- Variable; after one seizure patient may not have another, or others may have intractable seizures

Complications
- Status epilepticus, airway obstruction, injury during seizure activity

HEADACHE
Description
- Head pain that arises from extracranial structures such as the muscles, skin, arteries; from the posterior fossa; or from the dura, intracranial arteries, and cranial nerves at the base of the brain
- The brain itself is not sensitive to pain

Primary Headaches
- Tension headaches are described as squeezing, band-like pain; onset usually gradual and lasts days to years; is present when awaking; associated with anxiety or depression; no aura or associated neurological symptoms
- Migraines may be preceded by aura lasting hours to days with scotoma, paresthesias, and unilateral weakness; the headache is usually unilateral and associated with photophobia, sonophobia, and nausea and vomiting
- Unusual for new-onset primary headache syndromes to occur after age 50

Secondary Headaches Are a Symptom of an Underlying Disorder
- New-onset headache in the older adult may be a symptom of a serious illness requiring emergent intervention, especially in the presence of other neurological signs and symptoms

Etiology
Tension Headache
- Essentially unknown cause
- Studies have not supported "muscle tension" or increased muscle contractions
- Depression, anxiety, or stress may play a role

Migraines
- Believed to be caused by vascular constriction and dilation, possibly triggered by circulating estrogens, alcohol, and serotonin

Secondary Headaches Are Most Common in the Older Adult
- Neurologic causes include subarachnoid hemorrhage, trauma, brain tumors, and encephalitis
- Common diseases outside the CNS that cause headache include giant cell arteritis, sinusitis, intoxication, cervical spine arthritis, visual disturbances, fever, hypothyroidism, carbon monoxide poisoning, and infection

Incidence and Demographics
- Incidence of primary headaches declines in the sixth to tenth decade
- Migraines usually decrease in frequency with age; unusual to begin after age 50

Risk Factors
- Depends on etiology

Prevention and Screening
- None

Assessment
History
- Problem focused; organize to evaluate secondary causes
- Time frame of syndrome and of individual headaches including onset, duration, frequency, quality, location, intensity, change in pain, and provoking and alleviating factors
- Review of systems to include:
  - Neurologic: aura, paresthesias, paralysis, vertigo, mood, sleep changes
  - Visual symptoms: photophobia, diplopia, scotoma, tearing
  - Ear, nose, or throat symptoms; may indicate sinusitis
  - Gastrointestinal: nausea, vomiting, diarrhea, and constipation
- Constitutional symptoms: fever, chills, weight changes, appetite changes
- Suspected tension headaches with gradual onset lasting days to years without neurological symptoms; may be associated with anxiety, depression, and stress
- Suspected migraine with history of aura and neurological symptoms that resolve, followed by actual headache accompanied by photophobia and/or nausea and vomiting; usually a pattern and precipitating events
- History of head trauma, previous and current medical and nonpharmacologic management, diagnostic testing and referrals
- Family history of headache
- Functional history: is headache interfering with ADL and IADL?
- History of sudden onset, change in character, associated neurological symptoms, fever, neck pain, rash, or weight loss suggests a serious headache and potential emergency
- Also see brain tumor and stroke sections for pertinent history of these secondary causes of headache

Physical
- Primary—neurologic exam usually normal
- Focused physical exam as directed by history to rule out secondary causes of headache
- Funduscopic exam to rule out papilledema
- Neurological deficits suggest a secondary cause such as subarachnoid hemorrhage (SAH), CVA, tumor, or subdural hematoma
- Temporal artery tenderness and visual changes, particularly in patients over 50, suggests giant cell arteritis
- Rash over cranial nerve V with corresponding pain indicates herpes zoster

Diagnostic Studies
- Life-long history consistent with tension headache with normal physical exam usually does not require further diagnostic evaluation
- Brain CT if new headache in the older adult

- Immediate CT if:
  - Sudden, severe headache
  - Progressive headache
  - Headache with exertion, straining, sexual activity, or coughing
  - Change in mental state, focal neurological deficits, or fever
- ESR to rule out giant cell arteritis
- Other diagnostic testing as directed by history and physical exam to rule out infectious, metabolic, or autoimmune process
- Electroencephalogram is not useful in screening or diagnosing headaches

Differential Diagnosis
- Subarachnoid hemorrhage
- Cerebral aneurysm
- Brain tumor
- Giant cell arteritis
- Subdural hematoma
- Cervical spine arthritis
- Posttraumatic headache
- Meningitis
- Encephalitis
- Brain abscess
- Hydrocephalus
- Sinusitis
- Referred pain from ear, eyes, teeth
- TMJ
- Viral syndrome
- Drug-induced
- Caffeine withdrawal
- Depression and anxiety
- Intoxication
- Dehydration

Management
Nonpharmacologic Treatment
- Primary
  - Relaxation techniques, biofeedback, stress reduction
  - Adequate hydration

Pharmacologic Treatment

PRIMARY
- Analgesics: acetaminophen 650 to 1,000 mg 4 times a day as needed, or NSAIDs
- Use NSAIDs with caution; see Chapter 14, Musculoskeletal Disorders
- Opioids are not indicated for the treatment of headaches

SECONDARY
- Manage and treat the underlying cause
- Avoid opioids if level of consciousness needs to be monitored
- Opioids are not indicated for the treatment of headaches
- Acetaminophen for pain and fever if not contraindicated

How Long to Treat
- Treat acute attacks until headache resolves
- Opioids can be used to treat intractable pain

When to Consult, Refer, Hospitalize
- For sudden, severe headache or headache with change in level of consciousness or focal deficits, refer to emergency department for imaging and evaluation
- Refer to neurosurgeon if tumor, aneurysm, or AVM suspected
- Refer to neurologist for headaches that do not respond to medical management
- Refer to surgeon or ophthalmologist for temporal artery biopsy if giant cell arteritis is suspected
- Refer to ophthalmologist if a visual disorder is suspected cause or contributing factor
- Psychologist or psychiatry for relaxation therapy or psychotherapy or when suspected depression does not respond to trial of antidepressants
- Interdisciplinary pain center for chronic, intractable pain that interferes with daily life

Follow-up
Expected Course
- Tension headaches may be lifelong
- Migraines usually decrease in frequency or stop as the patient ages
- Secondary headaches depend on cause

Complications
- Unrecognized or mistreated serious headaches from secondary causes can lead to death

BRAIN TUMORS

Description
- Primary brain tumors: abnormal growth of cells arising from structures or tissues within the cranium (see Table 15–4)
- May be malignant or benign
- Secondary brain tumors most often metastasize from the lung, breast, kidney, or gastrointestinal tract

Etiology
- The exact cause of brain tumors is unknown
- Gliomas of supporting glial tissues account for 46% of all central nervous system tumors; higher grade has poorer prognosis
- Meningiomas develop from the covering of the brain and are rarely malignant

Incidence and Demographics
- Incidence of primary brain tumor is 8 per 100,000 in the United States
- Greatest incidence in 60- to 70-year-olds
- Gliomas more common in men; meningioma and pituitary adenomas more common in women

Risk Factors
- Meningiomas increase with age
- Primary cerebral lymphoma associated with AIDS

Prevention and Screening
- None; no recommended screening for relatively rare disease

Assessment
History
- Focused, complete neurological history including weakness, slurred speech, or word-finding difficulty; visual changes including diplopia or field cuts; hearing loss; cognitive changes; drowsiness; seizures; headache
- Tumors are suspected in patients with progressive deficits
- Deficit may suggest the location of the tumor
- Headache associated with tumor is dull and aching and increases over weeks
- Headaches are usually secondary to hydrocephalus or posterior fossa tumors that stretch pain-sensitive structures
- New-onset seizures in adulthood suggest a tumor, possibly in temporal lobe
- Review of systems include HEENT; loss of sense of smell or field cuts suggest pituitary adenoma, or craniopharyngioma; for unilateral hearing loss consider acoustic neuroma
- History of nausea and vomiting with deficits or headache suggests increased intracranial pressure
- Assess for symptoms of Cushing syndrome (see Chapter 17, Endocrine Disorders) if pituitary adenoma suspected

Physical
- Complete neurological exam may reveal focal cranial nerve or motor deficits
- Other systems as indicated by history
- If pituitary adenoma is suspected will need complete endocrine assessment; elevated blood pressure may be present
- Metastatic brain tumor: if primary tumor site unknown will need to evaluate for lung, breast, kidney, or colon cancer

Table 15-4. Primary Brain Tumors

Tumor	Structure	Treatment and Prognosis
Astrocytoma (Grade I, II glioma)	Glial tissue	Total excision usually not possible May respond to radiation Variable prognosis
Glioblastoma multiforme (Grade III, IV glioma)	Glial tissues	Total excision not possible, reoccurs Radiation and chemotherapy may slow growth Poor prognosis
Oligodendroglioma	Cerebral hemispheres	Successful surgical treatment Slow growing
Ependymoma	Glioma usually of the 4th ventricle	Presents with signs of increased intracranial pressure, shunt Surgical resection if possible Radiation therapy
Craniopharyngioma	Sella tunica Depresses optic chiasm	Surgical resection usually incomplete Bitemporal field cuts Endocrine dysfunction

continued

Table 15-4. Primary Brain Tumors (cont.)

Tumor	Structure	Treatment and Prognosis
Meningioma	Dura or arachnoid mater	Surgical excision, difficult to completely remove posterior fossa tumors Cure with complete resection
Acoustic neuroma	Nerve sheath Vestibular branch of 8th cranial nerve at the cerebellar pontine angle	Excision usually good outcome May have residual ipsilateral hearing loss, imbalance, facial weakness or numbness
Primary cerebral lymphoma	Reticuloendothelial system Immunocompromised patients	Shunt Prognosis depends on CD4 count

Diagnostic Studies
- CT scan
- Magnetic resonance imaging for suspected posterior fossa lesions and intrasellar lesions
- Angiography of intrasellar lesion with normal hormone levels to differentiate pituitary adenoma from an aneurysm
- Pituitary adenoma: ACTH, thyroid function test, and serum glucose and electrolytes
- Metastatic brain tumors: chest x-ray, mammogram, colonoscopy as appropriate to locate primary tumor if unknown

Differential Diagnosis
- Subdural hematoma
- Arteriovenous malformation
  - Aneurysm
  - Abscess
- CVA
- Hydrocephalus
  - Pseudotumor cerebri

Management
Nonpharmacologic Treatment
- Neurosurgical referral for excision
- Emotional support of patient and family
- Refer to social services, home health services, and spiritual counseling as needed

Pharmacologic Treatment
- Radiation and chemotherapy by neuro-oncologist
- Medical management of endocrine complications of pituitary adenoma
- Dexamethasone for cerebral edema: 4 to 20 mg every 6 hours
- Anticonvulsant therapy for seizure management (see sections on seizures and epilepsy)

How Long to Treat
- Defer to neurosurgeons, neurologists, oncologists, and endocrinologists

Special Considerations
- Malignant brain tumors
- Those under 45 live 3 times longer than those over 65
- Prognosis decreases with lower premorbid function

When to Consult, Refer, Hospitalize
- All patients with space-occupying lesions on imaging must be referred to neurosurgery
- Coordinate primary care with neuro-oncology team
- For pituitary adenomas with abnormal endocrine function tests, refer to endocrinologist
- Social work, home health services, hospice as needed

Follow-up
Expected Course
- Depends on type of tumor, location, age of patient
- For supratentorial meningioma expect complete cure
- Glioblastoma has 6- to 18-month life expectancy (see Table 15–4)

Complications
- New focal deficits as result of damage to normal brain tissue during surgery
- Usually complications associated with surgery and anesthesia
- Usual adverse effects of radiation and chemotherapy
- Death

TRIGEMINAL NEURALGIA

Description
- *Tic douloureux* is a paroxysmal lancinating pain of the face, usually unilateral; pain originates near mouth and shoots to nose, eye, or ear

Etiology
- Compression of the 5th cranial nerve root, usually by a blood vessel

Incidence and Demographics
- Most common in middle-aged to older women

Risk Factors
- Triggers for pain are touch, movement, drafts, chewing

Prevention and Screening
- None

Assessment
History
- Focused history if chief complaint is of facial pain
- Establish time frame, description of episode, any triggers, and pain management
- Review of systems to identify any neurological deficits such as weakness, numbness, or diplopia, indicating a space-occupying lesion
- Any ear, nose, throat, or dental symptoms indicating sinusitis, dental abscess, or otitis
- History of 5th cranial nerve herpes zoster or multiple sclerosis

Physical
- Examine head, eyes, ears, nose, throat, mouth, and neck, cranial nerves
- Complete neurological exam if cranial nerve abnormalities
- No physical findings with classic trigeminal neuralgia except possibly poor dental hygiene or lack of shaving or make-up on affected side

Diagnostic Studies
- CT or MRI if there are neurological deficits
- ESR if giant cell arteritis is suspected

Differential Diagnosis
- 5th cranial nerve tumor
- Multiple sclerosis, particularly in young or with bilateral pain
- Sinusitis, otitis, dental abscess, TMJ
- Herpes zoster; pain may present before vesicular rash
- Postherpetic neuralgia

Management
Nonpharmacologic Treatment
- Avoid triggers
- Surgical decompression, radiofrequency rhizotomy, gamma radiosurgery

Pharmacologic Treatment
- Carbamazepine 100 mg twice daily; increase by 200 mg daily up to 1,200 mg daily in divided doses; use lowest effective dose
- Phenytoin 100 to 300 mg/day
- Gabapentin 100 mg 3 times a day; titrate up to 1,800 mg divided/day; adjust for renal insufficiency
- Baclofen 50 to 60 mg/day in divided doses
- Start with lowest possible dose of medications; titrate up slowly

How Long to Treat
- Attempt to decrease or discontinue dose every 3 months

When to Consult, Refer, Hospitalize
- Refer to neurologist for confirmation of diagnosis and coordination of plan of care
- Refer to neurosurgeon if there is a 5th cranial nerve tumor or for surgical decompression if there is intractable pain with adequate trials of medication, or patient is unable to tolerate medication
- Surgery is inappropriate for trigeminal neuralgia secondary to multiple sclerosis

Follow-up
Expected Course
- Monitor CBC and liver function if patient is on anticonvulsant medication
- Attempt to wean and discontinue medications

Complications
- Secondary to medications, use with caution; these are not simple analgesics
- Cranial nerve paralysis secondary to 5th cranial nerve tumor

BELL'S PALSY

Description
- Acute onset of isolated, unilateral peripheral or lower motor neuron facial weakness due to inflammation of the 7th cranial nerve
- Paresis typically progresses over 7 to 10 days; most patients expect full recovery in 6 months

Etiology
- Unknown, although reactivation of herpes simplex virus has been implicated
- Cases are often preceded by an upper-respiratory infection
- There is an acute inflammatory response, causing swelling of the facial nerve and entrapment in the foramen of the temporal bone

Incidence and Demographics
- 20 to 30 per 100,000 individuals a year
- Median age is 40 years
- No gender or race predilection
- 10% of cases have a familial association

Risk Factors
- Diabetes mellitus
- Hypothyroidism
- AIDS
- Lyme disease
- Syphilis
- Sarcoidosis

Prevention and Screening
- None

Assessment
History
- Focused history with complete history of present illness; most important to establish time frame; sudden onset over hours to a few days suggests neuritis; progressive weakness over weeks indicates a tumor or other space-occupying lesion
- Past medical history including any recent upper respiratory infection, otitis, facial trauma, and history of chronic illness including diabetes, thyroid disease, multiple sclerosis, sarcoidosis, and AIDS
- Review of systems including visual pain and tearing, altered hearing or otalgia, altered taste, skin rash, history of tick bite or outdoor exposure, any other neurological symptoms

Physical
- Complete HEENT exam including all cranial nerves
- Bell palsy indicated by complete unilateral peripheral 7th nerve paresis or paralysis, with flattening of the forehead furrows, inability to completely close the ipsilateral eye, flattening of the nasolabial fold, drooping of the mouth
- A central 7th palsy or only drooping of the mouth, indicating damage only to the lower branch of the facial nerve, indicates an upper motor neuron lesion (stroke or tumor)
- Inspect eye for corneal abrasion, tearing
- Inspect ear canal and tympanic membrane for otitis or vesicular lesions
- Vesicular lesions indicate cephalic herpes zoster
- Palpate parotid glands for masses
- Check for lymphadenopathy and thyroid enlargement
- Inspect skin for rash, particularly bullseye lesion or erythema migrans of Lyme disease, although rash may not be present

- Complete neurological exam if indicated by history or presence of other cranial nerve abnormalities, although neuritis of multiple cranial nerves is not uncommon

Diagnostic Studies
- EMG and nerve conduction studies 5 to 10 days after onset of symptoms if complete paralysis or no improvement; to guide prognosis and treatment; if over 90% neural degeneration surgical decompression may be indicated
- X-ray if temporal bone fracture suspected
- MRI if tumor or space-occupying lesion suspected
- MRI also allows visualization of the facial nerve and temporal bone structures
- Complete blood count, chemistry panel, thyroid function tests if indicated by history to rule out associated chronic diseases
- ESR if giant cell arteritis suspected
- Lyme titer if indicated
- Syphilis and HIV serology if indicated by history and physical
- Audiology if hearing not improving after 1 week or acoustic neuroma suspected
- Cerebrospinal fluid analysis only if meningitis is suspected

Differential Diagnosis
- Tumor
- Stroke or TIA
- Herpes zoster
- Temporal bone fracture
- Giant cell arteritis
- Lyme disease
- HIV
- Infections
- Diabetic neuropathy
- Hypothyroidism
- Sarcoidosis
- Parotid gland obstruction or mass
- Multiple sclerosis or other demyelinating conditions
- Diabetic neuropathy
- Hypothyroidism
- Sarcoidosis

Management
Nonpharmacologic Treatment
- Protect eye, use artificial tears during the day; lubricant ointment at bedtime, patch eye
- No evidence that surgical decompression improves outcomes

Pharmacologic Treatment
- Medical treatment of Bell's palsy remains controversial
- 60% recover completely without treatment
- 10% may have permanent disfigurement and long-term consequences without treatment
- Possibly effective:
  - Prednisone 60 to 80 mg q.d. (divided doses) for 4 to 5 days, then taper over 10 days
  - Acyclovir 400 mg 5 times/day for 10 days

How Long to Treat
- Eye protection until patient can close and protect eye
- Steroid and antiviral therapy for 10 days

Special Considerations
- Poor prognosis is associated with complete paralysis, pain, or hyperacusis at presentation
- These characteristics combined with increased age and comorbidities should guide decision to treat with steroids and antiviral agents

When to Consult, Refer, Hospitalize
- Ophthalmology if corneal abrasion or significant prolonged decreased lacrimation
- Neurology if other neurologic deficits present, or recurrent paresis or paresis lasting over 6 months

Follow-up
Expected Course
- Facial weakness will generally get worse over 10 days, then begin to improve over 2 to 3 weeks, with expected complete improvement in 6 months or less

Complications
- Incomplete recovery or recurrent paresis or paralysis
- Corneal abrasion

PAIN

Description
- Unpleasant sensory and emotional experience associated with potential or actual tissue damage
- May be acute or persistent
- Accompanies many health conditions

Etiology
- Often more than one source of pain, so difficult to localize
- Need to identify source or sources of pain
- May nociceptive or neuropathic
- Common neuropathic pain syndromes in older adults include central post-stroke syndrome, diabetic neuropathy, postherpetic neuralgia, phantom limb pain, intracostal neuralgia following throracotomy, ilio-inguinal neuralgia following hernia repair, radicular spine pain, trigeminal neuralgia
- Common pain syndromes include osteoarthritis, spondylosis/spinal stenosis, degenerative disc disease, vertebral compression fractures, myofascial pain, fibromyalgia, trochanter bursitis

Incidence and Demographics
- 25% to 50% of community-dwelling older adults experience persistent pain
- 45% to 80% of older adults residing in long-term care facilities experience persistent pain

Risk Factors
- Inadequate treatment of acute pain

- Multiple chronic conditions
- Depression

Prevention and Screening
- Identifying pain source
- Adequate pain relief
- Multimodal treatment approach
- Assess for drug-seeking behaviors, diversion

Assessment
History
- Comprehensive pain assessment: McGill Pain Questionnaire, Geriatric Pain Measure, Verbal Descriptor Scale, Verbal Numeric Scale, Visual Analogue Scale
- Instruments for special older adult populations: Leeds Assessment of Neuropathic Symptoms and Signs, Neuropathic Pain Questionnaire, Arthritis Impact Measurement Scale, Discomfort in Dementia of the Alzheimer's Type, Checklist of Nonverbal Indicators, Noncommunicative Patient's Pain Assessment Instrument
- Assessment of pain behaviors
- Mood assessment
- Assessment of other comorbidities
- Assessment of coping skills
- Social support
- Functional assessment
- Sleep assessment

Physical Exam
- Complete physical exam
- Identify pain source/sources
- Distinguish between nociceptive, neuropathic, acute, and chronic pain
- Examine gait, motor, and sensory function

Diagnostic Studies
- X-ray of targeted pain region
- MRI
- C-reactive protein (CRP), erythrocyte sedimentation rate (ESR), rheumatoid factor (RF), antinuclear antibody (ANA), vitamin D
- Urine toxicology
- Rheumatology consult, if indicated
- Orthopedic consult, if indicated
- Neurology/neurosurgery consult, if indicated

Management
Nonpharmacological
- Physical therapy
- Hot/cold therapy
- Aquatherapy
- Reconditioning
- Muscle strengthening, balance, and gait
- Chiropractic treatment
- Ultrasound

- Iontophoresis
- Soft-tissue mobilization
- Electrical stimulation (TENS, spinal cord stimulator)
- Guided imagery
- Relaxation
- Biofeedback
- Energy therapies: healing touch
- Therapeutic touch
- Interventional therapies: trigger point injections, botulinum toxin type A (Botox) injections, epidural steroid injections, medial branch blocks

Pharmacological
- Extended—release medications provide better therapeutic coverage than intermittent or PRN medications
- Avoid propoxyphene, meperidine, methadone, ketorolac, muscle relaxants, and long-term use of NSAIDs (Beers Criteria, 2002)
- Decreased albumin, and decreased renal and hepatic function can increase drug effect or result in drug accumulation
- Increased incidence of drug-drug interactions in older adults
- Nonopioid pain medications: NSAIDs (short-term, use gastric protection), tramadol
- Neuropathic pain medications: antidepressants, anticonvulsants, alpha-2 agonists (use cautiously), serotonin and norepinephrine reuptake inhibitors,
- Topical analgesics
- Opioids: hydrocodone, oxycodone, morphine, fentanyl
- Anticipate and treat side effects (such as constipation, pruritus) aggressively

Length of Treatment
- Treatment may be short-term or lifelong
- Exacerbations of persistent pain may occur

Special Considerations
- Assess for changes in gait, balance, fall risk
- Monitor closely if patient is on opioids for treatment
- Assess mental status
- Mood disorders often accompany persistent pain syndromes
- Standard urine toxicology screening for patients on opioids
- Assess for tolerance, dependence, and addiction

When to Consult, Refer, Hospitalize
- Pain specialist if interventional procedure indicated
- Emergency department for overdose
- May need to refer to rheumatology, orthopedics, neurology, neurosurgery for further assessment or intervention
- Spinal cord stimulator may be indicated for radicular pain
- Implantable infusion pumps for spasticity, terminal cancer pain, or pain not controlled with oral medicatons

Follow-up
- Follow up every 3 months or sooner if indicated
- Random urine toxicology screening for patients on opioids

Complications
- Altered mental status
- Sleep disturbances
- Iatrogenic effects
- Medication side effects
- Falls

CASE STUDIES

Case 1: A 72-year-old woman with 3 falls in the last 2 months without serious injury. Reports difficulty getting out of chair and poor balance. She feels stiff and slow. Has tremor at rest. She is otherwise healthy without significant past medical history. She takes 2 acetaminophen a day for aches.

1. What other history is needed?
2. What assessment tools would you use?
3. What part of the neurologic exam should be normal?
4. What abnormalities do you expect to find on neurologic exam?
5. What is your most likely diagnosis?

Case 2: A 66-year-old man presents in office for follow-up after evaluation in the emergency department for left hemiparesis lasting 30 minutes. Reported negative head CT, chemistry panel, CBC, and toxicology screen. History of "borderline" hypertension. No medications except over-the-counter ibuprofen.

1. What was the event he had?
2. What other history do you want to obtain?
3. What physical findings might you expect?
4. What further diagnostic tests would be indicated?
5. How will you initially manage this patient?

Case 3: A 78-year-old woman with left side headache for 2 days, no relief with 1,000 mg acetaminophen every 6 hours. History of headaches since age 16. Past medical history significant for hypertension controlled with atenolol 25 mg a day.

1. What other history is important?
2. What systems will you examine?
3. What diagnostic testing?
4. What is your differential diagnosis?

REFERENCES

Adams, H. P., del Zoppo, G., Alberts, M. J., Bhatt, D. L., Brass, L., Furlan, A., et al. (2007). Guidelines for the early management of adults with ischemic stroke. *Stroke, 38,* 1655–1711.

Adams, R. J., Albers, G., Alberts, M. J., Benavente, O., Furie, K., Goldstein, L. B., et al. (2008). Update to the AHA/ASA recommendations for the prevention of stroke in patients with stroke and TIAs. *Stroke, 39,* 1647–1652.

Albers, G. W., Amarenco, P., Easton, J. D., Sacco, R. L., & Teal, P. (2004). Antithrombotic and thrombolytic therapy for ischemic stroke: The seventh ACCP conference on antithrombotic and thrombolytic therapy. *Chest, 26*(Suppl 3), 483S–512S.

American Medical Directors Association. (2002). *Parkinson's disease in the long term care setting.* Columbia, MD: Author.

Antithrombotic Trialists' Collaboration. (2002). Collaborative meta analysis of randomized trials of antiplatelet therapy for prevention of death, myocardial infarction, and stroke in high risk patients. *British Medical Journal, 324,* 71–86.

Brodie, M. J., & French, J. A. (2000). Management of epilepsy in adolescents and adults. *Lancet, 356,* 323–329.

Brott, T., & Bogousslavsky, J. (2000). Treatment of acute ischemic stroke. *New England Journal of Medicine, 342,* 710–722.

Coull, A. J., Lovett, J. K., Rothwell, P. M.; Oxford Vascular Study. (2004). Population based study of early risk of stroke after transient ischemic attack or minor stroke: Implications for public education and organization of services. *British Medical Journal, 324,* 326–328

Goodin D. S., Frohman E. M., Garmany G. P., Halper, J., Likosky, W. H., Lublin, F. D., et al. (2002). Disease modifying therapies in multiple sclerosis: Report of the Therapeutics and Technology Assessment Subcommittee of the American Academy of Neurology and the MS Council for Clinical Practice Guidelines. *Neurology, 58,* 169–178.

Grogan, P. M, & Gronseth, G. S. (2001). Practice parameter: Steroids, acyclovir, and surgery for Bell's palsy (an evidence-based review): Report of the Quality Standards Subcommittee of the American Academy of Neurology. *Neurology, 56,* 830–836.

Heart Protection Study Collaborative Group. (2004). Effects of cholesterol lowering with simvastatin on stroke and other major vascular events in 20,536 people with cerebrovascular disease or other high risk conditions. *Lancet, 363,* 757–767.

Jansen, M. P. (2008). *Managing pain in the older adult.* New York: Springer.

Johnston, S. C. (2002). Clinical practice: transient ischemic attack. *New England Journal of Medicine, 347,* 1687–1692.

Sacco, R. L., Adams, R., Albers, G., Alberts, M. J., Benavente, O., Furie, K., et al. (2006). Guidelines for prevention of stroke in adults with ischemic stroke or transient ischemic attack. *Stroke, 37,* 577–617.

Smith, S. C. Jr., Jackson, R., Pearson, T. A., Fuster, V., Yusuf, S., Faergeman, O., et al. (2004). Principles for national and regional guidelines on cardiovascular disease prevention: A scientific statement from the World Heart and Stroke Forum. *Circulation, 109,* 3112–3121.

Straus, S. E., Majumdar, S. R., & McAlister, F. A. (2002). New evidence for stroke prevention. *JAMA, 288,* 1388–1395.

Velez, L., & Selwa, L. M. (2003). Seizure disorders in the elderly. *American Family Physician, 67,* 325–332.

Weaver, F. M., Follett, K., Stern, M., Hur, K., Harris, C., Marks, W. J., et al. (2009). Best medical therapy versus bilateral deep brain stimulation for patients with advanced Parkinson's disease: A randomized controlled trial. *JAMA, 301,* 63–73.

Hematologic Disorders

Vaunette Fay, PhD, RN, FNP-BC, GNP-BC

GERIATRIC APPROACH
Normal Changes of Aging
- Hematopoiesis is slowed and the number of progenitor cells declines

Clinical Implications
History
- Fatigue, weakness, dizziness, drowsiness, irritability, and loss of libido are all symptoms of all anemias.
- Diseases of the blood in the geriatric population are usually insidious and often go undetected.
- Chronic alcohol use is associated with a number of anemias.

Physical
- Pallor or sometimes jaundice of the skin, gums, and mucosal surfaces, as well as splenomegaly, are all signs of anemia.

Diagnostic Studies
- Most anemias in the elderly tend to present with normocytic, normochromic anemia. Mean corpuscular volume (MCV) increases slightly with age; therefore, categorization by MCV is less accurate than in younger adults.
- An elevated reticulocyte count, indirect hyperbilirubinemia, and elevated LDH are diagnostic of hemolytic anemia.

- A low reticulocyte count, elevated indirect bilirubin, and elevated LDH suggest ineffective erythropoiesis.
- Macrocytosis in the elderly strongly suggests vitamin B_{12} and folate deficiency.
- Infection in the elderly should not be excluded if the white blood cell count is normal or low—neutrophil response is blunted. Look for change from patient's baseline.

Assessment

- Anemias are classified by cell morphology or structure.
- 60% of all anemias are seen in people over age 65.
- Combined deficiencies are common in older adults.
- Do not assume that anemia in patient with chronic inflammatory disease is "anemia of chronic disease."
- Physical exam and lab tests for liver and kidney disease should be performed
- Nutritional deficiencies are major causes of anemia in the older adult.
- Do not begin treatment for B_{12} deficiency without assessing and treating folate deficiency.
- Malignancies in the elderly tend to present insidiously. Taking action to diagnose them early will improve the overall treatment and prognosis.
- It is important to identify the type of leukemia for appropriate treatment.

ANEMIAS—LOW RED BLOOD CELLS

Definitions

See Tables 16–1 and 16–2 for lab values

- **Anemia:** A reduction in the total number of circulating red blood cells. Measured by red blood cell (**RBC**) count; the percentage of red blood cells, by volume, in a blood sample (hematocrit, or **Hct**); or a decrease in the quality or quantity or hemoglobin (**Hgb**).
  - Hematocrit is calculated from the MCV and RBC count.
- **Mean corpuscular (cell) volume (MCV):** Represents the size of the RBC and is calculated from the hemoglobin, hematocrit, or RBC value. Used in differentiation of types of anemia.
  - **Macrocytic anemia:** Anemia with elevated MCV. An example is vitamin B_{12}, folate.
  - **Microcytic anemia:** Anemia with decreased MCV. Example is iron-deficiency anemia, which is also a hypochromic anemia.
  - **Normocytic anemia:** Anemia with normal MCV. Examples are anemia of chronic disease, aplastic anemia.
- **Mean corpuscular hemoglobin: MCH** represents the average amount of Hgb in the cells.
  - **Hypochromic (low MCH):** Erythrocytes containing a decreased level of hemoglobin, causing the cells to appear "paler" on smear. Example is iron-deficiency anemia.
  - **Hyperchromic (high MCH):** Erythrocytes containing an increased level of hemoglobin, causing the cells to appear "darker" on smear. These anemias are rare.
- **Mean corpuscular hemoglobin concentration (MCHC):** Ratio of the weight of hemoglobin to the volume of the cell expressed as a percentage; normal value means the cell has the proper amount of hemoglobin for its size.
- **RDW:** Red blood cell distribution width, a statistical index of the variation in red cell widths; elevated value indicates abnormal RBCs.
  - **Anisocytosis:** Measure of variation in red cell size; occurs frequently in leukemias and most anemias; may indicate severity.
  - **Poikilocytosis:** Variation of red cells from their normal shape.

- **Reticulocyte count:** Immature red blood cells in the peripheral blood; increased in a severe anemia; shows that bone marrow is functioning.
- **Iron Studies**
  - **Total iron binding capacity (TIBC):** An indirect measure of transferrin, the amount of iron that can be bound to transferrin. Decreased in anemia of chronic disease.
  - **Ferritin:** Represents iron storage in the serum. May be elevated during infection or chronic inflammation and decreased in iron deficiency.
  - **Transferrin:** Iron transport protein; binds with free iron; marker of nutritional status.

Table 16-1. Normal Ranges for RBC Studies

Test	Females	Males
Hematocrit	36%–48%	40%–53%
Hemoglobin	12–16 grams/dL	13.5–17.7 g/dL
RBC (10^6/mcL)	4.0–5.4	4.5–6.0
MCV	80–100 fL	80–100 fL
MCH	26–34 pg	26–34 pg
MCHC	31%–37% g/dL	31%–37% g/dL
Reticulocyte count	0.5%–1.5% of RBC	0.5%–1.5% of RBC
Serum Iron	50–170 µg/dL	65–175 µg/dL
TIBC	250–450 µg/dL	250–450 µg/dL
Ferritin	10–120 ng/mL (avg. 55)	20–250 ng/mL (avg. 125)

Table 16-2. Blood Values Helpful in Differentiating Anemias

Anemia	MCV	Appearance of Red Cell
Chronic disease	Normal	Normochromic, normocytic, or microcytic
Aplastic	Normal	Normocytic, normochromic
Drug induced	Normal	Normocytic, normochromic
Iron deficiency	< 80 fl	Normocytic or microcytic, hypochromic
Posthemorrhagic	Normal	Normocytic, normochromic
Vitamin B_{12}	> 100 fl	Macrocytic, hyperchromic
Folate deficiency	> 100 fl	Macrocytic, hyperchromic

NORMOCYTIC ANEMIAS

Anemia of Chronic Disease

Description

- The anemia of chronic disease is thought to be a consequence of long-term disease with a major inflammatory component
- A diagnosis made from excluding active blood loss or production abnormalities associated with iron or folate intake.

Etiology

- Inflammatory process

Incidence and Demographics

- The most common anemia in the elderly

- The second most common anemia in the world
- Incidence parallels the rate of chronic inflammatory disease

Risk Factors
- Renal disease, liver disease, endocrine disorders, rheumatoid arthritis, infection, protein calorie malnutrition, and some forms of cancer

Assessment
History
- Chronic disease
- Fatigue, dyspnea on exertion, irritability, listlessness

Physical
- Signs of the underlying disease
- Signs of anemia, depending on severity—pallor, tachycardia, tachypnea on exertion

Diagnostic Studies
- CBC, reticulocyte count, iron studies (serum iron, TIBC, ferritin); studies pertinent to underlying disorder
- Characteristic laboratory values: Hgb usually 8–12 g/dl, Hct 25%–35%, MCV 75 to 85 as Hgb falls < 10, often low serum iron, low total iron binding capacity (TIBC) and normal or increased ferritin (TIBC is increased and ferritin decreased in iron deficiency), serum erythropoietin normal or in end-stage renal disease, low

Differential Diagnosis
- Fe deficiency anemia
- Multifactorial anemia
- Chronic renal insufficiency
- Liver disease (usually alcohol related)
- Posthemorrhagic anemia
- Endocrine disorders: hypothyroidism
- HIV infection

Management
Nonpharmacologic Treatment
- Treat underlying disease
- Ensure appropriate nutrition
- Transfusion only in severe symptomatic cases—restoring Hgb to higher levels improves function, quality of life

Pharmacologic Treatment
- Recombinant erythropoietin (Epogen, Procrit) in symptomatic patients at 30,000 units once weekly may be effective; Epogen is very expensive
- Iron supplements with erythropoietin and otherwise as indicated by iron studies

How Long to Treat
- Treatment required as long as underlying disease and anemia persist

Special Considerations
- A similar profile as iron deficiency may eventually develop with patient becoming mildly microcytic and hypochromic as Hgb falls < 10 g/dl

- Anemia of renal disease relates to severity of renal failure, due to decreased erythropoietin production

When to Consult, Refer, Hospitalize
- Refer if diagnosis is questionable
- Refer to confirm underlying cause (e.g., to rheumatologist for collagen/vascular problem or oncologist for cancer; nephrologist for renal disease; infectious disease specialist for infections)

Follow-up
- Frequent monitoring of BP, CBC, iron studies with recombinant erythropoietin therapy
- CBC should improve in 2 to 4 weeks on Epogen; do not continue Epogen if not effective

Expected Course
- Anemia will improve as the underlying disease improves, or progress as underlying disease progresses, or remain static.
- Patient can often tolerate fairly low Hct and Hgb—as low as 30/10—if they develop gradually.

Complications
- Possible exacerbation of cardiopulmonary disease, particularly in the older adult. (Anemia results in less oxygen delivered to tissues; heart rate and cardiac output increase to compensate; heart may begin to fail.)

Aplastic Anemia
Description
- Intrinsic bone marrow dysfunction with defective red blood cell synthesis
- Produces pancytopenia: anemia, neutropenia, thrombocytopenia
- Normochromic, normocytic anemia

Etiology
- 50% idiopathic; 20% drug or chemical exposure; 10% viral
- Notably associated with chloramphenicol, but occurs only in 1:40,000 to 1:25,000 courses of chloramphenicol
- Autoimmune suppression, tumor or fibrotic marrow, drugs, radiation, infection

Incidence and Demographics
- Not common in United States
- Rate equivalent in men and women

Risk Factors
- Family history, viral illnesses, thymus tumors, some medications, radiation
- Increases in prevalence with age

Prevention and Screening
- Hepatitis A and B vaccination; avoid radiation exposure, causative agents

Assessment
History
- Insidious onset

- Fever, fatigue, weight loss, weakness
- Dyspnea, palpitations
- Rectal bleeding, epistaxis

Physical
- Pallor, petechiae, bruises, sore throat
- No hepatosplenomegaly, bone tenderness/pain, or lymph node enlargement

Diagnostic Studies
- CBC with differential, peripheral smear, bleeding studies, iron studies, urinalysis, bone marrow, liver function
- Lab results: normochromic, normocytic anemia, total iron binding capacity (TIBC) normal
- Hematuria, bone marrow shows hypoplasia, fatty infiltration
- Pancytopenia is pathognomonic

Differential Diagnosis
- Leukemia
- Hypersplenism
- Systemic lupus erythematosus (SLE)
- Myelodysplasia
- Sepsis

Management
Nonpharmacologic Treatment
- Education and supportive care
- A well-balanced diet decreases risk of infection
- Manage underlying cause

Pharmacologic Treatment
- Immunosuppression therapy, oxygen
- 50% respond to antithymocyte globulin and cyclosporine
- Mild cases: RBC and platelet transfusions, antibiotics
- Severe: bone marrow transplant possible, although many centers defer transplants for patients older than 35

How Long to Treat
- Lifelong treatment may be required unless effective bone marrow transplant is curative

Special Considerations
- Other forms of drug-induced anemia are similar in morphology of the RBC, but do not have the pancytopenia and will be less severe than aplastic anemia

When to Consult, Refer, Hospitalize
- Refer immediately to hematologist when diagnosis is suspected; work closely with hematologist throughout therapy

Follow-up
Expected Course
- Often favorable outcome depending on age and treatment response
- Untreated cases are fatal

Complications
- Infection, leukemia, heart failure, hemorrhage

HYPOCHROMIC ANEMIAS

Iron-Deficiency Anemia

Description
- Microcytic, hypochromic anemia due to decreased iron stores; poor iron utilization or reutilization; iron deficiency due to chronic blood loss
- Posthemorrhagic anemia due to acute blood loss; patient may not be iron deficient

Etiology
- Hemorrhage, chronic occult bleeding, usually from GI tract; occult malignancy; decreased absorption

Incidence and Demographics
- Seen in 7% to 10% of adult population
- Prevalent in all ages and populations in the United States

Risk Factors
- Inadequate diet (related to institutionalization, decrease in IADLs [cooking or shopping], decreased appetite)
- Impaired absorption (achlorhydria, gastric surgery, celiac disease)
- GI bleeding (related to neoplasm, duodenal/gastric ulcers, gastritis from medicines, diverticulosis, ulcerative colitis, hemorrhoids, arteriovenous malformations)
- Disorders of hemostasis

Prevention and Screening
- Adequate diet
- Dietary supplements if patient has risk factors

Assessment

History
- Initially asymptomatic
- Easily fatigued, dyspnea on exertion, irritable, listless
- Palpitations, infection history, neuralgia
- Diet low in iron
- Drug/chemical exposure

Physical
- Angular stomatitis, ulcerations or fissure of the mouth
- Chronic atrophy of the nasal mucosa
- Pallor
- Dry skin and mucous membranes
- Nails thin and flat
- Splenomegaly

Diagnostic Studies
- CBC with differential, iron studies
- Laboratory findings: low Hct, MCV, and MCH; RDW > 15; serum ferritin level < 10 ng/ml in women and < 20 ng/mL in men; increased TIBC

- Bone marrow aspiration if diagnosis in doubt, absent for iron stain
- Special tests to determine underlying bleeding even in cases of mild anemia, such as stool for occult blood

Differential Diagnosis
- Thalassemia
- Infection
- Cancer
- Chronic diseases
- Hypothyroidism
- Renal failure

Management
Nonpharmacologic Treatment
- Correct underlying cause
- Symptomatic care on treatment side effects (constipation, nausea, cramps, diarrhea)
- Dietary consideration: no dairy or antacid within 2 hours of oral iron, increase dietary iron intake
- Normal dietary intake meets only daily losses, not therapeutic; RDA iron = 10 mg/day for men and 15 mg/day for women

Pharmacologic Treatment
- Oral iron supplements; oral iron therapy is safer and less costly than IM or IV iron
- Parenteral iron if poor absorption or inability to tolerate oral iron

Other
- Blood transfusion is not recommended for iron supplementation

How Long to Treat
- Anemia should resolve within two months
- Treat iron deficiency until iron stores are replaced; often takes 6 months

When to Consult, Refer, Hospitalize
- Refer if patient is not responsive to treatment
- Refer if underlying cause is not determined

Follow-up
Expected Course
- Increase in Hgb of 1 g/week expected
- Cure expected
- Regular follow-up recommended

Complications
- May have unidentified underlying source of bleeding
- Prolonged course of treatment may be required because of noncompliance
- Excessive iron levels can be harmful to the older adult

MACROCYTIC ANEMIAS
Vitamin B$_{12}$ Deficiency
Description
- Macrocytic anemia in which MCV is more than 100 and blood level of vitamin B$_{12}$ is less than 200 pg/mL

Etiology
- Pernicious anemia
- Malabsorption conditions (GI parasites, GI surgery, Crohn's disease), chronic alcoholism, strict vegetarians (rare)
- Decrease in acid secretion in stomach of older adults—B$_{12}$ needs acid to be absorbed

Incidence and Demographics
- Onset between age 50 and 60; median age at diagnosis = 60
- Women slightly > men

Risk Factors
- Age
- Chronic alcoholism
- GI surgery
- Crohn's disease
- Family history pernicious anemia

Prevention and Screening
- Adequate dietary intake
- Avoid risk factors if possible

Assessment
History
- Insidious onset
- Alcohol consumption
- GI surgeries or disorders, anorexia
- Peripheral neuropathy
- Personality changes, memory loss
- Should be considered in the differential diagnosis of dementia

Physical
- Characteristic beefy red, shiny tongue; tongue may be sore
- Abdominal tenderness, organomegaly
- Numbness, sensory ataxia, limb weakness, spasticity

Diagnostic Studies
- CBC with differential, peripheral smear, and serum B$_{12}$ levels
- Laboratory results: serum B$_{12}$ levels < 200 pg/mL; Hct decreased; MCV markedly elevated; decreased reticulocyte count
- A large, nucleated, embryonic type of cell that is a precursor of erythrocytes in an abnormal erythropoietic process is visible on smear

Differential Diagnosis
- Folic acid deficiency

- Myelodysplasia
- Liver dysfunction
- Side effects of medications
- Alcoholism
- Bleeding/hemorrhage
- Hypothyroidism

Management
Nonpharmacologic Treatment
- Education and supportive therapy
- Dietary intake—vitamin B_{12} is found in meats, eggs, milk products, fortified cereals

Pharmacologic Treatment
- Initial: 1,000 mcg of vitamin B_{12} IM weekly for 4 weeks
- Maintenance: 1,000 mcg monthly

How Long to Treat
- Lifetime

Special Considerations
- B_{12} deficiency may cause peripheral neuropathy and dementia in the absence of anemia
- If patient presents with abnormal neurologic signs, the symptoms might be irreversible, even with treatment
- Patient might have hypokalemia in first week of treatment
- Do not begin treatment for B_{12} deficiency without also assessing for and treating folate deficiency, because treatment of B_{12} deficiency may mask the symptoms of folate deficiency, while the damage from low folate will continue

When to Consult, Refer, Hospitalize
- Refer as needed for underlying cause; refer for follow-up endoscopy every 5 years to rule out malignancy

Follow-up
Expected Course
- Response rapid; good prognosis if treatment within 6 months of neurological signs

Complications
- Stomach cancer
- Permanent CNS signs/symptoms

Folic Acid Deficiency
Description
- Macrocytic, normochromic anemia due to lack of folic acid

Etiology
- Folic acid–deficient diet
- Malabsorption syndromes

Incidence and Demographics
- All races and age groups
- Malnourished people
- Most common between ages 60 and 70 years

Risk Factors
- Advanced age
- Alcoholics
- Patients with malabsorption syndromes
- Hemodialysis patients

Prevention and Screening
- Adequate intake of folic acid (RDA = 200 mcg/day)
- Avoid medications that interfere with folic acid absorption (such as trimethoprim, phenytoin, oral estrogen, or progesterone supplements)
- Monitor level if patient is on above medications

Assessment
History
- Indigestion, constipation, diarrhea, anorexia, lethargy
- Fatigue, weakness, headache, dizziness, dyspnea on exertion
- There may be no complaints of neurologic deficits
- Renal failure on hemodialysis

Physical
- Pallor
- Atrophic glossitis (red, shiny tongue), stomatitis
- Mild confusion, depression, apathy, intellectual loss
- Tachycardia, wide pulse pressure, heart murmur
- Peripheral neuropathy

Diagnostic Studies
- CBC, RBC, serum folate, serum B_{12}, TIBC, LDH
- Abnormal laboratory results: serum folate < 3 ng/mL RBC folate < 150 ng/mL, Hct decreased, Hgb normal, RDW elevated
- TIBC normal, LDH and MCV elevated, MCHC normal, Schilling test normal, serum B_{12} normal

Differential Diagnosis
- Vitamin B_{12} deficiency
- Myelodysplastic syndromes
- Pernicious anemia

Management
Nonpharmacologic Treatment
- Education and supportive therapy
- Good oral hygiene
- Folate rich diet—good sources of folic acid include green leafy vegetables, red beans, wheat bran, fish, bananas, asparagus; prolonged cooking destroys folate
- Need for frequent rest

Pharmacologic Treatment
- Folic acid replacement: 1 mg p.o. q.d. for 2 to 4 weeks or until folic acid serum evaluations are normal, or can administer chronically if there is suspicion that the patient will not be able to maintain an appropriate diet or has a clinical situation demanding increased intake of folate, such as chronic hemodialysis

How Long to Treat
- Treat until anemia is corrected, usually about 2 months until folic acid stores are replenished
- Duration of treatment depends on elimination of underlying cause

Special Considerations
- Folic acid body stores can be depleted in about 4 months

When to Consult, Refer, Hospitalize
- Not usually needed
- Refer patients who do not improve with therapy

Follow-up
Expected Course
- Good prognosis

LEUKEMIAS—LOW WHITE BLOOD CELLS

Description
The leukemias are a collection of disorders:
- Malignancy of the hematopoietic progenitor cells (acute lymphoblastic leukemia [ALL])
- Acute myelogenous leukemia (AML)
- Clonal malignancy of B lymphocytes (chronic lymphocytic leukemia [CLL]) and an overproduction of myeloid cells (chronic myelogenous leukemia [CML])
- These diseases produce a variety of bone marrow and white blood cell abnormalities that can be imminently fatal or can remain asymptomatic for years—they are characterized by specific laboratory findings and symptom presentation

Malignant proliferation is seen in the following cells:
- Immature lymphocytes in acute lymphoblastic leukemia (ALL)
- Myeloid cells in acute myelogenous leukemia (AML) or acute nonlymphocytic leukemia (ANLL)
- Mature-appearing lymphocytes (CLL)
- Immature granulocytes (CML)
- Mature B cells with prominent projections (hairy cell leukemia)

Etiology
- Unknown; theorized to be caused by exposure to chemicals or ionizing radiation, genetic factors (chromosomal abnormalities), viral agents
- In AML: heredity, radiation, chemical and other occupational exposures, and anticancer drugs

Incidence and Demographics
- CLL: most common form of leukemia in Western countries; 75% of case in patients > 60 years
- AML: incidence increased in adults > 65 years
- Hairy cell leukemia; rare disease of old age

Risk Factors
- Chemical or radiation exposure, chromosomal abnormalities, immunodeficiency, cigarette smoking

Prevention and Screening
- None known

Assessment
History
- General: fever, malaise, weakness, bruising, bleeding, weight loss
- CLL: might be asymptomatic, dyspnea on exertion

Physical
- Lymphadenopathy
- CLL: hepatosplenomegaly, lymphadenopathy, sustained absolute peripheral lymphocytosis, and increased lymphocytes in bone marrow.
- AML: fever, splenomegaly, hepatomegaly, lymphadenopathy, sternal tenderness; may have evidence of hemorrhage or infection

Diagnostic Studies
- CBC with differential and platelet; chemistries as baseline—anemia is frequent at time of diagnosis
- Bone marrow aspiration and biopsy
- Consider chest x-ray, ultrasound or CT scan, coagulation profile

Differential Diagnosis
- Aplastic anemia
- Viral diseases
- Myelodysplastic syndromes

Management
Nonpharmacologic Treatment
- Patient and family education and supportive therapy
- Good diet, compliance with treatment, management of side effects and chronic effects of diagnosis

Pharmacologic Treatment
- Chemotherapy, medications to prevent infection

Other
- Hospitalization required for induction of chemotherapy
- Binet staging A – C for CLL
- Avoid activities that might cause injury; avoid medications that affect platelets (such as aspirin)

How Long to Treat
- Goal is remission

Special Considerations
- Patients with leukemia are prone to other infections

When to Consult, Refer, Hospitalize
- Refer to hematologist upon suspicion of diagnosis and consult frequently throughout therapy

Follow-up

Expected Course
- CLL: depends on stage at diagnosis; median survival approximately 9 years

Complications
- Infections, bleeding, side effects of chemotherapy or radiation, relapses

MULTIPLE MYELOMA

Description
- Malignant disease of the plasma cells characterized by replacement of bone marrow, bone destruction, and paraprotein formation

Incidence and Demographics
- Peak incidence during the seventh decade of life
- Median age at presentation is 65 years
- Slightly higher incidence in men and occurs twice as much in Blacks than in Whites

Risk Factors
- Exposure to radiation, asbestos, benzenes, herbicides, and insecticides
- Repeated antigenic exposure to the reticuloendothelial system
- Family history

Assessment

History
- Bone pain of the back, chest, or extremities
- Weakness and fatigue; symptoms of anemia
- Pathologic fractures
- Abnormal bleeding
- Frequent infections

Physical
- Pallor
- Palpable liver and spleen
- Radiculopathy

Diagnostic Studies
- CBC with differential; liver and renal functions; chemistry profile; erythrocyte sedimentation rate (ESR); immunoelectrophoresis (M band occurs in > 90%); urinalysis; and urine electrophoresis
- Lab results: elevated creatinine and calcium, proteinuria, normochromic RBCs, normocytic/microcytic RBCs, increased sedimentation rate
- Bone marrow aspiration and biopsy: bone marrow with infiltrates of plasma cells
- Bone radiographs: lytic lesions in axial skeleton (proximal long bones, ribs, spine, and skull)

Differential Diagnosis
- Metastatic carcinoma
- Connective tissue diseases
- Chronic infection
- Lymphoma

- Benign gamma clonopathy
- Primary hyperparathyroidism
- Polyclonal hypergammaglobulinemia

Management
Nonpharmacologic Treatment
- Psychosocial considerations for patient and family, monitoring

Pharmacologic Treatment
- Minimal disease palliation—observe without treatment
- Chemotherapy
- Autologous stem cell transplant

How Long to Treat
- Aim is to cure with minimal toxicity

When to Consult, Refer, Hospitalize
- Referral to specialist for suspected cases

Follow-up
Expected Course
- Median survival is 3 years without transplant; this number is variable depending on "tumor burden"

Complications
- Prone to frequent infections, especially from encapsulated organisms
- Hypercalcemia
- Renal insufficiency
- Fractures/pain

HODGKIN'S LYMPHOMA

Description
- Malignant disease characterized by lymphoreticular proliferation and presence of Reed-Sternberg cells

Incidence and Demographics
- 3.5/100,000; bimodal age distribution (15–34 [peak at 20] and over 50 [peak at 70])
- 8:1 male to female ratio

Risk Factors
- Immunodeficiency, autoimmune diseases, HIV, first-degree relatives with Hodgkin's disease

Prevention and Screening
- None

Assessment
History
- Persistent fever, night sweats, persistent dry cough
- Unexplained pruritus

- Substernal discomfort
- Supraclavicular, cervical, or axillary adenopathy
- Weight loss > 10%, anorexia

Physical

- Painless lymphadenopathy; mediastinal adenopathy; node biopsy will show characteristic Reed-Sternberg giant cell

Diagnostic Studies

- CBC with differential, liver and renal functions, chemistry profile, chest x-ray
- Lymph node biopsy (needle aspiration is not sufficient)
- Lab results: normochromic RBCs, increased sedimentation rate, increased serum alkaline phosphatase and LDH, lymphocytopenia, mild leukocytosis, thrombocytosis

Differential Diagnosis

- Non-Hodgkin's lymphoma
- Leukemia
- Toxoplasmosis
- Cat scratch disease
- Drug reaction
- AIDS/HIV

Management

Nonpharmacologic Treatment

- Psychosocial considerations for patient and family, monitoring
- Radiation is initial treatment only for patients with low-risk stage IA and IIA disease; short-course chemotherapy may substituted

Pharmacologic Treatment

- Chemotherapy

Other

- Treatment is determined by stage of disease

How Long to Treat

- Aim is to cure with minimal toxicity

When to Consult, Refer, Hospitalize

- Referral to specialist for suspected cases

Follow-up

Expected Course

- Prognosis is good depending on classification at diagnosis

Complications

- Leukemia; chemotherapy and radiation side effects including secondary malignancies, sterility, and gonad dysfunction; infections; anemia

NON-HODGKIN'S LYMPHOMA

Description

- Malignant disease of the lymphoreticular system with absence of giant Reed-Sternberg cells

Etiology
- Unknown, suggestions: virus, immunodeficiency, exposure to ionizing radiation or chemicals

Incidence and Demographics
- Median age is 50 years
- Most common neoplasm between ages 20 and 40
- Incidence in adults 60 years and older has increased 80% since 1970

Risk Factors
- Incidence increases with age; is the 6th most common malignancy among older adults

Prevention and Screening
- Avoid potential etiological factors, such as exposure to agricultural pesticides

Assessment
History
- Persistent cough, chest discomfort
- Fever, night sweats, weight loss possible
- Skin lesions, testicular mass possible
- If abdomen involved: chronic pain, fullness, easily satiated

Physical
- Early systemic findings usually absent
- Painless peripheral lymphadenoptahy—nodes are nontender, firm, and rubbery
- Throat should be examined for involvement of the oropharyngeal lymphoid tissue (Waldeyer ring)

Diagnostic Studies
- Lab results: mild anemia, elevated LDH and ESR, absence of giant Reed-Sternberg cells
- Lymph node aspiration and biopsy
- CBC with differential, sedimentation rate, UA, LDH, BUN, creatinine, liver function tests
- Chest x-ray, bone marrow evaluation

Differential Diagnosis
- Infectious mononucleosis
- CMV
- Other malignancies
- STD
- Tuberculosis
- HIV
- Toxoplasmosis

Management
Nonpharmacologic Treatment
- Patient and family education and supportive therapy

Pharmacologic Treatment
- Radiation therapy, chemotherapy

Other
- Treatment depends on histologic findings

How Long to Treat
- Intermediate and high-grade lymphomas should be treated with cure in mind; others are cared for with palliative therapy

Special Considerations
- International Prognostic Index to categorize into risk groups
- Prognosis not as good as for Hodgkin's disease

When to Consult, Refer, Hospitalize
- Immediate referral to hematologist when diagnosis is suspected

Follow-up
Expected Course
- Response to treatment depends on classification at diagnosis; usually progressive

Complications
- Chemotherapy and radiation side effects
- Recurrence

SECONDARY NEUTROPENIA

Description
Drug-induced neutropenia is most common form of neutropenia. Neutropenia can also be caused by bone marrow infiltration by leukemia, lymphoma, myeloma, or metastatic solid tumors. Infections can also cause neutropenia by imparing neutrophil production.
- A diagnosis of exclusion in patients receiving known or potentially bone marrow–suppressing drugs such as alkylating chemotherapeutic drugs, antimetabolites, colchicine, and agents that interfere with the synthesis or RNA or DNA
- Idiosyncratic reactions occur with a wide variety of drugs, including alternative preparations or extracts and toxins
- HIV infections can cause chronic secondary neutropenia arising from impaired production of neutrophils and accelerated destruction of neutrophils by antibodies

Etiology
- Drugs interfere with the cell division process in the marrow
- Infection can induce immune destruction or rapid utilization of neutrophils

Incidence and Demographics
- Occurs anytime and at any age, but older people seem to be more vulnerable

Risk Factors
- Exposure to any of the following:
  - Ionizing radiation
  - Alkylating agents
  - Antimetabolites
  - Colchicine
  - Anthracycline derivatives

- Long-term exposure to the following:
  - Analgesics
  - H2 blockers
  - Antihistamines
  - Antimicrobial agents
  - Anticonvulsants
  - Antithyroid agents
  - Phenothiazines or other tranquilizers
  - Sulfonamides as antibacterial agents, diuretics, or hypoglycemic agents
- HIV infection
- Cancers that infiltrate the bone marrow

Prevention and Screening
- Awareness of toxicities and screening of WBC as needed based on toxicities of drug therapies

Assessment
History
- Drug/s
- Infections, including HIV
- Past medical history of cancer

Physical
- Neutopenia is aymptomatic until infection develops
- With drug induced neutropenia that is due to hypersensitivity, may have rash, fever, and lymphadenopathy

Diagnostic Studies
- CBC with differential and platelet, chemistries, bone marrow aspiration and biopsy

Differential Diagnosis
- Leukemia
- Aplastic anemia
- Endotoxemia
- Myeloproliferative disorders
- Vitamin B or folate deficiencies
- Idiopathic

Management
Nonpharmacologic Treatment
- Patient and family education and supportive therapy

Pharmacologic Treatment
- Stop offending drug
- Support with cytokine therapy—granulocyte colony stimulating (GCSF) factor
- If infection is present always treat immediately
- If caused by autoimmune disorders, administer corticosteroids to increase blood neutrophils

When to Consult, Refer, Hospitalize
- Refer to hematologist

Follow-up
Expected Course
- Response to treatment with return of WBC to normal after stopping the offending drug and or with support of GCSF

HEMOSTASIS—DRUG-INDUCED THROMBOCYTOPENIA

Description
- Decrease in platelet count below 150,000 in response to a drug

Etiology
- IgG-mediated response to drug or drug metabolites

Incidence and Demographics
- Can occur at any age and in response to a variety of different agents

Risk Factors
- New or continued exposure to the following:
  - Quinine and quinine-like drugs
  - Valproic acid
  - Heparin
  - Antimicrobials: cephalosporins, penicillin, trimethoprim, sulfa agents
  - Anti-inflammatory drugs—acetaminopen, ibuprofen
  - Cardiac drugs such as digoxin
  - Antiarrhythmic drugs such as procainamide and amiodarone
  - Diuretics
  - H2 antagonists
  - Antihistamines
  - Antineoplastic drugs

Prevention and Screening
- High index of suspicion when new thrombocytopenia occurs
- Appropriate screening of platelet counts when using drugs known to cause thrombocytopenia, such as antineoplastic agents

Assessment
History
- Excessive bruising, bleeding hours or days after injury, hematuria, hemorrhage or hematoma after minor injury
- Complete medication history—prescription and over-the-counter

Physical
- Bruises, deep-tissue bleeding, intracerebral hemorrhage

Diagnostic Studies
- CBC with platelet count and differential; PT/PTT/bleeding time; Factor VIII, Factor IX, and vitamin K levels
- Laboratory results: platelet count normal, PT normal, PTT greatly prolonged; bleeding time usually normal (prolonged in hemophilia A 15%–20%); Factor VIII low in H-A; Factor IX low in H-B

Differential Diagnosis
- Von Willebrand disease
- Vitamin K deficiency or malabsorption
- Other platelet disorder
- Disseminated intravascular coagulation (DIC)

Management
Nonpharmacologic Treatment
- Patient and family education and supportive therapy
- Early treatment of any trauma or spontaneous bleed; avoid aspirin, NSAIDs
- Activities restricted in relation to amount of thrombocytopenia

Pharmacologic Treatment
- Stop the offending agent if possible
- Platelet transfusion support

How Long to Treat
- Until platelet count is steadily above 20,000

When to Consult, Refer, Hospitalize
- Refer to hematologist at time of diagnosis of thrombocytopenia, hospitalize for platelet count below 20,000

Follow-up
- As needed

Expected Course
- Patients will fully recover once offending drug is removed from the regimen

Complications
- Spontaneous bleeding in the brain

CASE STUDIES

Case 1. An 83-year-old White male with a chief complaint of fatigue for the past few months. The fatigue is gradually getting worse. He now is too tired to walk to the dining room in his assisted living residence.

PMH: Patient has hypertension, history of PUD with GI bleed, smoker, depression, hyperlipidemia, rheumatoid arthritis, chronic hepatitis C, renal insufficiency

Current medications: paroxetine (Paxil) 40 mg OD; atorvastatin (Lipitor) 20 mg OD; naproxen (Naprosyn) 250 mg p.o. b.i.d., amlodipine (Norvasc) 5 mg q.d., omeprazole (Prilosec), and lisinopril (Zestril) 10 mg

PE: BP 164/84; some pallor; conjunctiva slightly pale

1. What types of anemia is this patient at risk for? What puts him at risk?

Lab: CBC done 1 month ago, results: RBC 3.34, Hgb 10.6, Hct 31.8, MCV 95.5, MCHC 34.5, RBC morphology normal

2. How would you classify/describe this anemia?
3. Does the lab work tell you which kind of anemia he has?
4. What additional tests are needed?
5. What is your diagnosis?
6. What treatment do you recommend?
7. Will an iron supplement be helpful? Why?

Case 2. An 88-year-old Black female is noted to have anemia on routine screening. Last CBC was done 1 year ago and her H&H were 11 and 34. Patient uses a wheelchair; lives in nursing home; is a picky eater; likes sweets; eats 1 to 2 servings of fruit/vegetables daily. Patient recently had an acute exacerbation of her COPD and was treated with prednisone p.o. for 2 weeks. Patient was noted to have diarrhea last week.

PMH: diabetes mellitus, osteoarthritis, COPD, aortic stenosis, CHF, constipation

Medications: metformin (Glucophage) 500 mg b.i.d., nabumetone (Relafen) 500 p.o. b.i.d., Combivent inhaler, furosemide (Lasix) 40 mg, Senokot q.d.

CBC: hemoglobin 9.6, hematocrit 28.9, MCV 80

Iron studies: Ferritin low with increased TIBC

1. Classify/describe the anemia
2. What anemias present as microcytic hypochromic?

PE: Pulse is 100, 20; BP 130/80. Cardiac exam shows tachycardia, murmur of atrial stenosis. Abdomen diffusely tender. Lungs: distant lung sounds. Peripheral neuropathy present, 2 plus pedal edema.

3. What do you learn from the physical exam?
4. What risk factors for anemia does the patient have?
5. What lab tests would you order? Why?
6. The stools for occult blood come back positive. What is your diagnosis?

Case 3. The family brings their 94-year-old mother to clinic because she seems more confused and tired recently.

PMH: Irritable bowel syndrome, lactose intolerance, S/P cholecystitis, history of asthma, macular degeneration, history of alcoholism

Current medications: dicyclomine (Bentyl) 10 mg t.i.d., Metamucil 1 scoop q.d., LactAid with meals, omeprazole (Prilosec) 20 mg q.d.

PE: patient confused, has peripheral neuropathy

Lab: RBC 5.23, Hgb 10.1, Hct 31.8, MCV 104.0, MCH 23.1, MCHC 29.7

1. Classify/describe this anemia
2. What diagnoses are you considering?
3. What additional information do you need?

Lab: The B_{12} level is less than 250 and the folate level is 4 ng/mL

4. What is your diagnosis now?
5. What risk factors does she have for B_{12} deficiency?
6. Why is it necessary to screen for folate deficiency before treating B_{12} deficiency?
7. What is your treatment plan?
8. Will the peripheral neuropathy resolve?

REFERENCES

Allen, L. H. (2004). Folate and vitamin B$_{12}$ status in the Americas. *Nutritional Review, 62*(6 pt 2), S29–S33; discussion S34.

Andreoli, T. E. (Ed.). (2001). *Cecil essentials of medicine* (5th ed.). Philadelphia: W.B. Saunders.

Balducci, L. (2007). Cancer. In R. J. Ham, P. D. Sloane, G. A. Warshaw, M. A. Bernard, & E. Flaherty (Eds.), *Primary care geriatrics* (5th ed., pp. 533–545). New York: Mosby Elsevier.

Beers, M. H., Porter, R. S., & Jones, T. V. (Eds.). (2006). *Merck manual of diagnosis and therapy* (18th ed.). Whitehouse Station, NJ: Merck.

Beghe, C., Wilson, A., & Ershler, W. B. (2004). Prevalence and outcomes of anemia in geriatrics: A systematic review of the literature. *American Journal of Medicine, 116*(Suppl 7A), 3S–10S.

Blackwell, S., & Hendrix, P. C. (2001). Common anemias: What lies beneath. *Clinician Reviews, 11*(3), 52–64, 121–122.

Blackwell, S., Hendrix, P. C. (2001). Less common anemias: beyond iron deficiency. *Clinician Reviews, 11*(4), 57–65.

Dambro, M. R. (2004). *The 5 minute clinical consult.* St. Louis, MO: Lippincott, Williams & Wilkins.

Dodd, J., Dare, M., & Middleton, P. (2004). Treatment for women with postpartum iron deficiency anemia. *Cochrane Database Systematic Review, 18*(4), CD004222.

Fauci, A. S., Braunwald, E., Kasper, D. L., Hauser, S. L., Longo, D. L., Jameson, J. L., et al. (ed). (2006). *Harrison's principles of internal medicine* (17th ed.). New York: McGraw-Hill.

Ferri, F. F. (2003). *Ferri's clinical advisor* (6th ed.). St. Louis, MO: Mosby.

Fleming, M., Garrusm, S. J., & Harris, A. (2006). Ethanol. In L. Burnton (Ed.), *Goodman & Gilman's the pharmacologic basis for therapeutics.* New York: McGraw Hill. Available online at http://www.accessmedicine.com/content.aspx?aID=941376&searchStr=use+of+alcohol

Goodnough, L. T., Skikne, B., & Brugnara, C. (2000). Erythropoietin, iron, and erythropoiesis. *Blood, 96,* 823–833.

Lee, G., Foerster, J., Lukens, J,. Paraskevas, F., & Rodgers, G. (2003). *Wintrobe's clinical hematology* (11th ed.). Baltimore: Lippincott, Williams & Wilkins.

Paulman, P. M., Prest, L. A., & Abboud, C. (1998). Selected disorders of the blood and hematopoietic system. In R. B. Taylor (Ed.), *Family medicine: Principles and practice* (5th ed., pp. 1084–1096). New York: Springer.

Petz, L. A., & Garratty, G. (2003). *Immune hemolytic anemias* (2nd ed.). New York: Churchill-Livingston.

Provencio, M., Espana, P., Millan, I., Yebra, M., Sanchez, A. C., de la Torre, A., et al. (2004). Prognostic factors in Hodgkin's disease. *Leukemia & Lymphoma, 45*(6), 1133–1339.

Reuben, D. B., Herr, K. A., Pacala, J. T., Pollock, B. G., Potter, J. F., & Semla, T. P. (2007). *Geriatrics at your fingertips* (9th ed.). New York: American Geriatric Society.

Tierney, L. M., McPhee, S. J., & Papadakis, A. (2005). *Current medical diagnosis and treatment* (44th ed.). Stamford, CT: Appleton & Lange.

Wetzler, M., Byrd, J. C., & Bloomfield, C. D. (2006). Acute and chronic myeloid leukemia. In L. Burnton (Ed.), *Goodman & Gilman's the pharmacologic basis for therapeutics.* New York: McGraw Hill.

Young, N. S. (2002). Acquired aplastic anemia. *Annals of Internal Medicine, 136,* 534–546.

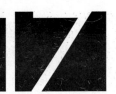

Endocrine Disorders

MJ Henderson, MS, RN, GNP-BC

GERIATRIC APPROACH

Normal Changes of Aging

- Reduced ability to maintain homeostasis, progressive loss of reserve capacity
- Occasionally, function of the system is maintained by increase in secretion of one hormone to offset decrease in another hormone
- Alteration frequently is undetected unless the patient is under stress

Specific Endocrine Function

- Thyroid gland becomes more fibrotic, nodular, and smaller, but generally circulating hormone levels remain within normal limits
- Parathyroid hormone levels increase, apparently to maintain calcium concentration
- Testicular testosterone secretion decreases: to compensate, pituitary luteinizing hormone (LH) increases
- Adrenal production of cortisol is unaffected
- Adrenal production of aldosterone and dehydroepiandrosterone (DHEA) declines
- Pancreatic function does not change significantly
- Postprandial glucose levels increase 5 mg/dL each decade after age 20, because of:
  - Increased fat and decreased muscle mass
  - Decrease insulin sensitivity
  - Sedentary lifestyle

Clinical Implications

History

- May present with no symptoms at all or as an abnormality in a system other than the endocrine system
- Patient presents with nonspecific signs and symptoms or with a functional decline
- Medications being administered for other problems can mask or change symptoms of existing illnesses and cause confusion

Physical

- Gynecomastia in older adult men is usually due to decreased testosterone levels, but also may be secondary to medications
- Endocrine disorders in older adults are often only detected with laboratory testing
- There are no age-adjusted normal ranges for endocrine test results

Assessment

- Endocrine dysfunction usually has multisystem effects
- Disorders ranging from hypertension to depression may originate from endocrine problems
- Regulation of hormone secretion is through a negative feedback system
- Basically three types of hormones:
    - Steroids such as cortisol (from the adrenal cortex); estrogen, progesterone (ovaries); and testosterone (testes)
    - Those derived from the amino acid tyrosine, such as thyroxine (thyroid) and catecholamines (adrenal medulla)
    - Proteins, peptides such as insulin (pancreas)

Treatment

- A key goal is to enhance or improve the individual's level of cognitive and physical functioning
- Consider other medical conditions when treating an endocrine problem
- Medications: "start low and go slow"; for example, a too-rapid increase in levothyroxine can precipitate angina
- Patients may need to carry or wear medical alert identification

DISORDERS OF THE PANCREAS

Diabetes Mellitus (DM)

Description

- Metabolic syndrome characterized by disorder in metabolism of carbohydrate, protein, and fat; results in high blood glucose level
- Fasting glucose level recommended for diagnosis of DM in the older adult
- American Diabetes Association diagnostic criteria

Diabetes Mellitus

- Fasting glucose levels 126 mg/dL or higher on two occasions
- Classic symptoms (polyuria, polydipsia, unexplained weight loss) plus random glucose of 200 mg/dL or higher
- Oral glucose tolerance test (OGGT): glucose of 200 mg/dL or more at 2 hours

Impaired Glucose Tolerance (common in the older adult)
- OGGT: glucose 140 to 199 mg/dL at 2 hours

Assessment
- Differentiate between types of DM by clinical history

History

> BOTH TYPE 1 AND 2
> - Polyuria, polydipsia, polyphagia, fatigue, slow-healing wounds, chronic skin infections, and recurrent infections (especially Candida and urinary tract infections)
> - Macrovascular changes more prominent than microvascular; for example, peripheral vascular insufficiency, cardiovascular/cerebrovascular disease, and atherosclerosis
> - History related to neurogenic and micro-/macrovascular changes
>   - Eyes: blurred vision, visual impairment
>   - Cardiovascular: postural dizziness
>   - GI: abdominal pain, nausea, vomiting, constipation, nocturnal diarrhea, gastroparesis
>   - GU: nocturia, bladder dysfunction, recurrent UTI, impotence, recurrent vaginal infections
>   - Neurological: memory loss, confusion, altered level of consciousness, paresthesias, cold extremities

Physical
- Skin infections, including cellulitis and lower-extremity ulcers
- Ptosis and visual changes seen on funduscopic exam: microaneurysms with soft exudates (cotton wool spots) and hard exudates, deep retinal hemorrhages, neovascularization, cataracts, glaucoma
- Oral and dental exam: oral Candida infections, dental caries, gingivitis
- Cardiovascular: orthostatic hypotension, resting tachycardia, silent myocardial infarction
- Abdominal: gastroparesis, incontinence, residual urine
- Peripheral vascular: decreased circulation, cool extremities, decreased pulses, edema, capillary refill greater than 3 seconds
- Neurologic: decreased sensation of pain, vibration, and light touch; decreased proprioception; absent lower-extremity reflexes; dysfunction in extraocular movements; weakness; ataxic gait

Follow-up
Complications
- Retinopathy, glaucoma, cataracts, blindness
- Nephropathy and renal failure, leads to dialysis
- Cardiovascular disease with lipid abnormalities, atherosclerosis, silent MI
- Peripheral neuropathy, foot and skin ulcerations, gangrene of lower extremities
- Infections
- Cerebrovascular disease, stroke
- Hyperglycemic hyperosmolar nonketotic coma, ketoacidosis

Diabetes Mellitus Type 1

Description
- Absolute deficiency or failure to produce insulin; type 1 diabetes mellitus is very rare in the older adult and will only be discussed briefly
- Without insulin therapy, ketoacidosis occurs rapidly

Etiology
- Destruction of beta-cells in pancreatic islets and absolute deficiency or failure to produce insulin

Incidence and Demographics
- Type 1 accounts for 10% to 12% of cases in the United States; generally occurs in puberty, between ages 8 and 14
- Can develop in adulthood; rare onset in geriatric patients
- Because of improvements in treatment, more people with type 1 diabetes are living to older age

Assessment
History
- Acute onset, weight loss, dehydration, ketotic episodes

Physical exam
- Ill looking, fruity odor to breath, ketoacidosis
- Weight loss, thin

Management
- Various insulins and synthetic human amylin analogues; best to refer to endocrinologist

When to Consult, Refer, Hospitalize
- Refer to endocrinologist to develop initial treatment plan

Table 17–1. Insulin Products

Preparation	Brand	Onset (hrs)	Peak (hrs)	Duration (hrs)	Administration
Rapid acting					
Insulin analogue Lispro	Humalog	< 1/4	1/2 to 3	2 to 5	SC before meals
Insulin aspart	Novolog	< 1/4	1/2 to 3	2 to 5	SC before meals
Insulin glulisine	Apidra	< 1/4	1/2 to 3	2 to 5	SC before meals
Short acting					
Regular (R)	Humulin R	1/4 to 1	2 to 4	3 to 8	SC before meals
Intermediate					
NPH	Humulin N Novolin N	1 to 4	4 to 12	12 to 18	SC b.i.d.

continued

Table 17–1. Insulin Products (cont.)

Preparation	Brand	Onset (hrs)	Peak (hrs)	Duration (hrs)	Administration
Long acting					
Insulin glargine	Lantus	1 to 10	none	24	SC q.h.s. or AM
Insulin detemir	Levemir	1 to 10	none	24	SC q.h.s. or AM
Humulin 70/30; 30/70*					SC b.i.d. AC breakfast and dinner
Novolin 70/30; 30/70; 50/50*					SC b.i.d. AC breakfsst and dinner

*These insulins are a mixture of 70% long-acting and 30% short-acting, or vice versa, or 50/50.

Add insulin for patients with type 2 DM who do not respond to oral medications.
Do not use sliding-scale insulin in nursing home patients. Better to use long-acting insulin q.d. and if necessary give short-acting insulin before meals. Get assistance from endocrinologist.

Diabetes Mellitus Type 2 (DM 2)
Description
- Metabolic disease causing hyperglycemia, characterized by resistance to the action of insulin in target tissues, decrease in insulin receptors, and/or impairment of insulin secretion
- Diabetes has been shown to be an important risk factor for cardiovascular disease, including hypertension and coronary artery disease; management of cardiovascular disease is important in the treatment of diabetes

Etiology
- Formally called non-insulin-dependent (NIDDM), adult- or maturity-onset, nonketotic
- Genetically and clinically a heterogeneous disorder with a familial pattern
- Insulin resistance with failure of adequate compensatory insulin secretion
- Influenced by environmental factors; see Risk Factors
- No HLA or islet cell antibodies

Incidence and Demographics
- Increases dramatically with increased age
- Approximately 20% of older adults over age 75 have DM2
- Increased prevalence in American Indian tribes, particularly Pima and Navajo; Mexican-Americans of southwest United States; in South Africa, and in Asian Indians

Risk Factors
- Obesity/inactivity: > 20% ideal body weight or body mass index (BMI) > 27 kg/m^2
- Diet: high in refined carbohydrates and fat, low in fiber
- Family history of diabetes, mostly Type 2
- Previously impaired glucose tolerance
- Older adults
- Black, Asian-American, Hispanic-American, American Indian, or Pacific Islander
- "Metabolic syndrome"; must have 3 or more of the following: fasting HDL < 50 mg/dL in women, < 40 mg/dL men; BP > 130/85; fasting glucose > 110 mg/dL; fasting triglycerides > 150 mg/dL; and central obesity (waist circumference) > 35 inches in women, > 40 inches in men

Prevention and Screening
- Adults > 45 years old screened every 3 years; more often with increased risk factors or borderline glucose
- Nonspecific recommendations for geriatric patients; many providers screen yearly
- Education regarding obesity, diet, exercise

Assessment
History
- Insidious onset
- No dehydration, no ketoacidosis
- May have polyuria, polydipsia, and weight loss
- History of macrovascular disease: MI, CAD, TIA, strokes, hypertension, hyperlipidemia

Physical
- Obesity, predominantly upper body fat with high waist-to-hip ratio
- Chronic skin infections and candidal vaginitis in women
- Usually discovered on routine exam with elevated glucose level
- Mildly hypertensive

Diagnostic Studies
- Other tests indicated
  - Urinalysis for protein, glucose, and ketones; microalbuminuria screening at initial diagnosis
  - BUN and urine and serum creatinine
  - Serum cholesterol and lipid profile
  - Glycosylated hemoglobin A1c—index of glycemic control over 2 to 3 months (5.5% to 7% indicates good control for geriatric patients)
  - EKG and chest x-ray for coronary and pulmonary pathology
  - Consider stress test

Differential Diagnosis
- Diabetes mellitus type 1
- Impaired glucose tolerance
- Diabetes insipidus
- Pancreatitis or pancreatic disease
- Pheochromocytoma
- Cushing syndrome
- Liver disease
- Secondary effects of corticosteroids, thiazides, phenytoin, nicotinic acid or severe stress from trauma, burns, or infection

Management
Nonpharmacologic Treatment
- Establish treatment goal
- For healthy older adults, goal is fasting glucose less than 120 mg/dL
- In frail, forgetful patients, hypoglycemia may precipitate falls, with potentially significant injury more likely; less strict control is indicated
- Patient education about condition and management to include diet, exercise, and medication

- Nutrition counseling for weight reduction if obese: loss of 5% to 10% increases insulin sensitivity
  - Regular meals with emphasis on balanced diet, avoiding simple sugars and refined carbohydrates
  - General diet guidelines: saturated fats < 7% of total calories; fiber 14 g/1000 kcal; avoid restrictive diets in nursing home patients
- Exercise recommended daily 30 minutes every day, to tolerance; exercise should be regular
- Limit alcohol to one drink for women and two for men daily; avoid smoking
- Foot care plan; use properly fitting shoes at all times
- Identification bracelet or necklace
- Annual influenza vaccine
- Referral to local support groups and American Diabetes Association

Pharmacologic Treatment
- Step approach, starting with diet and exercise, then medication; see Table 17–2 for list of medications available
- Begin oral antidiabetic agent with a low dose, increase dosage every 1 to 2 weeks on basis of glycemic control
- With failure to respond to first oral antidiabetic agent, add a second agent
- If second oral antidiabetic agents fail, add insulin or consult endocrinologist

  OBESE PATIENT
  - Step one: metformin for mild disease
  - Step two: add thiazolidinedione or sulfonylurea as appropriate; see Table 17–2
  - Step three: insulin

  NON-OBESE PATIENT
  - Step one: sulfonylurea for mild disease
  - Step two: metformin or thiazolidinedion; see restrictions, Table 17–2
  - Step three: insulin

  OTHER
  - Treat hypertension (BP > 135/85) with ACE inhibitor or angiotensin receptor blocker (ARB) unless contraindicated
  - Treat proteinuria, nephropathy with ACE inhibitor or ARB
  - Consider aspirin 81 to 325 mg p.o. q.d. to reduce risk for diabetic atherosclerosis
  - Treat hyperlipidemia with statins

Special Considerations
- Hypoglycemia
  - Plasma glucose concentration < 70 mg/dL
  - Cause: overmedication, poor or irregular nutrition, increased activity
  - Risk factors: kidney or liver disease, alcohol or sedative use, cognitive disorder
  - Classic symptoms: shakiness, tremors, nervousness, headache, sweating, weakness, dizziness, hunger, irritability, anxiety, visual changes, rapid heart rate, palpitations; symptoms typically last 15 to 30 minutes; less likely in the frail older adult
  - Older adults more likely to have CNS symptoms: confusion, headache, mental dullness, clumsiness, fatigue, visual disturbances, loss of consciousness, convulsions, coma

- Treatment
  - If able to take p.o., simple carbohydrate plus protein available in tablets, bars, or paste
  - For coma or mental confusion: glucagon injection, call 911, administer intravenous injection of 25 to 50 g glucose in 50% solution
  - Follow blood sugars closely
- Complications
  - Brain damage and tissue death from prolonged low glucose level
  - Older adults are susceptible to falls and fractures
- Hyperglycemic hyperosmolar nonketotic state
  - Syndrome: extreme hyperglycemia ($\geq$ 600), hyperosmolality, severe volume depletion, stupor, coma
  - High mortality rate: 12% to 46%
  - Often precipitated by severe illness such as infection
  - Emergent hospitalization: requires IV insulin, fluid replacement, treatment of underlying illness

When to Consult, Refer, Hospitalize

- Endocrinologist referral for uncontrolled hyperglycemia and follow-up
- Diabetic educator for further teaching for all patients
- Registered dietitian for further nutritional teaching
- Ophthalmologist for at least yearly checkups
- Podiatrist for routine foot care of older adults and foot problems as indicated
- Hospitalize for severe infections, hyperglycemic hyperosmolar nonketotic state

Table 17–2. Oral Antidiabetic Agents

Generic Class	Brand Name	Duration of Action	Dose	Administration	Precautions/Side Effects
Second-generation sulfonylureas: Increase endogenous insulin through stimulation of beta cells					
Glipizide	Glucotrol	12 to18 hours	2.5 to 10 mg q.d.– t.i.d.	Take ½ hour before meals	Good for postprandial hyperglycemia
	Glucotrol XL	24 hours	2.5 to10 mg q.d.	Take with breakfast	Risk for hypoglycemia
Meglitinides: Increase endogenous insulin					
Repaglinide	Prandin	Fast, short	0.5 to 4 mg b.i.d.– q.i.d.	Take before meals	Caution renal, liver disease malnourished older adults Greater risk of hypoglycemia

continued

Table 17-2. Oral Antidiabetic Agents (cont.)

Generic Class	Brand Name	Duration of Action	Dose	Administration	Precautions/Side Effects
Biguanides: decrease hepatic glucose production, increase action on muscle glucose uptake					
Metformin	Glucophage	Short-intermediate acting	500 to 1,000 mg q.d.–b.i.d.	Start with evening meal; if diarrhea, take just after the meal	Not for use in patients with unstable heart failure or hospitalized patients Contraindicated with creatinine > 1.5 in men, > 1.4 in women
	Glucophage XR	Long acting	500 mg q.d.–b.i.d.	Take with meals Take once a day	Use with caution in liver disease, alcohol use, or patients over age 80; can be used in patients with stable heart failure if renal function is normal Diarrhea common; lactic acidosis rare
Nateglinide	Starlix	Short acting	60 to 120 mg t.i.d., give within 30 minutes before meals	120 mg t.i.d.	Quick onset, which may be useful in individuals with irregular eating schedules; do not take if a meal is skipped; use with caution in severe renal disease; may be used as an adjunct with metformin
Thiazolidinediones: Reduce insulin resistance; not for use in patients with heart failure					
Pioglitazone	Actos	24 hr	15 to 45 mg q.d.	Timing not critical Actos may be used in combination with insulin and metformin, but must reduce dose of sulfonylureas to avoid hypoglycemia	**Black box warning of increased risk for heart failure** Headache, myalgia, edema are common effects **Black box warning: may cause or worsen heart failure and increase risk for MI;** do not use if there is renal or hepatic disease Does not cause hypoglycemia when used alone
Rosiglitazone	Avandia	24 hours	2 to 8 mg q.d.–b.i.d.		

continued

Table 17-2. Oral Antidiabetic Agents (cont.)

Generic Class	Brand Name	Duration of Action	Dose	Administration	Precautions/Side Effects
Alpha-glucosidase inhibitors: Delay cholesterol digestion and decrease postprandial glucose					
Acarbose	Precose	Very short acting	50 to 100 mg 3x/day	Take with first bite of meal	GI side effects: loose stool, flatulence. Does not cause hypoglycemia when used alone
Miglitol	Glyset	Very short acting	25 to 100 mg 3x/day		

New Products:

Exenitide (Byetta) is a synthetic peptide that mimics incretin, which is produced and released into the blood by the intestines in response to food. In DM2, GLP-1 increases secretion of insulin, slows gastric emptying and absorption of glucose, and reduces the action of glucagon; it is used with metformin and glyburide; 5 mcg SC b.i.d. within 60 mins of eating. Not for patients with end-stage renal dialysis or with creatinine clearance < 30 mL/min.

Sitagliptin phosphate (Januvia) is a dipeptidyl peptidase-4 enzyme (DPP-4) inhibitor. It blocks enzymes that degrade GLP-1; reduces action of glucagon; slows gastric emptying; given as monotherapy or used with metformin and pioglitazone or rosiglitazone; 25, 50, 100 mg tablets once daily depending on creatinine clearance.

Follow-up
Expected Course
- When first diagnosed or when adjusting medications, see weekly, then biweekly, monthly
- Well-controlled diabetics, see every 6 months
- Annual urine microalbumin, fasting blood sugar, and lipid profile; creatinine, EKG, full physical exam with funduscopic, neurologic exam; complete foot inspection
- If treated with medication, obtain hemoglobin A1c every 3 to 6 months; goal < 7%

THYROID DISORDERS

Table 17-3. Thyroid Function Tests

Condition	Test	Comments
Hypothyroidism	TSH elevated	Most sensitive screen for primary hypothyroidism
	Free T4 decreased	Confirmatory test, also excellent; may be normal in mild early, hypothyroidism
	Antithyroglobulin and antithyroid peroxidase antibodies	Elevated in Hashimoto thyroiditis

continued

Table 17-3. Thyroid Function Tests (cont.)

Condition	Test	Comments
Hyperthyroidism	Serum TSH decreased or undetectable	Most sensitive screen for primary hyperthyroidism
	Free T4 usually elevated	If normal FT4 and hyperthyroid is suspected, order free T3
	Free T3 elevated	Confirmatory
	Antithyroglobulin and antimicrosomal antibodies	Elevated in Graves' disease
Nodules	I-123 uptake and scan used to detect nodules	Cancer is usually "cold spots"; less reliable than fine needle aspiration
	Fine-needle aspiration (FNA)	Best diagnostic method for evaluating whether a nodule is cancer
	Ultrasound	Solid vs. cyst

- Nonthyroidal illnesses such as active hepatitis, cirrhosis, nephrotic syndrome, infections, malnutrition, and severe acute illness can affect serum thyroid function tests

Hypothyroidism

Description
- Decreased circulating thyroid hormone due to dysfunction in thyroid or pituitary glands

Etiology
- Primary: inability of thyroid gland to produce hormone
  - Hashimoto disease and other autoimmune thyroiditis
  - Ablation of gland through surgery, radiation, radioactive iodine, treatment of hyperthyroidism (Graves' disease)
- Secondary: lesions in pituitary gland—lack of pituitary TSH
  - Pituitary adenoma
- Tertiary: thyrotropin-releasing hormone (TRH) deficiency from hypothalamus
  - Certain drugs such as lithium, amiodarone, alpha interferon, coexisting autoimmune disorders
  - Iodide deficiency

Incidence and Demographics
- Primary: thyroid dysfunction > secondary > tertiary
- Females > males
- Increasing frequency in patients older than 60
- For > 60 years old, incidence is 10%

Risk Factors
- Family history of thyroid or autoimmune disorders
- There is some evidence that subclinical hypothyroidism confers increased risk for coronary heart disease

Prevention and Screening
- Routine screening is not recommended in healthy young-old patients
- Regular TSH screening in patients treated for hyperthyroidism
- Some recommend screening geriatric patients yearly, especially those with vague symptoms such as fatigue
- TSH should be ordered as part of the diagnostic study for change in mental status

Assessment
History
- Weight gain, fatigue, lethargy, memory loss, depression, weakness, arthralgias, myalgias, constipation, cold intolerance

Physical
- Weight gain
- Face: dull expression, swollen
- Skin: dry skin, coarse dry hair, brittle nails, hair loss, temporal thinning of eyebrows
- Eyes: periorbital edema
- Ears: decreased auditory acuity
- Mouth: swollen tongue, hoarseness
- Thyroid: enlarged gland (goiter) or atrophy, tender, nodules
- Cardiac: bradycardia, decreased heart sounds, mild hypotension or diastolic hypertension, cardiomegaly
- Respiratory: dyspnea, pleural effusion
- Abdominal: hypoactive bowel sounds, abdominal bloating
- Extremities: swollen hands/feet, leg edema
- Neurological: dementia, paranoid ideation, slow/delayed reflexes, cerebellar ataxia, carpal tunnel syndrome

Diagnostic Studies
- TSH, free T4
- CBC for anemia
- Electrolytes: hyponatremia, glucose (hypoglycemia), BUN, creatinine, calcium, albumin levels, urine protein, lipid studies (hypercholesterolemia)

Differential Diagnosis
- Depression
- Obesity
- Dementia
- Coronary heart disease
- Congestive heart failure
- Kidney failure
- Cirrhosis
- Nephrotic syndrome
- Chronic kidney disease
- Coexisting secondary cause

Management
Nonpharmacologic Treatment
- Education about thyroid disease
- Increase fluids and include fiber in diet for constipation
- Weight loss if obese with goal to lose if possible, or not gain anymore

Pharmacologic Treatment
- Primary hypothyroidism
  - Levothyroxine (T4) first-line therapy for primary hypothyroidism
  - Take on an empty stomach the first thing in morning to increase absorption, wait 30 minutes before taking other medications or food
  - Many potential drug interactions: calcium, cholestyramine, ferrous sulfate, aluminum hydroxide antacids, sucralfate
  - Concomitant use of CNS depressants, digoxin, insulin may decrease efficacy of thyroid replacement dosage
  - Starting dose: 25 mcg in frail older adults or 50 mcg in healthy older adults, p.o. daily with increase of 25 mcg every 6 to 8 weeks depending on patient's symptoms and labs

When to Consult, Refer, Hospitalize
- Refer developing myxedema coma, hypothermia, decreased mentation, respiratory acidosis, hypotension, hyponatremia, hypoglycemia, hypoventilation, significant cardiac disease, secondary hypothyroidism, or radically abnormal thyroid function tests to endocrinologist

Follow-up
Expected Course
- Older adults at risk for angina as thyroid levels increase
- Measure TSH 6 weeks after initial dosage then every 6–8 weeks until within normal limits and pt feels better, then every 6 to 12 months (TSH levels may remain elevated for several months despite effective treatment)
- If drug dosage changed, recheck TSH levels in 6 weeks
- Monitor for signs and symptoms of hyperthyroidism
- Improvement within 1 month of starting medication
- Symptoms resolve within 3 to 6 months of treatment
- Annual lipid levels
- Lifelong thyroid replacement therapy: maintain dosage where pt feels comfortable and to maintain euthyroidism

Complications
- Heart failure
- Psychoses
- Thyrotoxicity
- Myxedema coma—rare
- Complication of therapy—may precipitate angina palpitations

Hyperthyroidism
Description
- Clinical condition that occurs when the body's tissues are exposed to an increased level of thyroid hormones

Etiology
- Autoimmune response: Graves' disease (diffuse toxic goiter)
- Multinodular goiter (toxic nodular goiter)
- Solitary adenoma
- Transient thyroiditis (viral etiology)

- Drug induced, such as iodide and iodide-containing drugs (amiodarone) and contrast media

Incidence and Demographics
- Affects 2% of women and 0.2% of men
- Much less common in older adults than hypothyroidism

Risk Factors
- Family history of thyroid disorders and autoimmune disorders
- Thyroid replacement hormone overdosing

Prevention and Screening
- Monitor TSH and free T4 with thyroid replacement hormone

History
- Weight changes (older adults usually lose weight)
- Increased appetite, anxiety, palpitations, sweating, hypersensitivity to heat, fatigue, weakness, hand tremor
- Mental: confusion, severe depression, insomnia, irritability, anxiety, psychosis
- GI: increased frequency of bowel movements, diarrhea, anorexia in older adults

Physical
- Adrenergic: tachycardia, nervousness, sweating, palpitations, tremor, lid lag, excitability
- Skin: warm, moist hands, diaphoresis, thin/fine hair, spider angiomas, smooth skin on elbows, pretibial edema
- Eyes (Graves' disease only): periorbital edema, exophthalmos, lid lag, lid retraction, blurred vision, photophobia, diplopia
- Neck: goiter smooth or nodular, thyroid bruit or thrill
- Cardiac: arrhythmia such as atrial fibrillation, sinus tachycardia with resting rate > 90; angina; heart failure; systolic flow murmurs; widened pulse pressure
- Respiratory: dyspnea on exertion, tachypnea
- Muscle: proximal myopathy, periodic paralysis, progressive wasting of muscles
- Bone: osteoporosis, hypercalcemia
- Neurologic: hyperactive reflexes, tremors
- NOTE: In the older adult one more often sees cardiac problems such as heart failure and tachydysrhythmias, weakness, weight loss, and anorexia

Diagnostic Studies
- TSH, free T4, free T3

Differential Diagnosis
- Psychological disorders (such as anxiety, panic, psychosis)
- Pheochromocytoma
- Malignancy
- Heart failure
- New-onset or worsening angina
- Orbital tumors (cause exophthalmos)
- Myasthenia gravis (ophthalmoplegic changes)

Management
- Manage symptoms with beta-blockers to reduce tachycardia until patient can see endocrinologist and receives definitive therapy
- Immediately refer for definitive therapy

Nonpharmacologic Treatment
- Surgery last option because of possible complications of hypoparathyroidism and vocal cord paralysis

Pharmacologic Treatment
- Radioactive iodine (I-131) is treatment of choice in the older adult
- Euthyroid in 2 to 6 months
- Antithyroid medications
  - Propylthiouracil (PTU) 100 to 150 mg every 8 hours initially then 50 to 100 mg b.i.d. maintenance dose
  - Methimazole (Tapazole) 20 to 30 mg every 12 hours initially, then 50 mg q.d. or b.i.d. maintenance
  - 2 to 3 months to reach euthyroid
  - Patients usually remain on drug for 1 year, then it is gradually withdrawn
  - Relapses in older adults rarely occur
  - Agranulocytosis is a rare side effect of these drugs; order WBC before initiating antithyroid drugs and if patient gets an infection
- Symptomatic therapy
  - Catecholamine symptoms: beta-blocker (propranolol 10 to 60 mg every 6 hours; atenolol 50 to 100 mg q.d.); diltiazem for patients unable to take beta-blockers; gradually discontinue
  - Multivitamin; calcium replacement and vitamin D to maintain bone density
  - Ophthalmopathy: eye lubricants for mild cases; if severe refer to ophthalmologist

When to Consult, Refer, Hospitalize
- Endocrinologist for initial evaluation and management
- Ophthalmologist for evaluation of eye pathology

Follow-up
Expected Course
- Endocrinologist to monitor free T4 and TSH every 4 weeks until patient becomes euthyroid or hypothyroid
- Maintenance visits every 3 months, then every 6 months for 1 year, then wean off medications and see if patient becomes hyperthyroid again; if not, no medications, and monitor every month for 3 months then every 6 months, then annually or p.r.n. for S&S; If hyperthyroid again refer for I-131
- After radioactive iodine therapy order TSH every 6 weeks, 12 weeks, 6 months, then annually
- Baseline CBC; LFT every 3 to 6 months while patient is on antithyroid medications

Complications
- Thyroid storm: febrile, agitation, confusion, cardiac collapse
- Hypothyroidism due to treatment of Graves'
- Severe depression following treatment
- Visual disturbance from ophthalmopathy

- Weight gain if patient becomes hypothyroid with treatment
- Atrial fibrillation and other cardiac problems
- Osteoporosis

Thyroid Nodule
Description
- Single or multiple localized enlargements within thyroid gland; may function independently of pituitary gland
- Generally found on routine thyroid examination
- Critical assessment is whether or not it is cancerous

Etiology
- Unknown

Incidence and Demographics
- 90% of women over 60 have a nodular thyroid gland
- 60% of men over 80 have a nodular thyroid gland
- Less than 10% of solitary nodules are malignant
- Cysts comprise 15% to 25% of thyroid nodules

Risk Factors
- Female sex
- Increasing age; males have a higher risk for malignant nodules
- Family history of thyroid cancer
- Direct exposure to radiation of head, neck, chest; patients with radiation exposure have greater risk of developing thyroid disease
- Iodine deficiency—higher in parts of world where soil has low iodine, and there is no access to seafood or iodized salt

Assessment
History
- Hoarseness, dysphagia, obstruction, neck tenderness
- Benign or malignant nodules often asymptomatic but may have symptoms of hypo- or hyperthyroidism

Physical
- Malignant: hoarseness with cervical lymph nodes; dyspnea; tumors that are large, fixed, painless, hard, irregular in shape, do not move with swallowing, and are increasing in size
- Benign: multiple nodules that occur with Hashimoto thyroiditis; or thyroid nodule(s) that are nontender, soft, and multiple

Diagnostic Studies
- See Table 17–3

Differential Diagnosis
- Malignant nodules vs. benign nodules
- Cysts

Management
- Refer to endocrinologist

When to Consult, Refer, Hospitalize
- Refer to endocrinologist for all palpable nodules

Follow-up
Expected Course
- Good survival rate with malignant nodules unless they are due to follicular carcinoma or tumor has metastasized to the neck lymphatics

Complications
- Tumor recurrence
- Hypo- or hyperthyroidism

CUSHING'S SYNDROME
Description
- Syndrome of clinical abnormalities resulting from chronic excessive amounts of corticosteroids

Etiology
- In the older adult most commonly from chronic treatment with corticosteroids
- ACTH hypersecretion from pituitary gland due to benign pituitary microadenoma (most common)
- ACTH hypersecretion from adrenal adenomas or carcinomas
- Ectopic production of ACTH by malignant tumors, such as from lung

Incidence and Demographics
- Cushing's syndrome and primary adrenal tumors more common in women
- Pituitary tumors 5 times more frequent in women than in men

Risk Factors
- Adrenal tumor
- Pituitary tumor
- Long-term use of corticosteroids

Prevention and Screening
- Limit corticosteroid use

Assessment
History
- Mental changes, emotional lability, depression, psychosis, weakness, fatigue, poor wound healing, thin skin, polyuria, polydipsia, susceptibility to infections, loss of function
- Long-term use of corticosteroids

Physical
- High blood pressure
- Truncal obesity with thin extremities

- Skin: thin, atrophic, hirsutism, ecchymosis, hyperpigmentation, purple striae, poor healing
- Head: moon face
- Eyes: glaucoma, cataracts
- Abdomen: abdominal striae, protuberant
- Kidney: renal calculi
- Back: dorsal fat pad ("buffalo hump")
- Musculoskeletal: weakness, atrophy of muscles, osteoporosis

Diagnostic Studies
- Urine: glycosuria, elevated cortisol level
- Plasma cortisol level: elevated evening and 24-hour levels
- Screening tests: dexamethasone overnight suppression test if diagnosis questionable
- Elevated serum glucose, hypokalemia, hypernatremia, elevated triglycerides

Differential Diagnosis
- Alcoholism
- Obesity
- Depression
- Familial cortisol resistance
- Hirsutism

Management
Nonpharmacologic Treatment
- High-protein diet

Pharmacologic Treatment
- If due to prolonged use of steroids gradually discontinue therapy or change to alternate-day dosing schedule

When to Consult, Refer, Hospitalize
- Refer all cases to endocrinologist and coordinate primary care
- Hospitalize for acute illness as needed to hydrate and administer parenteral glucocortisol replacement

Follow-up
- If patient has recurrence of symptoms, measure urine free cortisol
- Once patient is taken off corticosteroid therapy, may need to restarted if he or she gets sick or stressed from any cause

Complications
- Hypertension
- Heart failure
- Osteoporosis with fractures
- Diabetes mellitus
- Susceptibility to infections
- Nephrolithiasis
- Psychosis
- Peptic ulcer disease
- If untreated, morbidity and death

OBESITY

Description
- Excess of total body fat

Etiology
- Genetic predisposition; 60% risk of obesity if one parent obese, 90% risk if both
- Environmental and psychological factors
- Secondary health problems such as adrenal problems, hypothyroid, polycystic ovarian disease occur in less than 1% of obese patients
- Medications that can increase weight include steroids, megestrol (Megace), mirtazapine (Remeron)

Incidence and Demographics
- New onset in older adults is rare, requires investigation
- Incidence and prevalence is increasing in both genders and all ages
- One-third of U.S. population is obese
- Prevalence rates higher in Hispanic and Black women, Asians and Pacific Islanders, American Indians, Native Hawaiians, and Alaska natives
- Over 50% of Mexican American and Black women are overweight

Risk Factors
- Overeating or other poor dietary habits
- Sedentary lifestyle
- Genetic predisposition
- Medications (e.g., antipsychotics, some antidepressants)

Prevention and Screening
- Balanced dietary intake throughout life span
- Regular exercise

Assessment
History
- Obtain weight history over life span
- Obtain 24-hour diet recall
- Collect comprehensive diet history including food categories, amount servings, number of meals per day, fluid intake, snacks
- Family history of obesity, overeating, metabolic disorders, cardiovascular disease, cerebral vascular disease, hypertension, diabetes mellitus
- Exercise history
- Motivation to lose weight and prior attempts to lose weight

Physical
- Height and weight, complete physical

Diagnostic Studies
- Calculate body mass index (BMI)=[704.5 × weight in pounds divided by height in inches squared] or go to http://www.cdc.gov/nccdphp/dnpa/bmi/bmi-adult.htm for BMI calculator
  - Healthy normal weight BMI between 18.5 and 25
  - Overweight BMI > 25

- Class I obesity: BMI 30 to 34.9
- Class II obesity: BMI 35 to 39.9
- Class III obesity: BMI > 40
- Regional fat distribution
  - Abdominal fat (visceral fat) associated with metabolic disorders (diabetes mellitus, Cushing's syndrome) and cardiovascular disease
  - Hip and thigh fat (visceral fat) more common in women and poses less medical risk than abdominal fat
  - Waist measurements > 35 inches in women and > 40 inches in men pose significant health risk for cardiovascular disease, and risk for death increases with BMI > 30

Differential Diagnosis
- Hypothalamic disease
- Thyroid disease
- Pituitary dysfunction
- Cushing syndrome

Management
Nonpharmacologic Treatment
- Long-term lifestyle changes
- Comprehensive multidisciplinary approach to weight reduction includes dietary control, exercise, eating behavior modifications, psychosocial modification

    DIET
    - Eating behavior modification: emphasize planning, regular weights, and food diary
    - Eat regular meals containing protein; control portion size
    - To lose 1 pound, 500 more calories must be expended than consumed per day, or 3,500 fewer per week
    - Calorie intake per day to maintain weight requires eating the same amount of calories that one's body is using daily. Limit fat to ≤ 30% of total calories; carbohydrate 55% to 60% of calories; the rest from protein
    - Recommend diet
      - Protein on a regular basis: meat, fish, poultry, eggs, beans, nuts
      - Fruit and vegetable groups to provide fiber and nutrients—3 to 5 servings/day
      - Carbohydrates in moderation: bread, rice, and cereals
      - Adequate calcium intake: milk, cheese, and yogurt or calcium supplement
      - Restrict consumption of sweets and fats
      - Limit or avoid alcohol

    EXERCISE
    - Patient may require stress test evaluation before beginning exercise plan depending on comorbid conditions
    - Exercise: for energy expenditure, exercise (walking, cycling, water walking) daily for 30 to 60 minutes; see health promotion interventions in Chapter 3 for more on exercise in the older adult
    - Must plan regular exercise sessions that fit into normal routine

PSYCHOSOCIAL MODIFICATION
- Support for losing weight essential, whether in the form of a close friend, peer, therapist, or formal organization of people (such as Overeaters Anonymous, TOPS, Weight Watchers)

Pharmacologic Treatment
- Fat blocker
  - Orlistat (Xenical) 120 mg 3 times a day with meals only; causes loose, oily stools; not recommended
  - May be used to help if patient has BMI > 30, not recommended in older adults because of decreased absorption of fat-soluble nutrients

Special Considerations
- Older adults at greater risk from being underweight than overweight

When to Consult, Refer, Hospitalize
- Nutritional counseling
- Counselor for behavior modification
- Refer people who are morbidly obese to specialists

Follow-up
- Frequently, at least initially, to evaluate progress
- Regular monitoring and reinforcement of progress until goal weight is reached
- Expected course for weight loss
  - Slow progress, with expected loss of ½ to 2 to 3 lbs per week maximum
  - Continue to monitor for obesity complications

Complications
- Cardiovascular disease: hypertension, coronary artery disease, peripheral vascular disease
- Metabolic disorders: hyperinsulinemia, type 2 diabetes, hyperlipidemia
- Cerebral vascular disease
- Pulmonary: sleep apnea syndrome, chronic respiratory infections, hypoventilation
- Degenerative joint disease, chronic orthopedic problems, impaired mobility
- Cholelithiasis
- Nephrotic syndrome
- Depression, loss of self-esteem
- Psychosocial disability
- Cancers: colon, rectum, prostate, uterine, biliary tract, breast, ovarian
- Skin disorders, especially candidal infections
- Increase perioperative morbidity and mortality

CASE STUDIES

Case 1. A 68-year-old overweight American Indian man comes to the office one afternoon with the complaint of a wound on his foot that has been there for 1 month and will not heal. Denies pain, fever. Admits to fatigue, blurred vision. Also complains of joint pain, especially in knees and hips.

1. What diagnostic studies would you order?
2. Which lab test is the best for diagnosing diabetes in the older adult?
3. What risk factors does the patient have for diabetes?
4. What is your management of this patient?
5. What complications are you worried about?

Case 2. An 82-year-old patient is brought in for geriatric assessment by her daughter. Patient is having difficulty sleeping, and complains of fatigue and constipation to her family. She does not get dressed in the morning, and is having difficulty balancing her checkbook. She has gained 10 pounds in the last year. She is otherwise reported to be healthy and has not seen a health care provider in years. She takes acetaminophen (Tylenol) for arthritis. Her family members state they think she is becoming more forgetful.

1. What other history do you need?
2. What physical exam would you do; what would you expect to find?
3. What diagnostic test would be conclusive?
4. What are your differential diagnoses? What should you rule out?

Case 3. A 74-year-old man comes to the office with a complaint of palpitations for about a month. He notices them especially at night when he is trying to sleep; he is having more trouble sleeping recently. The palpitations occur about 1 to 2 times a day. He sits and rests and they go away. He also complains of shortness of breath when walking. He has recently lost 15 pounds. Patient denies dieting.

1. What other body systems would you inquire about?
2. What physical exam is important?

Physical: This patient has atrial fibrillation, tachypnea, hyperactive reflexes, and a fine tremor.

3. What is your diagnosis?
4. What labs would confirm this diagnosis?
5. What would you do?
6. What is the preferred treatment?

REFERENCES

American Diabetes Association. (2003). Position statement: Prevention and management of diabetes complications Preventive foot care in people with diabetes. *Diabetes Care, 26*(Suppl 1): S23-24.

American Diabetes Association. (2007a). Position statement: Diabetes care in specific populations. Older individuals. *Diabetes Care, 30*(Suppl 1), S27.

American Diabetes Association. (2007b). Position statement: Physical activity. *Diabetes Care, 30*(Suppl 1), S12–S14.

American Diabetes Association. (2007c). Position statement: Prevention and management of diabetes complications. Diabetes nephropathy screening and treatment. *Diabetes Care, 30*(Suppl 1), S19.

American Diabetes Association. (2009). Clinical practice recommendations. *Diabetes Care, 32*(Suppl 1), S13–S61.

Brown, A. F., Mangione, C. M., Saliba, D., & Sarkisian, C. A. (2003). Guidelines for improving care of the older person with diabetes mellitus. California Health Care Foundation/American Geriatrics Society panel on improving care for elders with diabetes. *Journal of the American Geriatrics Society, 51*(5), S265–S280.

Burch, W. M. (1984). *Endocrinology for the house officer* (2nd ed.). Baltimore: Williams &Wilkins.

Cayea, D., & Durso, S. C. (2007). Management of diabetes mellitus in the nursing home. *Annals of Long Term Care, 15*(5), 27–33.

Collazo-Clavell, M. (2008). *Avandia: Is it a safe option?* Retrieved from from http://www. riversideonline.com/health_reference/Articles/DA00138.cfm

Cooper, D. S. (2001). Clinical practice. Subclinical hypothyroidism. *New England Journal of Medicine, 345*, 260–265.

Dayan, C. M. (2001). Interpretation of thyroid function tests. *Lancet, 357*, 619–624.

DeCoste, K. C., & Scott, L. K. (2004). Diabetes update: Promoting effective disease management. *AAPHN Journal, 52*(8): 344–353.

Doelle, G. C. (2004). The clinical picture of metabolic syndrome. An update on this complex of conditions and risk factors. *Postgraduate Medicine, 116*(1), 30–32, 35–38.

Harris, R., Donahue, K., Rathore, S. S., Frame, P., Woolf, S. H., & Lohr, K. N. (2003). Screening adults for type 2 diabetes: A review of the evidence for the U.S. Preventative Services Task Force. *Annals of Internal Medicine, 138*, 215–229.

Klein, I., & Ojamaa, K. (2001). Thyroid hormone and the cardiovascular system. *New England Journal of Medicine, 344*, 501–509.

Lavin, N. (Ed.). (2002). *Manual of endocrinology and metabolism* (3rd ed.). Philadelphia: Lipincott Williams & Wilkins.

Mayo Clinic Staff. (2008). *Insulin: Compare common options for insulin therapy.* Retrieved from http://www.mayoclinic.com/health/insulin/da00091

McCarren, M. (2003). American Diabetes Association Resource Guide 2003. Class action: Type 2 pills update. *Diabetes Forecast, 56*(1): 44–47.

Pandya, N., Thompson, S., & Sambamoorthi, U. (2008). The prevalence and persistence of sliding scale insulin use among newly admitted nursing home residents with diabetes mellitus. *Journal of the American Medical Directors Association, 11*, 663–669.

Skidmore Roth, L. (2008). *Mosby's nursing drug reference.* St. Louis, MO: Mosby Elsevier.

UK Prospective Diabetes Study Group. (1998). Intensive blood glucose control with sulfonylureas or insulin compared with conventional treatment and risk of complications in patients with type 2 diabetes. *Lancet, 352*, 837–853.

Psychiatric–Mental Health Disorders

Vaunette Fay, PhD, RN, FNP-BC, GNP-BC

GERIATRIC APPROACH

Mental illnesses are common. In a 1-year period, approximately 19.8% of people 55 years of age and older have a diagnosable mental disorder. This figure does not include older adults with Alzheimer's disease or other severe cognitive disorders. Mental illness is defined as serious brain disorders that affect thinking, motivation, emotions, and social interactions. Mental illness intrudes upon the elements of the self that define a person's humanity and can deprive a person of the most gratifying aspects of life. It can prevent people from taking pleasure in everyday events and rob them of what they have achieved or become.

Normal changes of aging do not cause mental illness, although they can be a risk factor. Dementia, another disease with malfunction of the brain, must be considered when diagnosing and treating mental illness in the older adult. Whatever diagnosis is being considered, dementia must specifically be ruled out. Dementia, delirium, and associated psychotic symptoms are discussed in Chapter 4. Dementia and depression frequently present in the same manner in older adults. They often coexist in the same patient, especially in the patient with early dementia. If you are not sure whether it is depression or dementia, treat for depression and observe for improvement.

Mental disorders are greatly underdiagnosed and undertreated in the older adult, causing much needless suffering. Primary care providers are a critical link in identifying and addressing mental health disorders, and they have not stressed recognition and treatment of these conditions.

Opportunities are missed to improve mental health and general medical outcomes when mental illness is under-recognized and undertreated in primary care settings.

Patients are reluctant to discuss mental illness because of social stigma. The use of psycho-therapy, medications, and other treatment interventions can greatly improve quality of life for older adults and their families. These interventions may need to be modified for age and health status.

Normal Changes of Aging

- The brain undergoes structural changes in later life; see Chapter 15, Neurological Disorders, for details
  - Neuronal death
  - Decrease in the neurotransmitters acetylcholine, dopamine, and serotonin
  - Changes in short-term memory, speed of processing
  - How these changes affect psychological problems in the older adult is poorly understood
- In general, personality remains stable over time, with decreases in levels of impulsivity, aggression, and activity
  - Many people still believe that the older mind is less able to change, but that
    - Critical age-related stresses include interpersonal loss; loss of social support such as loss of spouse, family, friends
    - Physical disability, loss of strength
    - Loss of youthful appearance and beauty
    - Change in social role, such as children caring for parent
    - Forced reliance on caregivers, other transportation
    - Change in living arrangements such as loss of house
    - Confrontation with death

Clinical Implications

History

- Obtain a complete psychosocial history
- May need to interview family members and other caregivers to obtain history
- Typical signs and symptoms of mental illness are disturbances of attention, consciousness, emotion, affect, mood, motor activity, thought processes, perceptions, and memory
- Assessment tools are frequently helpful in the older adult; see Chapter 3

Physical

- Observe demeanor, function, and interaction with family members or caregiver
- Is the older adult interactive, withdrawn, or agitated?
- Speech patterns
- Grooming, appearance
- Does the person appear physically ill or frail?

Assessment

- Distinguish between a mental disorder and a medical condition; need to do a complete history and physical
- History; emphasis on history of present illness, past history of similar symptoms, and review of systems

- Many older adults have medical conditions and are on medications that can confuse the diagnosis of mental conditions

Treatment
Most mild mental disorders can be effectively treated in a primary setting
- Relate to the patient in an optimistic, positive manner
- Treatment compliance is a special concern in individuals with cognitive deficits, physical problems, poor vision
- Consult, refer, or hospitalize when presenting symptoms are severe, chronic, or unresponsive to primary treatment
- Individuals with mental illness often self-medicate; when prescribing, always be aware of the potential for development of tolerance or dependence and the potential lethality of medications
- Older adults who represent a clear and present danger to themselves or others, including suicidal ideation or attempt, should never be left alone and should be immediately hospitalized even when it is contrary to their wishes

General guidelines for psychopharmacology in the elderly
- Identify target symptoms to treat; failure to do so is common cause of treatment failure
- Treat systematically and change one thing at a time, allowing adequate time to evaluate the change before making another change
- Avoid using medications for their side effects only; for example, giving a sedating antidepressant to a nondepressed patient with insomnia
- Titrate dosage slowly to avoid side effects, continue to increase until therapeutic response is achieved or maximum recommended dose is reached
- Allow adequate length of time to achieve best therapeutic effects (several weeks for antidepressants)
- Older adults generally require lower doses of psychotropic medications than do younger adults
- Mental illness (including depression) is not a normal process of aging; mental illness requires assessment and treatment.
- Addictions to alcohol, prescription sedatives, and prescription opioids often arise for the first time in patients after the age of 70
- Older adults can exhibit the full range of signs and symptoms of addiction using much smaller quantities of chemicals (alcohol, sedatives, opioids, cannabis) than younger adults
- Psychotropic medications commonly given to younger adults without complications can produce profound cognitive and emotional deterioration in older adults (benzodiazepines, medications for sleep, sedating antihistamines, corticosteroids, antispasmodics, anticholinergics)

DEPRESSION

Description
- The predominant feature of depression is a disturbance in mood—the sustained internal emotional state of an individual who is described as sad or blue
- Loss of interest or pleasure in nearly all activities is the second major symptom; either mood disturbance or loss of interest or pleasure must be present in order to diagnose depression
- Depression is a disorder with much variation

- Dementia frequently presents as depression
- The *Diagnostic and Statistical Manual of Mental Disorders*, 4th edition (DSM-IV-TR; American Psychiatric Association, 2000) classifies the types of depression; see Table 18–1

Table 18–1. DSM-IV-TR™ Differential Diagnosis of Depressive Symptoms in Late Life

Disorder	Description
Mood disorders	
Major Depression Major Depressive Disorder	Depressed mood and/or loss of interest or pleasure, with other symptoms (such as insomnia, significant weight loss or weight gain, fatigue, psychomotor agitation or retardation), present for at least 2 weeks
Dysthymia	Chronic, sustained depressed mood ongoing for a minimum of 2 years, more days than not
Bipolar Disorder	Recurrent episodes of depression with episodes of mania that are characterized by a lack of impulse control, excessive energy, grandiose or delusional thinking, elated mood, inappropriate behaviors, hyperactivity, pressured speech, and decreased need for sleep
Adjustment disorders	
Adjustment disorder with depressed mood	Significant emotional or behavioral symptoms in response to a clearly identifiable psychosocial stressor(s) Symptoms develop within 3 months of the onset of the stressor(s), last no longer than 6 months, and manifest themselves in a maladaptive response of impaired function and marked distress in excess of what would normally be expected
Uncomplicated bereavement	
Organic mood disorders	Primary degenerative dementia with associated major depression Secondary to physical illness (such as hypothyroidism, stroke, carcinoma of the pancreas) Secondary to pharmacologic agents (such as methyldopa, propranolol)
Psychoactive substance use disorders	Alcohol abuse and/or dependence Sedative, hypnotic, or anxiolytic abuse and/or dependence
Somatoform disorders	Hypochondriasis Somatization disorder

Etiology
- Biological
  - Genetic predisposition
  - Dysregulation of chemical neurotransmitters; abnormalities in neurotransmitters in the brain including serotonin, norepinephrine, dopamine, acetylcholine (cholinergic), epinephrine, and gamma-aminobutyric acid (GABA)
  - Environmental: stressful and traumatic life events such as the death of loved ones, major illness, divorce, financial difficulty, trouble with the law

Incidence and Demographics
- Depression is the most common mental illness seen in primary care practices
- Dysthymia is more common in older adults than major depression
- Depression occurs more frequently in women than in men
- The prevalence of depression does not differ among races
- Statistics depend on definition used in study
- 10% to 15% of older adults experience symptoms of depression; major depression disorder is relatively rare in older adults but can occur for the first time at any age, including in older adults.
- 25% of older adults with chronic illness or who are cognitively intact in a nursing home experience depression
- It is estimated that only 50% of all persons with major depression receive treatment
- NIH consensus panel found that a substantial proportion of older adult patients receive no treatment or inadequate treatment for depression in primary care settings
- Adjustment disorders
  - Common and vary widely as a function of the population and culture
- Bipolar disorder has an early onset, prior to age 30
  - Bipolar disorder persists into old age and becomes increasing difficult to treat
  - Bipolar disorder occurs equally in men and women
- Suicide is a major risk of depression in older adults
  - 15% of the individuals diagnosed with severe major depression die of suicide
  - 30% of individuals diagnosed with bipolar disorder die of suicide
  - Older adults are 12% of the population but account for 33% of suicides

Risk Factors for Depression
- Prior episodes of depression
- Family history, especially first-degree relative
- Alcohol and substance abuse
- Significant psychosocial stressors such as divorce, death of spouse or loved ones, financial difficulty, job loss, retirement, trauma, and sexual, emotional, or physical abuse
- Periods of prolonged stress
- Neuroanatomic changes in later life (see Normal Changes of Aging)
- Chronic medical conditions and disabilities
- Polypharmacy

Risk Factors for Suicide
- Older White men who are socially isolated have the highest suicide rate
- Social isolation
- Death or loss of spouse/loved one
- Chronic medical conditions and disabilities
- Decreased impulse control, impaired judgment
- Severe psychosocial stressors
- Prior suicide attempt(s)
- Recent purchase of a handgun
- Any alcohol use—50% of individuals dying from suicide were intoxicated at the time

Prevention and Screening
- Adequate family and social support systems
- Stress management and problem solving techniques

- Prevention of suicide: providers must be alert to symptoms
- Ask direct questions of patient and family about suicide risks

Assessment

History
- The DSM-IV-TR diagnostic symptoms of depression
  - Depressed mood, subjective or observed
  - Diminished interest or pleasure in activities
  - Weight loss or gain
  - Insomnia or hypersomnia
  - Psychomotor agitation or retardation
  - Fatigue or loss of energy
  - Feelings of worthlessness or excessive or inappropriate guilt
  - Diminished ability to think or concentrate, or indecisiveness
  - Recurrent thoughts of death, recurrent suicidal ideation
- Other symptoms common in the elderly
  - Difficulty getting along with others
  - Increased social isolation and withdrawal with increased solitary behavior
  - Inattention to self-hygiene and appearance
  - Increased oversensitivity to real or perceived rejections or failures
  - Self-destructive behaviors
  - Increased somatic complaints such as headache, abdominal pain

  ASSESSMENT TOOLS
  - Mental status: Mini-Mental Status Exam (MMSE), short, portable, can rule out dementia; however, depressed patients may have decreased MMSE scores because of inattention
  - Depression: Geriatric Depression Scale (GDS)—the 5-item short version
    - Are you basically satisfied with your life? (no)
    - Do you often get bored? (yes)
    - Do you often feel helpless? (yes)
    - Do you prefer to stay home rather than go out and do new things? (yes)
    - Do you feel pretty worthless the way you are now? (yes)

  SUICIDE ASSESSMENT
  - As many as 80% of patients who commit suicide had recently seen their primary care provider (within a month of their suicide), usually with physical complaints or hints of depression
  - Ask directly about suicidal thoughts, impulses; patient will not volunteer information, but frequently will admit upon questioning
  - Determine degree of risk of actual attempt
    - Plan, specificity of plan (access to method)
    - Feelings of hopelessness, helplessness
    - Giving away personal possessions, canceling future plans
    - History of prior attempts

Physical
- A complete physical exam with a mental status and neurological exam should be performed in order to rule out organic mood disorders
- Neurological exam: gait, focal neurological signs, frontal lobe signs—structural brain abnormalities

- Weight loss or gain, psychomotor retardation—slowed movements, thinking
- Look for sad affect, anxiety, disheveled personal appearance with poor grooming, neglected hygiene

Diagnostic Studies
- Labs to rule out medical causes—liver and kidney function
- CBC, thyroid profile, sedimentation rate, electrolytes, chemistry profile, vitamin B_{12}, folate levels
- Serum levels of current medications if appropriate, such as tricyclic antidepressants (TCA), anticonvulsants, or digoxin
- Toxicology screen if appropriate
- Cortisol levels have been used to identify depression and subtypes in research but not in primary care practice

Differential Diagnosis
- Medical illnesses
- Other mood disorders (see Table 18–1)

Endocrine disorders
- Diabetes
- Hypothyroidism
- Hyperthyroidism
- Male hypogonadism
- Addison's disease
- Cushing's syndrome

Neurological disorders
- Dementia
- Stroke
- Neoplasms
- Multiple sclerosis
- Seizure disorders
- Parkinson's disease
- Traumatic brain injury

Cardiac disorders
- Heart failure
- Myocardial infarction

Malnutrition
- B_{12}
- Protein/calorie deficiency
- Folate deficiency
- Autoimmune disorder (rheumatologic disorders)
- Electrolyte imbalances
- Chronic fatigue syndrome
- Chronic obstructive pulmonary disease (COPD)
- Infections
- Oncologic/hematologic disease

Table 18-2. Medications That May Contribute to Depression

Class of Medication	Examples
Cardiac medications	Digitalis, statins, beta blockers
Antihypertensives	Calcium channel blockers, methyldopa, thiazide diuretics
Hormones	Estrogens, progestins, corticosteroids
GI medications	Histamine blockers, metoclopramide
Anticonvulsants	Phenytoin, barbiturates, carbamazepine, clonazepam, valproic acid
Anti-infectives	Fluoroquinolones, isoniazid, metronidazole, sulfonamides
Anxiolytics/sedatives	Benzodiazepines, zolpidem, carisoprodol, all "muscle relaxants"
Anti-inflammatory agents	NSAIDs
Antineoplastic agents	Interferon, cancer chemotherapy, radiation therapy

Management
- Most cases of depression can be safely managed by a primary practitioner
- Major depression and dysthymia have similar treatment
- Adjustment disorders are usually managed successfully with cognitive behavioral therapy and adequate family and social support
- Patients diagnosed with bipolar disorder should be referred for treatment

Nonpharmacologic Treatment
- Psychosocial interventions have been proven highly effective
  - Pharmacological treatment should always be accompanied by some form of psychotherapy if patient accepts it; patient may be more amenable after medication starts working
  - Include patient, family, and support systems in treatment strategies and regime
  - A positive attitude on the part of the clinician encourages adherence to treatment
  - Choose type of therapy appropriate to individual patients needs
    - Cognitive behavioral therapy with a focus on cognitive distortions
    - Psychoanalysis or psychotherapy with a focus on intrapsychic phenomena
- Electroconvulsive therapy (ECT): only indicated for severely depressed or suicidal patients who do not respond to pharmacological agents; memory impairment and personality change following ECT may be permanent
- Patient and family education
  - Patient and family education concerning the nature of the illness, side effects, risks and benefits of treatment, and expected outcome
  - Depression is a medical illness like any other
  - Treatment with medication replaces depleted neurotransmitters in the brain, allowing it to function more normally

Pharmacologic Treatment
- Match the antidepressant and its side effects to the symptoms that are most troublesome to the patient
- In general, depressed patients can be categorized in one of two ways:
  - Patient is anxious, with insomnia and perhaps weight loss
  - Patient has psychomotor retardation, with hypersomnia and perhaps weight gain
- Predicting which medication will work on which patient is difficult
- Begin treatment with the agent that best fits the patient's needs; continue long enough and at a sufficient dosage to determine if the agent will be successful; length of treatment for most psychotherapeutic medications is more important than dose

- If treatment is not effective, changing to another agent in the same class may be effective
- Older adults experience increased side effects of the medications, and combining antidepressants can cause significant adverse effects
  - Drug interaction between antidepressants and other medications are common
  - Antidepressants or antianxiety agents may be given short term (1 to 3 months) for management of acute symptoms of adjustment disorder
- Treatment with an antidepressant may precipitate a manic episode in patients with bipolar disease unless the patient is also treated with a mood stabilizer

Table 18-3. Medications for Target Symptoms

Symptoms	Effective Medications
Psychomotor retardation	SSRI, venlafaxine, bupropion
Anxiety	SSRI*, paroxetine
Insomnia	Mirtazapine, trazodone
Weight loss	Mirtazapine
Weight gain	SSRI, bupropion

*Has anxiety indication, but has been found on occasion to cause/increase anxiety in the older adult.

Paxil has some histamine effect and may be more effective for anxiety.

Table 18-4. Classification of Medications by Affected Neurotransmitter(s)

Drug Category	Serotonin	Norepinephrine	Dopamine	Others
SSRI	Yes	No	No	Epinephrine
TCA	Yes	Yes	No	Acetylcholine Histamine, epinephrine
Bupropion (Wellbutrin)	Minimal	Yes	Yes	No
Mirtazapine (Remeron)	Yes	Yes	No	Histamine, epinephrine
Trazodone (Desyrel)	Yes	No	No	Acetylcholine, epinephrine
Venlafaxine (Effexor)	Yes	Yes	Yes	No
MAOI	Yes	Yes	Yes	No

Table 18-5. Effects According to Neurotransmitter

Neurotransmitter	Adverse Effects
Norepinephrine	Tachycardia, tremors, sexual dysfunction, augments sympathomimetics
Serotonin	Anxiety, agitation, anorexia, GI disturbances, headache, hypotension, sexual dysfunction
Dopamine	Extrapyramidal signs, increased prolactin levels, psychosis, insomnia, anorexia, psychomotor activation
Epinephrine	Orthostatic hypotension, cardiac conduction disturbance
Acetylcholine	Memory dysfunction, constipation, tachycardia, blurred vision, dry mouth, urinary retention
Histamine	Sedation, drowsiness, hypotension, weight gain

SELECTIVE SEROTONIN REUPTAKE INHIBITORS (SSRI)

- SSRI are usually the first-line drug of choice for the treatment of major depression because of their effectiveness and safety record
- SSRI can be effective for anxiety but can cause agitation in the older adult
- All SSRI are not alike
  - Fluoxetine has a long half-life (up to 72 hours), which is good if the patient forgets to take an occasional dose; however, in the older adult, fluoxetine can cause agitation, which will then last for several days
  - Sertraline (Zoloft) is among the least likely to cause adverse effects, either sedation or activation
  - Paroxetine (Paxil) also affects histamine and can cause sedation; it may help patients with anxiety or insomnia
  - Citalopram (Celexa) and escitalopram (Lexapro, the L-isomer of citalopram): dosage of escitalopram is half the dosage of citalopram; Aamong the least likely to cause adverse effects, either sedation or activation
  - Fluvoxamine (Luvox) indicated for obsessive-compulsive disorder; is associated with more drug-drug interactions than the others

Table 18-6. SSRI Therapy in Older Adult Patients

Medication	Initial Dose	Target Dose
Fluoxetine (Prozac)	10 mg q.d.	20 to 40 mg q.d.
Sertraline (Zoloft)	25 mg q.d.	50 to 150 mg q.d.
Paroxetine (Paxil)	10 mg q.d.	20 to 40 mg q.d.
Escitalopram (Lexapro)	5 mg q.d.	10 to 20 mg q.d.

OTHER ANTIDEPRESSANTS

- Some of the newer antidepressants are especially effective in the older adult
- Bupropion (Wellbutrin XR) is activating; avoid bedtime dosing; do not use with history of seizure
- Mirtazapine (Remeron) is useful in helping with insomnia, weight loss
- Venlafaxine (Effexor XR) may be activating; monitor for elevated blood pressure
- Trazodone is an older, heterocyclic medication; has been used for insomnia but is now largely replaced by Mirtazapine

Table 18-7. Other Commonly Used Antidepressants

Medication	Initial Dose	Target Dose
Bupropion (Wellbutrin SR)	100 mg p.o. QAM	150 to 400 mg p.o. QAM
Mirtazapine (Remeron)	7.5 to 15 mg q.h.s.	15 to 30 mg q.h.s.
Venlafaxine (Effexor XR)	37.5 mg q.d.	75 mg b.i.d.
Duloxetine (Cymbalta)	30 mg q.d.	60 mg q.d.
Trazodone (Desyrel)	25 q.h.s.	100 mg q.h.s.

TRICYCLICS

- Tricyclic antidepressants are also effective in the treatment and management of depression; however, their association with a greater incidence of side effects has reduced their use

- Tricyclics are contraindicated in patients at risk for adverse anticholinergic effects, such as with cardiac conduction disorders, narrow-angle glaucoma, and prostatic hypertrophy
- Can also be used for pain control, especially neuropathic pain; may be especially effective in depressed patients with chronic pain
- Amitriptyline is the most common one used for pain but has the highest side effects
- Nortriptyline has fewer side effects; also effective for pain
- Tricyclic medications have a high potential for lethality in overdose

Table 18–8. Commonly Used Tricyclic Antidepressants

Medication	Initial Dose	Target Dose
Amitriptyline (Elavil)	10 to 25 mg q.h.s.	50 to 100 mg q.h.s.
Desipramine (Norpramin)	25 mg q.h.s.	50 to 100 mg q.h.s.
Nortriptyline (Pamelor)	10 to 25 mg q.h.s.	50 to 75 mg q.h.s.

MONOAMINE OXIDASE INHIBITORS (MAOI)
- Because of the many potentially serious and lethal side effects associated with these antidepressants, such as hypertensive crisis, patients in need of these types of medications should always be referred to a psychiatrist
- MAOI such as phenelzine (Nardil) and tranylcypromine (Parnate) are used in the treatment of refractory or treatment-resistant depression

How Long to Treat
- Treatment can be divided into three phases
  - Acute: goal is symptom remission; lasts 4 to 8 weeks, or more
  - Continuation: goal is stabilization when risk of relapse is high; lasts 6 to 12 months; generally requires continuation of medication for 1 year in first episodes of depression
  - Maintenance: goal is prevention of recurrences; time will vary; may be lifetime, especially in recurrent depression

Special Considerations
- Depression is a chronic illness with frequent episodes of recurrence

When to Consult, Refer, Hospitalize
- All patients who present with suicidal ideation, plan, or recent attempt should immediately be referred to an emergency room or psychiatrist for further evaluation and treatment
- Refer patients to psychiatrist or other mental health specialist if:
  - They are severely impaired by their symptoms
  - The have psychotic symptoms such as delusions and hallucination
  - The have comorbid disorders such as obsessive-compulsive disorder, substance abuse
  - They lack social support
  - The diagnosis is bipolar disorder, depressed—these patients are at high risk for suicide and should be seeing a psychiatrist
- All patients should be referred to the appropriate mental health practitioner for therapy
- Patients with symptoms attributed to adjustment disorder that last more then 6 months must be re-evaluated and referred to a mental health specialist

Follow-up
- Patients should be followed weekly for the first 2 months while effective dosage is titrated and response to medication and side effects can be monitored
- Continue to follow monthly until the patient is stable
- Patients who are not responding to medication should be placed on another antidepressant
- When changing antidepressants, remember to first change to another class antidepressants; then refer out for TCA or MAOI

Expected Course
- Most older adult patients respond to antidepressants within 2 to 3 weeks of treatment; full effect many not be seen until several months of therapy
- Recurrences are frequent
- Prognosis is poor if combined with medical illness

Complications
- Depression in older adults leads to impairments in social, mental, and physical functioning
- Major depression in older adults is associated with higher morbidity and mortality rates
- Older primary care patients with depression make more emergency room and primary care provider visits, use more medication, incur higher outpatient charges. and experience longer hospital stays
- Suicide

GRIEF/BEREAVEMENT

Description
- The emotional and physiological reaction to the death or loss of a someone or something loved
- Grief and bereavement are the normal reaction to death or loss
- Uncomplicated grief presents as depressed mood that is situational and time limited
- Grief that lasts longer than 2 months should be evaluated for mood disorders

Etiology
- Frequently associated with death of a loved one
- Any loss can cause grief, including loss of a job, financial stability, health, a friendship; moving from one's home; illness of family member or friend

Incidence and Demographics
- Grief is a common phenomenon in older adults
- 10% to 20% of widows and widowers develop depression during the first year of bereavement

Risk Factors
- Old age
- Chronic illness

Prevention and Screening
- Ask about coping and depression in patients experiencing recent losses

Assessment
- Complete physical and neurologic exam with mental status, current medication, and over-the-counter products and supplements

History
- Determine nature and occurrence of the loss
- Determine type and degree of symptom, functional impairment
- Determine social and familial support systems
- Assess for suicidal ideation, risk of lethality
- Assess cognitive state, mood, and affect

Physical
- Clinical manifestations of grief
  - Feelings of sadness and profound loss
  - Crying spells
  - Insomnia
  - Loss of appetite and weight loss
  - Survivor guilt
  - Suicidal ideation, thoughts of mortality and one's own death

Diagnostic Studies
- Laboratory and diagnostic testing as indicated by presenting individual symptoms and general medical condition
- Mini-Mental Status Exam, GDS

Differential Diagnosis
- Depression
- Adjustment disorder with depressed mood
  - Normal grief reaction usually begins to show marked improvement within 8 weeks
  - The diagnosis of depression or adjustment disorder with depressed mood is not given unless symptoms are still present after 2 months and represent a significant change in function and impairment.

Management
Nonpharmacologic Treatment
- Encourage the expression of grief and mourning over loss
- Reassurance that grief is a normal, nonpathologic reaction to loss and is self-limited
- Encourage participation in support groups
- Encourage patient to talk to grief counselor or therapist
- Provide emotional support and encourage family and friends to spend time and listen
- Provide community resources
- Educate family and caregivers as to nature, normal course of bereavement process

Pharmacologic Treatment
- Consider mild antianxiety agents in lowest effective dose if patient is functionally impaired by grief
- Antidepressants if patient is impaired by depression
- Short-term treatment for up to 2 months

When to Consult, Refer, Hospitalize
- Individual verbalizes suicidal ideation, plan or desire to join deceased loved one

- Symptoms last longer than 2 months
- Symptoms intensify and severely impair daily function
- Patient has a history of major depressive illness, prior suicide attempts, or other mental illness
- Suicide attempts or suicidal ideation with a plan is always a psychiatric emergency and should immediately be referred to a mental health specialist or to the emergency department for evaluation and treatment

Follow-up
- Patients should be followed weekly during the acute phase with referral to a psychiatrist or mental health specialist for symptoms that last longer than 2 months

Expected Course
- The normal course of uncomplicated grief/bereavement is 2 months, but frequently lasts longer
- It is common for patients to exhibit some brief, limited symptoms close to the anniversary date of the loss of a loved one
- Cognitive behavioral therapy and social supports are associated with an improved prognosis

Complications
- Risk for depression continues to increase throughout second year of bereavement
- Older adults without adequate social/familial support are at high risk for developing major depression and suicidal ideation

ANXIETY DISORDERS

Description
- Excessive worry and feelings of apprehension, panic, or dread accompanied by symptoms of autonomic nervous system arousal (palpitations, muscle tension and restlessness, fatigue, sweating, difficulty concentrating)
- Symptoms occur more days than not, with the individual reporting little or no control, along with significant distress and impairment in social, occupational, and interpersonal areas

Subtypes
Generalized anxiety disorder (GAD): chronic, free-floating anxiety for at least 1 month
- Excessive worry; irrational, pervasive anxiety without apparent etiology or cause

Phobias: massive anxiety, sudden onset, no precipitating factor
- Social phobia: fear of situations in which the person is exposed to possible scrutiny by others and fears that he or she may do something humiliating or embarrassing
  - A severe, persistent fear of social or performance situations that provokes an immediate and intense anxiety response
  - Common examples are fear of speaking, urinating in public lavatory, saying foolish things
  - Patient then avoids social situations in which stimulus may occur
  - Patient realizes that the fear is excessive or unreasonable
- Specific phobia: persistent fear of a definite stimulus (object or situation)
  - Extreme, irrational fear of specific objects (such as elevators, snakes, or insects) that leads to avoidant behavior of that particular object

– Exposure to the stimulus provokes an immediate anxiety response
– Person recognizes that the fear is excessive or unreasonable

Panic disorder: massive anxiety, sudden onset, no precipitating factor
- Discrete episodes of recurrent and intense fear that occur without apparent warning accompanied by at least 4 symptoms of anxiety

Obsessive-compulsive disorder: persistent need to repeat either thoughts or behaviors
- Recurrent, repetitive, and intrusive thoughts and behaviors that are extremely difficult or impossible to control
- Thoughts and behaviors are excessive and unreasonable, resulting in significant anxiety, distress, and impairment in daily function

Posttraumatic stress disorder: anxiety following a major life stressor
- Exposure to an extreme traumatic stressor such as rape, sexual or physical abuse, natural disasters, war, or other perceived or actual threat to a person's physical being or self concept
- Results in delayed and persistent symptoms including nightmares, flashbacks, numbing of emotion, dissociative episodes, or inability to recall specific events

Etiology
- Behavioral
  - Conditioned behavioral response to earlier interpersonal or social experiences
- Biologic
  - Genetic predisposition
  - Overstimulated autonomic nervous system, stress response
  - Abnormalities of neurotransmitter receptors in the CNS, specifically GABA receptors

Incidence and Demographics
- Anxiety disorders are one of the most common mental illnesses in the United States
- Anxiety disorders account for 15% of the population seen in general practice settings
- Generalized anxiety disorder in older adults occurs more frequently than any other anxiety disorder
- Phobic disorders are the second most common type of anxiety in older adults
- Panic disorder and obsessive compulsive disorder have a low incidence in older adults
- Post-traumatic stress disorder is rare in older adults
- Anxiety disorders frequently coexist with depression in older adults

Risk Factors
- Family history
- Exposure to traumatic events
- Genetic predisposition

Prevention and Screening
- Public, patient, and caregiver education and awareness
- Strong familial, community, and social support systems

Assessment
History
- Determine onset, frequency, duration and type of symptoms

- Determine degree of distress and symptom interference with daily function (work, relationships, and leisure activities)
- Elicit predisposing factors
- Obtain complete medical history, current medications including OTC medications and supplements
- Obtain history and current patterns of use of caffeine, alcohol, and substances

Table 18-9. Symptoms of Anxiety Disorders

Symptom	Generalized Anxiety Disorder	Panic Attacks
Autonomic hyperactivity	Shortness of breath, smothering sensations Palpitations or tachycardia Sweating or cold, clammy hands Dry mouth Dizziness or lightheadedness Nausea, diarrhea, or other abdominal distress Flushes or chills Frequent urination Trouble swallowing or "lump in throat"	Sweating Nausea or abdominal distress Flushes or chills Choking
Motor tension	Trembling, twitching, or feeling shaky Muscle tension, aches, or soreness Restlessness Easy fatigability	Trembling or shaking Chest pain or discomfort
Vigilance and scanning	Feeling keyed up or on edge Exaggerated startle response Difficulty concentrating Trouble falling or staying asleep Irritability	
Psychological symptoms		Depersonalization or derealization Fear of dying Fear of going crazy or of doing something uncontrolled

Physical
- Complete physical with thorough neurologic exam to:
  - Rule out medical causes of symptoms
  - Observe signs of autonomic nervous system hyperactivity

Diagnostic Studies
- Routine diagnostic labs including CBC, metabolic panel, and thyroid function tests to rule out medical conditions that may present with anxiety
- EKG to evaluate tachyarrhythmias if indicated
- Holter monitor to evaluate episodes of palpitations to rule out arrhythmia
- Psychological testing: Mini-Mental Status Exam, Hamilton Anxiety Scale

Differential Diagnosis
Psychological Conditions
- Depression with anxiety

- Schizophrenia, atypical psychosis
- Bipolar disorder with mania
- Adjustment disorder with anxious mood
- Substance abuse

Medical Conditions
- Neurologic disorders
  - Neoplasms
  - Trauma
  - Migraine
  - Multiple sclerosis, seizure disorders
- Cardiac disorders
  - Arrhythmias
  - Myocardial Infarction
  - Heart failure
- Endocrine disorders
  - Cushing's disease
  - Hyper-/hypothyroidism
  - Hypoglycemia
- Pulmonary disorders
  - Hypoxia
  - Chronic obstructive pulmonary disease
  - Asthma
  - Pulmonary embolism
  - Pneumothorax
- Inflammatory
  - Systemic lupus erythematosus
  - Rheumatoid arthritis
  - Temporal arteritis

Medications/Substances Ingested
- Medications
  - Anticholinergics
  - Antihistamines
  - Corticosteroids
  - Antihypertensives
  - Antipsychotics
  - Antidepressants
  - Bronchodilators
  - Amphetamines
  - Anesthetics
  - Sympathomimetics
  - Vasopressors
- Substance abuse
  - Stimulants
  - Cannabis (acute withdrawal or intoxication)
  - Alcohol abuse
  - Caffeine
  - Nicotine

Management
- GAD is usually responsive to medical treatment in a primary care practice setting, but should be referred for psychological therapy
- Other anxiety disorders are usually referred to a mental health specialist for management
- Patient education is essential to ensure compliance and effective treatment
- Community resources and support should be provided as possible

Nonpharmacologic Treatment
- Cognitive behavioral therapy
- Psychotherapy and psychoanalysis
- Stress management education, courses, workshops
- Behavioral conditioning, biofeedback
- Community self-help and support groups
- Education of family members and caregivers as to behavioral techniques and interventions

Pharmacologic Treatment

ANTIDEPRESSANTS
- Antidepressants are commonly the first-line drug of choice in the treatment of anxiety disorders
- Potential for substance abuse and dependence is significantly less than with benzodiazepines
- Main therapeutic effect may take 3 to 4 weeks
- Patient education and awareness of length of time required to reach target dose and main effect of the drug is essential for greater likelihood of compliance
- Dosage is considerably higher than for major depressive disorder

ANTIDEPRESSANTS WITH FDA INDICATIONS FOR ANXIETY DISORDERS (SEE TABLES 18-10, 18-11, AND 18-12 FOR DOSING)
- Sertraline (Zoloft): OCD, panic disorder, post-traumatic stress disorder, social anxiety disorder
- Paroxetine (Paxil): OCD, panic disorder, social anxiety disorder
- Fluoxetine (Prozac): OCD
- Escitalopram (Lexapro): GAD
- Venlafaxine (Effexor): GAD
- Trazodone (Desyrel): depression with or without anxiety

BUSPIRONE (BUSPAR)
- Slower onset of action; may take up to 4 weeks for antianxiety effects
- Maximum therapeutic effect may not be reached for 4 to 8 weeks
- Significant adverse reactions are found in 20% to 30% of anxious older adults
- Most frequent side effects include gastrointestinal effects, dizziness, headache, sleep disturbance, fatigue, nausea/vomiting
- Less sedating than benzodiazepines
- Significant number of nonresponders

Table 18-10. Anxiolytic Drug for Anxiety Disorders

Anxiolytic	Starting Dose	Target Dose
Buspirone (BuSpar)	5 mg q.d.	15 to 30 mg divided t.i.d.

BENZODIAZEPINES
- Use with great caution in the older adult
- Use for shortest amount of time possible until other medication has reached therapeutic level
- All benzodiazepines are effective in treating the symptoms of anxiety disorders
- Benzodiazepines have rapid onset of action with quick symptom relief
- Benzodiazepines have significant potential for dependence and abuse
- Patients with substance abuse histories are at high risk for abuse
- Benzodiazepine toxicity in older adults often manifests as sedation, ataxia, dysarthria, cognitive impairment, psychomotor impairment, falls, mental confusion, memory impairment
- Half-life of benzodiazepines and their metabolites may be extended significantly in older adults
- Alprazolam and lorazepam are commonly used but have a high incidence of causing dependence and cognitive impairment; diazepam (Valium) has long half-life and should not be used in older adults
- Clonazepam (Klonopin) is FDA indicated for panic disorder and may be used long term with extreme caution in the older adult (adverse reactions include CNS effects, blood dyscrasias, liver disorders)

Table 18-11. Benzodiazepine Therapy for Anxiety Disorders

Benzodiazepines	Starting Dose	Usual Dose
Alprazolam (Xanax)	0.25 mg q.d.–b.i.d.	0.5 to 3 mg/day
Lorazepam (Ativan)	0.25 mg q.h.s.	0.5 mg q.d.–t.i.d.
Clonazepam (Klonopin)	0.25 mg q.d.–b.i.d.	1 to 2 mg/day

Table 18-12. Antidepressant Therapy for Anxiety Disorders

Medication	Initial Dose	Target Dose	Indications
Fluoxetine (Prozac)	10 mg q.d.	60 to 80mg q.d.	OCD, PD
Sertraline (Zoloft)	25 mg q.d.	50 to 250 mg q.d.	OCD, PD, GAD, PTSD
Paroxetine (Paxil)	10 mg q.d.	20 to 60 mg q.d.	OCD, PD, GAD, PTSD
Escitalopram (Lexapro)	5 mg q.d.	20 to 60 mg q.d.	OCD, PD, GAD, PTSD
Citalopram (Celexa)	10 mg q.d.	40 to 80 mg q.d.	OCD, PD, GAD, PTSD

How Long to Treat
- Length varies according to individual response and symptom management
- Mild anxiety usually resolves within 2 months

Special Considerations
- It is common for anxiety disorders to occur concomitantly with other disorders such as depression and substance abuse

- Anxiety disorders are also commonly seen with many physical, medical disorders
- Patients with anxiety disorders need reassurance that their disorder can be effectively treated
- The establishment of a trusting, safe therapeutic relationship with the primary practitioner is essential for compliance and effective treatment

When to Consult, Refer, Hospitalize
- Chronic, disabling anxiety requires a psychiatric consultation and referral
- Severe panic attacks, intense PTSD, and disabling OCD always require a psychiatric consult or referral and usually require a combination of pharmacotherapy and cognitive behavioral therapy

Follow-up
- Patients should be seen weekly during the acute phase of treatment
- Medications need to be monitored for effectiveness of symptom management, appropriate dose, and potential abuse

Expected Course
- Course of treatment varies according to degree of impairment and individual response

Complications
- Functional and social impairment

ALCOHOL AND OTHER SUBSTANCE ABUSE

Description
- The physiological dependence on a substance as indicated by evidence of tolerance, symptoms of withdrawal, and impairment of function in social, interpersonal, and occupational areas of one's life
- Addiction is often characterized by a preoccupation with the substance, loss of control over the amount and frequency of use, and physical and psychological dependence and tolerance
- The most common substance abuse problems are with alcohol and prescription medications such as benzodiazepines and opioids

Etiology
- Genetic predisposition
- Social and cultural conditioning

Incidence and Demographics
- The incidence of alcoholism is about the same in older adults as it is in younger adults
- Prevalence of heavy drinking in older adults estimated at 3% to 9%; it is frequently unrecognized
- Alcoholism rates are highest in Black and Hispanic males
- Overuse of alcohol and medications is associated with psychiatric disorders and chronic pain syndrome in older adults

Risk Factors
- Family history
- Abuse of other substances
- Cultural conditioning

- Domestic violence or abuse
- Presence of a psychiatric disorder
- Stressful events

Prevention and Screening
- Education and awareness by primary care providers of symptoms and special issues involving alcoholism and older adults
- Routinely ask questions to assess problem with alcohol

Assessment
History
- Nonspecific presentation: confusion, falls, decrease in ADL
- History of prior substance abuse treatment
- Psychiatric history
- Current use of prescribed and OTC medications
- Affect on function and social relationships
- Any physical symptoms secondary to alcohol
  - Neurologic: confusion, seizures, tremors, agitation, paresthesias
  - Cardiac: symptoms of alcohol cardiomyopathy
  - GI: vomiting blood, reflux symptoms, melena, jaundice, hypoglycemia
- Attitudes, thoughts, feelings, and observations of family and caregivers regarding use or abuse of alcohol by the older adult

Physical
- Clinical manifestations of alcoholism and alcohol abuse include:
  - Withdrawal symptoms that may begin with anxiety, decreased cognition, tremulousness, then to increased irritability and hyper-reactivity and to tremors, hallucinations, and seizures
  - Neurological: memory impairment, hyper-reflexia, ataxia, confabulation, sensory deficits
  - Cardiovascular: cardiomyopathy, hypertension, arrhythmias, generalized edema
  - Gastrointestinal: gastric distention, ascites, enlarged liver, icterus
  - Musculoskeletal: muscle wasting, falls, fractures, other injuries
  - Generally unkempt appearance, poor personal hygiene
  - Integumentary: cushingoid appearance, flushed face, spider nevi, ecchymosis, angiomas
  - HEENT: nystagmus, smell of alcohol on breath
  - Sexual dysfunction
  - Weight loss

Assessment Tools
- CAGE
  - Have you ever felt the need to **C**ut down on drinking?
  - Have you ever felt **A**nnoyed by criticism of your drinking?
  - Have you ever felt **G**uilty about your drinking?
  - Have you ever taken a morning **E**ye opener?
- MMSE (see Chapter 4 on dementia)

Diagnostic Studies
- Blood alcohol levels
  - Limited use in primary care, more useful in acute intoxication

- Normal level does not rule out abuse
- Blood concentration increases disproportionately to the amount consumed
- Drug levels in opioids, not available for benzodiazepines
- CBC to rule out infection, or anemia from GI bleed or macrocytic anemia indicative of B$_{12}$ and folate deficiency; MCV elevated in alcohol abuse
- Metabolic panel to assess kidney function and electrolytes and to rule out diabetes, hypoglycemia; alkaline phosphatase to rule out pancreatitis
- Liver function tests: GTT elevated early; AST twice as high as ALT is typical of alcoholic liver injury
- TSH, thyroid, T3, T4
- B$_{12}$ and folate
- Prothrombin time, PTT
- Lipid panel

Differential Diagnosis

The major differential to make is whether there are underlying psychiatric problems

- Schizophrenia
- Major depressive mood disorders
- Anxiety disorders
- Bipolar disorder
- Personality disorders
- Polysubstance abuse disorder
- B$_{12}$ and folate deficiency and malnutrition
- Endocrine disorders such as diabetes and Cushing's disease
- Neurological disorders, seizure disorders
- Cardiovascular disease

Management

Nonpharmacologic Treatment

- Substance abuse counseling
- Alcoholics Anonymous program
- Substance abuse treatment programs and halfway houses
- Cognitive behavioral therapy

Pharmacologic Treatment

ALCOHOL
- Detoxification for symptoms of withdrawal guided by specialist—can be done as outpatient or as inpatient in rehabilitation facility
- Titrate by monitoring symptoms (use the CIWA-Ar scale, found at http://www.agingincanada.ca/CIWA.HTM, which monitors nausea and vomiting, tremor, anxiety, agitation, tactile, visual and auditory disturbances, headache, and orientation)
- Evidence-based agents that reduce relapse to drinking include:
  - Disulfiram (Antabuse), causes toxic reaction if alcohol is consumed; rarely used
  - Acamprosate (Campral): reduces the urge to drink; requires 2 large tablets TID
  - Naltrexone (ReVia): opioid antagonist; reduces pleasure or satisfaction of drinking; available as a monthly deport injection (Vivitrol)

    – Topiramate (Topamax): reduces the appetite for alcholol

    – Thiamine, folic acid and B complex supplements

PRESCRIPTION SEDATIVE DEPENDENCE
- Use clonazepam or phenobarbital to slowly wean patient off medication
- Decrease dosage by smallest amount possible every 2 weeks to 1 month
- Usually requires a controlled setting as in a nursing home
- Add valproic acid to reduce the risk for seizures and make the withdrawal less difficult
- Pharmacologic and medical management of underlying medical disorders as appropriate by primary care provider

When to Consult, Refer, Hospitalize
- Patients diagnosed or suspected of alcoholism or substance abuse should always be referred to a substance abuse specialist for further evaluation and treatment
- Social issues need to be referred to a mental health specialist for long-term management

Follow-up
Expected Course
- Often chronic and relapsing

Complications
- Severe intoxication is a medical emergency and can lead to coma, respiratory depression, aspiration, and death
- Long-term use results in significant changes in brain function as well as severe impairment in social and interpersonal relations

TOBACCO USE AND SMOKING CESSATION

Description
- The repetitive use of tobacco and nicotine despite recurrent and significant adverse medical consequences
- Tobacco- and nicotine-seeking behaviors with accompanying physical dependence, tolerance, and withdrawal

Etiology
- Genetic predisposition
- Social, cultural, and behavioral influences
- Nicotine dependence

Incidence and Demographics
- Nicotine addiction is the leading health problem in the nation
- 430,000 individuals die each year of tobacco-related illnesses
- Deaths from cancer are 2 times greater for smokers than for nonsmokers

Risk Factors
- Family history of use
- Polysubstance abuse
- Psychiatric disorders

Prevention and Screening
- Smoking cessation programs

Assessment

History

- History of tobacco use including past attempts to quit, and techniques used, why unsuccessful
- Assess patient's desire to change behavior (see Trans-theoretical Model of Change, Chapter 3)
- Perform complete medical history to rule out all underlying medical problems
- Frequent upper-respiratory infections

Physical

- Hypertension
- Cigarette smell on breath, clothing, and hair
- Skin prematurely aged and wrinkled
- Stained teeth and fingers, dental caries
- Inflammation of sinuses, oropharynx, nasal cavities
- Respiratory impairment, infections
- Cardiovascular disease
- Peptic ulcer disease

Differential Diagnosis

- Polysubstance abuse
- Smokeless tobacco, snuff

Management

Nonpharmacologic Treatment

- The most important single intervention is to work with the patient to set a quit date
- Smoking cessation programs
- Behavioral therapy
- Hypnosis
- Reassure patient that relapses are normal, and encourage the patient to try again
- Provide educational literature and support

Pharmacologic Treatment

- Nicotine replacement therapies
  - Transdermal patch: most effective of all nicotine replacement therapies; most patients require the highest-dose patch and many will need two patches; available OTC
  - Nicotine gum
  - Nicotine nasal spray/nicotine inhaler
- Other effective agents
  - Varenicline (Chantix): partial agonist at the nicotine receptor site; blocks nicotine and partially stimulates the receptor, relieving craving; start while patient is still smoking; titrate up from 0.5 mg daily to 1 mg twice daily; primary adverse effect is nausea; some patients get depressed, so monitor for depression; continue for at least 3 to 6 months
  - Nortriptyline (Pamelor): start with 25 mg daily in the older adult, increase to 50 mg daily if tolerated; some patients get agitated; continue at least 3 to 6 months
  - Bupropion (Wellbutrin, Zyban): decreases craving and withdrawal; start with 100 mg of the SR form in the morning; can increase to 150 or 300 mg daily, and change to the XL form; continue for at least 3 to 6 month

Special Considerations
- Older adults with a history of smoking often present with severe, chronic medical problems as a consequence of chronic tobacco use
- It is never too late to stop; patient and family education and support are crucial, even with older adults with a history of chronic tobacco use and their caregivers

Follow-up
- Weekly visits during attempts to quit
- Monitor withdrawal symptoms, medication compliance, and effectiveness

Expected Course
- Relapses are frequent, commonly occurring during the first 2 weeks
- Most patients have relapses before they succeed; they should be encouraged to try again at each relapse

Complications: a major cause of morbidity and mortality
- Cardiovascular disease
  - Coronary artery disease
  - Stroke
  - Hypertension
  - Peripheral artery disease
  - Elevated cholesterol levels
- Cancer: lung, mouth, throat, esophagus, larynx, pancreas, bladder, and cervical
- Respiratory: chronic obstructive pulmonary disease, asthma, pneumonia
- Peptic ulcer disease
- Death

ABUSE AND NEGLECT OF THE ELDERLY

Description
- Physical, emotional, economic, or sexual pain and injury inflicted deliberately upon an elderly person by a person who has care or custody of the person or stands in a position of trust, with the express goal of manipulating, intimidating, and controlling that individual within the relationship
- Includes physical abuse, neglect, sexual assault, unreasonable physical restraint, physical abandonment, and deprivation of food, water, shelter, or medical treatment

Etiology
- See Risk Factors

Incidence and Demographics
- More than 2 million adults over the age of 60 are abused annually
- Greater incidence of abuse by family members than by paid provider

Risk Factors
- Over age 84
- Social isolation, lack of support
- Cognitively impaired
- Physical, emotional, and financial dependency

Prevention and Screening
- Public education and awareness
- Refer families to local department of aging or social worker for assistance with in-home care, adult day care, respite care, or long-term placement, or for financial counseling regarding long-term care
- Social programs such as Adult Protective Services

Assessment
History
- Determine primary caregivers, living arrangements, legal custodian, and power of attorney
- History of medical treatment, accidents, fractures, physical injuries, traumas, overdose of medications
- Determine environmental, psychosocial and financial stressors
- Any unusual or inappropriate activity in bank accounts, unpaid bills, lack of amenities, missing belongings
- Missed medical appointments
- Interview individual alone
- Mental status exam
- Document findings carefully
- Identify caregiver stress, interview caregivers and family members

Physical
- Monitor nutritional status and weight for dehydration, malnutrition
- Lacerations, bruises, wounds, burns, fractures inconsistent with explanation offered
- Delay between time of injury and treatment
- Poor skin and personal hygiene
- Fearful, evasive, guarded, depressed
- Sexually transmitted diseases, genital rash, trauma, discharge
- Rectal tissue swelling, discharge

Diagnostic Studies
- Specific to presenting symptoms
- Determine nutritional status (CBC, metabolic panel, cholesterol) and assess for unintentional weight loss

Differential Diagnosis
- Accidental injury
- Self neglect due to cognitive
- status or physical impairment
- Depression
- Dementia

Management
- Notify Protective Services if abuse is suspected
- Manage medical conditions

When to Consult, Refer, Hospitalize
- It is mandatory by law to report all older adult and disabled adult abuse and neglect to Adult Protective Service agencies
- Hospitalization or institutionalization when in the best interest of the individual

Follow-up
Expected Course
- Abuse will escalate unless there is intervention

Complications
- Death

CASE STUDIES

Case 1. A 72-year-old man presents to your office complaining of insomnia, generalized aches and pains, fatigue, and a 10-pound weight loss over the past 2 months. He states he has lost interest in his hobbies, doesn't go out of the house often except to buy groceries, and spends much of his day watching television.
Medications: ibuprofen (Advil) 2 to 6 tabs/day for pain

1. What additional questions would you ask?
2. What would you look for on physical examination?
3. What laboratory work would you order?
4. What treatment would you begin, assuming labs are normal?
5. What complications should you watch for?

Case 2. A 68-year-old woman presents to your office complaining of difficulty swallowing, diarrhea, dizzy spells, weakness in her legs, insomnia, feelings of impending doom, and a fear of loosing control.

1. What questions would you ask?
2. What would you look for on physical exam?
3. What laboratory tests would you order?
4. What treatment would you begin?
5. What complications might develop?

Case 3. Mr. Smith, 75 years old, comes for routine follow-up of diabetes. He reports his wife died 3 weeks ago. He joined AA at age 50. Medications: metformin (Glucophage) 500 mg b.i.d.

1. What questions would you ask?
2. What laboratory tests would you order?
3. What treatment would you begin?
4. What complications might develop?

REFERENCES

American Psychiatric Association. (2000). *Diagnostic and statistical manual of mental disorders* (4th ed., text rev.). Washington, DC: Author.

Dambro, M. R. (2004). *The 5 minute clinical consult.* St. Louis, MO: Lippincott, Williams & Wilkins.

Depp, C. A., & Jeste, D. V. (2004). Bipolar disorder in older adults: A critical review. *Bipolar Disorders, 6*(5), 343–367.

Dyer, C. B., Heisler, C. J., Hill, C. A., & Kim, L. C. (2005). Community approaches to elder abuse. *Clinical Geriatric Medicine, 21*, 429–447.

Ferri, F. F. (2003). *Ferri's clinical advisor* (6th ed.). St. Louis, MO: Mosby.

Hoyle, M. T., Alessi, C. A., Harker, J. O., Josephson, K. R., Pietruszka, F. M., Koelfgen, M., et al. (1999). Development and testing of a five-item version of the geriatric depression scale. *Journal of the American Geriatric Society, 47*, 873–878.

Lang, A. J., & Stein, M. B. (2001). Anxiety disorders and how to recognize and treat the medical symptoms of emotional illness. *Geriatrics, 56*(5), 24–27, 31–32, 34.

Lavretsky, H. (2000). Choosing appropriate treatment of geriatric depression. *Clinical Geriatrics, 8*(11), 99–108.

Medical Letter. (2003). Drugs for psychiatric disorders. *Treatment Guidelines, 1*(11), 69–76.

Mental health: Culture, race, and ethnicity, a supplement to mental health: a report of the Surgeon General. (2001). Retrieved from http://www.surgeongeneral.gov/library/mentalhealth/cre/

Mohlman, J., de Jesus, M., Gorenstein, E. E., Kleber, M., Gorman, J. M., & Papp, L. A. (2004). Distinguishing generalized anxiety disorder, panic disorder, and mixed anxiety states in older treatment-seeking adults. *Journal of Anxiety Disorders, 18*(3), 275–290.

Morse, J. Q., & Lynch, T. R. (2004). A preliminary investigation of self-reported personality disorders in life: Prevalence, predictors of depressive severity, and clinical correlates. *Aging and Mental Health, 8*(4), 307–315.

Quinn, M., & Tomita, S. (1997). *Elder abuse and neglect: Cause, diagnosis and intervention strategies.* New York: Springer.

Parker, G., & Hadzi-Pavlovic, D. (2004). Is the female preponderance in major depression secondary to a gender difference in specific anxiety disorders? *Psychological Medicine, 34*(3), 461–470.

Reuben, D. B., Herr, K. A., Pacala, J. T., Pollock, B. G., Potter, J. F., & Semla, T. P. (2007). *Geriatrics at your fingertips* (9th ed.). New York: The American Geriatrics Society.

Sandson, N. B., Marcucci, C., Bourke, D. L., & Smith-Lamacchia, R. (2006). An interaction between aspirin and valproate: the relevance of plasma protein displacement drug–drug interaction. *American Journal of Psychiatry, 163*(11), 1–6.

Satcher, D. (1999). *Mental health: A report of the Surgeon General.* Retrieved from http://www.surgeongeneral.gov/library/mentalhealth/home.html

Tierney, L. M., McPhee, S. J., & Papadakis, A. (2005). *Current medical diagnosis and treatment* (44th ed.). Stamford, CT: Appleton & Lange.

Unutzer, J., Katon, W., Callahan, C. M., Williams, J. W. Jr., Hunkeler, E., Harpole, L., et al. (2002). Collaborative care management of late-life depression in the primary care setting. *JAMA, 288*(22), 2836–2845.

Williams, J. W. Jr., Barrett, J., Oxman, T., Frank, E., Katon, W., Sullivan, M., et al. (2000). Treatment of dysthymia and minor depression in primary care. *JAMA, 284*(12), 1519–1526.

Discussion of Case Studies

CHAPTER 2—DIMENSIONS OF THE NP ROLE

Case 1. A 92-year-old female patient who lives alone at home has fallen several times in the past few months. She refuses to have physical therapy or to move to an assisted living or nursing home. Her daughter, who has not talked to her for the past 10 years, wants you to sign a document stating her mother is not competent so she can put her in a nursing home. The daughter also wants a copy of her mother's chart.

1. What are the legal issues involved?
   Competency and confidentiality

2. Should you tell the daughter about the patient's condition or give her a copy of the chart?
   No. This would violate the patient's confidentiality unless you got permission from the patient first.

3. Can you determine from the information given that the patient lacks the capacity to make healthcare decisions?
   No. Just because the patient makes decisions that you may not agree with does not mean that she is incompetent.

Case 2. An 82-year-old man is found to have lung cancer. This was an incidental finding on chest x-ray for admission to assisted living. He has no symptoms. He is a widower with one son.

1. What healthcare documents would you ask the patient about?
   Has he prepared a durable power of attorney for health care and living will? Who is named as the proxy? Are his finances are taken care of?

2. What healthcare decisions would you look for on his durable power of attorney?
   CPR, mechanical respiration, and feeding tubes for artificial nutrition and hydration. Should not just say "no heroic measures."

3. How would you decide how aggressively to manage this patient?
   Review durable power of attorney and explain the risks and benefits of treatment options to patient and proxy. Have a conference with the patient care team, including doctor, social worker, clergy, and nurse.

4. The patient becomes incompetent without writing down his wishes. You need to decide whether or not to put in a feeding tube. What question do you pose to the son?
   To the best of your knowledge, what would the patient have wanted if he were able to tell us? Not what the son wants.

Case 3. You just graduated from your nurse practitioner program.

1. What additional qualifications do you need in order to practice?
   You need a state nurse practitioner license. You must meet state requirements in order to practice; each state has laws establishing requirements, which vary from state to state. Most states require that you are certified by a national certifying organization. Some require a written agreement or other contract with a physician. Most have continuing education requirements.

CHAPTER 3—HEALTHCARE ISSUES

Case 1. You are asked to assess an 82-year-old man for admission to an assisted living facility.

1. What chronic conditions is he likely to have?
   Arthritis, heart disease (especially hypertension and hyperlipidemia), diabetes, stroke

2. What impairments is he likely to have?
   Hearing loss, visual impairment, decreased functional abilities, impaired nutrition, impaired safety, impaired taste

3. What kind of health insurance is he likely to have?
   Medicare, which will not pay for the assisted living facility

4. What cause is he most likely to die from?
   Heart disease, cancer, stroke, COPD, pneumonia/influenza, diabetes

Case 2. A 94-year-old nursing home patient with moderate dementia has had four falls in the past 2 days. She had not fallen in the past year.

1. What is this problem an example of?
   This is a nonspecific presentation of an illness

2. How would you begin the evaluation of this problem?
   Functional assessment of patient's mobility

3. What other aspects of the functional assessment would be important in this patient?
   ADLs, medical illnesses, cognitive function, medications

Case 3. You have a new patient in the nursing home, a 78-year-old woman with moderate dementia, impaired hearing, and impaired vision.

1. What would your initial approach be?
   See "Communicating With the Demented Patient"

2. How would you alter the environment to improve communication?
   See "How to Obtain a History"

3. How would you adjust your physical exam?
   See "The Physical Examination of the Older Adult"

CHAPTER 4—GERIATRIC MULTISYSTEM SYNDROMES

Case 1: An 82-year-old woman comes to clinic reporting "nearly fainting" 3 times in the last month.
History: States that several times in past month she has had episodes when she feels like she is going to faint. The spell lasts maybe a few minutes, and then she slowly feels better. If she is at home, she eats something then goes to lie down, relieving the sensation. She had a spell at church last Sunday and her friends insisted she come to the clinic for an evaluation.
PMH: Type 2 diabetes, osteoarthritis, hypertension, hypothyroidism, rheumatic fever as a child
Medications: Glipizide (Glucotrol XL) 10 mg q.d., hydrochlorothiazide 25 mg q.d., metoprolol (Lopressor) 100 mg q.d., levothyroxine sodium (Synthroid) 125 mg q.d., naproxen (Naprosyn) 250 mg b.i.d.

1. What part of the physical exam is appropriate?
   Complete, including orthostatic blood pressures

2. List the possible causes and contributing factors.
   Hypoglycemia, orthostatic hypotension secondary to BP medications, dehydration, normal changes of aging, anemia due to blood loss on NSAIDs, hypo- or iatrogenic hyperthyroid, brady-arrhythmia due to beta blocker, angina, cardiac valve disease, heart failure, polypharmacy

3. What diagnostic tests would you order?
   EKG, glucose, CBC, BUN, creatinine, electrolytes, hemoglobin A1C, TSH, fecal occult blood

Case 2. An 87-year-old man comes to your office reporting fatigue. Patient lives in an assisted living facility, needs help with bathing and dressing, walks with difficulty with walker, and becomes SOB walking 20 feet. He feels too tired to eat. Diagnoses include hypertension, depression, COPD, HF, Parkinson's disease, and osteoarthritis. He is on 10 medications, including atenolol 25 mg daily for hypertension, paroxetine 40 mg daily for depression, and oxycodone/acetaminophen (Percocet) 5/325 mg every 6 hours p.r.n. for pain related to osteoarthritis.

1. What further history would you want to assess?
   Onset, course, duration, daily pattern, exacerbating/relieving factors; impact on function and ability to complete activities of daily living; recent weight changes; impact of sleep or rest on symptoms; trouble concentrating, lack of interest in activities; input from family (may report weakness, decreased activity, or change in sleep patterns)

2. What diagnostic testing would you consider?
   CBC, ESR, chemistry panel including electrolytes, glucose, renal and liver function tests, TSH

3. List your differential diagnoses.
   Cancer, fatigue due to medication use (beta blocker, antidepressant, opioid), deconditioning, fatigue due to Parkinson's disease, HF, COPD, depression, pain, anemia, sleep disorder

Physical exam and diagnostic testing show patient has advanced colon cancer with metastasis to bone. The patient declines treatment and starts preparing to die. He complains that the pain in his low back will not let him sleep. You determine that he is competent to make his own decisions.

4. What is your initial plan?
   Comfort measures to include:
   - **Start pain management for musculoskeletal pain**
   - **For mild musculoskeletal pain, try acetaminophen or NSAIDs (with caution)**
   - **Increase doses and start opioids as soon as needed for pain control**
   - **Monitor closely for pain control and other symptoms**
   - **Offer hospice**
   - **Review advance directives**
   - **Make sure patient is able to get his affairs in order**
   - **Ensure that patient has someone to talk to and feels comfortable with his caregivers**

Over the next month, the pain becomes severe and the patient becomes bedbound. Because of the Parkinson's disease, he is having trouble handling his secretions. He is still able to take sips of p.o. liquids.

5. What is your next plan?
   Oral, personal hygiene; adequate opioids to avoid SOB; atropine or scopolamine to reduce secretions

6. What issues are likely to be the most important to this patient?
   Freedom from pain and respiratory distress, being kept clean, knowing what to expect, having someone he can trust, maintaining control and dignity as much as possible

Case 3. A daughter brings her 80-year-old mother with moderate Alzheimer's disease for a routine checkup. The daughter reports her mother is more easily distracted, increasingly irritable, and less aware of her surroundings. The daughter is not sure how long this has been going on. The patient is on multiple medications for cardiac disease and Alzheimer's disease.

1. What part of the history would be most important?
   Complete review of systems searching for symptoms of infectious processes, such as change in cardiac status (MI, angina, arrhythmia, HF), orthostasis, dehydration, bleeding or blood loss, loss of appetite or other GI symptoms; review medications for changes or missed medications, adverse reaction to medications; any environmental changes; MMSE for look for change in cognitive function

2. What would you look for on physical examination?
   Signs of infection, fever, clammy skin, pulmonary congestion, abdominal tenderness, cellulitis, signs of HF, edema, arrhythmia, or signs of dehydration

3. What laboratory and diagnostic tests would you consider?
   EKG, CXR, urinalysis and C&S, CBC, metabolic panel, medication levels if on digoxin, TSH B12, folate

4. What are your differential diagnoses?
   Progression of dementia versus delirium. Determine cause of delirium: change in environment, infection, any change in medication, exacerbation of heart disease such as HF, angina, or arrhythmia.

CHAPTER 5—INFECTIOUS DISEASE

Case 1. A 96-year-old woman resides in a nursing home. She usually gets up, dresses herself, and walks to breakfast in the dining room, but today the nursing assistant reports she won't get out of bed. She is agitated, trying to hit the staff, and crying out incoherently, and she was incontinent of urine overnight.
PMH: Moderate dementia, osteoporosis, type 2 DM, CHF
Medications: Metformin (Glucophage) 500 mg p.o. b.i.d., furosemide (Lasix) 20 mg p.o. q.d., lisinopril (Zestril) 10 mg p.o. q.d., digoxin (Lanoxin) 0.125 mg p.o. q.o.d., alendronate (Fosamax) 70 mg p.o. every week, donepezil (Aricept) 5 mg p.o. q.d.

1. What other history or review of systems would be needed?
   Pain, change in medications, any p.r.n. medications given, change in p.o. intake. Review of systems to include neurological, mental status, cardiac, endocrine, musculoskeletal.

2. What components of the physical exam would you perform?
   Complete physical with emphasis on control of existing conditions and look for infection in cardiac, respiratory, skin, musculoskeletal systems

3. What is your differential diagnosis?
   Pneumonia, UTI, dehydration, electrolyte imbalance, acute exacerbation of CHF, hyper- or hypoglycemia, medication, especially digoxin toxicity

4. What diagnostic tests are needed?
   Glucose fingerstick, CBC with differential, electrolytes, BUN, creatinine, digoxin level, urine for urinalysis and C&S; possibly CXR and EKG depending on physical

Case 2. A 68-year-old woman complains of diarrhea. It is soft to liquid and profuse. No nausea or vomiting. Patient was recently in the hospital for a cholecystectomy. Patient had Foley catheter during hospital stay. Was started on trimethoprim-sulfamethoxazole. Culture came back with resistant to TMP-SMZ, so patient was switched to ciprofloxacin. While on Cipro, she developed a pneumonia, so the Cipro was switched to clarithromycin (Biaxin).

1. What other history or review of system would be needed?
   Any change in medications or diet; review of intake of fluids and food because of diarrhea; any abdominal pain or fever; any odor to the stool; review when last large formed bowel movement was

2. What components of the physical exam would you perform?
   Abdominal and rectal, as well as cardiovascular to rule out acute changes secondary to infections; respiratory to check for resolution of the pneumonia

3. What is your differential diagnosis?
   C. *difficile*, infection versus antibiotic drug side effects

4. What diagnostic tests are needed?
   CBC may reveal an elevated WBC if there is C. *difficile*; stool *for* C. *difficile* should be sent x3

5. What treatment should be instituted pending diagnosis?
   Adequate hydration and electrolyte replacement. For superinfections with *Clostridium difficile*, see "Complications of Infections"

Case 3. A 74-year-old woman, living independently, presents with many vague complaints, including fatigue, weight loss, intermittent diarrhea, painful rash on trunk, numbness and tingling of toes, white coating in mouth. Patient's social history consists of 45 years unhappy marriage to distant husband, who died of mysterious illness in 2005 at age 80.
PE: Weight 108, down from 126 in past year, temporal wasting
- Rash vesicles on erythematous base in dermatome pattern on right side of trunk
- Decreased reflexes to LE
- White exudate that sticks to tongue in mouth, malodorous
- Normal abdominal and rectal exam

1. What is your differential diagnosis?
   Herpes zoster, thrush, diarrhea, peripheral neuropathy, AIDS

2. What diagnostic tests are needed?
   CBC for infection, electrolytes and BUN; for dehydration, fasting blood sugar, HIV screening, B$_{12}$, and folate in light of neuropathy

3. What treatment would you initiate?
   Counsel regarding HIV testing and provide emotional support, refer to specialist; antiviral for herpes zoster; oral antifungal for candidiasis, such as nystatin swish and swallow; monitor intake and output; pain management

CHAPTER 6—DERMATOLOGIC DISORDERS

Case 1. An 86-year-old female resident of long-term-care facility for 2 years secondary to advanced dementia has fallen and suffered a right hip fracture. She was sent to the hospital for open reduction–internal fixation and returned to the facility 2 days post-op. Upon readmission, she is noted to have a 3 x 3 cm bulla on her posterior right heel. Prior to the fall, she was underweight, needed assistance to ambulate, and had poor short-term memory and poor safety insight. Meds include multivitamin with minerals, docusate (Colace), and enoxaparin (Lovenox) injections.

1. What is the probable cause of the right heel bulla?
   Pressure sore due to decreased mobility from impaired mobility from surgery

2. What were her risk factors for pressure ulcers pre- and post-op?
   Pre-op: age, altered nutrition and mobility
   Post-op: more limited mobility, pain, decreased alertness/cognition secondary to surgery

3. How could this heel ulcer have been prevented?
   Increased skin inspections and care, nutritional support, pressure relief of bony prominences, pain relief

4. What are basics for treatment?
   Supplement nutrition to provide adequate vitamins and minerals, extra calories, and protein; provide tissue load management with repositioning and pressure relief; direct wound care to protect ulcer and avoid debridement if intact skin; adequate pain relief

5. What are possible complications of this pressure ulcer?
   Impaired rehabilitation from fracture due to decreased mobility, wound infection/ cellulitis, osteomyelitis, loss of limb

Case 2. A 75-year-old blond White male, former construction worker, complains of raised lump on the back of his neck that is irritated by his shirt collar. His wife has noticed that the lesion seems to be getting larger and darker in color over the past few months. He has no other significant medical history. Medications: safety coated aspirin (Ecotrin), atorvastatin (Lipitor), lisinopril.

1. How common are skin cancers?
   Basal cell cancer most commonly seen, and squamous cell cancer is the second most common type of skin cancer

2. How does this patient follow the demographics and risk factors for skin cancer?
   See "Incidence and Demographics" and "Risk Factors"; age > 40, male, fair skin with sun exposure

3. Does location of lesion help in assessment?
   See "Risk Factors" and "Assessment/History": sun-exposed area on back of neck

4. What diagnostic test is necessary?
   See under "Assessment/Diagnostic Studies": biopsy of lesion

5. What is appropriate treatment for lesions, and what is expected outcome?
   Refer to dermatology for excision; resolution expected; need to monitor for new lesions

Case 3. A 95-year-old nursing home patient has advanced dementia and is no longer ambulatory. She must be fed and is incontinent of urine. Chronic conditions include: obesity, diabetes mellitus, polymyalgia rheumatica, and gastroesophageal reflux. Medications: rosiglitazone (Avandia), prednisone, omeprazole (Prilosec), and acetaminophen (Tylenol) p.r.n. The nursing assistant involved with her care noticed red, inflamed skin on her abdomen and perineal area when cleaning her today. Upon exam, you find bright red, smooth macules with maceration and satellite lesions under her breasts and in the skin folds on her abdomen and perineal area.

1. What is your most likely diagnosis?
   Candida infection

2. What risk factors does she have?
   - **Chronic debilitation, inability to perform personal hygiene**
   - **Diabetes**
   - **Moisture from urine, sweat**
   - **Obesity with redundant skin folds**
   - **Occlusive clothing—adult incontinence briefs**
   - **Corticosteroid use**

3. What nonpharmacologic treatment would you order?
   Air exposure to affected areas, careful drying of skin, frequent changing of diapers, ideally weight loss (but not practical)

4. What pharmacologic treatment would you order?
   Better management of diabetes, attempt prednisone taper, topical antifungal cream such as clotrimazole 1%

5. How long would you expect to treat this condition?
   Several weeks

CHAPTER 7—EYE, EAR, NOSE, AND THROAT DISORDERS

Case 1. An 83-year-old female nursing home patient is observed to have crusting on both eyelashes in the mornings.

HPI: Patient diagnosed with Alzheimer's disease is a resident in a long-term-care (LTC) facility. You are told that there have been several cases of conjunctivitis in the facility in the past week. Patient is nonverbal, but has been observed rubbing her eyes in the past few days.

PMH: Resident in LTC for several years. Her personal care is provided by nurse aides. In general good health otherwise. Under treatment for seborrheic dermatitis. No food or drug allergies.

Medication: Hydrocortisone 1% cream sparingly to affected facial area daily; multivitamin daily.

1. Which are the most likely differential diagnoses for the presenting problem?
   Conjunctivitis, blepharitis

2. Review the risk factors for the possible diagnoses.
   Conjunctivitis: acute outbreak in LTC facility, with personal care provided by staff who may be caring for others with the infection
   Blepharitis: history of seborrheic dermatitis with facial area affected

3. What further history would you obtain?
   Character of drainage: continuous or worse at morning or night

4. What key findings would you look for in the physical exam?
   Condition of conjunctiva, eyelids, and surrounding skin surfaces

Exam: Eyelids are found to be inflamed, with broken and misdirected lashes. Scaling of lids noted. Conjunctiva are mildly injected. Golden crusting is noted along lid edges; drainage is reported to be worse in the morning, staying clear through the day.

5. What treatment plan would you develop, based on these findings?
   Discuss pharmacologic and nonpharmacologic plans, including any needed staff education
   - **Pharmacologic: topical ointment such as erythromycin or bacitracin ointment 1 to 4 times a day, depending upon severity of infection**
   - **Nonpharmacologic: warm soaks to remove crusts; lid hygiene b.i.d. with half-and-half baby shampoo and water**
   - **With staff: review rationale for bedtime lid hygiene (removing bacteria that will have overgrowth through the night), which should be an ongoing part of treatment plan**

6. What follow-up would you recommend?
   Maintenance of lid hygiene every evening at bedtime; assess for resolution of drainage

7. Under what circumstances would you make a referral?
   Failure of infection to resolve after 1 week, or worsening of infection in the meantime; refer to Tables 7–2 and 7–5 for review

Case 2. An 82-year-old man comes to clinic accompanied by his wife. He has not been back for his routine visits for 8 months. He has no complaints, says no to every question you ask. Wife states he is driving her nuts; she thinks he is getting senile or going crazy because he has lost interest in socializing and has stopped watching TV. Chart shows patient was a construction worker. He smoked and drank heavily for many years before quitting about 15 years ago. His medical diagnoses are hypertension, osteoarthritis, and COPD; medications are atenolol (Tenormin) 50 mg p.o. q.d., enalapril (Vasotec) 5 mg p.o. q.d., theophylline sustained release (Theo-Dur) 100 mg p.o. b.i.d., and aspirin as needed for arthritis pain.

1. What part of this history suggests hearing loss?
   Patient answers negatively to every question, denying everything; to test this, rephrase a question so that it requires a different answer. Wife thinking he is demented or mentally ill—hearing loss frequently presents as dementia or depression, loss of interest in events involving hearing

2. What risk factors for hearing loss does he have?
   Construction worker—probable exposure to loud noises, aspirin ingestion, alcohol abuse—he drank heavily for many years, hypertension and COPD can contribute to hearing loss

Exam: Shows that the patient can hear sound but cannot understand many of the words.

3. What kind of hearing loss does this suggest?
   Sensorineural

4. Would a referral for a hearing aid be appropriate for this kind of hearing loss?
   Yes, can be effective for sensorineural hearing loss, may improve quality of life

Case 3. A 65-year-old female patient presents with complaint of "a cold." States symptoms have been present for 6 days and include a "runny nose, cough, and just feel miserable." Has gotten worse in past 2 days. Gives history of "Allergies to pollen." No regular medications; has been taking ibuprofen and pseudoephedrine to control symptoms.
Exam: Patient appears mildly ill but not in distress; temp 100.2° F oral; pulse 100, respiration 20, mouth breathing, but no acute respiratory distress. Ears: canals clear, TMs bilaterally dull and retracted, nasal mucosa swollen, red, with green discharge. Palpable enlarged lymph nodes tender to palpation. Chest is clear, heart normal.

1. What further history would you like?
   Ear symptoms; throat symptoms characteristic of cough; nasal drainage, smell, or taste changes; visual changes; redness or swelling of face indicating cellulitis or other severe infection; past history of allergies, sinus infections, medication allergies

2. What else is included in your physical exam?
   Facial exam, looking for edema, tenderness over sinuses, mouth; looking for dental infections, throat for purulent drainage

3. What is your diagnosis?
   Sinusitis

4. What would you do for the patient on this visit?
    - Nonpharmacologic treatment—rest, and emphasize fluids and humidification
    - Prescribe an oral antibiotic: amoxicillin is first choice, followed by trimethoprim/sulfamethoxazole DS b.i.d.; first-generation macrolide (erythromycin) for patients with penicillin allergy
    - A nonsedating antihistamine may be indicated if seasonal allergies are a factor
    - Consider codeine if severe night cough
    - Add short course of nasal steroids if allergies an issue
    - Change pain medication to acetaminophen, as ibuprofen has been reported to be associated with hypertension
    - Schedule follow-up call in 4 days to report progress, sooner if increased pain or associated dyspnea or increased fever

CHAPTER 8—RESPIRATORY DISORDERS

Case 1. A 70-year-old male comes to clinic with productive cough, shortness of breath. Denies fever, upper-respiratory symptoms. Patient is a retired construction worker with history of asthma.
HPI: Medications include asthma medications: albuterol p.r.n., salmeterol (Serevent) 2 puffs b.i.d., triamcinolone (Azmacort) 2 puffs b.i.d., and loratadine (Claritin) p.r.n. allergies.

1. What additional history would you like?
   How much is he using his Alupent inhaler? How much is he coughing? What is he bringing up? Any SOB or wheezing?

Physical Exam: Vital signs stable. No acute respiratory distress, lungs without wheezes or rales (crackles), breath sounds are decreased bilaterally with prolonged expiration. Heart rate regular. Peak flow rate 300; his baseline is 350.

2. What is your assessment?
   Mild exacerbation of asthma, no evidence of infection

3. What do you think is happening?
   Forgetting to take inhalers or not using correctly; had a URI, exposure to his allergy trigger, exposure to environmental pollutants; any change in medication

4. What is your initial plan?
   Make sure he is using his inhalers correctly, with spacer if needed. Have patient use Alupent inhaler on regular basis 3 to 4 times a day until better.

Case 2. A 75-year-old female with complaints of productive cough, fever, chills, chest discomfort, and chest congestion; fatigue and headache for 3 days.
PMH: Bronchitis. Medications: Robitussin DM and Tylenol extra strength for headache. Allergic to penicillin.

1. What additional history would you ask?
   History of bronchitis, any history of pneumonia; color, amount of sputum, ability to mobilize sputum; fluid intake; whether cough is keeping her awake at night

Exam: Patient appears ill; temp 100.8° F, tachypnea with exertion, skin warm to touch; ENT exam normal; chest splinting with fremitus and rales (crackles) in right lower lobe.

2. What diagnostic tests will you order?
   CXR, CBC with differential, pulse oximetry

3. What are the most likely diagnoses?
   The most likely differential to consider: pneumonia, sinusitis, PE. Pneumonia most likely due to bacteria. *Streptococcus pneumoniae* is the most common. Next in frequency are *Mycoplasma pneumoniae*, and *Chlamydia*, and *Legionella* species. Not likely to be caused by Gram-negative bacilli because she is not severely ill.

4. Based on your current impression, what treatment will you order?
   Best first choice is a macrolide such as clarithromycin (Biaxin) or azithromycin (Zithromax); good also because of patient's allergy to penicillin. Doxycycline would also be an acceptable choice. Fluoroquinolone not as good a choice because of low probability of Gram-negative bacteria. Stop Robitussin DM; use Robitussin with codeine for cough suppression, expectorant, and analgesic effect.

Case 3. A 67-year-old male complains of shortness of breath, both at rest and on exertion. Unable to perform normal activities without becoming "winded." Notes occasional cough. **PMH:** Hypertension. Former smoker, 1½ packs per day for 40 years. Medications: OTC cough medicine, enalapril (Vasotec) 5 mg daily for hypertension.

1. What additional history would you ask?
   - **Timing of the worsening of the SOB, define cough in regard to daily, with activity only, with or without productive component, any hemoptysis history, number of episodes of URI**
   - **Any peripheral edema, chest pain or pressure**
   - **Amount of exercise, fluid intake**

Exam: Vital signs BP 152/90; no tachypnea; ENT, normal findings; chest, increased AP diameter, hyper-resonance on percussion, decreased expansion on respiration, no abnormal breath sounds; extremities, no edema, no nail clubbing.

2. What diagnostic tests would you order?
   Do peak flow rate in office. Diagnostic testing: CXR, CBC, chemistries, EKG, pulse oximetry

3. What is your differential diagnosis?
   Emphysema, COPD, CHF, cancer, ACE-inhibitor cough

4. What would you do for this patient on this visit?
   - **Ipratropium bromide (Atrovent) inhaler 2 inhalations q.i.d.**
   - **Ensure adequate hydration**
   - **This patient should have follow-up in 1 to 2 weeks**

CHAPTER 9—CARDIOVASCULAR DISORDERS

Case 1. A 68-year-old male is following up after consultation with an orthopedist for a recent fractured thumb. Orthopedist noted that the patient had a blood pressure of 166/104.

PMH: Chart shows that the patient had, at the last office visit, BP 144/92. Laboratory work was ordered. Review of chart shows labile blood pressure readings for the previous 2 years, which decreased after weight loss undertaken to treat hyperlipidemia. States he follows low-salt, low-fat diet and exercises 2 to 3 times a week. Nonsmoker.

Medications: Atorvastatin (Lipitor) 10 mg daily; ibuprofen (Motrin) 400 mg p.o. 3 times daily
FH: Diabetes type 2 and CAD

1. What cardiac risk factors does he have?
   - **Male**
   - **Previous readings of high blood pressure**
   - **Hyperlipidemia**
   - **Family history of CAD**
   - **Family history of DM**

Lab findings on previous visits:

BUN 22
Creatinine 0.8
Na+ 136
K+ 4.0
Glucose 162
Cholesterol 230
Triglycerides 250
LDL 148
HDL 32

2. What additional problem does this lab identify? Is this a significant coronary risk factor?
   Diabetes; yes

3. Is his hyperlipidemia well controlled?
   No, cholesterol is high, triglycerides are high, LDL (bad cholesterol) is high, HDL (good cholesterol) is low

Physical: Vital signs current visit: BP 160/102; pulse 98; resp 16; weight 205 lbs; height 5'9"
Cardiac: RRR, no murmur, no carotid bruits or pedal edema, no renal bruits
Resp: vesicular sounds throughout all lung fields
Funduscopic: clear disc, obvious arteriolar narrowing with focal areas of attenuation
UA: trace glucose and protein
ECG sinus rhythm

4. What is the significance of these findings?
   - Blood pressure elevated
   - BP in orthopedist's office could have been elevated due to acute illness/pain; however, you have two elevated readings, which defines hypertension
   - Urinalysis and funduscopic exam shows target organ damage
   - Protein in urine may be from hypertension or diabetes
   - Height and weight show patient is overweight

5. What stage hypertension does he have?
   Stage 2 hypertension with target organ damage

6. How would you manage this patient's hypertension? List steps.
   - **Nonpharmacologic: reinforce diet (patient obviously not following diet); needs low-fat, low-sodium and diabetic diet**
   - **Pharmacologic: discontinue ibuprofen**
   - **Start on medication**
   - **Would not start on diuretic or beta blocker because of compelling indication of diabetes with proteinuria**
   - **Start on ACE inhibitor**

Case 2. A 73-year-old White female complains of increasing shortness of breath and cough productive of frothy sputum over the last 24 hours. She has had trouble sleeping because of a cough she attributes to allergies, and has felt tired for the past 3 months. Two days ago she celebrated her 73rd birthday.
PMH: Two years ago she had an episode of weakness and dizziness. At that time, her EKG showed changes indicative of a mild MI. She was placed on atenolol (Tenormin) 100 mg and has remained stable. Has mild hypertension, hyperlipidemia; menopause 10 years ago. Smoking history ½ pack a day for 20 years; quit 5 years ago.
Lab: Chest x-ray showing mild cardiomegaly, otherwise unremarkable. An echocardiogram showing EF 40%, moderate left-ventricular dysfunction.

1. What is the most likely diagnosis?
   CHF

2. What factor(s) most likely to have precipitated this?
   Excess salt intake at birthday dinner—fluid overload, stress

3. What is the most likely the basic cause(s)?
   Myocardial damage; contributing—hypertension causing pressure overload over time

4. What over-the-counter drugs should you specifically ask about?
   NSAIDs

Exam: BP 142/94, pulse 88; resp 22; temp 98.8° F; weight: 180 lbs
Ht: 5'4"; general appearance: appears mildly short of breath
Resp: tachypnea, occasional nonproductive cough, bibasilar rales (crackles)
Extremities: 2+ edema extending halfway up lower legs

5. What other physical exam do you need to do and what would you look for?
   Cardiac—arrhythmias, murmur, S3, JVD
   Abdomen—ascites
   Extremities—circulation, cyanosis

Medications: Atenolol (Tenormin) 100 mg p.o. daily, lovastatin (Mevacor) 20 mg daily, aspirin 81 mg daily

6. What medications would you start today?
   Diuretic—furosemide (Lasix) 20 mg p.o. q.d.; ACE inhibitor—lisinopril (Zestril) 5 mg p.o. q.d.

7. What lab work would you need to check before starting these medications?
   Comprehensive lab—renal function, potassium level

8. What adverse reactions would you monitor for?
   Lasix—orthostatic hypotension, dizziness, weakness, GI upset; lisinopril—hyperkalemia, renal impairment, cough

Case 3. A 70-year-old White female presents for routine follow-up of lipids.
PMH: Her last visit she was started on a low-saturated-fat diet. Medical history significant for osteoporosis and hypercholesteremia. Ex-smoker with 15 pack-years, quit 7 years ago. Occasional ETOH with glass of wine once a week.
Medications: Fosamax 10 mg q.d.; calcium and vitamin D supplements
Exam: General appearance: alert, oriented, NAD; weight 130 lbs; height 5'5"
BP 138/82
Cardiac: RRR, no murmurs; no edema, peripheral pulses present
Resp: vesicular breath sounds throughout all lung fields
Abdomen: soft, no hepatosplenomegaly or masses

Labs:	Last Visit	This Visit
Cholesterol, total	275	230
Triglycerides	118	104
HDL	62	56
LDL	189	140

Basic metabolic panel, CBC, and LFT unremarkable

1. What is your assessment?
   Lipid panel improved significantly on lipid lowering diet in 2 months; borderline high blood cholesterol; HDL remains good; LDL borderline high risk; no signs of coronary artery disease

2. What cardiac risk factors does this patient have?
   Hyperlipidemia, smoking history, age

3. What other risk factors should you assess?
   Sedentary life style, other cardiac risk factors, diabetes, family history, history of smoking, stress, alcohol

4. What is your plan?

Nonpharmacologic intervention: weight-bearing exercise for osteoporosis and to increase HDL. Continue present diet for total of 6 months before considering medications; pharmacologic treatment considered controversial in this age group.

CHAPTER 10—GASTROINTESTINAL DISORDERS

Case 1. A 68-year-old male presents to your clinic with complaints of burning, epigastric pain after meals associated with nausea, especially when he lies down after eating. He has lost 15 lb over the past month, which he attributes to poor appetite.

HPI: The patient is a recovering alcoholic. He stopped drinking 8 months ago and has been going to AA meetings on a regular basis. The patient is also a heavy smoker and has frequent episodes of bronchitis. He continues to smoke but has cut back significantly. His past medical history includes treatment for a gastric ulcer 1 year ago. He is not taking any medication.

1. What other questions would you ask this patient?
   - **Any fevers or night sweats?**
   - **Any symptoms of cough, heartburn, regurgitation, vomiting, hematemesis, melena, rectal bleeding, or change in bowel pattern?**
   - **Does the pain radiate anywhere—chest, back, shoulder, or to the RUQ/LUQ of the abdomen?**
   - **Foods that may exacerbate symptoms—fatty meals, acidic foods?**
   - **NSAID use?**
   - **What treatment did he receive for the gastric ulcer? Was he re-evaluated after treatment?**
   - **Is there a past history of pancreatitis in this patient with history of alcoholism?**

Exam: Vital signs are stable. No lymphadenopathy. Heart and lung exams are normal. Abdomen is soft, nontender, normal bowel sounds, no hepatosplenomegaly, no masses, no abdominal bruits. Rectal exam is normal with guaiac-negative stools.

2. What laboratory tests would you order?
   CBC with differential, electrolytes, BUN/CR, calcium, liver function tests, amylase and lipase

3. What other studies would you order?
   The patient has weight loss with history of gastric ulcer, alcoholism, and heavy tobacco use. A nonhealing or recurrent gastric ulcer, as well as gastric cancer in this patient, should be ruled out. He should have an upper endoscopy.

4. What treatment would you provide?
   Referral to a gastroenterologist

Case 2. A 72-year-old male with HTN is in your office for a follow-up visit. He complains of being constipated.

HPI: The patient states that he's always had a regular bowel movement every morning. For the past month, bowel movements occur every 4 to 5 days only after he uses a laxative. Medications include a calcium-channel blocker and one aspirin a day.

1. Is a new onset of constipation in a 72-year-old concerning? Or is this a normal change related to the aging process?

    Constipation is more common in older adults because of decreased colonic motility in combination with poor dietary habits and medication side effects; however, any new onset of constipation would be concerning, as it could mean cancer of the colon

2. What other history would you obtain?
    - Character of stool, straining, incomplete evacuation, time to complete BM, digital evacuation, incontinence, hemorrhoids, or other anorectal disorders?
    - Fevers, night sweats, anorexia, weight loss, nausea, vomiting, abdominal pain, diarrhea, melena, rectal bleeding?
    - Dietary intake of fiber and fluids?
    - Physical activity?
    - Change in environment?
    - How long has he been taking his current medications? Name and dose of laxatives?
    - Is there a family history of colon cancer?
    - Has the patient ever had a flexible sigmoidoscopy for colon cancer screening?

Exam: The patient is alert and oriented x 3. Blood pressure and other vital signs are normal. His abdomen is mildly distended but nontender. Bowel sounds are present in all quadrants. No enlarged liver or spleen. No bruises. Rectal exam is normal, no impacted stool. The remainder of his examination is normal.

3. What laboratory tests would you order?
    - CBC with differential, electrolytes, calcium, BUN/creatinine, glucose, LFTs, alkaline phosphatase (evaluate for metastasis or increased alkaline phosphatase with cancer), thyroid function tests
    - Stool guaiac x 3 (for 3 days prior to and during collection: no ASA, red meat, vitamin C, or raw vegetables)

4. What other studies would you order?
    - Flat plate and upright of the abdomen
    - Refer for colonoscopy to rule out cancer

5. What treatment would you provide?
    - Increased fiber intake with bran supplement added to diet, or by using bulk-forming agents such as Metamucil or Citrucel
    - Increased fluid intake to 1.5 to 2 liters/day
    - Bowel training program
    - Regular physical activity
    - Re-evaluate the use of calcium-channel blocker for HTN management, especially if symptoms occurred with the initiation of this medication and laboratory and diagnostic data is within normal limits

Case 3. A 62-year-old obese White female presents with right upper quadrant pain, nausea, and vomiting. The onset of pain was sudden and occurred after eating at a restaurant. She has had similar episodes in the past but not as severe.

1. What additional history would you like?
   - Quality and duration of pain; radiation of pain to chest, shoulder, back, or other area of the abdomen
   - Fever, cough, heartburn, jaundice, hematemesis, diarrhea, melena, rectal bleeding
   - What foods precipitate symptoms? ETOH intake, NSAID use?
   - History of gallstones?

Exam: Temp is 99.5° F, with remaining vital signs normal. Abdomen is soft. Right upper quadrant pain increases when palpating the right upper quadrant during inspiration and there is localized guarding. There is no rebound tenderness. Bowel sounds are normal. No hepatosplenomegaly. There are no abdominal bruits. Rectal exam is normal with guaiac negative stool. The remainder of her exam is normal.

2. What diagnostic tests would you order?
   CBC with differential, electrolytes, BUN/creatinine, liver function tests, amylase and lipase, abdominal ultrasound

3. What is the most likely differential?
   Biliary colic, cholecystitis, pancreatitis, hepatitis, PUD, acute gastroenteritis

4. How would you treat her?
   Prompt surgical evaluation

CHAPTER 11—RENAL AND UROLOGIC DISORDERS

Case 1. A 94-year-old female patient with dementia returned home from the hospital for hip surgery with a Foley catheter. She complains of hip pain but not low back or pain or suprapubic tenderness. She has been incontinent of bowel and bladder for many years. She requires total care. Patient is afebrile.

1. What lab tests would you order?
   - CBC (to rule out anemia from post-surgical blood loss vs. anemia due to CRF) Comprehensive metabolic panel—BUN, creatinine, urinalysis
   - You do not order a urine culture and sensitivity. Patient has risk factors for asymptomatic bacteruria and has no symptoms or signs of UTI

Lab: Her creatinine is 1.2 and her BUN is 36.
Urinalysis shows many bacteria, no WBCs

2. How do you interpret this lab work?
   - Values are high but may demonstrate normal changes of aging
   - Urinalysis shows colonization but not infection based on lack of WBCs
   - No immediate action required except to ensure adequate hydration

3. What are your initial interventions?
   - Remove the Foley catheter
   - Assure adequate hydration
   - Review hygiene measures with nursing assistants

Lab: The nurse obtains a urine culture and sensitivity without your order. It shows 10,000 colonies each of 3 microorganisms, which are sensitive to ciprofloxacin (Cipro), sulfamethoxazole/trimethoprim, and levofloxacin (Levaquin).

4. Would you treat the patient with an antibiotic?
   No, the finding of three organisms is indicative of colonization, not infection

5. What would the urinalysis show if the patient did have a UTI?
   - **Leukocyte esterase might be positive**
   - **Urine would have WBCs and bacteria**
   - **There would be minimal epithelial cell**

6. What are the possible complications of a UTI in this patient?
   - **Urosepsis**
   - **Pyelonephritis**

Case 2. While talking to a 74-year-old female patient, you discover that she has stopped going downstairs for meals in her senior apartment building. She has also stopped going on trips and does not have enough groceries. She denies any pain or fatigue. Seems reluctant to talk about it. Admits to urinary frequency.

History: Upon questioning, patient is afraid she might not make it to the bathroom in time, so has restricted her activities. Urinates every 1 to 2 hours so she won't be incontinent. Still has occasional accidents in which she loses a large amount of urine.

1. What is the significance of loss of a large amount of urine?
   Indicates urge incontinence

2. What risk factors would you inquire about?
   - **Estrogen deficiency**
   - **Multiparity**
   - **Diseases such as diabetes, MS, CVA**
   - **Mobility**
   - **Medications such as diuretics**

3. What medications can contribute to incontinence?
   - **Anticholinergics**
   - **Tricyclics**
   - **Antispasmodics**
   - **Opioids, beta agonists**
   - **Alpha-adrenergic agents**
   - **Calcium-channel blockers**
   - **Diuretics**
   - **Caffeine**
   - **Psychotropics**
   - **Phenothiazines**
   - **Antiparkinsonian agents**
   - **Sedative hypnotics**
   - **ACE inhibitors**

4. What treatment is effective for her type of incontinence?
   - Bladder retraining
   - Timed voiding
   - Prompted voiding
   - Kegel exercises
   - Prevent constipation
   - Estrogen cream to urethra daily

5. What medications would you consider?
   - Oxybutynin HCL XL (Ditropan XL)
   - Tolterodine tartrate SR (Detrol SR)
   - Trospium chloride XR
   - Solifenacin
   - Darifenacin
   - (Fewer side effects from long-acting formulations and those taken once daily)

Case 3. An 83-year-old man has been taking ibuprofen for 20 years for degenerative joint disease. He also has hypertension, for which he takes hydrochlorothiazide. His blood pressure today is 160/94. He states that is what it usually is and that is fine with him. Routine screening lab shows BUN of 64 and creatinine of 1.8.

1. What is your initial assessment?
   Renal insufficiency, uncontrolled hypertension; renal insufficiency may be from longstanding hypertension, exacerbated by NSAID use

2. What other lab tests would you order? What would you look for?
   - Urinalysis—proteinuria and urinary sediment
   - Sodium level may be normal or low
   - Potassium may be elevated
   - Normochromic normocytic anemia

3. Which diuretic is most effective in patients with renal insufficiency?
   Furosemide, not HCTZ

4. What complications should you monitor for?
   - Anemia
   - CHF
   - Uremia
   - Infections
   - Bleeding
   - Death

CHAPTER 12—GYNECOLOGIC DISORDERS

Case 1. A 69-year-old female comes to your office for her annual physical exam. On exam, you note a lump in the upper outer aspect of the right breast. The lump is about 1 cm, mobile, firm, with regular borders. There is no dimpling, retraction, or other breast or chest wall lesions. There is no tenderness. There is no adenopathy. The remainder of the physical exam is normal. She was not aware of this lump or other changes in her breasts. However, she does not perform regular breast self exam. Her last mammogram was 3 years ago and last Papanicolau test was 1 year ago.

Breast History: The patient has no prior history of breast cancer or breast biopsies. Menarche: age 9. The patient is gravida 1, para 1, miscarriages/abortions 0. Age at first full-term pregnancy: 36. Age at menopause: 54. Hormones: HRT conjugated estrogen/medroxyprogesterone (Prempro) 10 years.

Past Medical History: Hypercholesterolemia, osteopenia

Medications: Prempro, atorvastatin (Lipitor) 20 mg, multivitamin, calcium

Habits: Diet—generally follows low-fat diet; exercise—walks 3 times a week for ½ hour; alcohol—3 to 4 drinks/week; tobacco—none

1. Based on the history and physical, what is your recommendation regarding diagnostic evaluation of the breast lump?
   Since the patient has a palpable mass on clinical breast exam, a diagnostic mammogram should be ordered. This test includes an ultrasound evaluation to determine if the lesion is solid or cystic.

2. The mammogram shows a small mass in the upper outer quadrant of the right breast. The sonogram shows a cystic lesion with a small solid component in the area of the palpable mass. What would be your next recommendation for follow-up of this mass?
   Refer to a surgeon for further evaluation. Although cysts are possible in women on hormone replacement therapy, large cysts are generally uncommon in postmenopausal women. Further, this lesion does not have the classic appearance of a simple cyst on ultrasound. The cyst may be secondary to obstruction of a duct by a malignant lesion. A complex mass that has a solid component within the cyst requires biopsy.

3. What aspects of the patient's history would be considered risk factors in assessing her risk for breast cancer?
   Age: There is an increased incidence of breast cancer in women over age 50. Menarche age 9: Early age of menarche is associated with increased risk for breast cancer. Some studies suggest that hormone levels may be higher throughout reproductive years in women with early menarche. The cumulative exposure to higher levels of estrogen may be associated with increased risk for developing breast cancer.
   First childbirth after age 35: The first pregnancy is associated with changes in the breast epithelium and properties of breast cells. The later the age of first pregnancy, the more likely that DNA errors have occurred that will be propagated during pregnancy.
   Use of hormone replacement therapy: Possibly a risk factor for breast cancer; remains controversial.

Case 2. A 70-year-old female comes to the clinic because she thinks she is shrinking. She is 5' 2", weighs 98 pounds, has smoked for 30 years, has COPD. Upon questioning, admits to having difficulty holding her urine because of frequency and urgency. She wears pads when she goes out, but she doesn't go out much because she is embarrassed.

1. What consequences of menopause does she have?
   Probable osteoporosis, vaginal atrophy with urge incontinence

2. What other consequence would you evaluate her for?
   Cardiovascular disease

3. What physical exam is indicated?
   - **Pelvic exam**
   - **Cardiac exam**
   - **Musculoskeletal exam**

4. What diagnostic tests would you order?
   - **Routine lab optional**
   - **Lipid profile for hyperlipidemia**
   - **Bone densitometry (DXA scan) for osteoporosis**

5. What is the single most important thing she can do to improve her health?
   Stop smoking

6. The pelvic exam shows moderate vaginal atrophy. How would you manage the vaginal atrophy?
   Estradiol vaginal cream (Estrace)

Case 3. A 78-year-old healthy female has a routine Pap results of CIN II.

1. What does the CIN II mean?
   Moderate dysplasia of 2/3 of lining to full thickness

2. What counseling would you give when you told her about the results?
   This is a precancerous condition

3. What would your actions be?
   Refer all abnormal Paps to gynecology

4. What would her life expectancy be if she were not treated?
   Cancer becomes invasive, and patient dies in 3 to 5 years

5. What follow-up would the patient need?
   Seek follow-up; repeat cytology every 3 to 4 months for the first year, then every 6 months for the next year, then annually once a pattern of normal readings has been established

CHAPTER 13—MALE REPRODUCTIVE SYSTEM DISORDERS

Case 1. An 83-year-old man complains of urinary hesitancy, dribbling, urinary frequency of small amounts, nocturia x 4/night. This has been gradually getting worse for the past few months.

1. What is the most likely diagnosis?
   - **BPH, classic symptoms**
   - **Not a UTI; no dysuria, gradual onset**
   - **Still have to rule out prostate cancer**

2. What physical exam is required?
   DRE, abdomen

3. If the symptoms are not troublesome, what is the usual approach?
   Watchful waiting

4. What symptoms would require referral for treatment?
   Urinary retention, recurrent UTIs, hematuria, bladder stone, or renal insufficiency

5. What nonpharmacologic treatment may be helpful?
   - **Avoid medications known to worsen symptoms**
   - **Avoid foods that can cause retention, as well as caffeine and alcohol**
   - **Avoid fluids at bedtime to lessen sleep interruption**

6. Which medications would you consider starting the patient on? What are their main disadvantages?
   - **Alpha-adrenergic blockers such as terazosin, doxazosin: orthostatic hypotension**
   - **Tamsulosin (Flomax): less risk for orthostatic hypotension**
   - **The 5-alpha-reductase inhibitor finasteride (Proscar): takes 6 months to take effect**

Case 2. A 78-year-old Black man comes to you feeling poorly. He complains of fatigue and low back pain, which has been gradually increasing for the past few months. He has had urinary symptoms, which he attributed to BPH for the past 6 years, gradually worsening so that he is now having hesitancy, dribbling, and a feeling of not emptying his bladder completely. He has never sought treatment for the BPH symptoms because he thought it was an inevitable consequence of aging.
PMH: 50 pack-year smoking, COPD, osteoarthritis, hypertension, and hyperlipidemia. Medications: ipratropium/albuterol (Combivent) inhaler, acetaminophen (Tylenol) p.r.n. for pain, hydrochlorothiazide 25 mg p.o. q.d., atorvastatin (Lipitor) 40 mg p.o. q.d.

1. What do his urinary symptoms indicate?
   Symptoms are obstructive; he could have urinary retention

2. What are the most likely possibilities for a differential diagnosis?
   BPH and prostate cancer

3. What lab work would you order?
   - **DRE—look for nodules, hardness**
   - **Renal functions to assess damage to kidneys**
   - **UA C&S to rule out hematuria, glycosuria, or infection**
   - **PSA**

4. Which would be most useful for deciding between the differential?
   PSA; DRE if it shows hard nodule, but the cancer may not be accessible to DRE

5. What risk factors does he have?
   Race and age

6. What would you do?
   Refer to urologist

7. What follow-up is required?
   Monitor PSA

Case 3. A 68-year-old man comes to your office with the complaint of insomnia. Says he is having some problems with his wife. She is not too happy with him. Patient seems reluctant to say what is really bothering him

1. How would you approach this situation?
   - **Maintain an open, trustworthy, and nonjudgmental approach**
   - **Openly ask about sex. Is he having sexual relations with his wife? Is it satisfactory to both of them?**
   - **Ask specifically about his sexual function.**

2. What normal changes of aging affect sexual function?
   Slowed arousal; erections less firm, shorter lasting; decreased forcefulness at ejaculation; longer interval to achieve subsequent erection.

History: Patient tells you he has a gradual loss of the ability to maintain an erection for the past year or so. His wife is upset about this and has been nagging him to do something about it. The problem became worse recently, after an argument with his wife.

3. Is this ED psychological or organic?
   Probably both: gradual onset is organic, argument with wife is psychological

PMH: Patient has hypertension, diabetes, lipid disorder, osteoarthritis.

4. How do these diseases affect ED?
   - **Hypertension; many medications can cause ED, contribute to vascular disorder**
   - **Diabetes leads to macrovascular changes that cause decreased circulation to penis and decreased erections**
   - **Lipid disorder contributes to vascular disorder**
   - **Arthritis causes pain, which contributes to ED**

5. What would be your initial approach?
   - Counseling to reassure patient, discuss relationship with wife
   - Optimal management of diabetes
   - Check hypertension medications to see if you can change to one less likely to cause ED

CHAPTER 14—MUSCULOSKELETAL DISORDERS

Case 1. A thin, petite 75-year-old Asian woman comes to clinic for sudden onset of thoracic back pain 2 days ago when she coughed.

1. What pertinent history is it important to ask?
   - Respiratory symptoms, any other joint pain, associated symptoms, any history of malignancy
   - Risk factors for osteoporosis: calcium, vitamin D, protein intake
   - Weight-bearing exercise, smoker or nonsmoker, alcohol intake
   - Family history of osteoporosis

2. What would you expect to find on PE?
   - Point tenderness over thoracic spine, pain with deep respiration, kyphosis
   - Lateral thoracic-spine x-ray shows wedging of vertebral body

3. How would you treat this patient?
   - Pain relievers; start with mild, may need opioid
   - Calcitonin (Miacalcin) nasal spray can help with pain control

4. How soon should the pain be relieved?
   6 weeks

5. What follow-up?
   - Monitor for resolution of pain, respiratory problems related to not taking deep breaths
   - Patient should have DXA scan to assess severity of osteoporosis
   - Patient has the risk factors, plus compression fracture is caused by osteoporosis; if not on bisphosphonates, should be started

Case 2. A 68-year-old woman complains of hip and knee pain for many years. She is overweight and unable to walk more than a half block because of pain. She spends her day in a recliner eating snacks and watching television. She has become incontinent because she cannot make it to the toilet on time. Every once in a while she thinks her knee is going to give out from under her. She notes loud cracking noises when she stands up. Her knees are enlarged with decreased ROM.

1. What history would you expect?
   - Gradual, progressive onset of joint pain over years
   - Stiffness in morning, lasting less than ½ hour
   - Pain worse with activity, relieved by rest

2. Which of her symptoms are indicative of advanced disease?
   - **Unable to walk more than ½ block because of pain**
   - **Every once in a while she thinks her knee is going to give out from under her**
   - **Her knees are enlarged with decreased ROM**

3. What is the most likely diagnosis?
   Osteoarthritis

4. What nonpharmacologic treatment would you institute?
   - **Physical activity/therapy is the cornerstone of treatment in the older adult**
   - **Occupational therapy**
   - **Social support**
   - **Help with daily activities may be needed**
   - **Arthritis self-help and water aquatics courses**
   - **Ambulation aids (canes, braces, walkers)**
   - **Weight loss programs**
   - **Heat/cold to affected joint**

5. What pharmacologic treatment would you order?
   - **Simple analgesics (acetaminophen up to 4,000 mg/day in divided doses is first-line therapy)**
   - **Topical analgesic creams such as capsaicin 0.025% b.i.d. to t.i.d., diclofenac (Voltaren) gel 1% q.i.d.**
   - **NSAIDs alone or combined with analgesics (ibuprofen up to 2,400 mg/day in divided doses, naproxen sodium up to 1,000 mg/day in divided doses, others)**
   - **Selective COX-2 inhibitors (Celecoxib 100 to 200 mg/day)**
   - **Tramadol (Ultram) 50 mg b.i.d. to t.i.d.**

6. What lab tests must be monitored if the patient is placed on a NSAID?
   Renal function

7. When should you refer?
   Patients with functional impairment (inability to perform normal activities of daily living) and with moderate to severe pain should be considered for joint replacement

Case 3. A 78-year-old man complains of low back pain (LBP) for the past 5 days. Pain is in his lower lumbar area radiating into the left buttock. Pain is worse when sitting up in hard chair; he has not been able to go out to the park and play checkers with his friends.
PMH: Has had episodes of LBP for past 5 years. Patient worked as a truck driver, delivering packages before he retired. Has not been active recently due to COPD from smoking; gets SOB easily and cannot walk long distances.

1. What risk factors does he have for low back pain?
   Physical deconditioning, poor body mechanics; cigarette smoking

2. What symptoms would prompt an emergency referral?
   Bilateral leg weakness, bladder and bowel incontinence seen with large central disk herniation or cauda equina

3. What simple physical exam maneuver will be the most useful?
Straight-leg raising

4. What is your most likely diagnosis?
Sciatica (likely related to either lumbosacral strain or degenerative changes of the lumbar spine)

5. If patient is compliant with therapy, how soon can he expect to have pain resolve?
4 to 6 weeks

CHAPTER 15—NEUROLOGICAL DISORDERS

Case 1. A 72-year-old female has 3 falls in the last 2 months without serious injury. Reports difficulty getting out of chair. She feels stiff and slow. Has tremor at rest. She is otherwise healthy without significant past medical history. She takes 2 acetaminophen (Tylenol) a day for aches.

1. What other history is needed?
   - **History surrounding the falls**
   - **Neurologic exam for focal neurologic deficits, other changes**
   - **Musculoskeletal problems**
   - **Medications**

2. What assessment tools would you use?
MMSE for cognitive changes; GDS for depression; get-up-and-go test for mobility

3. What part of the neurologic exam should be normal?
Sensory, motor, cranial nerves, reflexes

4. What abnormalities do you expect to find on neurologic exam?
Rigidity, difficulty initiating movement, shuffling gait, stooped posture, cogwheeling, tremor, fixed facial expression

5. What is your most likely diagnosis?
Parkinson's disease

Case 2. A 66-year-old male presents in office for follow-up after evaluation in the emergency department for left hemiparesis lasting 30 minutes. Reported negative head CT, chemistry panel, CBC, and toxicology screen. History of "borderline" hypertension. No medications except over-the-counter ibuprofen.

1. What was the event he had?
Probable TIA

2. What other history do you want to obtain?
Precipitating events, other neurologic symptoms, cardiovascular symptoms, cardiovascular risk factors, head trauma, alcohol or illicit drug use, family history of neurologic disorders and cardiovascular disease

3. What physical findings might you expect?
   May find elevated blood pressure, carotid bruit, normal neurologic and cardiac exam

4. What further diagnostic tests would be indicated?
   EKG, carotid Doppler studies

5. How will you initially manage this patient?
   * **Start patient on aspirin 325 mg p.o. q.d.**
   * **Counseling regarding cardiovascular risk reduction and antiplatelet therapy, alcohol use, and use of over-the-counter medications**

Case 3. A 78-year-old woman with left-side headache for 2 days, no relief with 1,000 mg acetaminophen every 6 hours. History of headaches since age 16. Past medical history significant for hypertension controlled with atenolol 25 mg a day.

1. What other history is important?
   Pattern of headaches, change in headaches, neurologic deficits, precipitating events, facial tenderness, rash, review of systems for other HEENT symptoms

2. What systems will you examine?
   Vital signs, HEENT, neurologic

3. What diagnostic testing?
   ESR; consider brain CT if change in headache or focal neurologic exam

4. What is your differential diagnosis?
   Giant cell arteritis, herpes zoster, sinusitis, tension or migraine headache, trigeminal neuralgia

CHAPTER 16—HEMATOLOGIC DISORDERS

Case 1. An 83-year-old White male with a chief complaint of fatigue for the past few months. The fatigue is gradually getting worse. He now is too tired to walk to the dining room in his assisted living residence.
PMH: Patient has hypertension, history of PUD with GI bleed, smoker, depression, hyperlipidemia, rheumatoid arthritis, chronic hepatitis C, renal insufficiency
Current medications: Paroxetine (Paxil) 40 mg once daily; atorvastatin (Lipitor) 20 mg once daily, naproxen (Naprosyn) 250 mg p.o. b.i.d., amlodipine (Norvasc) 5 mg q.d., omeprazole (Prilosec), and lisinopril (Zestril) 10 mg
PE: BP 164/84; some pallor; conjunctiva slightly pale

1. What types of anemia is this patient at risk for? What puts him at risk?
   * **Anemia of chronic disease—hepatitic C, rheumatoid arthritis**
   * **Iron deficiency—GI bleed due to PUD, naproxen**
   * **Anemia secondary to renal failure**

Lab: CBC done 1 month ago, results: RBC 3.34, Hgb 10.6, Hct 31.8, MCV 95.5, MCHC 34.5, RBC morphology normal

2. How would you classify/describe this anemia?
   Mild normocytic normochromic anemia

3. Does the lab work tell you which kind of anemia he has?
   - **No, but rules out iron deficiency; would be microcytic, microchromic**
   - **Anemia of renal disease and posthemorrhagic still possibilities**

4. What additional tests are needed?
   - **Comprehensive metabolic profile: glucose 96, BUN 46, creatinine 1.6, albumin 3.0, total protein low normal at 6.2, otherwise WNL**
   - **Iron studies: FE 60 (normal), TIBC 335 (normal), ferritin 37 (normal),**
   - **B$_{12}$ and folate levels were normal; stool guaiac for occult blood negative**

5. What is your diagnosis?
   Anemia of chronic disease

6. What treatment do you recommend?
   Optimal treatment of concurrent illnesses, no specific treatment for the anemia

7. Will an iron supplement be helpful? Why?
   Iron supplement is not helpful because the underlying defect is not iron deficiency; could be harmful

Case 2. An 88-year-old Black female is noted to have anemia on routine screening. Last CBC was done a year ago and her H&H were 11 and 34. Patient uses a wheelchair; lives in nursing home; is a picky eater; likes sweets; eats 1 to 2 servings of fruit/vegetables daily. Patient recently had an acute exacerbation of her COPD and was treated with prednisone p.o. for 2 weeks. Patient was noted to have diarrhea last week.
PMH: Diabetes mellitus, osteoarthritis, COPD, aortic stenosis, CHF, constipation
Medications: Metformin (Glucophage) 500 mg b.i.d., nabumetone (Relafen) 500 p.o. b.i.d., albuterol/ipratropium (Combivent) inhaler, furosemide (Lasix) 40 mg, senna laxative (Senokot) q.d.
CBC: Hemoglobin 9.6, hematocrit 28.9, MCV 80
Iron studies: Ferritin low with increased TIBC

1. Classify/describe the anemia
   Anemia is microcytic hypochromic

2. What anemias present as microcytic hypochromic?
   Iron deficiency anemia

PE: Pulse is 100, 20; BP 130/80; cardiac exam shows tachycardia, murmur of atrial stenosis; abdomen diffusely tender; distant lung sounds; peripheral neuropathy present, 2 plus pedal edema

3. What do you learn from the physical exam?
   - Tachycardia could have many causes: CHF, COPD, anemia
   - Murmur confirms aortic stenosis; lung sounds indicative of COPD
   - Bony enlargement of joints indicative of osteoarthritis
   - Peripheral neuropathy can be diabetes mellitus
   - Pedal edema from CHF
   - Abdominal tenderness is the only physical finding not readily explained by the patient's known diagnoses

4. What risk factors for anemia does the patient have?
   - Poor dietary intake
   - History of PUD, GI bleed; sudden drop indicative of posthemorrhagic anemia
   - NSAID ingestion
   - Recent prednisone treatment

5. What lab tests would you order? Why?
   - Iron studies because of poor diet, to determine need for iron supplementation
   - Stools for OB to rule out GI bleed due to Relafen and prednisone

6. The stools for occult blood come back positive. What is your diagnosis?
   Iron deficiency anemia secondary to GI bleed

Case 3. The family brings their 94-year-old mother to the clinic because she seems more confused and tired recently.
PMH: Irritable bowel syndrome, lactose intolerance, S/P cholecystitis, history asthma, macular degeneration, history of alcoholism
Current medications: dicyclomine (Bentyl) 10 mg t.i.d., Metamucil 1 scoop q.d., LactAid with meals, omeprazole (Prilosec) 20 mg q.d.
PE: patient confused, has peripheral neuropathy
Lab: RBC 5.23, Hgb 10.1, Hct 31.8, MCV 104.0, MCH 23.1, MCHC 29.7

1. Classify/describe this anemia
   Macrocytic anemia

2. What diagnoses are you considering?
   B_{12} deficiency, folate deficiency

3. What additional information do you need?
   B_{12} and folate levels

Lab: The B_{12} level is less than 250 and the folate level is 4 ng/mL

4. What is your diagnosis now?
   B_{12} deficiency

5. What risk factors does she have for B_{12} deficiency?
   - Poor diet
   - Malabsorption conditions, alcoholism
   - Age stomach less acidic, B_{12} needs acid to be absorbed
   - Omeprazole (Prilosec) decreases stomach acid

6. Why is it necessary to screen for folate deficiency before treating B_{12} deficiency?
   See special conditions: do not begin treatment for B_{12} deficiency without assessing for and treating folate deficiency also, as treatment of B_{12} deficiency may mask the symptoms of folate deficiency while the damage from low folate will continue

7. What is your treatment plan?
   B_{12} injections 1,000 mcg subcutaneously every week for 4 weeks, then every month

8. Will the peripheral neuropathy resolve?
   Perhaps but not likely; damage is usually permanent unless caught early

CHAPTER 17—ENDOCRINE DISORDERS

Case 1. A 68-year-old overweight American Indian man comes to the office one afternoon with the complaint of a wound on his foot that has been there for 1 month and will not heal. Denies pain, fever. Admits to fatigue, blurred vision. Also complains of joint pain, especially in knees and hips.

1. What diagnostic studies would you order?
   - **Random glucose, since patient has probably eaten today**
   - **Order fasting glucose for morning**
   - **CBC, ESR, BUN, creatinine, ALT/AST—for infection or anemia evidence, kidney function, and status of liver as a baseline before initiating treatment**

2. Which lab test is the best for diagnosing diabetes in the older adult?
   - **Fasting glucose: many older adults have impaired glucose tolerance; random glucose may be fairly high without patient having diabetes.**
   - **Hemoglobin A1C test is best for monitoring for control, *not for diagnosis***

3. What risk factors does the patient have for diabetes?
   - **Race**
   - **Obesity**
   - **Age**

4. What is your management of this patient?
   - **Nonpharmacologic treatment:**
   - **Treat foot wound**
   - **Foot care, including good shoes**
   - **Patient education about condition**
   - **Nutrition counseling for weight reduction, glucose control**
   - **Regular exercise**
   - **Teach how to do fingerstick blood sugar**
   - **Pharmacologic treatment:**
   - **Which categories of medications would be appropriate as initial treatment?**
   - **Biguanides**
   - **Thiazolidinediones**
   - **Second-generation sulfonylureas**
   - **Meglitinides**
   - **Alpha-glucosidase inhibitors**

5. What complications are you worried about?
    - **Infected foot with osteomyelitis, gangrene, amputation**
    - **Coronary artery disease**
    - **Peripheral vascular disease**
    - **Retina blindness (retinopathy)**
    - **Kidney: renal insufficiency (nephropathy)**
    - **Peripheral neuropathy**

Case 2. An 82-year-old patient is brought in for geriatric assessment by her daughter. Patient is having difficulty sleeping, and complains of fatigue and constipation to her family. She does not get dressed in the morning, and is having difficulty balancing her checkbook. She has gained 10 pounds in the last year. She is otherwise reported to be healthy and has not seen a health care provider in years. She takes acetaminophen (Tylenol) for arthritis. Her family members state they think she is becoming more forgetful.

1. What other history do you need?
    - **Weight history (gain/loss), cold intolerance, arthralgias, myalgias, lethargy, depression, weakness**
    - **Past history of thyroid disease**
    - **Family history of thyroid disease**

2. What physical exam would you do? What would you expect to find?
    - **Weight: gain**
    - **Face: dull expression; swollen, puffy eyelids**
    - **Skin: dry, coarse dry hair, hair loss, and loss of peripheral eye brows**
    - **Thyroid: enlarged gland, slightly firm, may be nodular**
    - **Cardiac: bradycardia, cardiomegaly**
    - **Respiratory: dyspnea, pleural effusion**
    - **Abdominal: hypoactive bowel sounds**
    - **Extremities: peripheral edema**
    - **Neurological: dementia, decreased/delayed reflexes**

3. What diagnostic test would be conclusive?
    TSH

4. What are your differential diagnoses? What should you rule out?
    - **Hypothyroidism**
    - **Depression**
    - **Dementia**
    - **Diabetes**
    - **Heart failure**
    - **Kidney failure**

Case 3. A 74-year-old man comes to the office with a complaint of palpitations for about a month. He notices them especially at night when he is trying to sleep; he is having more trouble sleeping recently. The palpitations occur about 1 to 2 times a day. He sits and rests and they go away. He also complains of shortness of breath when walking. He has recently lost 15 pounds. Patient denies dieting.

1. What other body systems would you inquire about?
   - **General: hypersensitivity to heat, fatigue, weakness**
   - **Mental: anxiety, irritability, psychosis, depression**
   - **Respiratory: cough, dyspnea**
   - **Cardiac: chest pain, orthopnea, racing heart**
   - **GI: increased appetite, increased frequency of bowel movements, diarrhea, vomiting, weight loss, anorexia**

2. What physical exam is important?
   - **Skin: velvety smooth, moist and warm hands, onycholysis**
   - **Eyes: exophthalmos, lid retraction, lid lag**
   - **Neck: thyroid enlarged goiter, bruit**
   - **Cardiac: tachycardia, arrhythmias such as atrial fibrillation**
   - **Respiratory**
   - **Musculoskeletal**
   - **Neurologic: hyperactive reflexes, tremors**

Physical: This patient has atrial fibrillation, tachypnea, hyperactive reflexes, and a fine tremor

3. What is your diagnosis?
   Hyperthyroidism

4. What labs would confirm this diagnosis?
   - **TSH decreased or undetectable**
   - **Free T4 usually elevated, but if normal order free T3**
   - **Free T3 elevated**

5. What would you do?
   - **Refer to endocrinologist**
   - **See cardiac chapter for management of the atrial fibrillation, which should resolve when hyperthyroidism is treated**
   - **Consider adjunctive therapy to control symptoms until patient sees endocrinologist, such as beta blocker, diltiazem**

6. What is the preferred treatment?
   Propylthiouracil (PTU) or methimazole (Tapazole)
   If condition does not resolve after a year of medication, radioactive iodine can be used to destroy the thyroid gland or subtotal thyroidectomy if gland is very large, causing problems with speech and swallowing

CHAPTER 18—PSYCHIATRIC–MENTAL HEALTH DISORDERS

Case 1. A 72-year-old man presents to your office complaining of insomnia, generalized aches and pains, fatigue and a 10-pound weight loss over the past 2 months. He states he has lost interest in his hobbies, doesn't go out of the house often except to buy groceries, and spends much of his day watching television.
Medications: ibuprofen (Advil) 2 to 6 tabs/day for pain.

1. What additional questions would you ask?
   Specifics about pain, appetite, sleep, complete review of systems to rule out physical causes including cardiopulmonary, neurologic, GI, GU, prior psychiatric history, recent losses, alcohol use, suicide intention, GDS, MMSE, current medications including OTC and herbal supplements

2. What would you look for on physical examination?
   General affect, facial expression, posture, hygiene, eye contact, signs of weight loss (serial weight, loose-fitting clothes), complete physical to look for clues to weight loss, fatigue (such as with cardiopulmonary, inflammatory, or neuromuscular disease), and cancer

3. What laboratory work would you order?
   CBC, metabolic panel, TFTs, LFTs, B$_{12}$, folate, possible ESR, RPR

4. What treatment would you begin, assuming labs are normal?
   Mirtazapine (Remeron) would be a good choice, as it helps with sleep and stimulates appetite; an SSRI would also be an acceptable choice

5. What complications should you watch for?
   Increased anxiety, insomnia, GI symptoms, suicidal intent

Case 2. A 68-year-old woman presents to your office complaining of difficulty swallowing, diarrhea, dizzy spells, weakness in her legs, insomnia, feelings of impending doom, and a fear of losing control.

1. What questions would you ask?
   Length of time, previous episodes, precipitating factors, review of systems (endocrine, cardiopulmonary), GDS, MMSE, current medications including OTC and herbal supplements, use of caffeine

2. What would you look for on physical exam?
   Affect, cardiopulmonary to rule out arrhythmia, neurovascular, GI, neck (thyroid)

3. What laboratory tests would you order?
   CBC, metabolic panel, TFTs, possible B$_{12}$ if signs of neuropathy or macrocytosis, urinalysis to rule out glycosuria, EKG, possible Holter monitor

4. What treatment would you begin?

   Paroxetine (Paxil) is the drug of first choice; consider another SSRI if patient unable to tolerate paroxetine's side effects; use lorazepam (Ativan) only if necessary for short-term relief, until paroxetine has time to take effect

5. What complications might develop?

   Sedation, fatigue, confusion, falls

Case 3. Mr. Smith, 75 years old, comes for routine follow-up of diabetes. He reports his wife died 3 weeks ago. He joined AA at age 50. Medications: Glucophage 500 mg b.i.d.

1. What questions would you ask?

   Coping skills and support systems (present and past, is hospice involved?), how much alcohol is he drinking, CAGE, GDS, MMSE, appetite, sleep, and activity patterns, hypo-/hyperglycemia symptoms, suicidal ideation, intention, and any plan

2. What laboratory tests would you order?

   BUN, creatinine, glucose, electrolytes, hemoglobin A1C, urinalysis
   Glucophage can cause lactic acidosis in the presence of alcohol use, dehydration, and renal failure

3. What treatment would you begin?

   Grief counseling, continue hospice/bereavement care for spouse

4. What complications might develop?

   Depression; resumption of alcohol use, which complicates diabetes management; suicide

Review Questions

1. The focus of the American Nurses Association's standards and scope of gerontological nursing practice is:

   a. The requisite knowledge base
   b. The assurance of safe practice
   c. Legal guidance for practice
   d. Quality of care

2. A 95-year-old woman in your nursing home had complained for about 3 days of pain and burning paresthesias over her right rib area. She now presents with a linear grouping of vesicles on an erythematous base along a dermatomal pathway extending from the sternum to the spine on the right side of the chest. What statement correctly describes this scenario?

   a. Probably a contact dermatitis from an incontinence brief
   b. Evidence of herpes zoster from the reactivation of the rubeola virus contracted as a child
   c. Result of untreated and repeated flea bites to trunk
   d. Signs and symptoms of herpes zoster, a varicella viral infection of a nerve ganglion

3. During cardiac auscultation, a soft S_1 with a pansystolic apical murmur that radiates to the left axilla suggests:

    a. Aortic stenosis
    b. Aortic regurgitation
    c. Mitral valve stenosis
    d. Mitral valve regurgitation

4. Which of the following is a potential complication of an inadequately treated urinary tract infection?

    a. Urolithiasis
    b. Renal insufficiency
    c. Reflex incontinence
    d. Poststreptococcal glomerulonephritis

5. Which of the following statements about sexual function in older people is true?

    a. Impotence is an inevitable consequence of aging
    b. Slower arousal and reaction times are normal signs of aging
    c. Moderate alcohol consumption can improve sexual dysfunction
    d. Hormonal replacements are necessary for sexual satisfaction

6. Which of the following is *not* recommended for primary prevention of stroke?

    a. Management of hypertension
    b. Diet counseling and exercise
    c. Warfarin
    d. Good glycemic control of diabetes

7. A 78-year-old patient with CAD has an elevated TSH with a low free T4. What medication would you give?

    a. Cytomel 5 mcg
    b. Levothyroxine (Synthroid) 25 to 50 mcg
    c. Amiodarone (Cordarone) 400 mg
    d. Atenolol 50 mg

8. You establish a program in your health clinic for the rehabilitation of stroke patients. This program would be an example of:

    a. Primary prevention
    b. Secondary prevention
    c. Tertiary prevention
    d. A screening test

9. Which is the most common symptom of infection in older adults?

    a. Fever
    b. Delirium or decrease in ADLs
    c. Symptoms specific to the system that is infected
    d. Classic symptoms of that particular infection

10. Which of the following lesions frequently found on or around the eyelids of the older adult patient will *not* require antibiotic treatment?

    a. Chalazion
    b. Hordeolum
    c. Blepharitis
    d. Xanthelasma

11. A 92-year-old woman comes for routine evaluation and has a blood pressure of 164/84. The chart reveals the patient's blood pressure at last visit was 158/82. What is the best advice?

    a. This is normal for the older adult, does not need treatment
    b. This is systolic hypertension, which needs to be treated
    c. Systolic BP is less important than diastolic BP in older adults
    d. Come back in 2 weeks for recheck of BP

12. Diabetes and hypertension are common etiologies for

    a. Renal insufficiency
    b. Bacteriuria
    c. Urolithiasis
    d. Pyelonephritis

13. A 69-year-old man comes to the clinic complaining of difficulty starting to urinate, hesitancy during urination, and dribbling after urinating. He has nocturia 4 or 5 times per night. He denies painful urination. His current medications include atenolol, isosorbide, diltiazem for CAD and HTN, and amitriptyline for insomnia. His residual urine volume is 100 ml. Your first action would be to:

    a. Discontinue amitriptyline
    b. Discontinue diltiazem, and replace with doxazosin to treat HTN
    c. Insert an indwelling catheter
    d. Refer the patient to a urologist for possible transurethral resection (TURP) of prostate

14. Which of the following is *not* a cause of aplastic anemia?

    a. Chloramphenicol
    b. Virus
    c. Allergies
    d. Radiation

15. A 74-year-old female presents complaining of palpitations, tachycardia, cold clammy hands, dizziness, insomnia, generalized aches and pains, and frequent urination. EKG is normal and all lab values are within normal ranges. The most likely diagnosis is:

    a. Posttraumatic stress disorder
    b. Anxiety disorder
    c. Major depression
    d. Substance abuse disorder

16. You have a new patient who is a 74-year-old male without major health problems. He has not consulted a healthcare provider for more than 10 years. What screening test would you recommend *most* highly for this patient?

    a. Blood pressure
    b. PSA
    c. Cholesterol
    d. TSH

17. 73-year-old Mrs. Adams has been treated for chronic xerosis, which seems to worsen every year and is particularly bothersome in the winter. Which of the following should be included in the patient education instructions you give to her?

    a. Do not use a humidifier in the home, especially when the heat is running
    b. Hot water and soap for a daily bath are effective aids to decrease scaling of skin
    c. Emollient lotions should be used regularly
    d. Hydrocortisone ointment should not be used if skin is inflamed or pruritic

18. An 85-year-old nonsmoker who has never been hospitalized develops fever and chills, productive cough, chest discomfort, and declining mental status. The physical exam shows temperature 101.4° F; pulse 100; respirations 24. Lungs have rhonchi and rales (crackles) in the LLL. The most likely causative organism is:

    a. *S. pneumoniae*
    b. *S. aureus*
    c. *Moraxella catarrhalis*
    d. Influenza A

19. Your 70-year-old patient has gastroesophageal reflux disease (GERD). After a trial of lifestyle modifications and antacids, the patient continues to have occasional mild heartburn after meals and at night. The most appropriate next action would be to use:

    a. Prokinetic agents
    b. H2 antagonists
    c. Proton-pump inhibitors
    d. Sucralfate

20. A 78-year-old woman comes to your office complaining of vague GI symptoms including nausea, loss of appetite, abdominal fullness, and pelvic pressure, which have gradually been worsening for the past 3 years. In the past year, she has experienced fatigue and weight loss of 15 pounds without dieting. What one action would the best for you to do?

    a. Discuss her diet with her
    b. Treat with omeprazole (Prilosec)
    c. Discuss hormone replacement therapy
    d. Refer to GYN oncology

21. Which patient is most likely to have osteoporosis?

    a. An 80-year-old underweight male who smokes and has been on steroids for psoriasis
    b. A 90-year-old female with no family history of osteoporosis who is on HRT
    c. A 68-year-old overweight female who drinks 1 to 2 alcoholic drinks/day
    d. An 82-year-old female who is ideal body weight, takes calcium and vitamins, has weight-bearing exercise daily

22. A patient's lab shows hemoglobin 10.1, Hct 31.3, low MCV and MCH, with low ferritin and increased TIBC. This is characteristic of:

    a. Iron deficiency
    b. B_{12} deficiency
    c. Folate deficiency
    d. Aplastic anemia

23. Which of the following psychiatric medications represents a class of drugs commonly prescribed in the older adult population that has a high incidence of abuse, misuse, and adverse reactions?

    a. Fluoxetine (Prozac)
    b. Nortriptyline (Pamelor)
    c. Risperidone (Risperdal)
    d. Lorazepam (Ativan)

24. Current recommendations for exercise in older adults suggest:

    a. Only those older adults who are overweight need to exercise
    b. Exercise should be done at least daily for at least 60 minutes
    c. Exercise programs ideally should combine aerobic, resistive, and stretching activities
    d. Older adults with any underlying chronic illnesses should not exercise

25. Which is *true* about HIV in older adults?

    a. Treatment is the same as for younger adults
    b. Older adult patients have a poorer prognosis than younger adults do
    c. Adverse reactions to the medications occur less frequently than with younger adults
    d. Viral burden and CD4 count do not predict prognosis

26. A patient presents with painful red eye. Which of the following is the most urgent ophthalmologic emergency?

    a. Keratitis
    b. Corneal abrasion
    c. Retinal tear
    d. Retinal venous occlusion

27. A 78-year-old client is seen with complaint of anorexia, nausea, and diarrhea. Also complains of weakness. He has a history of chronic heart failure. Which of his medications is most likely to cause these side effects?

    a. The ACE inhibitor quinapril (Accupril) 10 mg
    b. The diuretic furosemide (Lasix) 40 mg
    c. Digoxin (Lanoxin) 0.25 mg
    d. The beta blocker carvedilol (Coreg) 12.5 mg

28. Your 69-year-old postmenopausal patient describes involuntary loss of urine for the past 5 years. She reports that laughing or sneezing will cause her to leak urine. This is probably:

    a. Urge incontinence
    b. Stress incontinence
    c. Reflex incontinence
    d. Overflow incontinence

29. What is the most important adverse reaction to bisphosphonates?

    a. Increased risk for breast cancer
    b. Esophagitis
    c. Dizziness and falls
    d. Headache

30. Which of the following foods are *not* good sources of folic acid?

    a. Green leafy vegetables
    b. Red meat
    c. Red beans
    d. Bananas

31. A recently widowed (1 month) 76-year-old male presents stating he is very despondent. He complains of insomnia, generalized anxiety, and crying spells. He states he thinks about his own mortality frequently and feels guilty that his wife expired before he did. What about this man would make you worry that he was suicidal?

    a. He is an avid hunter and has guns in the home
    b. He says he has difficulty concentrating
    c. He says he plans to see his attorney and revise his will
    d. He says he is looking forward to joining his wife

32. Which of the following individuals would you want to screen for alcohol abuse?

    a. Those individuals who deny ever drinking
    b. Those individuals who frequently fall, have a sudden change in functional status and/or cognition, present with weight loss or malnutrition, and have experienced recent losses
    c. Those individuals who already take other medications
    d. Those individuals who are middle to upper middle class

33. Which of the following is true about influenza vaccine?

    a. Provides immunity to all those immunized
    b. Protection begins about 2 weeks after vaccination
    c. Protection lasts for a few months to a year after vaccination
    d. Adverse reactions occur in about 20%

34. A 72-year-old retired schoolteacher complains of dizziness, ringing in the ear, and not being able to hear in his right ear. It came on rather suddenly over a couple days about a week ago. Denies any recent acute illness. What is the most likely cause?

    a. Acoustic neuroma
    b. Ménière disease
    c. Labyrinthitis
    d. Benign positional vertigo

35. Which medication would be the *least* optimal for a patient with chronic stable coronary heart disease?

    a. Nitroglycerin
    b. Aspirin
    c. Verapamil (Calan)
    d. Metoprolol (Lopressor)

36. Which of the following is true regarding the Women's Health Initiative study of hormone replacement therapy (HRT)?

    a. HRT has a beneficial effect on coronary artery disease
    b. HRT decreases the risk for breast cancer
    c. HRT increases the risk for colon cancer
    d. HRT increases the risk for thromboembolic events and stroke

37. Which joint is the most common site of an initial gout attack

    a. First MTP joint
    b. Ankle
    c. Knee
    d. Wrist

38. A 75-year-old Black male is seen for fever, malaise, weakness, bruising, and weight loss. The physical shows hepatosplenomegaly and lymphadenopathy. Laboratory tests show proliferation of mature-appearing lymphocytes. What is the most likely diagnosis?

    a. Chronic lymphocytic leukemia
    b. Aplastic anemia
    c. Bacteria infection
    d. Hairy cell leukemia

39. You suspect your 84-year-old patient is being abused. What are you legally required to do?

    a. Confront the patient
    b. Confront perpetrator
    c. Notify authorities
    d. Refer to social worker

40. A patient has a bacterial infection. You would expect the following to be elevated:

    a. Neutrophils
    b. Eosinophils
    c. Basophils
    d. Mast cells

41. Which medication causes rebound rhinitis?

    a. Oxymetazoline (Afrin)
    b. Azelastine HCL 0.1% (Astelin)
    c. Phenylephrine HCL (Neo-Synephrine)
    d. Intranasal corticosteroids

42. Which of the following medications is *not* used for primary prevention of CHD?

    a. Aspirin
    b. Folic acid
    c. ACE inhibitors
    d. Beta blockers

43. Low back pain that is worse lying down is characteristic of:

    a. Osteoarthritis
    b. Compression fracture
    c. Spinal stenosis
    d. Sciatica

44. Which of the following is *not* a DSM-IV symptom of depression?

    a. Weight loss
    b. Insomnia
    c. Diminished interest in activities
    d. Social isolation

45. A patient has herpes zoster on the tip of the nose. What do you do?

    a. Treat with acyclovir (Zovirax) ointment 5%
    b. Refer to ophthalmologist
    c. Treat with valacyclovir (Valtrex) 1000 mg t.i.d.
    d. Monitor for infection

46. Your patient has high blood pressure with episodes of flushing, palpitations, pallor, tremor, profuse perspiration, angina, and diaphoresis. This picture is most likely produced by:

    a. Renal parenchymal disease
    b. Pheochromocytoma
    c. Hyperaldosteronism
    d. Cushing disease

47. Cardiac complications of diabetes do *not* include:

    a. Orthostatic hypotension
    b. Resting tachycardia
    c. Silent myocardial infarction
    d. Heart murmur

48. A patient has a gait characterized by diminished arm swing and difficulty initiating movement and turns. It is most likely due to:

    a. Normal pressure hydrocephalus
    b. Parkinson's disease
    c. Frontal lobe gait apraxia
    d. Cerebellar disease

49. Which of the following is *not* a significant adverse reaction to statins?

    a. Elevated CPK
    b. Rhabdomyolysis
    c. Renal dysfunction
    d. Blood dyscrasias

50. Which is one of the most common fractures from falls in older adults?

    a. Hip
    b. Vestibular compression
    c. Torn rotator cuff
    d. Ankle

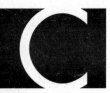

Answers to the Review Questions

1. **Correct Answer: D.** NONPF helps determine knowledge base, assurance of safe practice is the responsibility of the NP, and the ANA cannot offer legal advice. The scopes and standards focus on quality of care.

2. **Correct Answer: D.** Contact dermatitis would not be painful. It's not the rebeola virus, and untreated flea bites would not have burning paresthesias. This is classic presentation of herpes zoster.

3. **Correct Answer: D.** Aortic stenosis has no radiation to the axilla; aortic regurgitation is not likely to radiate; and mitral valve stenosis is not pansystolic.

4. **Correct Answer: B.** Early treatment of urinary tract infections in older adults can prevent deterioration of renal function; ascending infections can damage renal parenchyma irreversibly.

5. **Correct Answer: B.** The first and third choices are persistent myths; the problem is usually psychological or due to an underlying condition. Hormonal replacements are not necessary.

6. **Correct Answer: C.** Warfarin is not primary prevention; the others are important steps to prevent stroke.

7. **Correct Answer: B.** Start with a low dose of Levothyroxine. Cytomel is not recommended, amiodarone causes hypothyroidism, and atenolol is used for symptoms of hyperthyroidism.

8. **Correct Answer: C.** Tertiary prevention is treatment to avoid or postpone complications of the illness.

9. **Correct Answer: B.** Fever is frequently absent, and older adults typically present nonspecific, atypical symptoms.

10. **Correct Answer: D.** This yellow plaque found along the nasal aspect of the eyelids is benign and does not require treatment.

11. **Correct Answer: B.** Systolic hypertension is a risk factor for cardiovascular disease.

12. **Correct Answer: A.** Both of these conditions cause renal damage when not controlled well or present for long periods of time.

13. **Correct Answer: A.** Anticholinergics can cause urinary retention.

14. **Correct Answer: C.** Chloramphenicol, viruses, and radiation all cause aplasic anemia.

15. **Correct Answer: B.** Posttraumatic stress disorder would be associated with a specific event and the symptoms wouldn't indicate substance abuse unless the patient is in withdrawal. The symptoms are characteristic of anxiety.

16. **Correct Answer: A.** Blood pressure screens are well-documented to be beneficial. The efficacy of PSA and cholesterol remain controversial, and TSH provides a low yield, especially in men.

17. **Correct Answer: C.** Emollient lotions are an important treatment. A humidifier and hydrocortisone ointment are useful; hot water and soap are very drying and should not be used.

18. **Correct Answer: A.** *S. pneumonia* is the most prevalent cause of community-acquired pneumonia.

19. **Correct Answer: B.** H2 antagonists are a good second-line treatment of mild symptoms.

20. **Correct Answer: D.** The patient has signs and symptoms of ovarian cancer.

21. **Correct Answer: A.** Men get osteoporosis around age 70, and he has risk factors.

22. **Correct Answer: A.** Iron deficiency indicates microcytic hypochronic anemia.

23. **Correct Answer: D.** Fluoxetine is generally safe and effective and nortriptyline and risperidone have low abuse potential. Lorazepam should be used with caution.

24. **Correct Answer: C.** A variety of exercises is beneficial to older adults and should be individualized according to ability.

25. **Correct Answer: B.** Older adults have a much poorer prognosis.

26. **Correct Answer: C.** Retinal tears require emergency referral to prevent blindness.

27. **Correct Answer: C.** The patient is on a high dose and these are common signs of digitalis toxicity.

28. **Correct Answer: B.** *Stress incontinence* is defined as the involuntary loss of urine associated with activities that increase intra-abdominal pressure.

29. **Correct Answer: B.** The patient must remain sitting or standing or will have severe esophagitis.

30. **Correct Answer: B.** Red meat is not a source; folic acid is found in vegetable sources.

31. **Correct Answer: D.** This is a danger signal potentially requiring emergency management. Revising his will is rational, difficulty concentrating is a common symptom of grief, and many people own guns.

32. **Correct Answer: B.** Patients with those symptoms should be screened for alcohol abuse. The others are not uncommon, and alcohol abuse is equally represented in all economic groups.

33. **Correct Answer: C.** The protection is short-term.

34. **Correct Answer: B.** Vertigo, tinnitus, and hearing loss are the classic triad for making this diagnosis.

35. **Correct Answer: C.** Verapamil is used only for vasospastic angina.

36. **Correct Answer: D.** HRT increases the risk for CHD and breast cancer and decreases the risk for colon cancer.

37. **Correct Answer: A.** The first MTP joint is the classic presentation of an initial gout attack. The others are affected later.

38. **Correct Answer: A.** Chronic lymphocytic leukemia is most common in older adults. The other options would present with different findings.

39. **Correct Answer: C.** Notifying the authorities is legally required. Confronting the patient is not legally required; confronting the perpetrator could be dangerous to the patient; and referring to a social worker may be an intervention, but is not legally required.

40. **Correct Answer: A.** Neutrophils become elevated early in infection as they fight bacterial infection.

41. **Correct Answer: A.** Oxymetazoline causes rebound rhinitis if used for longer than recommended.

42. **Correct Answer: D.** Beta blockers are used for secondary prevention.

43. **Correct Answer: B.** Compression fractures get worse when lying down. The others are relieved by rest or get better when lying down.

44. **Correct Answer: D.** Social isolation, though not a DSM-IV symptom, is common in older adults.

45. **Correct Answer: B.** Herpes zoster on the tip of the nose may cause blindness if not treated.

46. **Correct Answer: B.** These are characteristic symptoms of pheochromocytoma.

47. **Correct Answer: D.** Diabetes does not affect valves.

48. **Correct Answer: B.** A patient with Parkinson's disease would exhibit these symptoms due to stiffness.

49. **Correct Answer: D.** The other symptoms are significant; blood dyscrasias are not a problem.

50. **Correct Answer: A.** Hip fractures are a common cause of disability.

Index